lifetime physical fitness & wellness

A PERSONALIZED PROGRAM

THIRTEENTH EDITION

Werner W. K. Hoeger
Professor Emeritus (Active)
Department of Kinesiology
Boise State University

Sharon A. Hoeger
Fitness & Wellness, Inc.
Boise, Idaho

Australia • Brazil • Mexico • Singapore • United Kingdom • United States

Lifetime Physical Fitness & Wellness:
A Personalized Program, **Thirteenth Edition**
Werner W.K. Hoeger and Sharon A. Hoeger

Product Director: Yolanda Cossio

Product Manager: Aileen Berg

Content Developer: Alexis Glubka

Content Coordinator: Kellie Petruzzelli

Product Assistant: Chelsea Joy

Media Developer: Stefanie Beeck

Marketing Manager: Lindsy Lettre

Content Project Manager: Tanya Nigh

Art Director: John Walker

Manufacturing Planner: Karen Hunt

Rights Acquisitions Specialist: Dean Dauphinais

Production Service and Compositor:
  Graphic World Inc.

Photo and Text Researchers: PreMedia Global

Copy Editor: Graphic World Inc.

Illustrator: Graphic World Inc.

Text Designer: RHDZ/Graphic World Inc.

Cover Designer: Denise Davidson

Cover Image: Poncho/Digital Vision/
  Getty Images

© 2015, 2013 Cengage Learning

ALL RIGHTS RESERVED. No part of this work covered by the copyright herein may be reproduced, transmitted, stored, or used in any form or by any means, graphic, electronic, or mechanical, including but not limited to photocopying, recording, scanning, digitizing, taping, Web distribution, information networks, or information storage and retrieval systems, except as permitted under Section 107 or 108 of the 1976 United States Copyright Act, without the prior written permission of the publisher.

> For product information and technology assistance, contact us at
> **Cengage Learning Customer & Sales Support, 1-800-354-9706.**
> For permission to use material from this text or product,
> submit all requests online at **www.cengage.com/permissions.**
> Further permissions questions can be e-mailed to
> **permissionrequest@cengage.com.**

Library of Congress Control Number: 2013950066

ISBN-13: 978-1-285-73314-2

ISBN-10: 1-285-73314-2

Cengage Learning
200 First Stamford Place, 4th Floor
Stamford, CT 06902
USA

Cengage Learning is a leading provider of customized learning solutions with office locations around the globe, including Singapore, the United Kingdom, Australia, Mexico, Brazil, and Japan. Locate your local office at **www.cengage.com/global.**

Cengage Learning products are represented in Canada by Nelson Education, Ltd.

To learn more about Cengage Learning Solutions, visit **www.cengage.com.**

Purchase any of our products at your local college store or at our preferred online store **www.cengagebrain.com.**

Printed in the United States of America
2 3 4 5 6 7 17 16 15 14

contents

CHAPTER 1
Physical Fitness and Wellness 1

Life Expectancy 4
Leading Health Problems in the United States 5
Diseases of the Cardiovascular System 5
Cancer 5
Chronic Lower Respiratory Disease (CLRD) 6
Accidents 6
Lifestyle as a Health Problem 6
Physical Activity and Exercise Defined 7
    Importance of Increased Physical Activity 7
National Initiatives to Promote Healthy and Active Lifestyles 8
    Federal Guidelines for Physical Activity 8
    Adults between 18 and 64 years of age 9
    Older adults (ages 65 and older) 9
    Children 6 years of age and older and adolescents 9
    Pregnant and postpartum women 9
National Health Objectives for the Year 2020 10
National Physical Activity Plan 10
    Monitoring Daily Physical Activity 11
"Sitting Disease": A 21st Century Chronic Disease 13
Wellness 14
    The Seven Dimensions of Wellness 14
Physical Wellness 17
Emotional Wellness 17
Mental Wellness 17
Social Wellness 18
Environmental Wellness 18
Occupational Wellness 18
Spiritual Wellness 18
    Wellness, Fitness, and Longevity 19
Types of Physical Fitness 20
Fitness Standards: Health versus Physical Fitness 21
    Health Fitness Standards 21
    Physical Fitness Standards 22
Which Program Is Best? 24
    Benefits of a Comprehensive Fitness Program 24
Health Benefits 24
Exercise and Brain Function 25
    Economic Benefits 26

The Wellness Challenge for Our Day 27
Wellness Education: Using This Book 29
    A Personalized Approach 29
    Exercise Safety 29
Assessment of Resting Heart Rate and Blood Pressure 30
Mean Blood Pressure 31
Assess Your Behavior 31
Assess Your Knowledge 32

CHAPTER 2
Behavior Modification 41

Living in a Toxic Health and Fitness Environment 43
    Environmental Influences on Physical Activity 44
Environmental Influence on Diet and Nutrition 46
Values and Behavior 47
Your Brain and Your Habits 50
Barriers to Change 51
Self-Efficacy 52
    Sources of Self-Efficacy 52
Motivation and Locus of Control 53
Changing Behavior 54
    Behavior Change Theories 54
The Process of Change 58
    Consciousness-Raising 58
    Social Liberation 58
    Self-Analysis 59
    Emotional Arousal 59
    Positive Outlook 59
    Commitment 59
    Behavior Analysis 59
    Goals 59
    Self-Reevaluation 59
    Countering 59
    Monitoring 59
    Environment Control 59
    Helping Relationships 60
    Rewards 60
Techniques of Change 61
Goal Setting and Evaluation 61
    SMART Goals 61
    Goal Evaluation 68
Assess Your Behavior 68
Assess Your Knowledge 69

CHAPTER 3
Nutrition for Wellness 71

Nutrients 76
- Carbohydrates 76
- Fats (Lipids) 78
- Proteins 82
- Vitamins 84
- Minerals 85
- Water 85

Balancing the Diet 86
- Nutrition Standards 86
- Nutrient Analysis 88

Achieving a Balanced Diet 92
- Choosing Healthy Foods 96
- Vegetarianism 100

Nutrient Concerns 101
- Diets from Other Cultures 103

Nutrient Supplementation 105
- Antioxidants 106
- Benefits of Foods 109
- Functional Foods 109
- Organic Foods 110
- Genetically Modified Crops 111

Energy Substrates for Physical Activity 112

Energy (ATP) Production 112

Nutrition for Athletes 113
- Carbohydrate Loading 113
- Hyponatremia 114
- Creatine Supplementation 114

Bone Health and Osteoporosis 115

Iron Deficiency 117

2010 Dietary Guidelines for Americans 118
- Balancing Calories to Manage Weight 118
- Foods and Nutrients to Increase 119
- Recommendations for Specific Population Groups 119

Proper Nutrition: A Lifetime Prescription for Healthy Living 119

Assess Your Behavior 120

Assess Your Knowledge 120

CHAPTER 4
Body Composition 123

Essential and Storage Fat 126

Techniques to Assess Body Composition 126
- Dual Energy X-ray Absorptiometry 126
- Hydrostatic Weighing 127
- Air Displacement 127
- Skinfold Thickness 128
- Girth Measurements 128
- Bioelectrical Impedance 129
- Body Mass Index 130
- Waist Circumference 133
- Waist-to-Height Ratio: "Keep your waist circumference to less than half your height." 137

Determining Recommended Body Weight 139
- Importance of Regular Body Composition Assessment 141

Assess Your Behavior 142

Assess Your Knowledge 143

CHAPTER 5
Weight Management 147

Overweight versus Obesity 151

Tolerable Weight 152

The Weight Loss Dilemma 153
- Diet Crazes 153
- Low-Carb Diets 154

Eating Disorders 158
- Anorexia Nervosa 158
- Bulimia Nervosa 159
- Binge-Eating Disorder 160
- Emotional Eating 160
- Treatment 161

Physiology of Weight Loss 161
- Energy-Balancing Equation 161
- Setpoint Theory 162

Diet and Metabolism 164

Hormonal Regulation of Appetite 165

Sleep and Weight Management 165

Monitoring Body Weight 165

Exercise and Weight Management 166
- The Role of Exercise Intensity and Duration in Weight Management 168
- Overweight and Fit Debate 170
- Healthy Weight Gain 171
- Weight Loss Myths 171

Losing Weight the Sound and Sensible Way 172
- Monitoring Your Diet with Daily Food Logs 176
- Low-Fat Entrees 177
- Protein Intake 177
- Effect of Food Choices on Long-Term Weight Gain 177
- Behavior Modification and Adherence to a Weight Management Program 177

The Simple Truth 182

Assess Your Behavior 191

Assess Your Knowledge 191

CHAPTER 6
Cardiorespiratory Endurance 193

Basic Cardiorespiratory Physiology: A Quick Survey 196

Aerobic and Anaerobic Exercise 197
    Benefits of Aerobic Training 197

Physical Fitness Assessment 199
    Responders versus Nonresponders 199

Assessment of Cardiorespiratory Endurance 201
    Components of Oxygen Uptake (VO_2) 201
    Tests to Estimate VO_{2max} 202
    Interpreting the Results of Your Maximal Oxygen Uptake 206

Principles of CR Exercise Prescription 206
    Readiness for Exercise 206

Guidelines for CR Exercise Prescription 213
    Intensity of Exercise 213
    Duration (Time) of Exercise 219
    Excessive Sitting: A Deadly Proposition 221
    Exercise Volume 221
    Rate of Progression 221

Fitness Benefits of Aerobic Activities 222
    Getting Started and Adhering to a Lifetime Exercise Program 224

A Lifetime Commitment to Fitness 224

Assess Your Behavior 228

Assess Your Knowledge 228

CHAPTER 7
Muscular Fitness: Strength and Endurance 231

Strength-Training Benefits 233
    Muscular Fitness and Aging 233
    Gender Differences 234
    Changes in Body Composition 236

Assessment of Muscular Strength and Endurance 236
    Muscular Strength: Hand Grip Strength Test 237
    Muscular Endurance Test 237
    Muscular Strength and Endurance Test 238

Strength-Training Prescription 244
    Factors That Affect Muscular Fitness 244

Principles Involved in Strength Training 245
    Mode of Training 245
    Resistance (Intensity) 248
    Frequency 250
    Exercise Variations 250

Plyometrics 251
    Strength Gains 251

Strength-Training Exercises 251
    Dietary Guidelines for Strength Development 251
    Core Strength Training 253
    Pilates Exercise System 253
    Stability Exercise Balls 254
    Elastic-Band Resistive Exercise 254

Exercise Safety Guidelines 254

Setting Up Your Own Strength-Training Program 256

Assess Your Behavior 261

Assess Your Knowledge 261

Strength-Training Exercises without Weights 262

Strength-Training Exercises with Weights 266

Stability Ball Exercises 276

CHAPTER 8
Muscular Flexibility 279

Benefits of Good Flexibility 281

Flexibility in Older Adults 282

Factors Affecting Flexibility 282

Assessment of Flexibility 283
    Interpreting Flexibility Test Results 283

Principles of Muscular Flexibility Prescription 287
    Modes of Training 287
    Physiological Response to Stretching 288
    Intensity 288
    Repetitions 289
    Frequency of Exercise 289
    When to Stretch? 289

Flexibility Exercises 290
    Contraindicated Exercises 290

Preventing and Rehabilitating Low Back Pain 290
    Effects of Posture 295
    Effects of Stress 295
    Proper Body Mechanics for Back Care 295
    Personal Flexibility and Low-Back Conditioning Program 295

Assess Your Behavior 299

Assess Your Knowledge 299

Flexibility Exercises 300

Exercises for the Prevention and Rehabilitation of Low Back Pain 303

CHAPTER 9
Comprehensive Fitness Programming 305

Choices of Aerobic Activities 307
    Traditional Fitness Activities 307
    Walking 307
    Jogging 308

Strength Training 308
Hiking 308
Aerobics 308
Swimming 309
Water Aerobics 310
Cycling 310
Cross-Training 312
Cross-Country Skiing 312
Rowing 312
Elliptical Training/Stair Climbing 312
Racquet Sports 313
Yoga 313

New Fitness Trends 313
High-Intensity Interval Training (HIIT) 313
Stability Exercise Balls 313
Core Training 314
Fitness Boot Camp 314
Bodyweight Training 314
Circuit Training 314
Functional Fitness 315
Zumba 315

Specific Exercise Considerations 315

Exercise-Related Injuries 322
Acute Sports Injuries 323
Muscle Soreness and Stiffness 323
Exercise Intolerance 324
Side Stitch 324
Shin Spints 324
Muscle Cramps 324

Exercise and Aging 324
Physical Training in the Older Adult 324

Preparing for Sports Participation 326
Base Fitness Conditioning 326
Sport-Specific Conditioning 326
Overtraining 327
Periodization 328

Personal Fitness Programming: An Example 330
Cardiorespiratory Endurance 331
Muscular Fitness (Strength and Endurance) 331
Muscular Flexibility 331
Body Composition 331
You Can Get It Done 332

Assess Your Behavior 333
Assess Your Knowledge 333

CHAPTER 10
Preventing Cardiovascular Disease 339

Prevalence of Cardiovascular Disease 342

Stroke 342

Coronary Heart Disease 342
Coronary Heart Disease Risk Profile 343
Leading Risk Factors for CHD 343
Physical Inactivity 347
Abnormal Electrocardiograms 348
Abnormal Cholesterol Profile 349
Elevated Triglycerides 356
Elevated Homocysteine 356
Inflammation 357
Diabetes 358
Metabolic Syndrome 360
Hypertension 361
Excessive Body Fat 365
Cigarette Smoking 365
Tension and Stress 366
Personal and Family History 367
Age 367
Other Risk Factors for Coronary Heart Disease 367

Cardiovascular Risk Reduction 368

Assess Your Behavior 368

Assess Your Knowledge 368

CHAPTER 11
Cancer Prevention 371

Incidence of Cancer 374

Guidelines for Preventing Cancer 377
Dietary Changes 377
Abstaining from Tobacco 381
Avoiding Excessive Exposure to Sun 381
Monitoring Estrogen, Radiation Exposure, and Potential Occupational Hazards 382
Physical Activity 382
Early Detection 383
Other Factors 383

Warning Signals of Cancer 384

Cancer: Assessing Your Risks 384

Common Sites of Cancer 384
Lung Cancer 384
Colon/Rectum Cancer 384
Skin Cancer 389
Breast Cancer 390
Cervical Cancer (Women) 393
Endometrial Cancer (Women) 394
Prostate Cancer (Men) 395
Testicular Cancer (Men) 395
Pancreatic Cancer 396
Kidney and Bladder Cancer 396
Oral Cancer 396
Esophageal and Stomach Cancer 396
Ovarian Cancer (Women) 397

Thyroid Cancer 397
Liver Cancer 397
Leukemia 397
Lymphoma 397

What Can You Do? 398

Assess Your Behavior 399

Assess Your Knowledge 399

CHAPTER 12
Stress Assessment and Management Techniques 401

The Mind–Body Connection 403
   The Brain 403
   The Immune System 403
   Sleep and Wellness 404
   Stress 405

Stress Adaptation 406
   Alarm Reaction 406
   Resistance 406
   Exhaustion/Recovery 406

Perceptions and Health 406
   Self-Esteem 407

Fighting Spirit 408

Sources of Stress 408

Behavior Patterns 408

Vulnerability to Stress 412

Time Management 413
   Five Steps to Time Management 413
   Time Management Skills 416

Coping with Stress 417
   Physical Activity 422
   Relaxation Techniques 424
   Visual Imagery 427
   Autogenic Training 428
   Meditation 428
   Yoga 430
   Tai Chi 431

Which Technique Is Best? 431

Assess Your Behavior 434

Assess Your Knowledge 434

CHAPTER 13
Addictive Behavior 435

Addiction 437
   Risk Factors for Addiction 438

Drugs and Dependence 438
   Nonmedical Use of Prescription Drugs 439
   Marijuana 439
   Cocaine 440
   Methamphetamine 441
   MDMA (Ecstasy) 442
   Heroin 443
   Spice 444
   Inhalant Abuse 444
   Alcohol 444

Treatment of Addictions 449

Tobacco Use 450
   Morbidity and Mortality 450
   Effects on Cardiovascular System 451
   Smoking and Cancer 451
   Other Forms of Tobacco 452
   Health Care Costs of Tobacco Use 453
   Trends 453

Why People Smoke 454
   Smoking Addiction and Dependency 454
   "Why Do You Smoke?" Test 454
   Smoking Cessation 455
   "Do You Want to Quit?" Test 455
   Breaking the Habit 456
   Quitting Cold Turkey 459
   Cutting Down Gradually 460
   Nicotine-Substitution Products 460
   Electronic Cigarettes 460
   Life after Cigarettes 460

Assess Your Behavior 466

Assess Your Knowledge 466

CHAPTER 14
Preventing Sexually Transmitted Infections 467

Chlamydia 470

Gonorrhea 470

Pelvic Inflammatory Disease 470

Human Papillomavirus and Genital Warts 471

Genital Herpes 472

Syphilis 473

Trichomoniasis 473

HIV and AIDS 474
   Transmission of HIV 477
   Risky Behaviors 478
   Myths about HIV Transmission 478
   Wise Dating 479
   Trends in HIV Infection and AIDS 479
   HIV Testing 479
   HIV Treatment 480

Guidelines for Preventing Sexually Transmitted Infections 481

Assess Your Behavior 483

Assess Your Knowledge 484

CHAPTER 15
Lifetime Fitness and Wellness 485

Life Expectancy and Physiological Age 487

Conventional Western Medicine 488

Complementary and Alternative Medicine 490
- Integrative Medicine 497

Quackery and Fraud 497

Looking at Your Fitness Future 500
- Health/Fitness Club Memberships 500
- Personal Trainers 501

Purchasing Exercise Equipment 502

Self-Evaluation and Behavioral Goals for the Future 502
- Self-Evaluation 505
- Behavioral Goals for the Future 505

The Fitness/Wellness Experience and a Challenge for the Future 505

Assess Your Behavior 511

Assess Your Knowledge 511

Appendix A: Physical Fitness and Wellness Profile 513

Appendix B: Nutritive Value of Selected Foods 515

Notes and Suggested Readings 527

Answer Key 537

Glossary 539

Index 547

Preface

The American lifestyle does not provide the human body with sufficient physical activity to enhance or maintain adequate health. In reality, our way of life is such a serious threat to our health that it increases the deterioration rate of the human body and leads to premature illness and mortality.

People in the United States say they believe that physical activity and positive lifestyle habits promote better health, but most do not reap these benefits because they simply do not know how to implement and maintain a sound physical fitness and wellness program that will yield the desired results. About one-half of the adults in the United States do not achieve the recommended amount of daily physical activity, thereby placing themselves at risk for premature morbidity and early death.

A regular exercise program is as close as we get to the miracle pill that people look for to enjoy good health and quality of life over a now longer lifespan. Myriad benefits of exercise include enhanced functional capacity; increased energy; weight loss; improved mood, self-esteem, and physical appearance; and decreased risk for many chronic ailments, including obesity, cardiovascular disease, cancer, and diabetes. As stated as far back as 1982 in the prestigious *Journal of the American Medical Association,* "There is no drug in current or prospective use that holds as much promise for sustained health as a lifetime program of physical exercise."

The benefits of exercise along with healthy lifestyle habits are only reaped through action. Along with the most up-to-date health, fitness, and nutrition guidelines, the information in this book provides extensive behavior modification strategies to help you abandon negative habits and adopt and maintain healthy behaviors. The contents of this book will be of little value to you if you are unable to abandon your negative habits and adopt and maintain healthy behaviors.

Many of the behaviors we adopt are a product of our environment. Unfortunately, we live in a "toxic" health/fitness environment. Becoming aware of how the environment affects our health is vital if we wish to achieve and maintain wellness. Yet we are so habituated to this modern-day environment that we miss the subtle ways it influences our behaviors, personal lifestyle, and health every day. As you study and assess physical fitness and wellness parameters, you will need to take a critical look at your behaviors and lifestyle—and most likely make selected lifetime changes to promote overall health and wellness.

The book is organized in the most efficient manner possible for students to derive the greatest benefit from its contents. Each chapter starts with the chapter objectives, followed by *Frequently Asked Questions (FAQ)* and *Real Life Stories* that will pique the students' interest in the chapter's topic. The chapter contents are presented next, with extensive use of graphs, charts, tables, activities, critical thinking questions, informational boxes, behavior modification boxes, definitions of key terms, and photographs to maximize student learning, content retention, and motivation for healthy lifetime behavioral change. As no other textbook, the Hoegers' *Fitness & Wellness* series makes exceptional use of these special pedagogical aids and high-interest features.

A unique feature of *Lifetime Physical Fitness & Wellness* is the activity experiences provided as key information is addressed in each chapter. These activities allow each student to develop *A Personalized Program* according to individual needs. All chapters conclude with *Assess Your Behavior* and *Assess Your Knowledge* sections so that students may evaluate the impact of the subject matter on their personal lifestyles and their understanding of the chapter contents through 10 multiple-choice questions.

Scientific evidence has clearly shown that improving the quality—and most likely the longevity—of our lives is a matter of personal choice. The biggest challenge we face in the 21st century is to learn how to take control of our personal health habits to ensure a better, healthier, happier, and more productive life. The information presented in this book has been written with this goal in mind, and provides the student with the necessary tools and guidelines to implement and adhere to a *Lifetime Physical Fitness and Wellness Program.* The emphasis throughout the book is on teaching the students how to take control of their personal lifestyle habits so that they can do what is necessary to stay healthy and realize their highest potential for well being.

New in the 13th Edition

All 15 chapters in the 13th edition of *Lifetime Physical Fitness & Wellness: A Personalized Program* have been revised and updated according to recent advances and recommendations in the field, including information reported in the literature and at professional health, fitness, and sports medicine conferences.

Chapter Updates

- All the statistics related to health and fitness in Chapter 1, "Physical Fitness and Wellness," have been brought up to date according to the latest figures available from national organizations. A new section on "Sitting Disease," the term for a 21st century ailment coined by the scientific community to reflect the detrimental effects of excessive sitting on health and well-being (independent of meeting daily recommended guidelines for moderate- or vigorous-intensity physical activity) is also provided in this introductory chapter. The contents on *Exercise and Brain Function* have also been enhanced in the chapter.

- A new section on *Values and Behavior* was added to the "Behavior Modification" chapter, Chapter 2, to emphasize the critical role core values play in human behavior. Values explain why people look to conduct themselves in a manner that is conducive to living and attaining goals consistent with their beliefs and what's important to them.

- The topic of Chapter 3, "Nutrition for Wellness," was updated and revised to include new material on sugar-sweetened beverages, energy drinks, unsaturated fatty acids (including omega-9s), olive oil and canola oil, the key role of adequate protein intake throughout the day, complementary proteins for vegetarian diets, red-meat intake and premature death, the Harvard Healthy Eating Plate, and the latest advances for the prevention and treatment of osteoporosis.

- Data and figures for the different obesity classes (I, II, and III) and the new waist-to-height ratio (WHtR) have been included in Chapter 4, "Body Composition." The WHtR is a new health risk assessment tool to ascertain the health risks of obesity and appears to predict disease risk (including multiple coronary heart disease risk factors) and premature mortality more effectively than body mass index and waist circumference.

- Important changes related to the recommendations and advances in the field regarding weight loss and proper weight management were added to Chapter 5, "Weight Management." The data on the obesity epidemic in the United States now include obesity prevalence estimates based on gender, level of education, and cultural ethnicity. Enhancements were also made to the *Physiology of Weight Loss* and *Weight Loss Strategies* sections; including a better explanation on the rule of thumb that one pound of fat represents 3,500 calories, popular diets on the market today; a new section on the *Overweight and Fit Debate* (fit and fat); the value of having three regular meals and two healthy snacks daily; the importance of adequate amount of lean protein sources with each meal; the benefits of exercise-intensity, interval training, and cold-water swimming on weight loss; and information on the fat mass and obesity-associated gene.

- Chapters 6, 7, and 8, "Cardiorespiratory Endurance," "Muscular Fitness: Strength and Endurance" (previously muscular strength and endurance), and "Muscular Flexibility," have been revised to ensure they conform with the American College of Sports Medicine (ACSM) position paper on the "Quantity and Quality of Exercise for Developing and Maintaining Cardiorespiratory, Musculoskeletal, and Neuromotor Fitness in Apparently Healthy Adults," and the newly released ninth edition (2014) of the ACSM's Guidelines for Exercise Testing and Prescription.
  - The "Cardiorespiratory Endurance" chapter also includes updates on the number of people who meet the 2008 Federal Guidelines for Physical Activity and additional information on energy drinks, the new FITT-VP acronym used for exercise prescription, exercise volume, and fitness apps.

- The title of Chapter 7 has been changed to "Muscular Fitness: Strength and Endurance," a new term that describes the general health, strength, and endurance of a person's muscular system. Updates were also made to the benefits of strength-training section, effects on aging and lean body mass, free weights versus strength-training machines, dietary protein guidelines for strength development, and exercise safety guidelines.

- Minor updates were made to the section on preventing and rehabilitating low back pain in the "Muscular Flexibility" chapter, including new information on bacterial infections as a possible cause among individuals suffering from long-term back pain.

- Chapter 9, "Comprehensive Fitness Programming," has been reorganized to incorporate many of the 2013 fitness trends in the United States, including functional fitness, bodyweight training, and the resurgence of circuit training and high-intensity circuit training (HICT).

- Statistics on the prevalence of cardiovascular disease have been updated in Chapter 10, "Preventing Cardiovascular Disease." Content updates have also been made to several individual risk factors and the information provided under "other risk factors for coronary heart disease." Facts on sudden cardiac death and the ever-increasing role of exercise in preventing premature death have been expanded in the chapter. As a result of several requests from colleges and universities, Activity 10.1, Self-Assessment Coronary Heart Disease Risk Factor Analysis, has been simplified for student use without basic medical testing.

- In addition to an update on the incidence and mortality rates for cancer in the United States provided in Chapter 11, "Cancer Prevention," the guidelines and questionnaire for cancer prevention have been brought up to date for several of the cancer sites. A new questionnaire on *Early Signs of Illness* is also included in the chapter.

- Information on the damaging effects of stress on the body has been added to Chapter 12, "Stress Assessment and Management Techniques." The concept of mindfulness meditation for stress management has been added to section on meditation.

- Data on the most recent trends in substance abuse reported in the *National Survey on Drug Use and Health* by the U.S. Department of Health and Human Services have been extensively updated in Chapter 13, "Addictive Behavior." The detrimental effects of illicit drug use and the alarming increase in the abuse of prescription-type psychotherapeutic drugs used nonmedically has been enhanced in the chapter. A brief introduction to e-cigarettes as a nicotine-substitution treatment modality has been added to the chapter.

- Important changes are included in Chapter 14, "Preventing Sexually Transmitted Infections." The most recent data on STIs released in 2013 by the Centers for Disease Control and Prevention (CDC), along with the ever-increasing risks of developing an STI, are more thoroughly emphasized in the chapter. The CDC STI screening guidelines are also provided, and major updates are provided on facts and information related to the human papillomavirus (HPV), genital herpes, HIV and AIDS, and new content is presented on trichomoniasis. Because STIs are preventable, significant reductions in new infections are not only possible, they are urgently needed. Prevention can minimize the negative, long-term consequences of STIs. Currently, one in four college students has had or has an STI; thus, college students are at substantial risk of exposure to STIs, underscoring the need for STI prevention.

- Chapter 15, "Lifetime Fitness and Wellness," now includes information on the importance of selecting a primary care physician while you are in good health and how to choose a hospital, should you need one for a medical procedure.

Ancillaries

- **Health MindTap for *Lifetime Physical Fitness & Wellness*.** Instant Access Code, ISBN-13: 9781285776422. MindTap is well beyond an e-Book, a homework solution or digital supplement, a resource center website, a course delivery platform, or a learning management system. More than 70 percent of students surveyed said it was unlike anything they have seen before. MindTap is a new personal learning experience that combines all your digital assets—readings, multimedia, activities, and assessments—into a singular learning path to improve student outcomes.

- **Diet & Wellness Plus.** The Diet & Wellness Plus App in MindTap helps you gain a better understanding of how nutrition relates to your personal health goals. It enables you to track your diet and activity, generate reports, and analyze the nutritional value of the food you eat! It includes more than 55,000 foods in the database, custom food and recipe features, the latest dietary references, as well as your goal and actual percentages of essential nutrients, vitamins, and minerals. It also helps you to identify a problem behavior and make a positive change. After completing a wellness profile questionnaire, Diet & Wellness Plus will rate the level of concern for eight different areas of wellness, helping you determine the areas where you are most at risk. It then helps you put together a plan for positive change by helping you select a goal to work toward—complete with a reward for all your hard work.

   The Diet & Wellness Plus App is accessed from the App dock in MindTap and can be used throughout the course for students to track their diet and activity and behavior change.

   There are activities and labs in the course that have students access the App to further extend learning and integrate course content.

- **Instructor Companion Site.** Everything you need for your course in one place! This collection of book-specific lecture and class tools is available online via www.cengage.com/login. Access and download PowerPoint presentations, images, instructor's manual, videos, and more.

- **Cengage Learning Testing Powered by Cognero.** Cengage Learning Testing Powered by Cognero is a flexible, online system that allows you to:
  - author, edit, and manage test bank content from multiple Cengage Learning solutions
  - create multiple test versions in an instant
  - deliver tests from your LMS, your classroom or wherever you want

- **Global Health Watch.** Instant Access Code, ISBN-13: 9781111377335. Printed Access Card, ISBN-13: 9781111377311. Updated with today's current headlines, Global Health Watch is your one-stop resource for classroom discussion and research projects. This resource center provides access to thousands of trusted health sources, including academic journals, magazines, newspapers, videos, podcasts, and more. It is updated daily to offer the most current news about topics related to your health course.

- **Behavior Change Workbook.** ISBN-13: 9780495011453. The Behavior Change Workbook includes a brief discussion of the current theories behind making positive lifestyle changes along with exercises to help students make these changes in their everyday lives.

- **Careers in Health, Physical Education, and Sports, 2e.** ISBN-13: 9780495388395. This unique booklet takes students through the complicated process of picking the type of career they want to pursue; explains how to prepare for the transition into the working world; and provides insight into different career paths, education requirements, and reasonable salary expectations. A designated chapter discusses some of the legal issues that surround the workplace, including discrimination and harassment. This supplement is complete with personal development activities designed to encourage students to focus on and develop better insight into their futures.

- **Walk4Life® Pedometer.** ISBN-13: 9780495013150. Provided through an alliance with Walk4Life, the Walk4Life Elite Model pedometer tracks steps, elapsed time, and distance. A calorie counter and a clock are included in this excellent class activity and tool to encourage students to track their steps and walk toward better fitness awareness.

- **Readings for a Healthy Living.** ISBN-13: 9780759359444. This reader features 12 articles written by author Dianne Hales and published in *PARADE* magazine. Readings include "Take Your Meds—The Right Way," "You Can Think Yourself Thin," "Getting Yourself Back on Track," "Too Tough to Seek Help," and "The Best Medical Help Online."

Brief Author Biographies

Werner W.K. Hoeger is a Professor Emeritus of the Department of Kinesiology at Boise State University. He remains active in research and continues to lecture in the areas of exercise physiology, physical fitness, health, and wellness.

Dr. Hoeger completed his undergraduate and Master's degrees in physical education at the age of 20 and received his Doctorate degree with an emphasis in exercise physiology at the age of 24. He is a *Fellow* of the *American College of Sports Medicine* and also of the *Research Consortium* of the *American Alliance for Health, Physical Education, Recreation, and Dance.* In 2002, he was recognized as the *Outstanding Alumnus* from the *College of Health and Human Performance* at *Brigham Young University.* He is the recipient of the first *Presidential Award for Research and Scholarship* in the *College of Education* at *Boise State University* in 2004.

In 2008, he was asked to be the *keynote speaker* at the *VII Iboamerican Congress of Sports Medicine and Applied Sciences* in Mérida, Venezuela, and was presented with the *Distinguished Guest of the City* recognition. In 2010, he was also honored as the *keynote speaker* at the *Western Society for Kinesiology and Wellness* in Reno, Nevada.

Dr. Hoeger uses his knowledge and personal experiences to write engaging, informative books that thoroughly address today's fitness and wellness issues in a format accessible to students. Since 1990, he has been the most widely read fitness and wellness college textbook author in the United States. He has published a total of 56 editions of his 9 fitness and wellness-related titles. Among the textbooks written for Cengage Learning are *Principles and Labs for Fitness and Wellness,* twelfth edition; *Fitness and Wellness,* eleventh edition; *Principles and Labs for Physical Fitness,* ninth edition; *Wellness: Guidelines for a Healthy Lifestyle,* fourth edition; and *Water Aerobics for Fitness and Wellness,* fourth edition (with Terry-Ann Spitzer Gibson).

Dr. Hoeger was the first author to write a college fitness textbook that incorporated the "wellness" concept. In 1986, with the release of the first edition of *Lifetime Physical Fitness & Wellness,* he introduced the principle that to truly improve fitness, health, and quality of life, and to achieve wellness, a person needed to go beyond the basic health-related components of physical fitness. His work was so well received that every fitness author immediately followed his lead.

As an innovator in the field, Dr. Hoeger has developed many fitness and wellness assessment tools, including fitness tests such as the Modified Sit-and-Reach, Total Body Rotation, Shoulder Rotation, Muscular Endurance, and Muscular Strength and Endurance, and Soda Pop Coordination Tests. Proving that he "practices what he preaches," he was the oldest male competitor in the 2002 Winter Olympics in Salt Lake City, Utah, at the age of 48. He raced in the sport of luge along with his then 17-year-old son Christopher. It was the first time in Winter Olympics history that father and son competed in the same event. In 2006, at the age of 52, he was the oldest competitor at the Winter Olympics in Turin, Italy. In 2011, Dr. Hoeger raced in the 800-, 1,500-, and 5,000-meter events in track and field at the World Masters Athletic Championships held in Sacramento, California. In 2012, he reached All-American standards for his age group by USA Track and Field in the 1,500-meter event.

Sharon A. Hoeger is Vice-President of Fitness & Wellness, Inc. of Boise, Idaho. Sharon received her degree in computer science from Brigham Young University. She is extensively involved in the research process used in retrieving the most current scientific information that goes into the revision of each textbook. She is also the author of the software written specifically for the fitness and wellness textbooks. Her innovations in this area since the publication of the first edition of *Lifetime Physical Fitness & Wellness* set the standard for fitness and wellness computer software used in this market today.

Sharon is a co-author in five of the seven fitness and wellness titles. She also served as Chef de Mission (Chief of Delegation) for the Venezuelan Olympic Team at the 2006 Olympic Winter Games in Turin, Italy. Husband and wife have been jogging and strength training together for more than 37 years. They are the proud parents of five children, all of whom are involved in sports and lifetime fitness activities. Their motto: "Families that exercise together, stay together."

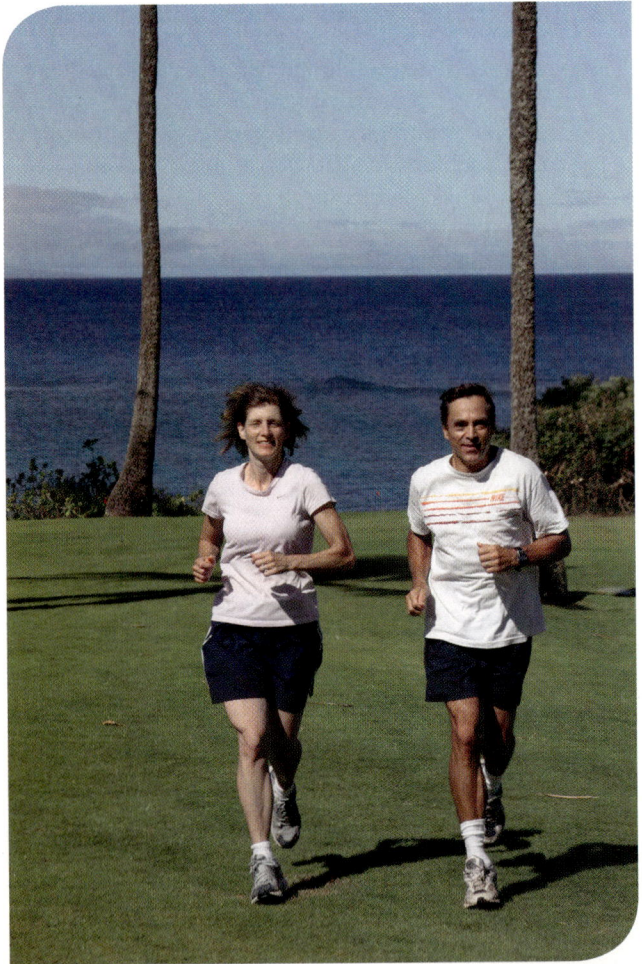

Acknowledgments

This book is dedicated to Dr. LaVon Johnson—coach, professor, mentor, colleague, and lifetime friend—for believing in me, guiding me, and providing me with the opportunities to make the most out of my athletic and professional career. For your unconditional help and support, I am forever grateful.

                                        Werner W. K. Hoeger

The completion of the 13th edition of *Lifetime Physical Fitness & Wellness: A Personalized Program* was made possible through the contributions of many individuals. In particular, we would like to express our gratitude to the reviewers of the 12th edition; their valuable comments and suggestions are most sincerely appreciated.

Reviewers for the 13th edition:

Chip Darracott, Georgia Regents University

Kathy Gieg, Missouri Baptist University

Laurelia Hardy, Georgia Regents University

Candace Hendershot, University of Findlay

Kevin B. Kinser, Tarrant County College

Linda J. Romaine, Raritan Valley Community College

William Russell, Missouri Western State University

Staci Jo Smith, Tarrant County College

Physical Fitness and Wellness

The human body is extremely resilient during youth—not so during middle and older age. The power of prevention, nonetheless, is yours: It enables you to make healthy lifestyle choices today that will prevent disease in the future and increase the quality and length of your life.

Objectives

- **Understand** the health and fitness consequences of physical inactivity.
- **Identify** the major health problems in the United States.
- **Learn** how to monitor daily physical activity.
- **Learn** the Federal Physical Activity Guidelines for Americans.
- **Define** wellness and list its dimensions.
- **Define** physical fitness and list health-related and skill-related components.
- **State** the differences among physical fitness, health promotion, and wellness.
- **Distinguish** between health fitness standards and physical fitness standards.
- **Understand** the benefits and significance of participating in a comprehensive wellness program.
- **List** key national health objectives for the year 2020.
- **Determine** if you can safely initiate an exercise program.
- **Learn** to assess resting heart rate and blood pressure.

CENGAGEbrain.com

Visit www.cengagebrain.com to access course materials and companion resources for this text, including a daily exercise log, the Physical Activity Readiness Questionnaire (PAR-Q), the health history questionnaire, quiz questions designed to check your understanding of the chapter contents, and more! See the preface on page ix for more information.

FAQ

Why should I take a fitness and wellness course?

Most people go to college to learn how to make a living, but a fitness and wellness course will teach you how to *live*—how to truly live life to its fullest potential. Some people seem to think that success is measured by how much money they make. Making a good living will not help you unless you live a wellness lifestyle that will allow you to enjoy what you earn. You may want to ask yourself: Of what value are a nice income, a beautiful home, and a solid retirement portfolio if at age 45 I suffer a massive heart attack that will seriously limit my physical capacity or end life itself?

Is the attainment of good physical fitness sufficient to ensure good health?

Regular participation in a sound physical fitness program will provide substantial health benefits and significantly decrease the risk of many chronic diseases. And although good fitness often motivates toward adoption of additional positive lifestyle behaviors, to maximize the benefits for a healthier, more productive, happier, and longer life we have to pay attention to all seven dimensions of wellness: physical, social, mental, emotional, occupational, environmental, and spiritual. These dimensions are interrelated, and one frequently affects the other. A wellness way of life requires a constant and deliberate effort to stay healthy and achieve the highest potential for well-being within all dimensions of wellness.

If a person is going to do only one thing to improve health, what would it be?

This is a common question. It is a mistake to think, though, that you can modify just one factor and enjoy wellness. Wellness requires a constant and deliberate effort to change unhealthy behaviors and reinforce healthy behaviors. Although it is difficult to work on many lifestyle changes all at once, being involved in a regular physical activity program, proper nutrition, and avoidance of addictive behavior are lifestyle factors to work on first. Others should follow, depending on your current lifestyle behaviors.

Modern-day conveniences lull people into a sedentary lifestyle.

Scientific findings have shown that physical inactivity and a negative lifestyle seriously threaten health and hasten the deterioration rate of the human body. Movement and physical activity are basic functions for which the human organism was created.

Advances in technology, however, have almost completely eliminated the necessity for physical exertion in daily life. Physical activity is no longer a natural part of our existence. We live in an automated society, where most of the activities that used to require strenuous exertion can be accomplished by machines with the simple pull of a handle or push of a button.

Most industrialized nations in the world are experiencing an epidemic of physical inactivity. In the United States,

Real Life Story | Jim's Experience

I am pretty athletic and played baseball and basketball in high school. I also grew up eating well, since my dad is a chef who specializes in healthy cuisine. So when I got to college, I was sure that I was already doing everything necessary to be healthy. However, at the same time that I was congratulating myself for my healthy lifestyle, I was practicing some very unhealthy habits without even thinking about it. My sleep schedule was horrible. I would sometimes only get three to four hours of sleep a night. At times I would pull an "all-nighter" and other times I would crash and sleep for twelve hours. I drank huge amounts of black coffee, diet soda, or energy drinks to stay alert. I was under a lot of stress—I was pre-med and I was struggling in some of my classes. My two roommates and I did not get along, so there was constant fighting and tension between us. I felt isolated and unhappy and I questioned whether I had made a mistake choosing the college I did. In order to blow off steam, I started going to frat parties and drinking too much. I would often get sick and then suffer a hangover the next morning. I didn't see this as a problem because it seemed to be something a lot of students were doing. And to add to all that, after months of high-impact running on concrete surfaces, I ended up injuring my knee. I was barely able to move around, let alone work out. I was only in my second year of college when I took a fitness and wellness class. It was then that I really thought about how my lifestyle was affecting my health and wellness. During the course of the class, I made several changes. I tried to even out my sleep schedule and get seven to eight hours a night. To do so, I had to work on my procrastination. I could no longer wait to write a paper until the night before it was due and still expect to get eight hours of sleep. This change actually helped me do better in my classes, which relieved some of my stress. The times when I still felt stressed out, I started meditating or listening to relaxing music instead of going out and drinking. I also learned about how to exercise safely and prevent injuries. I took up swimming, since it is a good, low-impact workout. I feel like just how sometimes problems can snowball and lead to more problems, small changes for the better can sometimes snowball too; and once you improve one habit, other things in your life become easier to fix. Because of the changes I have made, the rest of my college career has been much healthier and happier than my first year!

---

physical inactivity is the second greatest threat to public health and has been termed "**Sedentary Death Syndrome**" or **SeDS** (the number-one threat is tobacco use—the largest cause of preventable deaths).

Widespread interest in **health** and preventive medicine in recent years, nonetheless, is motivating people to participate in organized fitness and wellness programs. The growing number of participants is attributed primarily to scientific evidence linking regular physical activity and positive lifestyle habits to better health, longevity, quality of life, and overall well-being.

At the beginning of the 20th century, **life expectancy** for a child born in the United States was only 47 years. The most common health problems in the Western world were infectious diseases, such as tuberculosis, diphtheria, influenza, kidney disease, polio, and other diseases of infancy. Progress in the medical field largely eliminated these diseases. Then, as more people started to enjoy the "good life" (**sedentary** living, alcohol, fatty foods, excessive sweets, tobacco, drugs), we saw a parallel increase in the incidence of **chronic diseases** such as cardiovascular disease, cancer, diabetes, and chronic respiratory diseases (Figure 1.1). According to the World Health Organization (WHO), chronic diseases account for 60 percent of all deaths worldwide.[1]

As the incidence of chronic diseases climbed, we recognized that prevention is the best medicine. Consequently, a fitness and wellness movement developed gradually in the 1980s. People began to realize that good health is mostly self-controlled and that the leading causes of premature death and illness could be prevented by adhering to positive lifestyle habits. We all desire to live a long life, and wellness programs seek to enhance the overall quality of life—for as long as we live.

There are three basic factors that determine our health and longevity: genetics, the environment, and our behavior (Figure 1.2). Although we cannot change our genetic pool, we can exert control over the environment and our health behaviors so that we may reach our full physical potential based on our genetic code. How we accomplish this goal will be thoroughly discussed through the chapters of this book.

> **Sedentary Death Syndrome (SeDS)** Cause of deaths attributed to a lack of regular physical activity.
>
> **Health** A state of complete well-being—not just the absence of disease or infirmity.
>
> **Life expectancy** Number of years a person is expected to live based on the person's birth year.
>
> **Sedentary** Description of a person who is relatively inactive and whose lifestyle is characterized by a lot of sitting.
>
> **Chronic diseases** Illnesses that develop as a result of an unhealthy lifestyle and last a long time.

PERSONAL PROFILE: General Understanding of Fitness and Wellness

To the best of your ability, please answer the following questions. If you do not know the answer(s), this chapter will guide you through them.

I. Physical fitness implies making a constant and deliberate effort to stay healthy and achieve the highest potential for well-being. ___ True ___ False

II. The minimum requirement in the U.S. Federal Physical Activity Guidelines is that you accumulate ___ minutes of moderate-intensity aerobic activity or ___ minutes of vigorous-intensity aerobic activity on a weekly basis.

III. Agility, balance, coordination, reaction time, power, and speed are the basic components of health-related fitness. ___ True ___ False

IV. My current blood pressure is ___ / ___ mm Hg.

V. I am aware of risk factors in my life that can increase my chances of developing chronic diseases. ___ Yes ___ No

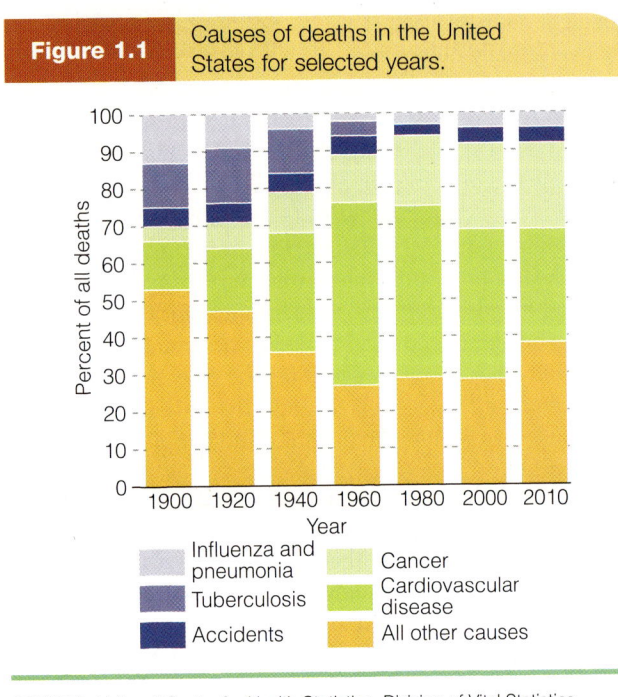

Figure 1.1 Causes of deaths in the United States for selected years.

SOURCE: National Center for Health Statistics, Division of Vital Statistics.

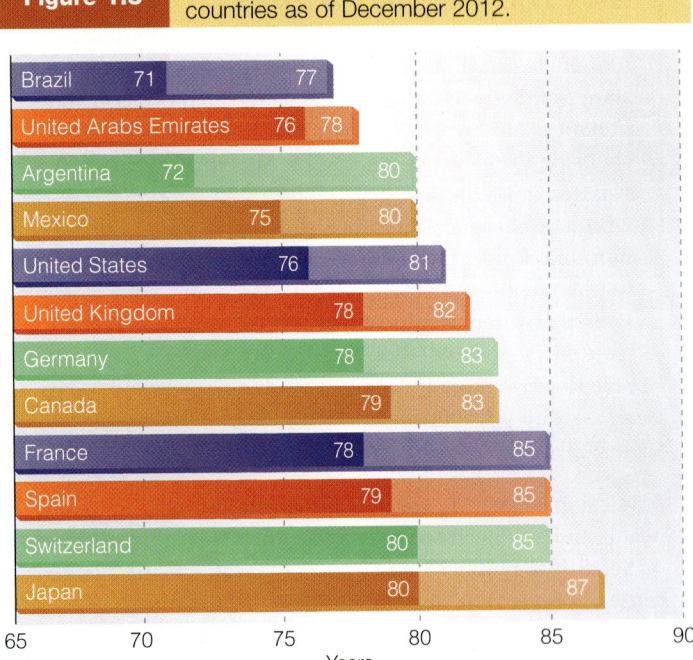

Figure 1.3 Life expectancy at birth for selected countries as of December 2012.

*Dark color is men; light color is women.

SOURCE: United Nations, Social Indicators: Indicators on Health, http://unstats.un.org/unsd/demographic/products/socind/default.htm. Downloaded May 20, 2013.

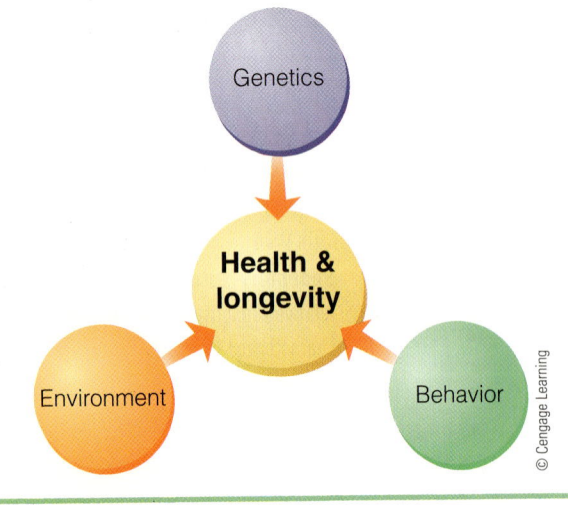

Figure 1.2 Factors that determine health and longevity.

1.1 Life Expectancy

Currently, the average life expectancy in the United States is 78.7 years (76.3 years for men and 81.1 years for women). In the past decade alone, life expectancy has increased by 1 year—the news, however, is not all good. The data show that people now spend an extra 1.2 years with a serious illness and an extra 2 years of disability. Mortality has been postponed because medical treatments allow people to live longer with various chronic ailments (cardiovascular disease, cancer, diabetes).

Based on the WHO data, the United States ranks 28th in the world for life expectancy (see Figure 1.3). Between 2000 and 2010, U.S. male life expectancy slipped from 18th to 24th in the world and female life expectancy from 28th to 35th. Japan ranks first in the world with an overall life expectancy of 82.6 years.

Several factors may account for the current U.S. life expectancy ranking: the extremely poor health of some groups (such as Native Americans, rural African Americans, and the inner-city poor), the obesity epidemic, the low level of daily physical activity, the high incidence of tobacco use and coronary heart disease, and fairly high levels of violence (notably homicides).

Life expectancy for men in the United States is almost five years lower than in women. For years it has been assumed that the difference is based on biology, but most likely the gender gap is related to lifestyle behaviors most commonly observed in men. Around 1980, the gender gap in life expectancy was almost eight years. The decrease in the gender gap is thought to be due to the fact that women are increasingly taking on jobs, habits, and stressors of men such as smoking, drinking, and employment outside the home.

Men, nonetheless, still report higher stress on the job and are less likely to engage in stress management programs. Also, 95 percent of employees in the 10 most dangerous jobs are men. Furthermore, men's health is not given the same degree of attention in terms of public health policies. Fewer programs are available that specifically target men's health issues. Thus, men need to take a more proactive role for their own health and public health policies.

"Masculinity" itself is also partially to blame. Men are less likely to visit a physician when something is wrong and are less likely to heed preventive care visits to be screened for potential risk factors such as hypertension, elevated cholesterol, diabetes, obesity, substance abuse, and depression or anxiety. Chronic diseases in men are often diagnosed at a later stage, when a cure or adequate management is more difficult to achieve. Men also drive faster than women and are more likely to engage in risk-taking activities.

Although life expectancy in the United States gradually increased by 30 years over the past century, scientists from the National Institute of Aging believe that in the coming decades the average lifespan may decrease by as much as 5 years. This decrease in life expectancy will be related primarily to the growing epidemic of obesity. According to estimates from the Centers for Disease Control and Prevention, 34 percent of the adult population in the United States is obese. If the current trend continues, the current generation of children may not outlive their parents. Additional information on the obesity epidemic and its detrimental health consequences is given in Chapter 5.

1.2 Leading Health Problems in the United States

The leading causes of death in the United States today are largely lifestyle related (Figure 1.4). The U.S. Surgeon General has stated that 7 of 10 Americans die of preventable chronic

Healthy Habits That Cut the Risk for Serious Disease

According to the Centers for Disease Control and Prevention, four health habits can reduce your risk of chronic diseases such as heart disease, cancer, and diabetes by almost 80 percent:

- Get at least 30 minutes of daily moderate-intensity physical activity.
- Don't ever smoke.
- Eat a healthy diet (ample fruits and vegetables, whole grain products, and low meat consumption).
- Maintain a body mass index (BMI) less than 30.

diseases.[2] Specifically, about 52 percent of all deaths in the United States are caused by cardiovascular disease and cancer.[3] Almost 80 percent of the latter deaths could be prevented through a healthy lifestyle program. The third and fourth leading causes of death, respectively, are chronic lower respiratory disease and accidents.

1.3 Diseases of the Cardiovascular System

The most prevalent degenerative diseases in the United States are those of the cardiovascular system. About 30 percent of all deaths in this country are attributed to diseases of the heart and blood vessels (about 800,000 total deaths). According to the American Heart Association (AHA), 83.6 million people in the United States are afflicted with diseases of the cardiovascular system, including 77.9 million with hypertension (high blood pressure) and 15.4 million with coronary heart disease (CHD). (Many of these people have more than one type of cardiovascular disease.) The estimated direct and indirect cost of cardiovascular disease in 2010 exceeded $312.6 billion.[4] A complete cardiovascular disease prevention program is outlined in Chapter 10.

1.4 Cancer

The second leading cause of death in the United States is cancer. Even though cancer is not the number-one killer, it is the number-one health fear of the American people. About 23 percent of all deaths in the United States are attributable to cancer. More than 580,000 people died from this disease in 2013, and more than 1.6 million new cases were reported the same year.[5] The major contributor to the increase in the incidence of cancer during the past five decades is lung cancer, of which 87 percent is caused by tobacco use. Furthermore, smoking accounts for more than 30 percent of all deaths from cancer. More than 30 percent of deaths are related to nutrition, physical inactivity, excessive body weight, and other faulty lifestyle habits.

The American Cancer Society maintains that the most influential factor in fighting cancer today is prevention through health education programs. Evidence indicates that as much as 80 percent of all human cancer can be prevented through positive lifestyle behaviors. A comprehensive cancer-prevention program is presented in Chapter 11.

1.5 Chronic Lower Respiratory Disease (CLRD)

CLRD, the third leading cause of death, is a general term that includes chronic obstructive pulmonary disease, emphysema, and chronic bronchitis (all diseases of the respiratory system). Although CLRD is related mostly to tobacco use (see Chapter 13 for discussion on how to stop smoking), lifetime nonsmokers also can develop CLRD.

Precautions to prevent CLRD include consuming a low-fat, low-sodium, nutrient-dense diet; staying physically active; not smoking and not breathing cigarette smoke; getting a pneumonia vaccine if older than age 50 and a current or ex-smoker; and avoiding swimming pools for individuals sensitive to chlorine vapor.

1.6 Accidents

Accidents are the fourth leading cause of death. Even though not all accidents are preventable, many are. Fatal accidents are often related to abusing drugs and not wearing seat belts. Furthermore, with the advent of cell phones, 1.6 million car accidents each year are caused by drivers using cell phones or reading/sending text messages.

Most people do not perceive accidents as a health problem. Even so, accidents affect the total well-being of millions of Americans each year. Accident prevention and personal safety are part of a health-enhancement program aimed at achieving a better quality of life. Proper nutrition, exercise, stress management, and abstinence from cigarette smoking are of little help if the person is involved in a disabling or fatal accident as a result of distraction, a single reckless decision, or not wearing seat belts properly.

Accidents do not just happen. We cause accidents, and we are victims of accidents. Although some factors in life, such as earthquakes, tornadoes, and airplane accidents, are completely beyond our control, more often than not, personal safety and accident prevention are a matter of common sense. Most accidents stem from poor judgment and confused mental states, which occur when people are upset, are not paying attention to the task at hand, or are abusing alcohol or other drugs.

Alcohol abuse is the number-one cause of all accidents. About half of accidental deaths and suicides in the United States are alcohol related. Further, alcohol intoxication is the leading cause of fatal automobile accidents. Other commonly abused drugs alter feelings and perceptions, generate mental confusion, and impair judgment and coordination, greatly enhancing the risk for accidental **morbidity** and mortality (Chapter 13).

1.7 Lifestyle as a Health Problem

The underlying causes of death attributable to leading risk factors in the United States (Figure 1.5) indicate that most factors are related to lifestyle choices we make. Of the approximately 2.4 million yearly deaths in the United States, the "big five" factors—tobacco smoking, high blood pressure, overweight and obesity, physical inactivity, and high blood glucose—are responsible for almost 1.5 million deaths each year.

As the incidence of chronic diseases rose, it became obvious that prevention was—and remains—the best medicine. According to the U.S. Surgeon General's office, more than half of the people who die in this country each year die because of what they do. Based on estimates, more than half of disease is lifestyle related, a fifth is attributed to the environment, and a tenth is influenced by the health care the individual receives. Only 16 percent is related to genetic factors (Figure 1.6). Thus, the individual controls as much as 84 percent of his or her vulnerability to disease—and thus quality of life. The same data indicate that 83 percent of deaths before age 65 are preventable. In essence, most people in the United States are threatened by the very lives they lead today.

Because of the unhealthy lifestyles that many young adults lead, their bodies may be middle-aged or older! Many school physical fitness programs do not emphasize the skills necessary for young people to maintain a high level of fitness and health throughout life. The intent of this book is to provide those skills and help to prepare you for a lifetime of physical fitness and wellness. A healthy lifestyle is self-controlled, and you can learn how to be responsible for your own health and fitness. Healthy choices made today influence health for decades.

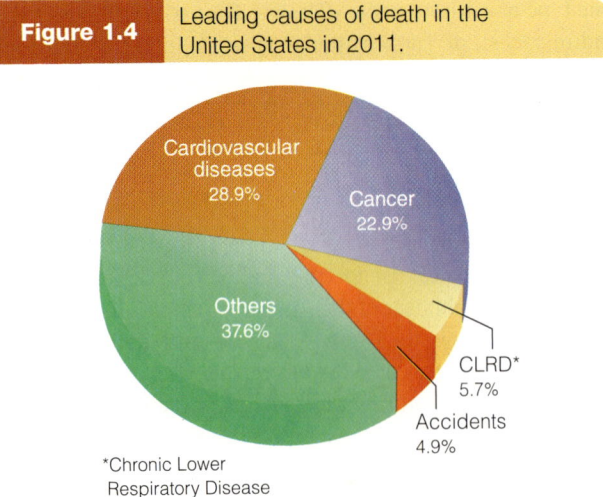

Figure 1.4 Leading causes of death in the United States in 2011.

Cardiovascular diseases 28.9%
Cancer 22.9%
Others 37.6%
CLRD* 5.7%
Accidents 4.9%

*Chronic Lower Respiratory Disease

SOURCE: U.S. Department of Health and Human Services, Centers for Disease Control and Prevention, National Center for Health Statistics, National Vital Statistics reports, *Deaths: Preliminary Data for 2011,* 61:6 (October 10, 2012).

Figure 1.5 Death from all causes attributable to lifestyle-related risk factors for men and women in the United States.

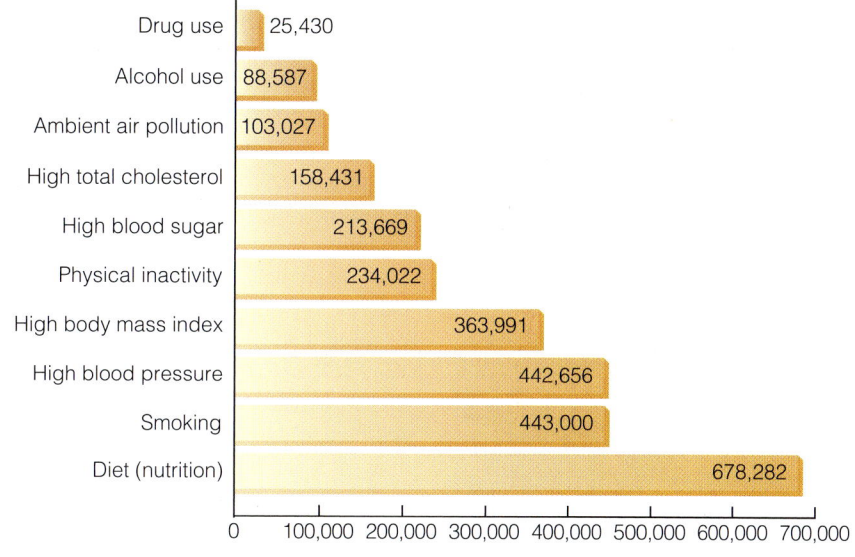

Risk Factor	Deaths
Drug use	25,430
Alcohol use	88,587
Ambient air pollution	103,027
High total cholesterol	158,431
High blood sugar	213,669
Physical inactivity	234,022
High body mass index	363,991
High blood pressure	442,656
Smoking	443,000
Diet (nutrition)	678,282

SOURCE: Adapted from G. Danaei, et al., "The Preventable Causes of Death in the United States: Comparative Risk Assessment of Dietary, Lifestyle, and Metabolic Risk Factors," *PLoS Med* 6, no. 4 (2009): e1000058.doi:10.1371/journal.pmed.1000058.

1.8 Physical Activity and Exercise Defined

Abundant scientific research over the past three decades has established a distinction between physical activity and exercise. **Physical activity** is bodily movement produced by skeletal muscles. It requires energy expenditure and produces progressive health benefits. Physical activity typically requires only a low to moderate intensity of effort. Examples of physical activity include walking to and from work, taking the stairs instead of elevators and escalators, gardening, doing household chores, dancing, and washing the car by hand. Physical inactivity, by contrast, implies a level of activity that is lower than that required to maintain good health.

Exercise is a type of physical activity that requires planned, structured, and repetitive bodily movement to improve or maintain one or more components of physical fitness. Examples of exercise are walking, running, cycling, aerobics, swimming, and strength training. Exercise is usually viewed as an activity that requires a vigorous-intensity effort.

Importance of Increased Physical Activity

The U.S. Surgeon General has stated that poor health as a result of lack of physical activity is a serious public health problem that must be met head-on at once. Regular **moderate physical activity** provides substantial benefits in health and well-being for the vast majority of people who are not physically active. For those who are already moderately active, even greater

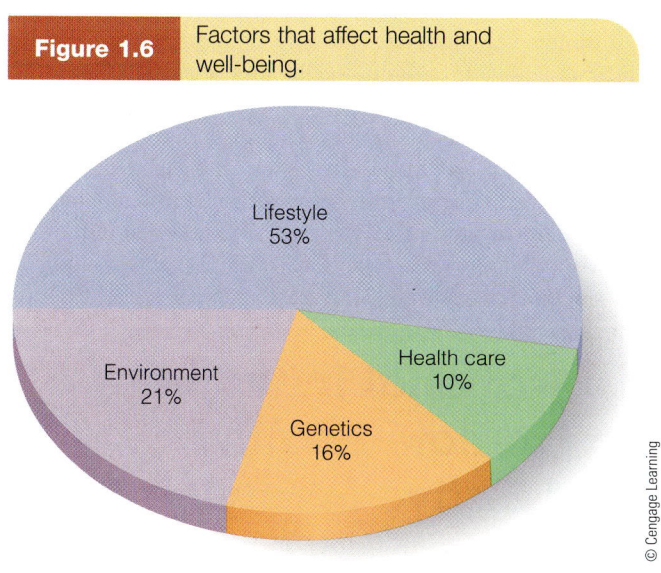

Figure 1.6 Factors that affect health and well-being.

- Lifestyle 53%
- Environment 21%
- Genetics 16%
- Health care 10%

Morbidity A condition related to or caused by illness or disease.

Physical activity Bodily movement produced by skeletal muscles; requires expenditure of energy and produces progressive health benefits. Examples include walking, taking the stairs, dancing, gardening, yard work, house cleaning, snow shoveling, washing the car, and all forms of structured exercise.

Exercise A type of physical activity that requires planned, structured, and repetitive bodily movement with the intent of improving or maintaining one or more components of physical fitness.

Moderate physical activity Activity that uses 150 calories of energy per day, or 1,000 calories per week.

health benefits can be achieved by increasing the level of physical activity.

Among the benefits of regular physical activity and exercise are a significant reduction in premature mortality and decreased risks for developing heart disease, stroke, metabolic syndrome, type 2 diabetes, obesity, osteoporosis, colon and breast cancers, high blood pressure, and depression.[6] Regular physical activity also is important for the health of muscles, bones, and joints, and it improves cognitive function, mood, and enhances one's ability to perform daily tasks throughout life. It also can help control health care costs and maintain a high quality of life into old age.

Moderate physical activity has been defined as any activity that requires an energy expenditure of 150 calories per day, or 1,000 calories per week. The general health recommendation is that people strive to accumulate at least 30 minutes of physical activity a minimum of 5 days per week (Table 1.1). Whereas 30 minutes of continuous activity is preferred, on days when time is limited, 3 activity sessions of at least 10 minutes each still provide substantial health benefits. Examples of moderate physical activity are brisk walking or cycling, playing basketball or volleyball, swimming, water aerobics, dancing fast, pushing a stroller, raking leaves, shoveling snow, washing or waxing a car, washing windows or floors, and even gardening. Light-intensity activities of daily living such as casual walking, self-care, shopping, or moderate activities lasting less than 10 minutes in duration cannot be included as part of the moderate physical activity recommendation.

Although accumulating 30 minutes of moderate- or vigorous-intensity physical activity provides substantial health benefits, new data indicate that most of these benefits may be voided if people spend most of the rest of the day in a sedentary condition. Sitting for long periods of time seems to be an independent risk factor for premature morbidity and mortality. This topic is discussed under the heading *"Sitting Disease": A 21st Century Chronic Disease* on page 13 in this chapter.

Because of the ever-growing epidemic of obesity in the United States, the Institute of Medicine of the National Academy of Sciences increased the recommendation to 60 minutes of moderate-intensity physical activity every day.[7] This recommendation was based on evidence indicating that people who maintain healthy weight typically accumulate 1 hour of daily physical activity.

Subsequently, the Dietary Guidelines for Americans by the U.S. Department of Health and Human Services and the Department of Agriculture recommend that up to 60 minutes of moderate- to vigorous-intensity physical activity per day may be necessary to prevent weight gain, and between 60 and 90 minutes of moderate-intensity physical activity daily is recommended to sustain weight loss for previously overweight people.[8]

In sum, although health benefits are derived from 30 minutes of physical activity per day, people with a tendency to gain weight need to be physically active for an hour to an hour and a half daily to prevent weight gain. And 60 to 90 minutes of activity per day provides additional health benefits, including a lower risk for cardiovascular disease and diabetes.

An active lifestyle increases health, quality of life, and longevity.

1.9 National Initiatives to Promote Healthy and Active Lifestyles

Federal Guidelines for Physical Activity Because of the importance of physical activity to our health, the

Table 1.1 Physical Activity Guidelines

Benefits	Duration	Intensity	Frequency per Week	Weekly Time
Health	30 min	MI*	5 times	150 min
Health and fitness	20 min	VI*	3 times	75 min
Health, fitness, and weight gain prevention	60 min	MI/VI†	5–7 times	300 min
Health, fitness, and weight regain prevention	60–90 min	MI/VI†	5–7 times	450 min

*MI = moderate intensity, VI = vigorous intensity
†MI/VI = You may use MI or VI or a combination of the two
© Cengage Learning

U.S. Department of Health and Human Services has issued the Federal Physical Activity Guidelines for Americans. These guidelines complement the Dietary Guidelines for Americans (Chapter 3, pages 118-119) and further substantiate previous recommendations issued by the American College of Sports Medicine (ACSM) and the AHA in 2007,[9] and the U.S. Surgeon General in 1996.[10]

The federal guidelines provide science-based guidance on the importance of being physically active to promote health and reduce the risk for chronic diseases. The federal guidelines include the following recommendations[11]:

Adults between 18 and 64 years of age

- Adults should do 2 hours and 30 minutes a week of moderate-intensity aerobic (cardiorespiratory) physical activity, 1 hour and 15 minutes (75 minutes) a week of vigorous-intensity aerobic physical activity, or an equivalent combination of moderate- and vigorous-intensity aerobic physical activity (also see Chapter 6). When combining moderate- and vigorous-intensity activities, a person could participate in moderate-intensity activity twice a week for 30 minutes and high-intensity activity for 20 minutes on another 2 days. Aerobic activity should be performed in episodes of at least 10 minutes long each, preferably spread throughout the week.
- Additional health benefits are provided by increasing to 5 hours (300 minutes) a week of moderate-intensity aerobic physical activity, 2 hours and 30 minutes a week of vigorous-intensity physical activity, or an equivalent combination of both.
- Adults should also do muscle-strengthening activities that involve all major muscle groups, performed on two or more days per week.

Older adults (ages 65 and older)

- Older adults should follow the adult guidelines. If this is not possible due to limiting chronic conditions, older adults should be as physically active as their abilities allow. They should avoid inactivity. Older adults should do exercises that maintain or improve balance if they are at risk of falling.

Children 6 years of age and older and adolescents

- Children and adolescents should do 1 hour (60 minutes) or more of physical activity every day. Most of the 1 hour or more a day should be either moderate- or vigorous-intensity aerobic physical activity.
- As part of their daily physical activity, children and adolescents should do vigorous-intensity activity at least three days per week. They also should do muscle-strengthening and bone-strengthening activities at least three days per week.

Pregnant and postpartum women

- Healthy women who are not already doing vigorous-intensity physical activity should get at least 2 hours and 30 minutes (150 minutes) of moderate-intensity aerobic activity a week. Preferably, this activity should be spread throughout the week. Women who regularly engage in vigorous-intensity aerobic activity or high amounts of activity can continue their activity provided that their condition remains unchanged and they talk to their health care provider about their activity level throughout their pregnancy.

In a previous 2007 report, the ACSM and the AHA also released a joint statement on physical activity recommendations for healthy adults.[12] The ACSM/AHA report states that a greater amount of physical activity that exceeds the minimum recommendations provided earlier for adults between 18 and 64 years of age provides even greater benefits and is recommended for individuals who wish to further improve personal fitness, reduce the risk for chronic disease and disabilities, prevent premature mortality, or prevent unhealthy weight gain.

In conjunction with the previously described report, the ACSM and the American Medical Association (AMA) have launched a nationwide "Exercise Is Medicine" program.[13] The goal of this initiative is to improve the health and wellness of the nation through exercise prescriptions from physicians and health care providers. It calls on all physicians to assess and review every patient's physical activity program at every visit.

"Exercise is medicine and it's free." All physicians should be prescribing exercise to all patients and participate in exercise themselves. Exercise is considered to be the much-needed vaccine of our time to prevent chronic diseases. Physical activity and exercise are powerful tools for both the treatment and the prevention of chronic diseases and premature death. Additional information on this program can be obtained by consulting the following Web site: www.exerciseismedicine.org/.

> **Critical Thinking**
>
> Do you consciously incorporate physical activity throughout the day into your daily lifestyle? • Can you provide examples? • Do you think you get sufficient daily physical activity to maintain good health?

1.10 National Health Objectives for the Year 2020

Every 10 years, the U.S. Department of Health and Human Services releases a list of objectives for preventing disease and promoting health. Since 1979, the Healthy People initiative has set and monitored national health objectives to meet a broad range of health needs, encourage collaborations across sectors, guide individuals toward making informed health decisions, and measure the impact of our prevention activity. Currently, Healthy People is leading the way to achieve increased quality and years of healthy life and to seek to eliminate health disparities among all groups of people. The objectives address three important points[14]:

1. *Personal responsibility for health behavior.* Individuals need to become ever more health conscious. Responsible and informed behaviors are the keys to good health.
2. *Health benefits for all people and all communities.* Lower socioeconomic conditions and poor health often are interrelated. Extending the benefits of good health to all people is crucial to the health of the nation.
3. *Health promotion and disease prevention.* A shift from treatment to preventive techniques will drastically cut health care costs and help all Americans achieve a better quality of life.

Developing these health objectives involves more than 10,000 people representing 300 national organizations, including the Institute of Medicine of the National Academy of Sciences, all state health departments, and the federal Office of Disease Prevention and Health Promotion. Figure 1.7 summarizes the key 2020 objectives. Living the fitness and wellness principles provided in this book will enhance the quality of your life and also will allow you to be an active participant in achieving the Healthy People 2020 Objectives.

1.11 National Physical Activity Plan

Established in 2010, the National Physical Activity Plan calls for policy, environmental, and cultural changes to help all Americans enjoy the health benefits of physical activity. It aims to in-

Figure 1.7 Selected health objectives for the year 2020.

- Increase the proportion of persons with health insurance, a usual primary care provider, and coverage for clinical preventive services.
- Ensure that all people, including those with illnesses and chronic disability, participate daily in meaningful and freely chosen recreation, leisure, and physical activity, which directly influences well-being and quality of life.
- Reduce the proportion of adults who engage in no leisure-time physical activity.
- Increase the proportion of adolescents and adults who meet current Federal Physical Activity Guidelines.
- Increase the proportion of adults who are at a healthy weight, and reduce the proportion of children, adolescents, and adults who are overweight or obese.
- Reduce coronary heart disease and stroke deaths.
- Reduce the mean total blood cholesterol levels among adults and the proportion of persons in the population with hypertension.
- Increase the proportion of adults aged 20 years and older who are aware of, and respond to, early warning symptoms and signs of a heart attack and stroke.
- Reduce the overall cancer death rate and provide counseling about cancer prevention.
- Reduce the diabetes death rate and the annual number of new cases of diagnosed diabetes in the population.
- Reduce infections caused by key pathogens commonly transmitted through food.
- Increase the proportion of sexually active persons who use condoms.
- Reduce the rate of HIV transmission among adults and adolescents, and reduce the number of deaths resulting from HIV infection.
- Increase the proportion of substance-abuse treatment facilities that offer HIV/AIDS education, counseling, and support.
- Increase school-based health promotion programs available to youth between the ages of 14 and 22 to decrease the rate of sexually transmitted diseases and teen pregnancy and to increase the proportion of adolescents who abstain from sexual intercourse or use condoms if sexually active.
- Reduce tobacco use by adults and adolescents, and reduce the initiation among children, adolescents, and young adults.
- Reduce average annual alcohol consumption, and increase the proportion of adolescents who disapprove of substance abuse.
- Increase the proportion, among persons who need alcohol and/or illicit drug treatment, of those who receive specialized treatment for abuse or dependence.
- Reduce drug-induced deaths.

crease physical activity among all segments of the population. The plan is a comprehensive private/public sector joint effort to create a culture that supports active lifestyles and enables everyone to meet physical activity guidelines throughout life.

The vision of the plan is that one day all Americans will be physically active, and they will live, work, and play in environments that facilitate regular physical activity. The plan complements the Federal Physical Activity Guidelines and the Healthy People 2020 objectives and comprises recommendations organized in eight sectors of societal influence: education; business and industry; health care; mass media; parks recreation, fitness, and sports; public health; volunteer and non-profit; and transportation, land use, and community design. Strategies to implement the plan include:

- Developing and implementing policies requiring school accountability for quality and quantity of physical education and physical activity.
- Encouraging early childhood education programs to have children as physically active as possible.
- Providing access to and opportunities for physical activity before and after school.
- Making physical activity a patient "vital sign" (tracking activity levels) that all health care providers assess and discuss with patients.
- Using routine performance measures by local, state, and federal agencies to set benchmarks for active travel (walking, biking, public transportation).
- Enhancing the existing parks and recreation infrastructure with effective policy and environmental changes to promote physical activity.
- Identifying and disseminating best practice models for physical activity in the workplace.
- Providing tax breaks for building owners or employers who provide amenities in workplaces and support active commuting, including showers in buildings, secure bicycle parking, free bicycles, or transit subsidies.
- Encouraging businesses to implement work policies that allow employees to get some physical activity before, during, or after work hours.

The implementation of the National Physical Activity Plan requires cooperation among school officials, city and county council members, state legislators, corporations, and Congress.

Monitoring Daily Physical Activity

The majority of U.S. adults are not sufficiently physically active to promote good health. The most recent data released in 2013 by the Centers for Disease Control and Prevention (CDC) indicate that only 19.4 percent of U.S. adults 18 and over meet the Federal Physical Activity Guidelines for both aerobic and muscular fitness (strength and endurance) activities, whereas 46.1 percent meet the guidelines for aerobic fitness and just 23 percent do so for muscular fitness. Another 34 percent of Americans are completely inactive during their leisure time (Figure 1.8).

Other than carefully monitoring actual time engaged in activity, an excellent tool to monitor daily physical activity is a **pedometer**. A pedometer is a small mechanical device that senses vertical body motion and is used to count footsteps. Wearing a pedometer throughout the day allows you to determine the total steps you take in a day. Some pedometers also record distance, cal-

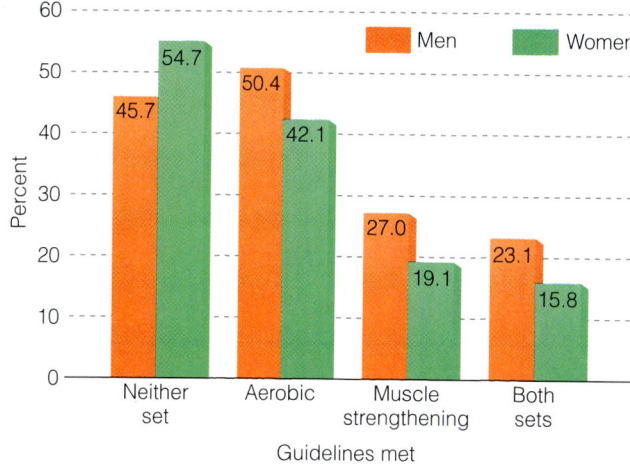

Figure 1.8 Percentage of adults who did not meet and meet the 2008 federal guidelines for physical activity by gender.

SOURCE: http://www.cdc.gov/nchs/data/series/sr_10/sr10_257.pdf (downloaded July 9, 2013)

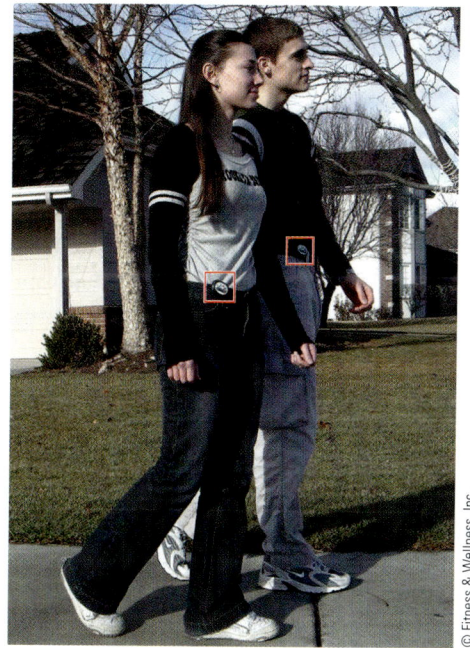

Pedometers are used to monitor daily physical activity; the recommendation is a minimum of 10,000 steps per day.

Pedometer An electronic device that senses body motion and counts footsteps. Some pedometers also record distance, calories burned, speeds, "aerobic steps," and time spent being physically active.

Table 1.2 Adult Activity Levels Based on Total Number of Steps Taken per Day

Steps per Day	Category
<5,000	Sedentary lifestyle
5,000–7,499	Low active
7,500–9,999	Somewhat active
10,000–12,499	Active
12,500	Highly active

SOURCE: C. Tudor-Locke and D. R. Basset, "How Many Steps/Day Are Enough? Preliminary Pedometer Indices for Public Health," *Sports Medicine* 34 (2004):1-8.

ories burned, speeds, and actual time of activity each day. A pedometer is a great motivational tool to help increase, maintain, and monitor daily physical activity that involves lower-body motion (walking, jogging, running).

Before purchasing a pedometer, be sure to verify its accuracy. Many of the free and low-cost pedometers provided by corporations for promotion and advertisement purposes are inaccurate, so their use is discouraged. Pedometers also tend to lose accuracy at a very slow walking speed (slower than 30 minutes per mile) because the vertical movement of the hip is too small to trigger the spring-mounted lever arm inside the pedometer to properly record the steps taken.

You can obtain a good pedometer for about $25, and ratings are available online. The most accurate pedometer brands are Walk4Life, Yamax, Kenz, and New Lifestyles. To test the accuracy of a pedometer, follow these steps: Clip the pedometer on the waist directly above the kneecap, reset the pedometer to zero, carefully close the pedometer, walk exactly 50 steps at your normal pace, carefully open the pedometer, and look at the number of steps recorded. A reading within 10 percent of the actual steps taken (45 to 55 steps) is acceptable.

The typical male American takes about 6,000 steps per day, in comparison to women, who take about 5,300 steps. The general recommendation for adults is 10,000 steps per day, and Table 1.2 provides specific activity categories based on the number of daily steps taken.

All daily steps count, but some of your steps should come in bouts of at least 10 minutes, so as to meet the national physical activity recommendation of accumulating 30 minutes of moderate-intensity physical activity in at least three 10-minute sessions five days per week. A 10-minute brisk walk (a distance of about 1,200 yards at a 15-minute per mile pace) is approximately 1,300 steps. A 15-minute-mile (1,770 yards) walk is about 1,900 steps.[15] Thus, new pedometer brands have an "aerobic steps" function that records steps taken in excess of 60 steps per minute over a 10-minute period of time.

If you do not accumulate the recommended 10,000 daily steps, you can refer to Table 1.3 to determine the additional walking or jogging distance required to reach your goal. For example, if you are 5'8" tall, female, and you typically accumulate 5,200 steps per day, you would need an additional 4,800 daily steps to reach your 10,000-steps goal. You can do so by jogging 3 miles at a 10-minute-per-mile pace (1,602 steps × 3 miles = 4,806 steps) on some days, and you can walk 2.5 miles at a 15-minute-per-mile pace (1,941 steps × 2.5 = miles = 4,853 steps) on other days. If you do not find a particular speed (pace) that you typically walk or jog at in Table 1.3, you can estimate the number of steps at that speed using the prediction equations at the bottom of this table.

Table 1.3 Estimated Number of Steps to Walk, Jog, or Run a Mile Based on Pace, Height, and Gender

	Pace (min/mile)											
	Walking								Jogging/Running			
	20		18		16		15		12	10	8	6
Height	Women	Men	Women	Men	Women	Men	Women	Men	(both men and women)			
5'0"	2,371	2,338	2,244	2,211	2,117	2,084	2,054	2,021	1,997	1,710	1,423	1,136
5'2"	2,343	2,310	2,216	2,183	2,089	2,056	2,026	1,993	1,970	1,683	1,396	1,109
5'4"	2,315	2,282	2,188	2,155	2,061	2,028	1,998	1,965	1,943	1,656	1,369	1,082
5'6"	2,286	2,253	2,160	2,127	2,033	2,000	1,969	1,937	1,916	1,629	1,342	1,055
5'8"	2,258	2,225	2,131	2,098	2,005	1,872	1,941	1,908	1,889	1,602	1,315	1,028
5'10"	2,230	2,197	2,103	2,070	1,976	1,943	1,913	1,880	1,862	1,575	1,288	1,001
6'0"	2,202	2,169	2,075	2,042	1,948	1,915	1,885	1,852	1,835	1,548	1,261	974
6'2"	2,174	2,141	2,047	2,014	1,920	1,887	1,857	1,824	1,808	1,521	1,234	947

Prediction equations (pace in min/mile and height in inches):

Walking
Women: Steps/mile = $1,949 + [(63.4 \times pace) - (14.1 \times height)]$
Women: Steps/mile = $1,916 + [(63.4 \times pace) - (14.1 \times height)]$

Jogging
Women: Steps/mile = $1,084 + [(63.4 \times pace) - (14.1 \times height)]$

Adapted from Werner W. K. Hoeger et al., "One-Mile Step Count at Walking and Running Speeds," *ACSM's Health & Fitness Journal*, Vol 12(1):14-19, 2008.

The first practical application that you can undertake in this course is to determine your current level of daily activity. The log provided in Activity 1.1 will help you do this. Keep a 4-day log of all physical activities that you do daily. On this log, record the time of day; type and duration of the exercise/activity; and, if possible, steps taken while engaged in the activity. The results will indicate how active you are and serve as a basis to monitor changes in the next few months and years.

1.12 "Sitting Disease": A 21st Century Chronic Disease

The human body requires time to recover (sit and sleep) from labor, tasks, and other typical daily activities. Most Americans, however, sit way too many hours than ever before. On *average* people spend about eight hours per day or more of their waking time sitting. Prolonged sitting is unnatural to the body and research now indicates that too much sitting is hazardous to human health.[16] Although not recognized by the medical community as a diagnosable illness, the scientific community has coined the term "**sitting disease**" as a chronic 21st century disease that reflects the detrimental effects of excessive sitting on health and well-being.

The data indicate that even if people exercise five times per week for at least 30 minutes but otherwise spend most of the rest of the day sitting, they are canceling out all the health benefits of the exercise sessions. Death rates are still high for people who spend most of their day sitting, even though they meet the minimum physical activity recommendations on a weekly basis. The data show that:

- Time spent sitting correlates to overall health: The more time you spend sitting throughout the day, the greater the risk for adverse health effects.
- Sitting for more than three hours per day cuts off two years of life, even if you regularly exercise and avoid unhealthy habits like smoking.
- Physically inactive women and men who sit more than 6 hours a day have an almost 100 percent and 50 percent greater chance, respectively, of dying during a span of a little more than a decade than their physically active peers who sit less than 3 hours per day.
- People who spend most of their day sitting have as much as a 50 percent greater risk of dying prematurely from all causes and an 80 percent greater risk of dying from cardiovascular disease.
- Among many other conditions, excessive sitting leads to weaker muscles, a sluggish central nervous system, decreased cognitive function, increased fatigue, obesity, decreased insulin sensitivity, higher blood pressure, decreased activity of lipoprotein lipase (an enzyme that breaks down fats in the blood); and increased cholesterol, LDL cholesterol, and triglycerides.
- Excessive sitting is the "new smoking." The risk of a heart attack in people who sit most of the day is almost the same as that of smokers.
- Prolonged daily sitting time, independent of the daily physical activity/exercise routine, is an underestimated risk factor for cancer and has an effect on overall risk of premature death. Too much sitting has been estimated to cause 92,000 cancer deaths each year in the United States alone (49,000 breast cancers and 42,000 colon cancers).
- Americans who decrease their sitting time by half can expect a 2-year increase in life expectancy. Furthermore, reducing TV viewing to less than 2 hours per day adds another 1.4 years of life.

Most people do not realize how much time they spend sitting on a given day. On any given day, consider the amount of time that you spend driving to and from school or work (1 hour); sitting in classes or working at the office (8 hours); eating meals (1 to 1.5 hours); doing homework (2 to 4 hours); or your typical recreational hours watching TV, at the movies, or at the computer surfing the net, checking email, playing games, and social networking sites (2 to 6 hours). You can easily accumulate 8 to 12 or more sitting hours.

You can fight sitting disease by taking actions to become more physically active. The key is to sit less and move more. To minimize inactivity, look to enhance daily nonexercise activity thermogenesis (NEAT) or the energy expended doing daily activities not related to exercise. Aim to achieve NEAT for 10 minutes every waking hour. Examples of such activities include:

1. Walk instead of drive when you only need to go short distances.
2. Park farther away or get off the subway, train, or bus several blocks from the campus or office.
3. Take a short walk right after each meal or snack.
4. Walk faster than usual.
5. Move about whenever you take a break.
6. Take the stairs as often as you can. Walk up and down the escalators when you don't have a choice of stairs.
7. When watching TV, stand up and move during each commercial break, or even better, workout during TV time.
8. Do not shy away from housecleaning chores or yard work.
9. Stand more while working/studying. Place your computer on an elevated stand or shelf and stand while doing work, writing emails, or surfing the Internet. Standing triples the energy requirement of doing a similar activity sitting.
10. Always stand while talking on the phone.
11. When reading a book, get up and move after every 6-10 pages of the book.

> **Sitting disease** A term coined by the scientific community to refer to the detrimental health effects caused by excessive sitting throughout most days of the week.

12. Use a stability ball for a chair. Such use enhances body stability; balance; and abdominal, low-back, and leg strength.
13. Whenever feasible, walk while conversing or holding meetings.
14. Walk to classmates' homes or coworkers' offices to study or discuss matters with them instead of using the phone, e-mail, or computer.
15. Take intermittent 10-minute breaks for every hour that you are at the computer or studying. Stretching, walking around, or talking to others while standing or walking is beneficial.

1.13 Wellness

Most people recognize that participating in fitness programs improves their quality of life. At the end of the 20th century, however, we came to realize that physical fitness alone was not always sufficient to lower the risk for disease and ensure better health. For example, individuals who run 3 miles (about 5 km) a day, lift weights regularly, participate in stretching exercises, and watch their body weight might be easily classified as having good or excellent fitness. Offsetting these good habits, however, might be risk factors, including high blood pressure, smoking, excessive stress, drinking too much alcohol, and eating too many foods high in saturated fat. These factors place people at risk for cardiovascular disease and other chronic diseases of which they may not be aware. Thus, a new concept that is rapidly gaining popularity is **primordial prevention** or the prevention of the development of risk factors for disease.

Even though most people are aware of their unhealthy behaviors, they seem satisfied with life as long as they are free from symptoms of disease or illness. They do not contemplate change until they incur a major health problem. Nevertheless, present lifestyle habits dictate the health and well-being of tomorrow.

Good health should not be viewed simply as the absence of illness. The notion of good health has evolved considerably and continues to change as scientists learn more about lifestyle factors that bring on illness and affect wellness. Furthermore, once the idea took hold that fitness by itself would not always decrease the risk for disease and ensure better health, **health promotion** programs and the **wellness** concept followed.

Wellness implies a constant and deliberate effort to stay healthy and achieve the highest potential for well-being. Wellness requires implementing positive lifestyle habits to change behavior and thereby improve health and quality of life, prolong life, and achieve total well-being. Living a wellness way of life is a personal choice, but you may need additional support to achieve wellness goals. Thus, health promotion programs have been developed to educate people regarding healthy lifestyles and provide the necessary support to achieve wellness.

For example, you may be prepared to initiate an aerobic exercise program, but if you are not familiar with exercise prescription guidelines or places to exercise safely, or if you lack peer support or flexible scheduling to do so, you may have difficulty accomplishing your goal. Similarly, if you want to quit smoking but do not know how to do it and everyone else around you smokes, the chances for success are limited. To some extent, the environment limits your choices. Hence, the availability of a health promotion program would provide the much-needed support to get started and implement a wellness way of life.

Figure 1.9 Dimensions of wellness.

The Seven Dimensions of Wellness Wellness has seven dimensions: physical, emotional, mental, social, environmental, occupational, and spiritual (Figure 1.9). These dimensions are interrelated: one frequently affects the others. For example, a person who is emotionally "down" often has no desire to exercise, study, socialize with friends, or attend church, and he or she may be more susceptible to illness and disease.

The seven dimensions show how the concept of wellness clearly goes beyond the absence of disease. Wellness incorporates factors such as adequate fitness, proper nutrition, stress management, disease prevention, spirituality, not smoking or abusing drugs, personal safety, regular physical examinations, health education, and environmental support.

For a wellness way of life, individuals must be physically fit and manifest no signs of disease and they also must be free of risk factors for disease (such as hypertension, hyperlipidemia, cigarette smoking, negative stress, faulty nutrition, careless sex). The relationship between adequate

Primordial prevention Prevention of the development of risk factors for disease.

Health promotion The science and art of enabling people to increase control over their lifestyle to move toward a state of wellness.

Wellness The constant and deliberate effort to stay healthy and achieve the highest potential for well-being. It encompasses seven dimensions—physical, emotional, mental, social, environmental, occupational, and spiritual—and integrates them all into a quality life.

Activity 1.1: Daily Physical Activity Log

Name _____ Date _____

Course _____ Section _____ Gender _____ Age _____

Date: [   ]   Day of the Week: [   ]

Time of Day	Exercise/Activity	Duration	Number of steps	Comments

Totals: [   ] [   ]

Activity category based on steps per day (use Table 1.2, page 12): [   ]

Date: [   ]   Day of the Week: [   ]

Time of Day	Exercise/Activity	Duration	Number of steps	Comments

Totals: [   ] [   ]

Activity category based on steps per day (use Table 1.2, page 12): [   ]

Lifetime Physical Fitness and Wellness

Date: _____ Day of the Week: _____

Time of Day	Exercise/Activity	Duration	Number of steps	Comments

Totals: _____ _____

Activity category based on steps per day (use Table 1.2, page 12): _____

Date: _____ Day of the Week: _____

Time of Day	Exercise/Activity	Duration	Number of steps	Comments

Totals: _____ _____

Activity category based on steps per day (use Table 1.2, page 12): _____

Briefly evaluate your current activity patterns, discuss your feelings about the results, and provide a goal for the weeks ahead.

_____
_____
_____
_____
_____
_____
_____

Figure 1.10 Wellness continuum.

fitness and wellness is illustrated in the continuum in Figure 1.10. Even though an individual tested in a fitness center may demonstrate adequate or even excellent fitness, indulging in unhealthy lifestyle behaviors will still increase the risk for chronic diseases and diminish the person's well-being.

1.14 Physical Wellness

Physical wellness is the dimension most commonly associated with being healthy. It entails confidence and optimism about one's ability to protect physical health and take care of health problems.

Physically well individuals are physically active, exercise regularly, eat a well-balanced diet, maintain recommended body weight, get sufficient sleep, practice safe sex, minimize exposure to environmental contaminants, avoid harmful drugs (including tobacco and excessive alcohol), and seek medical care and exams as needed. Physically well people also exhibit good cardiorespiratory endurance, adequate muscular strength and flexibility, proper body composition, and the ability to carry out ordinary and unusual demands of daily life safely and effectively.

1.15 Emotional Wellness

Emotional wellness involves the ability to understand your own feelings, accept your limitations, and achieve emotional stability. Furthermore, it implies the ability to express emotions appropriately, adjust to change, cope with stress in a healthy way, and enjoy life despite its occasional disappointments and frustrations.

Emotional wellness brings with it a certain stability, an ability to look both success and failure squarely in the face and keep moving along a predetermined course. When success is evident, the emotionally well person radiates the expected joy and confidence. When failure seems evident, the emotionally well person responds by making the best of circumstances and moving beyond the failure. Wellness enables you to move ahead with optimism and energy instead of spending time and talent worrying about failure. You learn from it, identify ways to avoid it in the future, and then go on with the business at hand.

Emotional wellness also involves happiness—an emotional anchor that gives meaning and joy to life. Happiness is a long-term state of mind that permeates the various facets of life and influences our outlook. Although there is no simple recipe for creating happiness, researchers agree that happy people are usually participants in some category of a supportive family unit where they feel loved. Healthy, happy people enjoy friends, work hard at something fulfilling, get plenty of exercise, and enjoy play and leisure time. They know how to laugh, and they laugh often. They give of themselves freely to others and seem to have found deep meaning in life.

An attitude of true happiness signals freedom from the tension and depression that many people endure. Emotionally well people are obviously subject to the same kinds of depression and unhappiness that occasionally plague us all, but the difference lies in the ability to bounce back. Well people take minor setbacks in stride and have the ability to enjoy life despite it all. They don't waste energy or time recounting the situation, wondering how they could have changed it, or dwelling on the past.

1.16 Mental Wellness

Mental wellness, also referred to as intellectual wellness, implies that you can apply the things you have learned, create opportunities to learn more, and engage your mind in lively interaction with the world around you. When you are mentally well, you are not intimidated by facts and figures with which you are unfamiliar, but you embrace the chance to learn something new. Your confidence and enthusiasm enable you to approach any learning situation with eagerness that leads to success.

Mental wellness brings with it vision and promise. More than anything else, mentally well people are open-minded and accepting of others. Instead of being threatened by people who are different from themselves, they show respect and curiosity without feeling they have to conform. They are faithful to their own ideas and philosophies and allow others the same privilege. Their self-confidence guarantees

> **Physical wellness** Good physical fitness and confidence in your personal ability to take care of health problems.
>
> **Emotional wellness** The ability to understand your own feelings, accept your limitations, and achieve emotional stability.
>
> **Mental wellness** A state in which your mind is engaged in lively interaction with the world around you.

that they can take their place among others in the world without having to give up part of themselves and without requiring others to do the same.

1.17 Social Wellness

Social wellness, with its accompanying positive self-image, endows you with the ease and confidence to be outgoing, friendly, and affectionate toward others. Social wellness involves a concern for oneself and also an interest in humanity and the environment as a whole.

One of the hallmarks of social wellness is the ability to relate to others and to reach out to other people, both within one's family and outside it. Similar to emotional wellness, it involves being comfortable with your emotions and thus helps you understand and accept the emotions of others. Your own balance and sense of self allow you to extend respect and tolerance to others. Healthy people are honest and loyal. This dimension of wellness leads to the ability to maintain close relationships with other people.

1.18 Environmental Wellness

Environmental wellness refers to the effect that our surroundings have on our well-being. Our planet is a delicate **ecosystem**, and its health depends on the continuous recycling of its elements. Environmental wellness implies a lifestyle that maximizes harmony with the earth and takes action to protect the world around us.

Environmental threats include air pollution, chemicals, ultraviolet radiation in the sunlight, water and food contamination, secondhand smoke, noise, inadequate shelter, unsatisfactory work conditions, lack of personal safety, and unhealthy relationships. Health is affected negatively when we live in a polluted, toxic, unkind, and unsafe environment.

Unfortunately, most first-year college students are not concerned about the health of the environment. To enjoy environmental wellness, we are responsible for educating and protecting ourselves against environmental hazards and also protecting the environment so that we, our children, and future generations can enjoy a safe and clean environment.

Steps that you can take to live an environmentally conscious life include conserving energy (walk to your destination or ride public transportation, do not drive unless absolutely necessary, turn off lights and computers when not in use); not littering and politely asking others not to do it either; recycling as much as possible (paper, glass, cans, plastics, cardboard); conserving paper and water (take shorter showers, don't let the water run while brushing your teeth); not polluting the air, water, or Earth if you can avoid doing so; not smoking; planting trees and keeping plants and shrubs alive; evaluating purchases and conveniences based on their environmental impact; donating old clothes to Goodwill, veterans' groups, or other charities; and enjoying, appreciating, and spending time outdoors in natural settings.

1.19 Occupational Wellness

Occupational wellness is not tied to high salary, prestigious position, or extravagant working conditions. Any job can bring occupational wellness if it provides rewards that are important to the individual. To one person, salary might be the most important factor, whereas another might place much greater value on creativity. Those who are occupationally well have their own "ideal" job, which allows them to thrive.

People with occupational wellness face demands on the job, but they also have some say over demands placed on them. Any job has routine demands, but in occupational wellness, routine demands are mixed with new, unpredictable challenges that keep a job exciting. Occupationally well people are able to maximize their skills, and they have the opportunity to broaden their existing skills or gain new ones. Their occupation offers the opportunity for advancement and recognition for achievement. Occupational wellness encourages collaboration and interaction among coworkers, which fosters a sense of teamwork and support.

1.20 Spiritual Wellness

Spiritual wellness provides a unifying power that integrates all dimensions of wellness. Basic characteristics of spiritual people include a sense of meaning and direction in life and a relationship to a higher being. Pursuing these avenues may lead to personal freedom, including prayer, faith, love, closeness to others, peace, joy, fulfillment, and altruism.

Several studies have reported positive relationships among spiritual well-being, emotional well-being, and satisfaction with life. Spiritual health is somehow intertwined with physical health. People who attend church and regularly participate in religious organizations enjoy better health, have a lower incidence of chronic diseases, are more socially integrated, handle stress more effectively, and appear to live longer.[17] Other studies have shown that spirituality strengthens the immune system, is good for mental health, prevents age-related memory loss, decreases the incidence of depression, leads to fewer episodes of chronic inflammation, and decreases the risk of death and suicide.

Prayer is a signpost of spirituality at the core of most spiritual experiences. It is communication with a higher power. At least 200 studies have been conducted on the effects of prayer on health. About two-thirds of these studies have linked prayer to positive health outcomes—as long as these prayers are offered with sincerity, humility, love, empathy, and compassion. Some studies have shown faster healing time and fewer complications in patients who didn't even know they were being prayed for, compared with patients who were not prayed for.[18]

Altruism, a key attribute of spiritual people, seems to enhance health and longevity. Studies indicate that people who regularly volunteer live longer. Research has found that health benefits of altruism are so powerful that doing good for others is good for oneself, especially for the immune system.

Researchers believe that there seems to be a strong connection among the mind, spirit, and body. As one improves, the others follow. The relationship between spirituality and wellness is meaningful in our quest for a better quality of life. As with the other dimensions, development of the spiritual dimension to its fullest potential contributes to wellness. Wellness requires a balance among all seven dimensions.

> **Critical Thinking**
>
> Now that you understand the seven dimensions of wellness, rank them in order of importance to you and explain your rationale in doing so.

Wellness, Fitness, and Longevity During the second half of the 20th century, scientists began to realize the importance of good fitness and improved lifestyle in the fight against chronic diseases, particularly those of the cardiovascular system. Because of more participation in wellness programs, cardiovascular mortality rates dropped. The decline began in about 1963, and between 1960 and 2000, the incidence of cardiovascular disease dropped by 28 percent, with another 10 percent drop between 2000 and 2010. This decrease is credited to higher levels of wellness and better treatment modalities in the United States.

Furthermore, several studies showed an inverse relationship between physical activity and premature mortality rates. The first major study in this area was conducted in the 1980s among 16,936 Harvard alumni, and the results linked physical activity habits and mortality rates.[19] As the amount of weekly physical activity increased, the risk for cardiovascular deaths decreased. The largest decrease in cardiovascular deaths was observed among alumni who used more than 2,000 calories per week through physical activity.

A landmark study subsequently conducted at the Aerobics Research Institute in Dallas upheld the findings of the Harvard alumni study.[20] Based on data from 13,344 people followed over an average of eight years, the study revealed a graded and consistent inverse relationship between physical activity levels and mortality, regardless of age and other risk factors. As illustrated in Figure 1.11, the higher the level of physical activity, the longer the lifespan.

The death rate during the eight-year study from all causes for the low-fit men was 3.4 times higher than that of the high-fit men. For the low-fit women, the death rate was 4.6 times higher than that of high-fit women. A most significant finding of this landmark study was the large drop in all-cause, cardiovascular, and cancer mortality when individuals went from low fitness to moderate fitness—a clear indication that moderate-intensity physical activity, achievable by most adults, does provide considerable health benefits and extends life. The data also revealed that the participants attained more protection by combining higher fitness levels with reduction in other risk factors such as hypertension, serum cholesterol, cigarette smoking, and excessive body fat.

Two additional studies reported in 2009 confirm that fitness improves wellness, quality of life, and longevity. The first study included 4,384 subjects and the results showed that the least-fit group had an almost twofold greater risk of all-cause and cardiovascular mortalities as compared with the moderately fit groups and a fourfold increased risk in comparison to the most-fit group.[21] The researchers concluded that the mortality rates between the least-fit and the other groups was most likely related to their **sedentary** lifestyle rather than differences in other health parameters.

The second study looked at four health-related factors among a group of more than 23,000 people.[22] These factors included lifetime nonsmoker, not considered obese (body mass index less than 30), engaging in a minimum of 3.5 hours of weekly physical activity, and adher-

Altruism enhances health and well-being.

> **Social wellness** The ability to relate well to others, both within and outside the family unit.
>
> **Environmental wellness** The capability to live in a clean and safe environment that is not detrimental to health.
>
> **Ecosystem** A community of organisms interacting with each other in an environment.
>
> **Occupational wellness** The ability to perform your job skillfully and effectively under conditions that provide personal and team satisfaction and adequately reward each individual.
>
> **Spiritual wellness** The sense that life is meaningful, that life has purpose, and that some power brings all humanity together; the ethics, values, and morals that guide you and give meaning and direction to life.
>
> **Prayer** Sincere and humble communication with a higher power.
>
> **Altruism** Unselfish concern for the welfare of others.

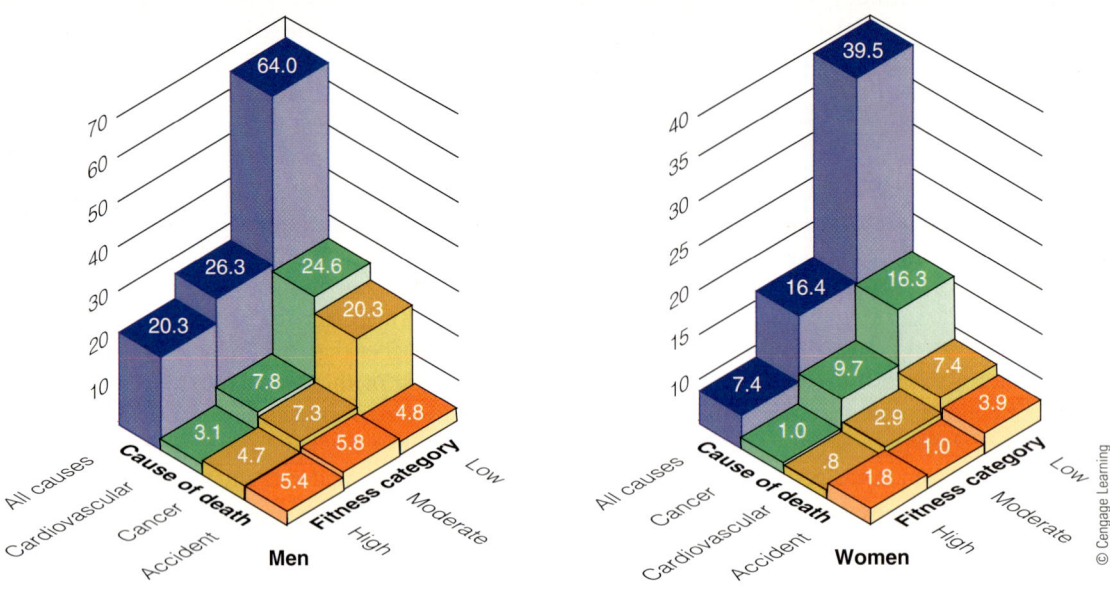

Figure 1.11 Death rates by physical fitness groups.

ence to healthy nutrition principles (high consumption of whole-grain breads, fruits, and vegetables and low consumption of red meat). Those who adhered to all four health habits were 78 percent less likely to develop chronic diseases (diabetes, heart disease, stroke, and cancer) during the almost eight-year study. Furthermore, the risk for developing a chronic disease progressively increased as the number of health factors decreased.

Currently, research on the benefits of physical activity and exercise on health and longevity is far too impressive to be ignored. A 2010 analysis of 33 studies involving more than 180,000 people quite clearly concluded that better aerobic fitness is associated with a substantial lower risk of all-cause mortality and cardiovascular disease.[23] In today's society, a person cannot afford not to participate in a lifetime physical fitness program.

While it is clear that moderate-intensity exercise does provide substantial health benefits, research data also show a dose-response relationship between physical activity and health. That is, greater health and fitness benefits occur at higher duration and/or intensity of physical activity. **Vigorous activity** and longer duration are preferable to the extent of one's capabilities because they are most clearly associated with better health and longer life.

Vigorous-intensity exercise seems to provide the best benefits.[24] As compared with prolonged moderate-intensity activity, vigorous-intensity exercise has been shown to provide the best improvements in aerobic capacity, coronary heart disease risk reduction, and overall cardiovascular health.[25]

Further, a comprehensive review of research studies found a lower rate of heart disease in vigorous-intensity exercisers as compared with those who exercised at moderate intensity.[26] While no differences were found in weight loss between the two groups, greater improvements are seen in cardiovascular risk factors in the vigorous-intensity groups, including aerobic fitness, blood pressure, and blood glucose control.

A word of caution, however, is in order. Vigorous exercise should be reserved for healthy individuals who have been cleared to do so (Activity 1.3) and who have been participating regularly in at least moderate-intensity activities.

A series of studies published in 2012 in the British medical journal *The Lancet* further substantiate the importance of regular physical activity worldwide. In one of the studies[27] it was determined that 1 in 10 deaths is caused by physical inactivity, accounting for more than 5.3 million deaths worldwide. If the inactivity rate were to go down by only 20 percent, more than 1 million lives could be saved on a yearly basis and global life expectancy would increase by almost a year. Currently, 1.5 billion adults have a 20 percent to 30 percent increased risk of heart disease, diabetes, and some types of cancers.[28]

1.21 Types of Physical Fitness

As the fitness concept grew at the end of the past century, it became clear that several specific components contribute to an individual's overall level of fitness. **Physical fitness** is classified into health-related and skill-related.

Health-related fitness relates to the ability to perform activities of daily living without undue fatigue and is conducive to a low risk of premature **hypokinetic diseases**. The health-related fitness components are cardiorespiratory (aerobic) endurance, muscular fitness (muscular strength and endurance), muscular flexibility, and body composition (Figure 1.12).

Skill-related fitness components consist of agility, balance, coordination, reaction time, speed, and power (Figure 1.13). These components are related primarily to successful sports and motor skill performance. Participating in skill-related activities contributes to physical fitness, but in terms of general health

Chapter 1 Physical Fitness and Wellness

Figure 1.12 Health-related components of physical fitness.

promotion and wellness, the main emphasis of physical fitness programs should be on the health-related components.

> **Critical Thinking**
>
> What role do the four health-related components of physical fitness play in your life? Rank them in order of importance to you and explain the rationale you used.

1.22 Fitness Standards: Health versus Physical Fitness

A meaningful debate regarding age- and gender-related fitness standards has resulted in two standards: health fitness (also referred to as *criterion referenced*) and physical fitness.

Figure 1.13 Motor skill–related components of physical fitness.

Following are definitions of both. The assessment of health-related fitness is presented in Chapters 4, 6, 7, and 8; where appropriate physical fitness standards are included for comparison.

Health Fitness Standards

The **health fitness standards** proposed here are based on data linking minimum fitness values to disease prevention and health. Attaining the health fitness standard requires only moderate physical activity. For example, a 2-mile walk in less than 30 minutes, 5 or 6 times a week, seems to be suffi-

Vigorous activity Any exercise that requires a MET level equal to or greater than 6 METs (21 mL/kg/min). One MET is the energy expenditure at rest, 3.5 mL/kg/min, and METs are defined as multiples of this resting metabolic rate. (Examples of activities that require a 6-MET level include aerobics, walking uphill at 3.5 mph, cycling at 10 to 12 mph, playing doubles in tennis, and vigorous strength training.)

Physical fitness The ability to meet the ordinary as well as unusual demands of daily life safely and effectively without being overly fatigued and still have energy left for leisure and recreational activities.

Health-related fitness Fitness programs that are prescribed to improve the individual's overall health.

Hypokinetic diseases "Hypo" denotes "lack of"; therefore, illnesses related to lack of physical activity.

Skill-related fitness Fitness components important for success in skillful activities and athletic events; encompasses agility, balance, coordination, power, reaction time, and speed.

Health fitness standards The lowest fitness requirements for maintaining good health, decreasing the risk for chronic diseases, and lowering the incidence of muscular-skeletal injuries.

Figure 1.14 Health and fitness benefits based on the type of lifestyle and physical activity program.

Good health-related fitness and skill-related fitness are required to participate in highly skilled activities.

heart, lungs, and muscles can operate during aerobic exercise (Chapter 6). VO_{2max} is commonly expressed in milliliters (mL) of oxygen (volume of oxygen) per kilogram (kg) of body weight per minute (mL/kg/min). Individual values can range from about 10 mL/kg/min in cardiac patients to more than 80 mL/kg/min in world-class runners, cyclists, and cross-country skiers.

Research data from the study presented in Figure 1.11 reported that achieving VO_{2max} values of 35 and 32.5 mL/kg/min for men and women, respectively, may be sufficient to lower the risk for all-cause mortality significantly. Although greater improvements in fitness yield an even lower risk for premature death, the largest drop is seen between the least fit and the moderately fit. Therefore, the 35 and 32.5 mL/kg/min values could be selected as the health fitness standards.

cient to achieve the health-fitness standard for cardiorespiratory endurance.

As illustrated in Figure 1.14, significant health benefits can be reaped with such a program, although fitness improvements, expressed in terms of maximum oxygen uptake, or VO_{2max} (explained next and in Chapter 6), are not as notable. Nevertheless, health improvements are quite striking. These benefits include reduction in blood lipids, lower blood pressure, weight loss, stress release, less risk for diabetes, and lower risk for disease and premature mortality.

More specifically, improvements in the **metabolic profile** (measured by insulin sensitivity, glucose tolerance, and improved cholesterol levels) can be notable despite little or no weight loss or improvement in aerobic capacity. Metabolic fitness can be attained through an active lifestyle and moderate-intensity physical activity.

An assessment of health-related fitness uses **cardiorespiratory endurance** measured in terms of the maximal amount of oxygen the body is able to utilize per minute of physical activity (VO_{2max})—essentially, a measure of how efficiently the

Physical Fitness Standards Physical fitness standards are set higher than health fitness standards and require a more intense exercise program. Physically fit people of all ages have the freedom to enjoy most of life's daily and recreational activities to their fullest potentials. Current health fitness standards may not be enough to achieve these objectives.

> **Metabolic profile** A measurement of plasma insulin, glucose, lipid, and lipoprotein levels to assess risk for diabetes and cardiovascular disease.
>
> **Cardiorespiratory endurance** The ability of the lungs, heart, and blood vessels to deliver adequate amounts of oxygen to the cells to meet the demands of prolonged physical activity.
>
> **Physical fitness standards** A fitness level that allows a person to sustain moderate-to-vigorous physical activity without undue fatigue and the ability to closely maintain this level throughout life.

Behavior Modification Planning

Financial Fitness Prescription

Although not one of the components of physical fitness, taking control of your personal finances is critical for your success and well-being. The sooner you start working on a lifetime personal financial plan, the more successful you will be in becoming financially secure and being able to retire early, in comfort, if you choose to do so. Most likely, you have not been taught basic principles to improve personal finance and enjoy "financial fitness." Thus, start today using the following strategies:

1. *Develop a personal financial plan.* Set short-term and long-term financial goals for yourself. If you do not have financial goals, you cannot develop a plan or work toward that end.

2. *Subscribe to a personal finance magazine or newsletter.* In the same way that you should regularly read reputable fitness/wellness journals or newsletters, you should regularly peruse a "financial fitness" magazine. If you don't enjoy reading financial materials, then find a periodical that is quick and to the point; there are many available. You don't have to force yourself to read the *Wall Street Journal* to become financially knowledgeable. Many periodicals have resources to help you develop a financial plan. Educate yourself and stay current on personal finances and investment matters.

3. *Set up a realistic budget and live on less than you make.* Pay your bills on time and keep track of *all* expenses. Then develop your budget so that you spend less than you earn. Your budget may require that you either cut back on expenses and services or figure out a way to increase your income. Balance your checkbook regularly and do not overdraft your checking account.

4. *Learn to differentiate between wants and needs.* It is fine to reward yourself for goals that you have achieved (see Chapter 2), but limit your spending to items that you truly need. Avoid simple impulse spending because "it's a bargain" or something you just want to have.

5. *Pay yourself first; save 10 percent of your income each month.* Before you take any money out of your paycheck, put 10 percent of your income into a retirement or investment account. If possible, ask for an automatic withdrawal at your bank from your paycheck to avoid the temptation to spend this money. This strategy may allow you to have a solid retirement fund or even provide for an early retirement. If you start putting away $100 a month at age 20, and earn a modest 6 percent interest rate, at age 65 you will have more than $275,000.

6. *Set up an emergency savings fund.* Whether you ultimately work for yourself or for someone else, there may be uncontrollable financial setbacks or even financial disasters in the future. So, as you are able, start an emergency fund equal to 3 to 6 months of normal monthly earnings. Additionally, start a second savings account for expensive purchases such as a car, a down payment on a home, or a vacation.

7. *Use credit, gas, and retail cards responsibly and sparingly.* As soon as you receive new cards, sign them promptly and store them securely. Due to the prevalence of identity theft (someone stealing your creditworthiness), cardholders should even consider a secure post office box, rather than a regular mailbox, for all high-risk mail. Shred your old credit cards, monthly statements, and any and all documents that contain personal information to avoid identity theft. Pay off all credit card debt monthly, and do not purchase on credit unless you have the cash to pay it off when the monthly statement arrives. Develop a plan at this very moment to pay off your debt if you have such. Credit card balances, high interest rates, and frequent credit purchases lead to financial disaster. Credit card debt is the worst enemy to your personal finances!

8. *Understand the terms of your student loans.* Do not borrow more money than you absolutely need for actual educational expenses. Student loans are not for wants but needs (see item 4). Remember, loans must be repaid, with interest, once you leave college. Be informed regarding the repayment process and do not ever default on your loan. If you do, the entire balance (principal, interest, and collection fees) is due immediately and serious financial and credit consequences will follow.

9. *Eat out infrequently.* Besides saving money that you can then pay to yourself, you will eat healthier and consume fewer calories.

10. *Make the best of tax "motivated" savings and investing opportunities available to you.* For example, once employed, your company may match your voluntary 401(k) contributions (or other retirement plan), so contribute at least up to the match (you may use the 10 percent you "pay yourself first"—see item 5—or part of it). Also, under current tax law, maximize your Roth IRA contribution personally. Always pay attention to current tax rules that provide tax incentives for investing in retirement plans. If at all possible, *never* cash out a retirement account early. You may pay penalties in addition to tax, in most situations. As you are able, employ a tax professional or financial planner to avoid serious missteps in your tax planning.

11. *Stay involved in your financial accumulations.* You may seek professional advice, but you stay in control. Ultimately, no

(continued)

Behavior Modification Planning

one will look after your interests as well as you. Avoid placing all your trust (and assets) in one individual or institution. Spreading out your assets is one way to diversify your risk.

12. *Protect your assets.* As you start to accumulate assets, get proper insurance coverage (yes, even renter's insurance) in case of an accident or disaster. You have disciplined yourself and worked hard to obtain those assets, now make sure they are protected.

13. *Review your credit report.* The best way to ensure that your credit "identity" is not stolen and ruined is to regularly review your credit report, at least once a year, for accuracy.

14. *Contribute to charity and the needy.* Altruism (doing good for others) is good for heart health and emotional well-being. Remember the less fortunate and donate regularly to some of your favorite charitable organizations and volunteer time to worthy causes.

The Power of Investing Early

Jon and Jim are both 20 years old. Jon begins investing $100 a month starting on his 20th birthday. He stops investing on his 30th birthday (he has set aside a total of $12,000). Jim does not start investing until he's 30. He chooses to invest $100 a month as Jon had done, but he does so for the next 30 years (Jim invests a total of $36,000). Although Jon stopped investing at age 30, assuming an 8 percent annual rate of return in a tax-deferred account, by the time both Jon and Jim are 60, Jon will have accumulated $199,035, whereas Jim will have $150,029. At a 6 percent rate of return, they would both accumulate about $100,000, but Jim invested three times as much as Jon did.

Post these principles of financial fitness in a visible place at home where you can review them often. Start implementing these strategies as soon as you can and watch your financial fitness level increase over the years.

© David Johnson, CPA and Fitness & Wellness, Inc.

Sound physical fitness gives the individual a degree of independence throughout life that many people in the United States no longer enjoy. Most adults should be able to carry out activities similar to those they conducted in their youth, though not with the same intensity. These standards do not require being a championship athlete, but activities such as changing a tire, chopping wood, climbing several flights of stairs, playing basketball, mountain biking, playing soccer with children or grandchildren, walking several miles around a lake, and hiking through a national park do require more than the current "average fitness" level of most Americans.

1.23 Which Program Is Best?

Your own personal objectives will determine the fitness program you decide to use. If the main objective of your fitness program is to lower the risk for disease, attaining the health fitness standards will provide substantial health benefits. If, however, you want to participate in vigorous fitness activities, achieving a high physical fitness standard is recommended. This book gives both health fitness and physical fitness standards for each fitness test so that you can personalize your approach.

Benefits of a Comprehensive Fitness Program

An inspiring story illustrating what fitness can do for a person's health and well-being is that of George Snell from Sandy, Utah. At age 45, Snell weighed approximately 400 pounds, his blood pressure was 220/180, he was blind because of undiagnosed diabetes, and his blood glucose level was 487.

Snell had determined to do something about his physical and medical condition, so he started a walking/jogging program. After about 8 months of conditioning, he had lost almost 200 pounds, his eyesight had returned, his glucose level was down to 67, and he was taken off medication. Just 2 months later—less than 10 months after beginning his personal exercise program—he completed his first marathon, a running course of 26.2 miles!

1.24 Health Benefits

Most people exercise because it improves their personal appearance and makes them feel good about themselves. Although many benefits accrue from participating in a regular fitness and wellness program, and active people generally live longer, *the greatest benefit of all is that physically fit individuals enjoy a better quality of life.* These people live life to its fullest, with far fewer health problems than inactive individuals.

The benefits derived by regularly participating in exercise are so extensive that it is difficult to compile an all-inclusive list. Many of these benefits are summarized in Table 1.5. As far back as 1982, the American Medical Association indicated that *"there is no drug in current or prospective use that holds as much promise for sustained health as a lifetime program of physical exercise."* Furthermore, researchers and sports medicine leaders have stated that *if the benefits of exercise could be packaged in a pill, it would be the most widely prescribed medication throughout the world today.*

While most of the chronic (long-term) benefits of exercise are well established, what many people fail to realize is that there are *immediate benefits* derived by participating in just one single bout of exercise. Most of these benefits dissipate within 48 to 72 hours following exercise. The *immediate benefits*, summarized in Table 1.4, are so striking that it prompted Dr. William L. Haskell of Stanford University to state: *"Most of the health benefits of exercise are relatively short term, so people should think of exercise as a medication and take it on a daily basis."* Of course, as you regularly exercise a minimum of 30 minutes 5 times per week and maintain a certain amount of physical activity throughout the day, you will realize the impressive long-term benefits listed in Table 1.5.

1.25 Exercise and Brain Function

If the previous benefits of exercise still have not convinced you to start a regular exercise program, you may want to consider the effects of exercise on brain function and academic performance. Physical activity is related to better cognitive health and effective functioning across the lifespan.

While much of the research is still in its infancy, even in 400 years BC, the Greek philosopher Plato stated: *"In order for man to succeed in life, God provided him with two means, education and physical activity. Not separately, one for the soul and the other for the body, but for the two together. With these two means, man can attain perfection."*

Data on more than 2.4 million students in the state of Texas have shown consistent and significant associations between physical fitness and various indicators of academic achievement; in particular, higher levels of fitness were associated with better academic grades. Cardiorespiratory fitness was shown to have a dose-response association with academic performance (better fitness, better grades), independent of other sociodemographic and fitness variables.[29]

Emerging research shows that exercise allows the brain to function at its best because it increases blood and oxygen flow to the brain and leads to biological processes that instigate the growth of new cells (neurons) and for these cells to bind one to another. These connections are critical for learning to take place. Exercise provides the necessary stimulus for brain neurons to interconnect, creating the perfect environment in which the brain is ready, willing, and able to learn.[30]

Second, muscular activity generates growth factors (e.g., vascular endothelial growth factor and insulin-like growth factor) that are used to create new nerve cells, to increase the strength of the synaptic transmission (transmission between neurons), and in the mechanisms involved in the highest thought processes. Exercise also has an effect on the hippocampus in the brain, a key component to memory forming, organizing, and storing. The hippocampus tends to shrink in late adulthood, leading to memory impairment. In older adults, aerobic exercise has been shown to increase the size of the hippocampus. Other studies have shown that regular physical activity decreases the rate of brain shrinkage and white matter lesions, processes linked to declines in thinking, memory skills, dementia, and Alzheimer's disease (a form of dementia). Exercise also increases the levels of brain's derived neurotrophic factor, a compound involved with learning and memory.

The strongest data from research so far show that regular physical activity is the most important lifestyle change a person can make to prevent dementia and Alzheimer's later in life. Aerobics, strength training, and even stretching and toning are beneficial. In terms of the type and optimal amount of activity to prevent cognitive decline, more research will be required, but hints are emerging that strength training might be the best exercise intervention.

Keeping the mind engaged with proactive cognitive challenges like reading, studying, playing games, and doing puzzles is critical (but not passive TV watching). Physical activity and exercise, nonetheless, provide better protection than intellectual challenges themselves. Even light-intensity

Table 1.4 Immediate (Acute) Benefits of Exercise

You can expect a number of benefits as a result of a single exercise session. Some of these benefits last as long as 72 hours following your workout. Exercise:

- increases heart rate, stroke volume, cardiac output, pulmonary ventilation, and oxygen uptake.
- begins to strengthen the heart, lungs, and muscles.
- enhances metabolic rate or energy production (burning calories for fuel) during exercise and recovery (for every 100 calories you burn during exercise, you can expect to burn another 15 during recovery).
- uses blood glucose and muscle glycogen.
- improves insulin sensitivity (decreasing the risk of type 2 diabetes).
- immediately enhances the body's ability to burn fat.
- lowers blood lipids.
- improves joint flexibility.
- reduces low-grade (hidden) inflammation (see pages 357-358 in Chapter 10).
- increases endorphins (hormones), which are naturally occurring opioids that are responsible for exercise-induced euphoria.
- increases fat storage *in muscle,* which can then be burned for energy.
- improves endothelial function (endothelial cells line the entire vascular system, which provides a barrier between the vessel lumen and surrounding tissue—endothelial dysfunction contributes to several disease processes, including tissue inflammation and subsequent atherosclerosis).
- enhances mood and self-worth.
- provides a sense of achievement and satisfaction.
- decreases blood pressure the first few hours following exercise.
- decreases arthritic pain.
- leads to muscle relaxation.
- decreases stress.
- improves brain function.
- promotes better sleep (unless exercise is performed too close to bedtime).
- improves digestion.
- boosts energy levels.
- improves resistance to infections.

© Cengage Learning

Table 1.5 Long-Term Benefits of Exercise

Regular participation in exercise:

- improves and strengthens the cardiorespiratory system.
- maintains better muscle tone, muscular strength, and endurance.
- improves muscular flexibility.
- enhances athletic performance.
- helps maintain recommended body weight.
- helps preserve lean body tissue.
- increases resting metabolic rate.
- improves the body's ability to use fat during physical activity.
- improves posture and physical appearance.
- improves functioning of the immune system.
- lowers the risk for chronic diseases and illnesses (including heart disease, stroke, and certain cancers).
- decreases the mortality rate from chronic diseases.
- thins the blood so that it doesn't clot as readily, thereby decreasing the risk for coronary heart disease and stroke.
- helps the body manage blood lipid (cholesterol and triglycerides) levels more effectively.
- prevents or delays the development of high blood pressure and lowers blood pressure in people with hypertension.
- helps prevent and control type 2 diabetes.
- helps achieve peak bone mass in young adults and maintain bone mass later in life, thereby decreasing the risk for osteoporosis.
- helps people sleep better.
- helps prevent chronic back pain.
- relieves tension and helps in coping with life stresses.
- raises levels of energy and job productivity.
- extends longevity and slows the aging process.
- improves and helps maintain cognitive function, decreasing the risk for dementia and Alzheimer's disease.
- promotes psychological well-being, including higher morale, self-image, and self-esteem.
- reduces feelings of depression and anxiety.
- encourages positive lifestyle changes (improving nutrition, quitting smoking, controlling alcohol and drug use).
- speeds recovery time following physical exertion.
- speeds recovery following injury or disease.
- regulates and improves overall body functions.
- improves physical stamina and counteracts chronic fatigue.
- reduces disability and helps to maintain independent living, especially in older adults.
- enhances quality of life: People feel better and live a healthier and happier life.

© Cengage Learning

No current drug or medication provides as many health benefits as a regular physical activity program.

activities of daily living appear to provide protection against cognitive impairment. The research further shows that as the amount of activity increases, the rate of cognitive decline decreases. And the amount of daily activity performed appears to be more important than the intensity itself in terms of warding off dementia. Of course, greater protection is obtained by combining both physical and cognitive challenges.

Exercise also increases the neurotransmitters dopamine, glutamate, norepinephrine, and serotonin, all of which are vital in the generation of thought and emotion. Low levels of serotonin have been linked to depression, and exercise has repeatedly been shown to be effective in treating depression. Furthermore, physical activity, and aerobic exercise in particular, protect against age-related loss of cognitive function (memory, thought process, and information processing).

Economic Benefits Sedentary living can have a strong impact on a nation's economy. As the need for physical exertion in Western countries decreased steadily during the past century, health care expenditures increased dramatically. One of the biggest challenges we face in America is the overwhelming rising cost of medical expenses. Health care costs in the United States rose from $12 billion in 1950 to $2.6 trillion in 2010 (Figure 1.15), or about 16 percent of the gross domestic product (GDP). This figure represents the highest of any country in the Organisation for Economic Co-operation and Development (OECD). The next closest country is France at 11.0 percent and Canada ranks sixth at 10.1 percent of the GDP (Figure 1.16). In 1980, health care costs in the United

States represented 8.8 percent of the GDP, and if the current trend continues, they are projected to reach 19.3 percent by the year 2019. According to the Institute of Medicine, up to a third of health care costs is wasteful or inefficient.

In terms of yearly health care costs per person, the United States spends more per person than any other industrialized nation. Per capita U.S. health care costs exceed $8,200 per year. These costs are about 2.5 times the OECD average (Figure 1.17). Furthermore, in terms of health care value, the consumer does not have the needed information to make rational decisions. Costs (prices) and care quality are not readily available as in other markets (automobile, housing, groceries). Once sick or ill, the individual seeks medical care without the needed knowledge to make an informed decision. Most often the person does not understand or question unfair medical costs because he/she trusts that health insurance companies will take care of the matter.

One of the reasons for the low overall ranking is the overemphasis on state-of-the-art cures instead of prevention programs. The United States is the best place in the world to treat people once they are sick, but the system does a poor job of keeping people healthy in the first place. Ninety-five percent of our health care dollars are spent on treatment strategies, and less than five percent is spent on prevention.

Unhealthy behaviors also contribute to the staggering U.S. health care costs. Risk factors for disease such as obesity and smoking carry a heavy price tag. Half of the people use up about 97 percent of health care dollars. Without reducing the current burden of disease, real health care reform will most likely be impossible. True health care reform will require a nationwide call for action by everyone against chronic disease.

Scientific evidence links participation in fitness and wellness programs to better health, in addition to lower medical costs and higher job productivity. As a result of the staggering rise in medical costs, many organizations offer health-promotion programs, because keeping employees healthy costs less than treating them once they are sick.

1.26 The Wellness Challenge for Our Day

Because a better and healthier life is something that every person should strive for, our biggest health challenge today is to teach people how to take control of their personal health

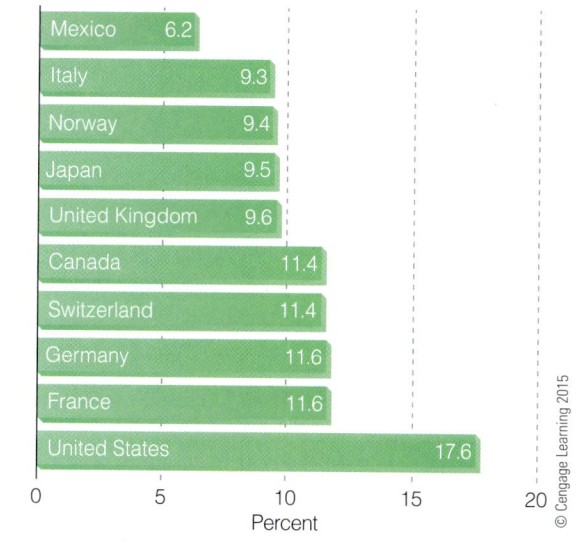

Figure 1.16 Health care expenditures for selected countries as a percentage of the gross domestic product (GDP), 2010.

Figure 1.15 U.S. health care cost increments since 1950.

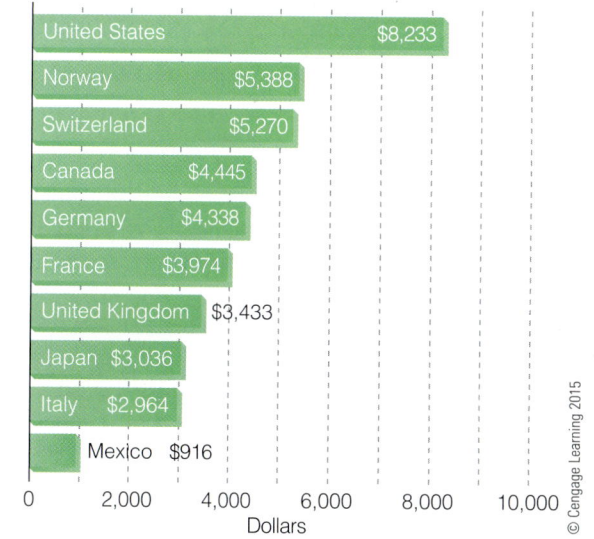

Figure 1.17 Health care expenditure per capita for selected countries, 2010.

Behavior Modification Planning

Healthy Lifestyle Habits

Research indicates that adherence to the following 12 lifestyle habits will significantly improve health and extend life:

1. **Participate in a lifetime physical activity program.** Attempt to accumulate 60 minutes of moderate-intensity physical activity most days of the week. The 60 minutes should include 20 to 30 minutes of aerobic exercise (vigorous-intensity) at least 3 times per week, along with other routine activities of daily living, and strengthening and stretching exercises two to three times per week. Avoid excessive periods of sitting throughout most days of the week.

2. **Do not smoke cigarettes.** Cigarette smoking is the largest preventable cause of illness and premature death in the United States. If we include all related deaths, smoking is responsible for about 443,000 unnecessary deaths each year.

3. **Eat right.** Eat a good breakfast and two additional well-balanced meals every day. Avoid eating too many calories, processed foods, and foods with a lot of sugar, saturated fat, trans fat, and salt. Increase your daily consumption of fruits, vegetables, and whole-grain products.

4. **Avoid snacking.** Refrain from frequent high-sugar snacks between meals. Insulin is released to remove sugar from the blood, and frequent spikes in insulin may contribute to the development of diabetes and heart disease.

5. **Maintain recommended body weight through adequate nutrition and exercise.** This is important in preventing chronic diseases and in developing a higher level of fitness.

6. **Sleep seven to eight hours every night.**

7. **Lower your stress levels.** Reduce your vulnerability to stress and practice stress management techniques as needed.

8. **Be wary of alcohol.** Drink alcohol moderately or not at all. Alcohol abuse leads to mental, emotional, physical, and social problems.

9. **Surround yourself with healthy friendships.** Unhealthy friendships contribute to destructive behaviors and low self-esteem. Associating with people who strive to maintain good fitness and health reinforces a positive outlook in life and encourages positive behaviors. Mortality rates are much higher among people who are socially isolated.

10. **Be informed about the environment.** Seek clean air, clean water, and a clean environment. Be aware of pollutants and occupational hazards: asbestos fibers, nickel dust, chromate, uranium dust, and so on. Take precautions when using pesticides and insecticides.

11. **Increase education.** Data indicate that people who are more educated live longer. As education increases, so do the number of connections between nerve cells. An increased number of connections help the individual make better survival (i.e., healthy lifestyle) choices.

12. **Take personal safety measures.** Although not all accidents are preventable, many are. Taking simple precautionary measures—such as using seat belts and keeping electrical appliances away from water—lessens the risk for avoidable accidents.

Try It Look at the previous list and indicate which habits are already a part of your lifestyle. What changes could you make to incorporate some additional healthy habits into your daily life?

---

habits and adhere to a positive lifestyle. A wealth of information on the benefits of fitness and wellness programs indicates that improving the quality and possible length of our lives is a matter of personal choice.

Even though people in the United States believe a positive lifestyle has a great impact on health and longevity, most people do not reap the benefits because they simply do not know how to implement a safe and effective fitness and wellness program. Others are exercising incorrectly and, therefore, are not reaping the full benefits of their program. How, then, can we meet the health challenges of the 21st century? That is the focus of this book—to provide the necessary tools that will enable you to write, implement, and regularly update your personal lifetime fitness and wellness program.

Critical Thinking

What are your thoughts about lifestyle habits that enhance health and longevity? • How important are they to you? • What obstacles keep you from adhering to these habits or incorporating new habits into your life?

1.27 Wellness Education: Using This Book

Although everyone would like to enjoy good health and wellness, most people don't know how to reach this objective. Lifestyle is the most important factor affecting personal well-being. Granted, some people live long because of genetic factors, but quality of life during middle age and the "golden years" is more often related to wise choices initiated during youth and continued throughout life. In a few short years, lack of wellness can lead to a loss of vitality and gusto for life, as well as premature morbidity and mortality.

A Personalized Approach Because fitness and wellness needs vary significantly from one individual to another, all exercise and wellness prescriptions must be personalized to obtain the best results. The Wellness Lifestyle Questionnaire in Activity 1.2 will provide an initial rating of your current efforts to stay healthy and well. Subsequent chapters of this book and their respective activities discuss the components of a wellness lifestyle and set forth the necessary guidelines that will allow you to develop a personal lifetime program to improve fitness and promote your own preventive health care and personal wellness.

The activities in this book have been prepared on tear-out sheets so that they can be turned in to class instructors. As you study this book and complete the worksheets, you will learn to:

- Implement motivational and behavior modification techniques to help you adhere to a lifetime fitness and wellness program
- Determine whether medical clearance is needed for your safe participation in exercise
- Conduct nutritional analyses and follow the recommendations for adequate nutrition
- Write sound diet and weight-control programs
- Assess the health-related components of fitness
- Write exercise prescriptions for cardiorespiratory endurance, muscular fitness, and muscular flexibility
- Understand the relationship between fitness and aging
- Determine your levels of tension and stress, reduce your vulnerability to stress, and implement a stress management program if necessary
- Determine your potential risk for cardiovascular disease and implement a risk-reduction program
- Follow a cancer risk-reduction program
- Implement a smoking cessation program, if applicable
- Avoid chemical dependency and know where to find assistance if needed
- Learn the health consequences of sexually transmitted infections (STIs), including human immunodeficiency virus (HIV)/acquired immune deficiency syndrome (AIDS), and guidelines for preventing STIs
- Write goals and objectives to improve your fitness and wellness and learn how to chart a wellness program for the future
- Differentiate myths from facts about exercise and health-related concepts

Exercise Safety Even though testing and participation in exercise are relatively safe for most apparently healthy individuals, the reaction of the cardiovascular system to higher levels of physical activity cannot be totally predicted. Consequently, a small but real risk exists for exercise-induced abnormalities in people with a history of cardiovascular problems, certain chronic conditions, and those who are at higher risk for disease. Among the exercise-induced abnormalities are abnormal blood pressure; irregular heart rhythm; fainting; and, in rare instances, a heart attack or cardiac arrest.

Before you engage in an exercise program or participate in any exercise testing, at a minimum you should fill out the Physical Activity Readiness Questionnaire (PAR-Q & YOU) found in Activity 1.3. Additional information can be obtained by filling out the Health History Questionnaire also given in Activity 1.3. Exercise testing and participation are not wise under some of the conditions listed in this activity and may require a medical evaluation, including a stress electrocardiogram (ECG) test for a few individuals. If you have any questions regarding your current health status, consult your doctor before initiating, continuing, or increasing your level of physical activity.

Now that you are about to embark in a wellness lifestyle program, sit down and subjectively determine where you are at on each of the seven dimensions of wellness. Use Activity 1.5 to help you with this exercise. Record the date at the top of the respective column. Next, write a goal for each wellness dimension to accomplish prior to the end of this course. Also, list three specific objectives that will help you accomplish each goal.

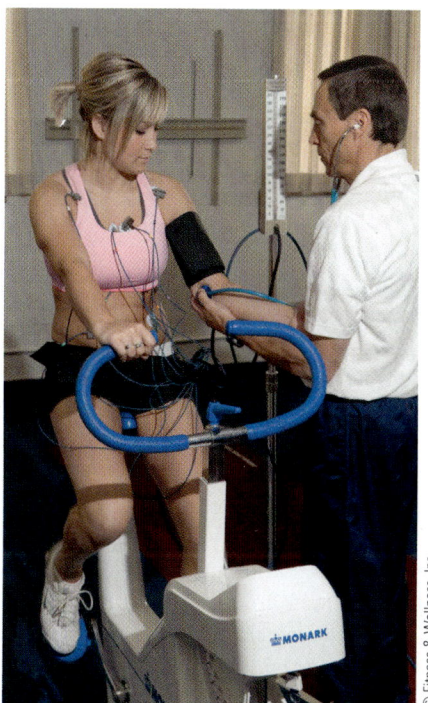

An exercise tolerance test with 12-lead electrocardiographic monitoring (stress ECG test) may be required of some individuals prior to initiating an exercise program.

Table 1.6 **Resting Heart Rate Ratings**

Heart Rate (bpm)	Rating
59	Excellent
60–69	Good
70–79	Average
80–89	Fair
≥90	Poor

© Cengage Learning

As you continue to study the content of this book, use this same form to monitor your progress. About once a month reassess your status and make adjustments in your specific objectives so you may reach the desired goals. Modifying unhealthy behaviors and developing new positive habits take time. The plan of action that you are about to develop will help you achieve the desired outcomes.

1.28 Assessment of Resting Heart Rate and Blood Pressure

Heart rate can be obtained by counting your pulse either on the wrist over the radial artery or over the carotid artery in the neck (Chapter 6, page 203). In Activity 1.4 you will have an opportunity to determine your heart rate and blood pressure and calculate the extra heart rate life years an increase in exercise may produce.

You may count your pulse for 30 seconds and multiply by 2 or take it for a full minute. The heart rate usually is at its lowest point (resting heart rate) late in the evening after you have been sitting quietly for about half an hour watching a relaxing TV show or reading in bed, or early in the morning just before you get out of bed. Your pulse should have a consistent (regular) rhythm. A pulse that misses beats or speeds up or slows down may be an indication of heart problems and should be followed up by a physician.

Unless you have a pathological condition, a lower resting heart rate indicates a stronger heart. To adapt to cardiorespiratory or aerobic exercise, blood volume increases, the heart enlarges, and the muscle gets stronger. A stronger heart can pump more blood with fewer strokes.

Resting heart rate categories are given in Table 1.6. Although resting heart rate decreases with training, the extent of **bradycardia** depends not only on the amount of training but also on genetic factors. Although most highly trained athletes have a resting heart rate around 40 beats per minute, occasionally one of these athletes has a resting heart rate in the 60s or 70s even during peak training months of the season. For most individuals, however, the resting heart rate decreases as the level of cardiorespiratory endurance increases.

Blood pressure is assessed using a **sphygmomanometer** and a stethoscope. Use a cuff of the appropriate size to get accurate readings. Size is determined by the width of the inflatable bladder, which should be about 80 percent of the circumference of the midpoint of the arm.

Blood pressure usually is measured while the person is in the sitting position, with the forearm and the manometer at the same level as the heart. The arm should be flexed slightly and placed on a flat surface. At first, the pressure is recorded from each arm, and after that from the arm with the highest reading.

The cuff should be applied approximately an inch above the antecubital space (natural crease of the elbow), with the center of the bladder directly over the medial (inner) surface of the arm. The stethoscope head should be applied firmly, but with little pressure, over the brachial artery in the antecubital space.

To determine how high the cuff should be inflated, the person recording the blood pressure monitors the subject's radial pulse with one hand and, with the other hand, inflates the manometer's bladder to about 30 to 40 mm Hg above the point at which the feeling of the pulse in the wrist disappears. Next, the pressure is released, followed by a wait of about one minute, then the bladder is inflated to the predetermined level to take the blood pressure reading. The cuff should not be overinflated, as this may cause blood vessel spasm, resulting in higher blood pressure readings. The pressure should be released at a rate of 2 to 4 mm Hg per second.

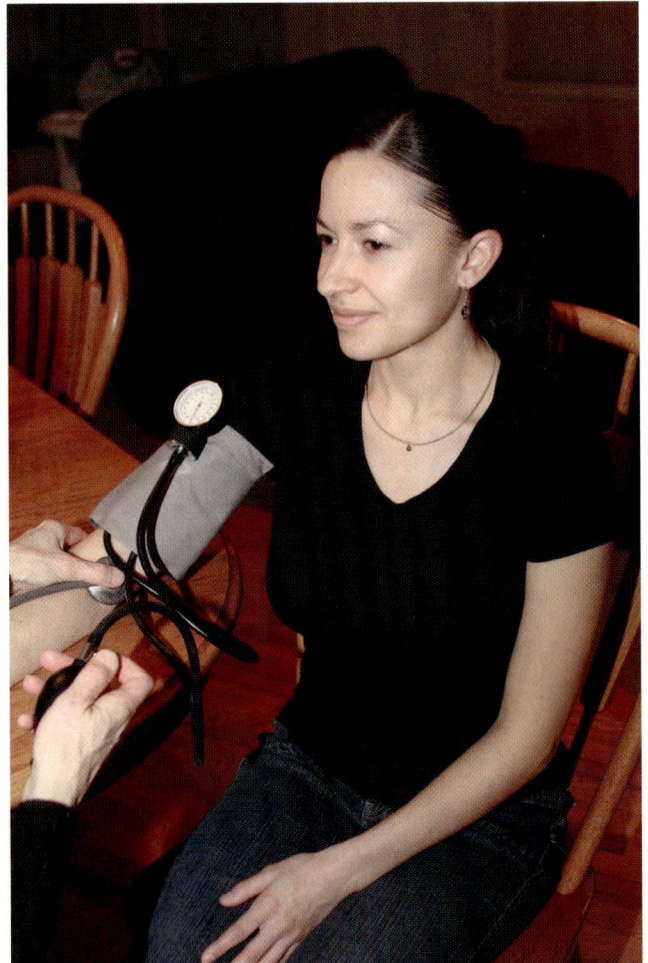

Assessment of resting blood pressure with an aneroid manometer.

Table 1.7 Resting Blood Pressure Guidelines (expressed in mm Hg)

Rating	Systolic	Diastolic
Normal	≤120	≤80
Prehypertension	120–139	80–89
Hypertension	≥140	≥90

SOURCE: National Heart, Lung, and Blood Institute.

As the pressure is released, **systolic blood pressure (SBP)** is recorded as the point where the sound of the pulse becomes audible. The **diastolic blood pressure (DBP)** is the point where the sound disappears. The recordings should be expressed as systolic over diastolic pressure—for example, 124/80.

If you take more than one reading, be sure the bladder is completely deflated between readings and allow at least a full minute before making the next recording. The person measuring the pressure also should note whether the pressure was recorded from the left or the right arm. Resting blood pressure ratings are given in Table 1.7.

In some cases, the pulse sounds become less intense (point of muffling sounds) but still can be heard at a lower pressure (50 or 40 mm Hg) or even all the way down to zero. In this situation, the diastolic pressure is recorded at the point of a clear, definite change in the loudness of the sound (also referred to as fourth phase) and at complete disappearance of the sound (fifth phase) (e.g., 120/78/60 or 120/82/0).

1.29 Mean Blood Pressure

During a normal resting contraction/relaxation cycle of the heart, the heart spends more time in the relaxation (diastolic) phase than in the contraction (systolic) phase. Accordingly, mean blood pressure (MBP) cannot be computed by taking an average of the SBP and DBP blood pressures. The equations used to determine MBP are shown in Activity 1.4.

When measuring blood pressure, be aware that a single reading may not be an accurate value because of the various factors (rest, stress, physical activity, food) that can affect blood pressure. Thus, if you are able, ask different people to take several readings at different times of the day to establish the real values. You can record the results of your resting heart rate and your SBP, DBP, and MBP assessments in Activity 1.4. You can also calculate the effects of aerobic activity on resting heart rate in this activity.

Bradycardia Slower heart rate than normal.

Sphygmomanometer Inflatable bladder contained within a cuff and a mercury gravity manometer (or aneroid manometer) from which blood pressure is read.

Systolic blood pressure (SBP) Pressure exerted by blood against walls of arteries during forceful contraction (systole) of the heart.

Diastolic blood pressure (DBP) Pressure exerted by the blood against the walls of the arteries during the relaxation phase (diastole) of the heart.

ASSESS YOUR BEHAVIOR

CENGAGE**brain** To access course materials, including companion resources, please visit www.cengagebrain.com.

1. Are you aware of your family health history and lifestyle factors that may negatively impact your health?
2. Do you accumulate at least 30 minutes of moderate-intensity physical activity 5 days per week and avoid excessive periods of daily sitting?
3. Do you make a constant and deliberate effort to stay healthy and achieve the highest potential for well-being?

ASSESS YOUR KNOWLEDGE

Evaluate how well you understand the concepts presented in this chapter using the chapter-specific quizzing available in the online materials at www.cengagebrain.com.

1. Advances in modern technology
   a. help people achieve higher fitness levels.
   b. have led to a decrease in chronic diseases.
   c. have almost completely eliminated the necessity for physical exertion in daily life.
   d. help fight hypokinetic disease.
   e. make it easier to achieve good aerobic fitness.

2. Most activities of daily living in the United States help people
   a. get adequate physical activity on a regular basis.
   b. meet health-related fitness standards.
   c. achieve good levels of skill-related activities.
   d. Choices a, b, and c are correct.
   e. None of the choices is correct.

3. The leading cause of death in the United States is
   a. cancer.
   b. accidents.
   c. CLRD.
   d. diseases of the cardiovascular system.
   e. drug abuse.

4. Bodily movement produced by skeletal muscles is called
   a. physical activity.
   b. kinesiology.
   c. exercise.
   d. aerobic exercise.
   e. muscle strength.

5. Among the long-term benefits of regular physical activity and exercise are significantly reduced risks for developing or dying from
   a. heart disease.
   b. type 2 diabetes.
   c. colon and breast cancers.
   d. osteoporotic fractures.
   e. All are correct choices.

6. To be ranked in the "active" category, an adult has to take between
   a. 3,500 and 4,999 steps per day.
   b. 5,000 and 7,499 steps per day.
   c. 7,500 and 9,999 steps per day.
   d. 10,000 and 12,499 steps per day.
   e. 12,500 and 15,000 steps per day.

7. The constant and deliberate effort to stay healthy and achieve the highest potential for well-being is defined as
   a. health.
   b. physical fitness.
   c. wellness.
   d. health-related fitness.
   e. physiological fitness.

8. Research on the effects of fitness on mortality indicates that the largest drop in premature mortality is seen between
   a. the average and excellent fitness groups.
   b. the low and moderate fitness groups.
   c. the high and excellent fitness groups.
   d. the moderate and good fitness groups.
   e. The drop is similar among all fitness groups.

9. Metabolic fitness can be achieved through
   a. a moderate-intensity exercise program.
   b. a high-intensity speed-training program.
   c. an increased basal metabolic rate.
   d. anaerobic training.
   e. an increase in lean body mass.

10. What is the greatest benefit of being physically fit?
    a. absence of disease
    b. a higher quality of life
    c. improved sports performance
    d. better personal appearance
    e. maintenance of recommended body weight

Correct answers can be found at the back of the book.

Activity 1.2: Wellness Lifestyle Questionnaire

Name _____ Date _____

Course _____ Section _____ Gender _____ Age _____

> The purpose of this questionnaire is to analyze current lifestyle habits and help determine changes necessary for future health and wellness. Check the appropriate answer to each question, and obtain a final score according to the guidelines provided at the end of the questionnaire.

	ALWAYS	NEARLY ALWAYS	OFTEN	SELDOM	NEVER
1. I participate in vigorous-intensity aerobic activity for 20 minutes on 3 or more days per week, and I accumulate at least 30 minutes of moderate-intensity physical activity on a minimum of 2 additional days per week.	5	4	3	2	1
2. I participate in strength-training exercises, using a minimum of eight different exercises, two or more days per week.	5	4	3	2	1
3. I perform flexibility exercises a minimum of two days per week.	5	4	3	2	1
4. I maintain recommended body weight (includes avoidance of excessive body fat, excessive thinness, or frequent fluctuations in body weight).	5	4	3	2	1
5. Every day, I eat three regular meals that include a wide variety of foods.	5	4	3	2	1
6. I limit the amount of saturated fat and trans fats in my diet on most days of the week.	5	4	3	2	1
7. I eat a minimum of five servings of fruits and vegetables and six servings from grain products daily.	5	4	3	2	1
8. I regularly avoid snacks, especially those that are high in calories and fat and low in nutrients and fiber.	5	4	3	2	1
9. I avoid cigarettes or tobacco in any other form.	5	4	3	2	1
10. I avoid alcoholic beverages. If I drink, I do so in moderation (one daily drink for women and two for men), and I do not combine alcohol with other drugs.	5	4	3	2	1
11. I avoid addictive drugs and needles that have been used by others.	5	4	3	2	1
12. I use prescription drugs and over-the-counter drugs sparingly (only when needed), and I follow all directions for their proper use.	5	4	3	2	1
13. I readily recognize and act on it when I am under excessive tension and stress (distress).	5	4	3	2	1
14. I am able to perform effective stress-management techniques.	5	4	3	2	1
15. I have close friends and relatives with whom I can discuss personal problems and approach for help when needed, and with whom I can express my feelings freely.	5	4	3	2	1
16. I spend most of my daily leisure time in wholesome recreational activities.	5	4	3	2	1
17. I sleep seven to eight hours each night.	5	4	3	2	1
18. I floss my teeth every day and brush them at least twice daily.	5	4	3	2	1

		ALWAYS	NEARLY ALWAYS	OFTEN	SELDOM	NEVER
19.	I get "safe sun" exposure (that is, 10–20 minutes unprotected sun exposure to the face, neck, and arms, on most days of the week between hours of 10:00 a.m. and 4:00 p.m.), I avoid overexposure to the sun, and I use sunscreen and appropriate clothing when I am out in the sun for an extended time.	5	4	3	2	1
20.	I avoid using products that have not been shown by science to be safe and effective. (This includes drugs and unproven nutrient and weight loss supplements.)	5	4	3	2	1
21.	I stay current with the warning signs for heart attack, stroke, and cancer.	5	4	3	2	1
22.	I practice monthly breast/testicle self-exams, get recommended screening tests (blood lipids, blood pressure, Pap tests), and seek a medical evaluation when I am not well or disease symptoms arise.	5	4	3	2	1
23.	I have a dental checkup at least once a year, and I get regular medical exams according to age recommendations.	5	4	3	2	1
24.	I am not sexually active. / I practice safe sex.	5	4	3	2	1
25.	I can deal effectively with disappointments and temporary feelings of sadness, loneliness, and depression. If I am unable to deal with these feelings, I seek professional help.	5	4	3	2	1
26.	I can work out emotional problems without turning to alcohol, other drugs, or violent behavior.	5	4	3	2	1
27.	I associate with people who have a positive attitude about life.	5	4	3	2	1
28.	I respond to temporary setbacks by making the best of the circumstances and by moving ahead with optimism and energy. I do not spend time and talent worrying about failures.	5	4	3	2	1
29.	I wear a seat belt whenever I am in a car, I ask others in my vehicle to do the same, and I make sure that children are in an infant seat or wear a shoulder harness.	5	4	3	2	1
30.	I do not drive under the influence of alcohol or other drugs, and I make an effort to keep others from doing the same.	5	4	3	2	1
31.	I avoid being alone in public places, especially after dark; I seek escorts when I visit or exercise in unfamiliar places.	5	4	3	2	1
32.	I seek to make my living quarters accident-free, and I keep doors and windows locked, especially when I am home alone.	5	4	3	2	1
33.	I try to minimize environmental pollutants, and I support community efforts to minimize pollution.	5	4	3	2	1
34.	I use energy conservation strategies and encourage others to do the same.	5	4	3	2	1
35.	I study and/or work in a clean environment (including avoidance of secondhand smoke).	5	4	3	2	1
36.	I participate in recycling programs for paper, cardboard, glass, plastic, and aluminum.	5	4	3	2	1

How to Score

Enter the score you have marked for each question in the spaces provided below. Next, total the score for each specific wellness lifestyle category and obtain a rating for each category according to the criteria provided below.

Health-Related Fitness	Nutrition	Avoiding Chemical Dependency	Stress Management	Personal Hygiene/Health	Disease Prevention	Emotional Well-being	Personal Safety	Environmental Health & Protection
1.	5.	9.	13.	17.	21.	25.	29.	33.
2.	6.	10.	14.	18.	22.	26.	30.	34.
3.	7.	11.	15.	19.	23.	27.	31.	35.
4.	8.	12.	16.	20.	24.	28.	32.	36.
Total:								
Rating:								

Category Rating

Excellent (E) = ≥17 Your answers show that you are aware of the importance of this category to your health and wellness. You are putting your knowledge to work for you by practicing good habits. As long as you continue to do so, this category should not pose a health risk. You are also setting a good example for family and friends to follow. Because you got a very high score on this part of the test, you may want to consider other categories in which your score indicates room for improvement.

Good (G) = 13–16 Your health practices in this area are good, but you have room for improvement. Look again at the items you answered with a 4 or lower and identify changes that you can make to improve your lifestyle. Even small changes often can help you achieve better health.

Needs Improvement (NI) = ≤12 Your health risks are showing. You may be taking serious and unnecessary risks with your health. Perhaps you are not aware of the risks or what to do about them. Most likely you need additional information and help in deciding how to successfully make the changes you desire. You can easily get the information that you need to improve, if you wish. The next step is up to you.

Please note that no final overall rating is provided for the entire questionnaire, because it may not be indicative of your overall wellness. For example, an excellent rating in most categories will not offset the immediate health risks and life-threatening consequences of using addictive drugs or not wearing a seat belt.

Activity 1.3: PAR-Q and Health History Questionnaire

Name _____ Date _____ Grade _____
Instructor _____ Course _____ Section _____

NECESSARY LAB EQUIPMENT
None.

OBJECTIVE
To determine the safety of exercise participation.

Physical Activity Readiness
Questionnaire - PAR-Q
(revised 2002)

PAR-Q & YOU
(A Questionnaire for People Aged 15 to 69)

Regular physical activity is fun and healthy, and increasingly more people are starting to become more active every day. Being more active is very safe for most people. However, some people should check with their doctor before they start becoming much more physically active.

If you are planning to become much more physically active than you are now, start by answering the seven questions in the box below. If you are between the ages of 15 and 69, the PAR-Q will tell you if you should check with your doctor before you start. If you are over 69 years of age, and you are not used to being very active, check with your doctor.

Common sense is your best guide when you answer these questions. Please read the questions carefully and answer each one honestly: check YES or NO.

YES	NO	
☐	☐	1. Has your doctor ever said that you have a heart condition <u>and</u> that you should only do physical activity recommended by a doctor?
☐	☐	2. Do you feel pain in your chest when you do physical activity?
☐	☐	3. In the past month, have you had chest pain when you were not doing physical activity?
☐	☐	4. Do you lose your balance because of dizziness or do you ever lose consciousness?
☐	☐	5. Do you have a bone or joint problem (for example, back, knee or hip) that could be made worse by a change in your physical activity?
☐	☐	6. Is your doctor currently prescribing drugs (for example, water pills) for your blood pressure or heart condition?
☐	☐	7. Do you know of <u>any other reason</u> why you should not do physical activity?

If you answered

YES to one or more questions

Talk with your doctor by phone or in person BEFORE you start becoming much more physically active or BEFORE you have a fitness appraisal. Tell your doctor about the PAR-Q and which questions you answered YES.
- You may be able to do any activity you want — as long as you start slowly and build up gradually. Or, you may need to restrict your activities to those which are safe for you. Talk with your doctor about the kinds of activities you wish to participate in and follow his/her advice.
- Find out which community programs are safe and helpful for you.

NO to all questions

If you answered NO honestly to all PAR-Q questions, you can be reasonably sure that you can:
- start becoming much more physically active – begin slowly and build up gradually. This is the safest and easiest way to go.
- take part in a fitness appraisal – this is an excellent way to determine your basic fitness so that you can plan the best way for you to live actively. It is also highly recommended that you have your blood pressure evaluated. If your reading is over 144/94, talk with your doctor before you start becoming much more physically active.

DELAY BECOMING MUCH MORE ACTIVE:
- if you are not feeling well because of a temporary illness such as a cold or a fever – wait until you feel better; or
- if you are or may be pregnant – talk to your doctor before you start becoming more active.

PLEASE NOTE: If your health changes so that you then answer YES to any of the above questions, tell your fitness or health professional. Ask whether you should change your physical activity plan.

<u>Informed Use of the PAR-Q:</u> The Canadian Society for Exercise Physiology, Health Canada, and their agents assume no liability for persons who undertake physical activity, and if in doubt after completing this questionnaire, consult your doctor prior to physical activity.

> No changes permitted. You are encouraged to photocopy the PAR-Q but only if you use the entire form.

NOTE: If the PAR-Q is being given to a person before he or she participates in a physical activity program or a fitness appraisal, this section may be used for legal or administrative purposes.

"I have read, understood and completed this questionnaire. Any questions I had were answered to my full satisfaction."

NAME _____
SIGNATURE _____ DATE _____
SIGNATURE OF PARENT _____ WITNESS _____
or GUARDIAN (for participants under the age of majority)

> Note: This physical activity clearance is valid for a maximum of 12 months from the date it is completed and becomes invalid if your condition changes so that you would answer YES to any of the seven questions.

© Canadian Society for Exercise Physiology   Supported by: Health Canada / Santé Canada   continued on other side...

Public Health Agency of Canada and the Canadian Society for Exercise Physiology, reproduced by permission of the Canadian Society for Exercise Physiology.

SOURCE: Physical Activity Readiness Questionnaire (PAR-Q) © 2002. Used with permission from the Canadian Society for Exercise Physiology www.csep.ca.

HEALTH HISTORY QUESTIONNAIRE

INTRODUCTION

Although exercise testing and exercise participation are relatively safe for most apparently healthy individuals, the reaction of the cardiovascular system to increased levels of physical activity cannot always be totally predicted. Consequently, there is a small but real risk of certain changes occurring during exercise testing and participation. Some of these changes may be abnormal blood pressure, irregular heart rhythm, fainting, and in rare instances a heart attack or cardiac arrest. Therefore, you must provide honest answers to this questionnaire. Exercise may be contraindicated under some of the conditions listed below; others may simply require special consideration. **If any of the conditions apply, consult your physician before you participate in an exercise program.** Also, promptly report to your instructor any exercise-related abnormalities that you may experience during the course of the semester.

A. Have you ever had or do you now have any of the following conditions?

- [ ] 1. A myocardial infarction
- [ ] 2. Coronary artery disease
- [ ] 3. Congestive heart failure
- [ ] 4. Elevated blood lipids (cholesterol and triglycerides)
- [ ] 5. Chest pain at rest or during exertion
- [ ] 6. Shortness of breath
- [ ] 7. An abnormal resting or stress electrocardiogram
- [ ] 8. Uneven, irregular, or skipped heartbeats (including a racing or fluttering heart)
- [ ] 9. A blood embolism
- [ ] 10. Thrombophlebitis
- [ ] 11. Rheumatic heart fever
- [ ] 12. Elevated blood pressure
- [ ] 13. A stroke
- [ ] 14. Diabetes
- [ ] 15. A family history of coronary heart disease, syncope, or sudden death before age 60
- [ ] 16. Any other heart problem that makes exercise unsafe

B. Do you have any of the following conditions?

- [ ] 1. Arthritis, rheumatism, or gout
- [ ] 2. Chronic low-back pain
- [ ] 3. Any other joint, bone, or muscle problems
- [ ] 4. Any respiratory problems
- [ ] 5. Obesity (more than 30 percent overweight)
- [ ] 6. Anorexia
- [ ] 7. Bulimia
- [ ] 8. Mononucleosis
- [ ] 9. Any physical disability that could interfere with safe participation in exercise

C. Do any of the following conditions apply?

- [ ] 1. Do you smoke cigarettes?
- [ ] 2. Are you taking any prescription drugs?

D. Do you have any other concern regarding your ability to safely participate in an exercise program? If so, explain:

_____

_____

_____

Student's Signature: _____ **Date:** _____

Activity 1.4: Resting Heart Rate and Blood Pressure

Name _____ Date _____

Course _____ Section _____ Gender _____ Age _____

Resting Heart Rate and Blood Pressure
Determine your resting heart rate and blood pressure in the right and left arms while sitting comfortably in a chair.

Resting Heart Rate: [ ]   Rating: [ ] (see Table 1.6, page 30)

Blood Pressure:	Right Arm	Rating (from Table 1.7, page 31)	Left Arm	Rating (from Table 1.7, page 31)
Systolic	[ ]	[ ]	[ ]	[ ]
Diastolic	[ ]	[ ]	[ ]	[ ]

Mean Blood Pressure Computation
The following equation is used to determine MBP:

$MBP = DBP + \frac{1}{3} PP$ Where PP = pulse pressure or the difference between the systolic and diastolic pressures.

1. Compute your MBP using your own blood pressure results:

   PP = _____ (systolic) − _____ (diastolic) = _____ mm Hg

   MBP = _____ (DBP) + $\frac{_____ (PP)}{3}$ = _____ mm Hg

2. Determine the MBP for a person with a BP of 130/80 and a second person with a BP of 120/90.

   _____
   _____
   _____
   _____

   Which subject has the lower MBP? _____

Computing the Effects of Aerobic Activity on Resting Heart Rate
Using your actual resting heart rate (RHR) from Part I of this lab, compute the total number of times your heart beats each day and each year:

A. Beats per day = _____ (RHR bpm) × 60 (min per hour) × 24 (hours per day) = _____ beats per day

B. Beats per year = _____ (heart rate in beats per day, use item A) × 365 = _____ beats per year

If your RHR dropped 20 bpm through an aerobic exercise program, determine the number of beats that your heart would save each year at that lower RHR:

C. Beats per day = _____ (your current RHR − 20) × 60 × 24 = _____ beats per day

D. Beats per year = _____ (heart rate in beats per day, use item C) × 365 = _____ beats per year

E. Number of beats saved per year (B − D) _____ − _____ = _____ beats saved per year

Assuming that you will reach the average U.S. life expectancy of 81 years for women or 76 for men, determine the additional number of "heart rate life years" available to you if your RHR were 20 bpm lower:

F. Years of life ahead = _____ (use 81 for women and 76 for men) − _____ (current age) = _____ years

G. Number of beats saved = _____ (use item E) × _____ (use item F) = _____ beats saved

H. Number of heart rate life years based on the lower RHR = _____ (use item G) ÷ _____ (use item D) = _____ years

Activity 1.5: Dimension of Wellness–Setting Your Goal

Name _____ Date _____

Course _____ Section _____ Gender _____ Age _____

Instructions

1. In the Wellness Dimension chart below, record the date at the top of the first column, then fill in that column using the following scale to indicate your wellness rating for each dimension:
   poor = 5, fair = 4, average = 3, good = 2, excellent = 1
2. Next, write a goal that you want to accomplish prior to the end of this course for each wellness dimension, and list three specific objectives that will help you accomplish each goal.
3. Once a month, review this form, fill in another column of self-evaluation, and adjust your objectives as necessary.

Here's an example:

Social goal: | To improve my social life at school |

Specific objectives

1. Find study buddies. Ask each instructor and counselor about study groups.
2. Attend Friday night discussion groups in Student Center.
3. Locate activities I enjoy—basketball, chess, dancing—and start a conversation.

Date

Wellness Dimension					
Physical					
Emotional					
Social					
Environmental					
Mental					
Spiritual					
Occupational					

Goals and Objectives

Physical goal: _____

Specific objectives

1. _____
2. _____
3. _____

Emotional goal: _____

Specific objectives

1. _____
2. _____
3. _____

Social goal: _____

Specific objectives

1. _____
2. _____
3. _____

Environmental goal: _____

Specific objectives

1. _____
2. _____
3. _____

Mental goal: _____

Specific objectives

1. _____
2. _____
3. _____

Spiritual goal: _____

Specific objectives

1. _____
2. _____
3. _____

Occupational goal: _____

Specific objectives

1. _____
2. _____
3. _____

Behavior Modification

2

"To reach a goal you have never before attained, you must do things you have never before done."
—Richard Scott

Objectives

- **Learn** the effects of environment on human behavior.
- **Understand** obstacles that hinder the ability to change behavior.
- **Explain** the concepts of motivation and locus of control.
- **Identify** the stages of change.
- **Describe** the processes of change.
- **Explain** techniques that will facilitate the process of change.
- **Describe** the role of SMART goal setting in the process of change.
- **Be able** to write specific actions for behavioral change.
- **Prepare** for a healthy change in lifestyle.

CENGAGEbrain.com

Visit **www.cengagebrain.com** to access course materials and companion resources for this text, including quiz questions designed to check your understanding of the chapter contents. See the preface on page ix for more information.

FAQ

Why is it so hard to change?

Change is incredibly difficult for most people. Our behaviors are based on our core values and actions that are rewarded. Whether we are trying to increase physical activity, quit smoking, change unhealthy eating habits, or reverse heart disease, it is human nature to resist change that isn't immediately rewarded, even when we know that change will provide substantial benefits in the near future. Furthermore, Dr. Richard Earle, managing director of the Canadian Institute of Stress and the Hans Selye Foundation, explains that people have a tendency toward pessimism. In every spoken language, there is a ratio of three pessimistic adjectives to one positive adjective. Thus, linguistically, psychologically, and emotionally, we focus on what can go wrong and we lose motivation before we even start. That's why we have the saying, "The only person who truly welcomes a change is a baby with a full diaper."

What triggers the desire to change?

Motivation comes from within. In most instances, no amount of pressure, reasoning, or fear will inspire people to take action. Change in behavior is most likely to occur when people either receive instant gratification for their actions or when people's feelings are addressed. People pursue change when it's rewarded (for example, lower health care premiums if you quit smoking) or they start contemplating change when there is a change in core values that will make them feel uncomfortable with the present behavior(s) or lack thereof (e.g., a long and healthy life is more important than smoking). Core values change when feelings are addressed. The challenge is to find ways that will help people understand the problems and solutions in a manner that will influence emotions and not just the thought process. Once the problem behavior is understood and "felt," the person may become uncomfortable with the situation and will be more inclined to address the problem behavior or adopt a healthy behavior.

Dr. Jan Hill, a Toronto-based life skills specialist, stated that discomfort is a great motivator. People tolerate any situation until it becomes too uncomfortable for them: "Then they have to take steps to make changes in their lives." It is at this point that the skills presented in this chapter will help you implement a successful plan for change. Keep in mind that as you make lifestyle changes, your relationships and friendships also need to be addressed. You need to distance yourself from those individuals who share your bad habits (e.g., smoking, drinking, sedentary lifestyle) and associate with people who practice healthy habits. Are you prepared to do so?

Adapted from K. Jenkins, "Why Is Change So Hard?" http://www.healthnexus.ca/projects/articles/change.htm, downloaded March 12, 2011.

The benefits of regular physical activity and living a healthy lifestyle to achieve wellness are well documented. Nearly all Americans accept that exercise is beneficial to health and see a need to incorporate it into their lives. Seventy percent of new and returning exercisers, however, are at risk for early dropout.[1] As the scientific evidence continues to mount each day, most people still are not adhering to a healthy lifestyle program.

Let's look at an all-too-common occurrence on college campuses. Most students understand that they should be exercising, and they contemplate enrolling in a fitness course. The motivating factor might be improved physical appearance, health benefits, or simply fulfillment of a college requirement. They sign up for the course, participate for a few months, finish the course, and stop exercising! They offer a wide array of excuses: too busy, no one to exercise with, already have the grade, inconvenient gym hours, job conflicts, and so on. A few months later they realize once again that exercise is vital, and they repeat the cycle (Figure 2.1).

The information in this book will be of little value to you if you are unable to abandon your negative habits and adopt and maintain healthy behaviors. Before looking at any physical fitness and wellness guidelines, you will need to take a critical look at your behaviors and lifestyle—and most likely make some permanent changes to promote your overall health and wellness.

Figure 2.1 Exercise/exercise dropout cycle.

Real Life Story | Sharon's Experience

Prior to my marriage, I had never really tried jogging. But then I became convinced that aerobic exercise would improve my fitness and help me maintain a healthy weight. My fiancé was really serious about fitness and had been jogging regularly for several years. We wrote out an exercise prescription and started jogging together. Exercise helped me to accomplish my health goals through my first two pregnancies. The feeling of being physically fit was a reward in itself, but jogging two consecutive miles was rarely truly enjoyable. With young children at home, my husband and I were forced to take turns jogging so that one of us would always be home. My jogging program consisted of a 20-minute jog: 1 mile out and 1 mile back, 5 to 6 times per week.

Five years later, on one particular day, 25 minutes went by and I wasn't ready to stop jogging. At 30 minutes, I went and knocked on the door: "Honey, I feel great I'll be back in 10 minutes." I did this again at 40 and 50 minutes.

I ended up jogging for a full 60 minutes for the first time in my life, and the experience was genuinely joyful! That day, I finally reached "the top of the mountain" (the termination/adoption stage of change) and truly experienced the joy of being physically fit. Jogging became as easy as a "bird in flight." I have not stopped jogging in more than 37 years! It wasn't easy at first, but knowledge, commitment, support, action, and perseverance paid off.

Fitness also was the factor that led to improvements in other wellness components in our lives (continuing health education, good nutrition, stress reduction, and chronic disease prevention). Fitness is the daily "bread and butter" that enhances our quality of life. Our children now also follow our active lifestyle. We always say: "A family that exercises together stays together."

PERSONAL PROFILE: Personal Behavior Modification Profile

Are you able to answer the following questions regarding behavior change? If you are unable to do so, the chapter contents will help you do so.

I. Can you identify behavioral changes that you have consciously made in your life and the process that you went through to do so?

II. Would you categorize yourself as having an internal or external locus of control?

III. Can you identify your current stage of change for physical activity? How about exercise?

IV. A person precontemplating a change in behavior is said to be ready to start the process of change. ___True ___False

V. SMART goals enhance the odds of success. ___True ___False

VI. Can you list the processes of change that most helped Sharon adhere to her fitness program?

2.1 Living in a Toxic Health and Fitness Environment

Most of the behaviors we adopt are a product of our environment—the forces of social influences we encounter and the thought processes we go through (also see self-efficacy on pages 52–53). This environment includes families, friends, peers, homes, schools, workplaces, television, radio, and movies, as well as our communities, country, and culture in general.

Unfortunately, when it comes to fitness and wellness, we live in a "toxic" environment. Becoming aware of how the environment affects us is vital if we wish to achieve and maintain wellness. Yet, we are so habituated to the environment that we miss the subtle ways it influences our behaviors, personal lifestyle, and health each day.

From a young age, we observe, we learn, we emulate, and without realizing it, we incorporate into our own lifestyle the behaviors of people around us. We are transported by parents, relatives, and friends who drive us nearly any place we need to go. We watch them drive short distances to run errands. We see them take escalators and elevators and ride moving sidewalks at malls and airports. They use remote controls and cell phones. We observe them stop at fast-food restaurants and pick up supersized, calorie-dense, high-fat meals. They watch television and surf the Internet for hours at a time. Some smoke, some drink heavily, and some have hard-drug addictions. Others engage in risky behaviors by not wearing seat belts, by drinking and driving, and by having unprotected sex. All of these unhealthy habits can be passed along, unquestioned, to the next generation.

Environmental Influences on Physical Activity

Among the leading underlying causes of death in the United States are physical inactivity and poor diet. This is partially because most activities of daily living, which a few decades ago required movement or physical activity, now require almost no effort and negatively affect health, fitness, and body weight. Small movements that have been streamlined out of daily life quickly add up, especially when we consider their loss over 7 days a week and 52 weeks a year.

We can examine the decrease in the required daily energy (caloric) expenditure as a result of modern-day conveniences that lull us into physical inactivity. For example, short automobile trips that replace walking or riding a bike decrease energy expenditure by 50 to 300 calories per day; automatic car window and door openers represent about 1 calorie at each use; automatic garage door openers, 5 calories; drive-through windows at banks, fast-food restaurants, dry cleaners, and pharmacies add up to about 5 to 10 calories each time; elevators and escalators, 3 to 10 calories per trip; food processors, 5 to 10 calories; riding lawnmowers, about 100 calories; automatic car washes, 100 calories; hours of computer use to e-mail, surf the Internet, text, and conduct Internet transactions represent another 50 to 300 calories; and excessive television viewing can add up to 200 or more calories. Little wonder that we have such a difficult time maintaining a healthy body weight.

Health experts recommend five to six miles of walking per day. This level of activity equates to about 10,000 to 12,000 daily steps. If you have never clipped on a pedometer, try to do so. When you look at the total number of steps it displays at the end of the day, you may be shocked by how few steps you took.

With the advent of now-ubiquitous cell phones, people are moving even less. Family members call each other on the phone even within the walls of their own home. Some people don't get out of the car anymore to ring a doorbell. Instead, they wait in front and send a text message to have the person come out.

Even modern-day architecture reinforces unhealthy behaviors. Elevators and escalators are often of the finest workmanship and located conveniently. Most of our shopping centers and convention centers don't provide accessible stairwells, so people are all but forced to ride escalators. If they want to walk up the escalator, they can't because the people in front of them obstruct the way. Entrances to buildings provide electric sensors and automatic door openers. Without a second thought, people walk through automatic doors instead of taking the time to push a door open.

At work, most people have jobs that require them to sit most of the day. We don't even get up and walk a short distance to talk to coworkers. Instead, we use e-mail, IM, and telephones.

For individuals who spend an excessive amount of daily time sitting (riding in a car, sitting at a desk, watching TV and movies, playing computer games, surfing the Internet), research data indicate that the amount of daily sitting time is associated with an increased risk for all-cause and cardiovascular disease mortality, independent of leisure-time physical activity and excessive body weight.[2] The greater the amount of sitting time per day, the greater the risk of premature mortality. As expected, the highest mortality rates were seen in obese individuals who sit almost all of the time.

Our environment is not conducive to a healthy, physically active lifestyle.

Of particular interest, this study and others have shown that death rates are still higher for people who spent a large portion of their day sitting, even though they meet current minimum 30 minutes of either moderate or vigorous physical activity recommendations five days per week. The researchers concluded that for better health and a longer life people should avoid sedentarism and, most importantly, decrease total daily sitting time.

A subsequent study published in 2010 linked excessive TV watching and earlier death.[3] A total of 8,800 adults with no history of heart disease were followed for more than 6 years. As compared to individuals who only watched 2 hours of TV per day, those who watched 4 or more daily hours were 80 percent more likely to die from heart disease and 46 percent more likely to die from all causes. The authors also indicated that exercise does not make up for long TV sessions. Sitting is the "default position" for TV viewing, and such an action minimizes tasks such as standing, walking, and moving about during the course of the day. Excessive TV viewing may also be more detrimental than other sedentary activities such as reading, studying, or doing homework.

Leisure time is no better. When people arrive home after work, they surf the net, play computer games, or watch television for hours at a time. The first thing people consider when setting up a family room is where to put the television. This little (or big-screen) box has truly lulled us into inactivity. Excessive TV viewing is directly linked to obesity, and the amount of time people choose to spend watching television programs and DVDs is climbing. The average household watches close to 8 hours of programming each day—up 1 hour from 1982 and 2 from 1970.[4]

Television viewing is more than just a sedentary activity. Think about people's habits before they sit down to watch a favorite show. They turn on the television, then stop by the kitchen for a box of crackers and processed cheese. They return to watch the show, start snacking, and are bombarded with commercials about soft drinks, beer, and unhealthy foods. Viewers are enticed to purchase and eat unhealthy, calorie-dense foods in an unnecessary and mindless "snacking setting." Television viewing even has been shown to reduce the number of fruits and vegetables some people consume, most likely because people are eating the unhealthy foods advertised on television.[5]

Our communities aren't much help either. Walking, jogging, and bicycle trails are too sparse in most cities, further discouraging physical activity. Places for safe exercise are hard to find in many metropolitan areas, motivating many people to remain indoors during leisure hours for fear of endangering their personal safety and well-being.

In addition to sitting most of the day at work and at home, we also sit in our cars. We are transported or drive everywhere we have to go. Safety concerns also keep people in cars instead of on sidewalks and in parks. Communities are designed around the automobile. City streets make driving convenient and walking or cycling difficult, impossible, or dangerous. Streets typically are rated by traffic engineers according to their "level of service"—that is, based on how well

Walking and cycling are priority activities in many European communities.

they facilitate motorized traffic. A wide, straight street with few barriers to slow motorized traffic gets a high score. According to these guidelines, pedestrians are "obstructions." Only recently have a few local governments and communities started to devise standards to determine how useful streets are for pedestrians and bicyclists.

For each car in the United States, there are seven parking spaces.[6] Drivers can almost always find a parking spot, but walkers often run out of sidewalks and crosswalks in modern streets. Sidewalks have not been a priority in city, suburban, or commercial development. Whereas British street design manuals recommend sidewalks on both sides of the street, American manuals recommend sidewalks on one side of the street only.

One measure that encourages activity is the use of "traffic-calming" strategies: intentionally slowing traffic to make the pedestrian's role easier. These strategies were developed and are widely used in Europe. Examples include narrower streets, rougher pavement (cobblestone), pedestrian islands, and raised crosswalks.

Many European communities place a high priority on walking and cycling, which makes up 40 to 54 percent of all daily trips taken by people in Austria, the Netherlands, Denmark, Italy, and Sweden. By contrast, in the United States, walking and cycling account for 10 percent of daily trips, whereas the automobile accounts for 84 percent.[7]

Granted, many people drive because the distances to cover are vast. We live in bedroom communities and commute to work. When people live near frequently visited destinations, they are more likely to walk or bike for transportation. Neighborhoods that mix commercial and residential land use encourage walking over driving because of the short distances among home, shopping, and work.

Children also walk or cycle to school less frequently than in the past. The reasons? Distance, traffic, weather, perceived crime, and school policy. Distance is a significant barrier because the trend during the past few decades has been to build larger schools on the outskirts of communities instead of small schools within neighborhoods.

2.2 Environmental Influence on Diet and Nutrition

The present obesity epidemic in the United States and other developed countries has been getting worse every year. We are becoming a nation of overweight and obese people. You may ask why. Let's examine the evidence.

According to the U.S. Department of Agriculture's Center for Nutrition Policy and Promotion, the amount of daily food supply available in the United States is about 3,900 calories per person, before wastage. This figure represents a 700-calorie rise over the early 1980s,[8] which means that we have taken the amount of food available to us and tossed in a Cinnabon for every person in the country.

The overabundance of food increases pressure on food suppliers to advertise and try to convince consumers to buy their products. The food industry spends more than $33 billion each year on advertising and promotion, and most of this money goes toward highly processed foods. The few ads and campaigns promoting healthy foods and healthful eating simply cannot compete. Most of us would be hard-pressed to recall a jingle for brown rice or kale. The money spent advertising a single food product across the United States is often 10 to 50 times more than the money the federal government spends promoting MyPlate nutrition guidelines (the recommended daily food and nutrient amounts according to a person's caloric requirement) or encouraging us to eat fruits and vegetables.[9]

Coupled with our sedentary lifestyle, many activities of daily living in today's culture are associated with eating. We seem to be eating all the time. We eat during coffee breaks, when we socialize, when we play, when we watch sports, at the movies, during television viewing, and when the clock tells us it's time for a meal. Our lives seem to be centered on food, a nonstop string of occasions to eat and overeat. And much of the overeating is done without a second thought. For instance, when people rent a video, they usually end up in line with the video and also with popcorn, candy, and soft drinks. Do we really have to eat while watching a movie?

As a nation, we now eat out more often than in the past, portion sizes are larger, and we have an endless variety of foods to choose from. We also snack more than ever before. Unhealthy food is relatively inexpensive and is sold in places where it was not available in the past.

Increasingly, people have decided that they no longer require special occasions to eat out. Mother's Day, a birthday, or someone's graduation are no longer the only reasons to eat at a restaurant. Eating out is part of today's lifestyle. In the late 1970s, food eaten away from home represented about 18 percent of our energy intake. In the mid-1990s, this figure rose to 32 percent. Almost half of the money Americans spend on food today is on meals away from home.[10]

Eating out would not be such a problem if portion sizes were reasonable or if restaurant food were similar to food prepared at home. Compared with home-cooked meals, restaurant and fast-food meals are higher in fat and calories and lower in essential nutrients and fiber.

Food portions in restaurants have increased substantially in size. Patrons consume huge amounts of food, almost as if this were the last meal they would ever have. They drink entire pitchers of soda pop or beer instead of the traditional 8-ounce cup size. Some restaurant menus may include selections that are called healthy choices, but these items may not provide nutritional information, including calories. In all likelihood, the menu has many other choices that look delicious but provide larger serving sizes with more fat and calories and fewer fruits and vegetables. Making a healthy selection is difficult, because people tend to choose food for its taste, convenience, and cost instead of nutrition.

Restaurant food is often less healthy than we think. Trained dietitians were asked to estimate nutrition information for five restaurant meals. The results showed that the dietitians underestimated the number of calories and amount of fat by 37 and 49 percent, respectively.[11] Findings such as these do not offer much hope for the average consumer who tries to make healthy choices when eating out.

Most restaurants are also pleasurable places to be: colorful, well-lit, and thoughtfully decorated. These intentional features are designed to enhance comfort, appetite, and length of stay, with the intent to entice more eating. Employees are formally trained in techniques that urge patrons to eat more and spend more. Servers are prepared to approach the table and suggest specific drinks, with at least one from the bar. When the drink is served, they recommend selected appetizers. Drink refills are often free while dining out. Following dinner, the server offers desserts and coffee. A person could literally get a full day's worth of calories in one meal without ever ordering an entree.

Fast-food restaurants do not lag far behind. Menu items frequently are introduced at one size and, over time, popular items are increased in size two to five times.[12] Large portion sizes are a major problem because people tend to eat what they are served. A study by the American Institute for Cancer Research found that with bigger portion sizes, 67 percent of Americans ate the larger amount of food they were served.[13] The tendency of most patrons is to "clean the plate."

Individuals seem to have the same disregard for hunger cues when snacking. Participants in one study were randomly given an afternoon snack of potato chips in different bag sizes. The participants received bags from 1 to 20 ounces for 5 days. The results showed that the larger the bag, the more the person ate. Men ate 37 percent more chips from the largest than the smallest bag. Women ate 18 percent more. Of significant interest, the size of the snack did not change the amount of food the person ate during the next meal.[14] Another study found no major difference in reported hunger or fullness after participants ate different sizes of sandwiches that were served to them, even though they ate more when they were given larger sandwiches.[15]

Other researchers set out to see if the size of the package—not just the amount of food—affects how much people eat. Study participants received two different-sized packages with the same number of spaghetti strands. The larger package was twice the size of the smaller package. When participants were asked to take out enough spaghetti to prepare a meal for two adults, they took out an average of 234 strands from the small package versus 302 strands from the larger package.[16] In our own kitchens, and in restaurants, we seem to have taken away from our internal cues the decision of how much to eat. Instead we have turned that choice over to businesses that profit from our overindulgence.

Also working against our hunger cues is our sense of thrift. Many of us consider cost ahead of nutrition when we choose foods. Restaurants and groceries often appeal to this sense of thrift by using "value marketing," meaning that they offer us a larger portion for only a small price increase. Customers think they are getting a bargain, and the food providers turn a better profit because the cost of additional food is small compared with the cost of marketing, production, and labor.

The National Alliance for Nutrition has further shown that a little more money buys a lot more calories. Ice cream upsizing from a kid's scoop to a double scoop, for example, adds an extra 390 calories for only an extra $1.62. A medium-sized movie theater popcorn (unbuttered) provides 500 additional calories over a small-size popcorn for just an extra 71 cents. Equally, king-size candy bars provide about 230 additional calories for just another 33 cents over the standard size.[17] We often eat more simply because we get more for our money without taking into consideration the detrimental consequences to our health and waistline.

Another example of financial but not nutritional sense is free soft-drink refills. When people choose a high-calorie drink over diet soda or water, the person does not compensate by eating less food later that day.[18] Liquid calories seem to be difficult for people to account for. A 20-ounce bottle of regular soda contains the equivalent of one-third cup of sugar. One extra can of soda (160 calories) per day represents an extra 16.5 pounds of fat per year (160 calories × 365 days ÷ 3,500 calories). Even people who regularly drink diet sodas tend to gain weight. In their minds, they may rationalize that a calorie-free drink allows them to consume more food.

A larger variety of food also entices overeating. Think about your own experiences at parties that have a buffet of snacks. Do you eat more when everyone brings something to contribute to the snack table? When unhealthy choices outnumber healthy choices, people are less likely to follow their natural cues to choose healthy food.

The previously mentioned environmental factors influence our thought processes and hinder our ability to determine what constitutes an appropriate meal based on actual needs. The result: On average, American women consume 335 more daily calories than they did 20 years ago and men an additional 170 calories.[19]

Now you can analyze and identify the environmental influences on your behaviors. Activity 2.1 provides you with the opportunity to determine whether you control your environment or the environment controls you.

Living in the 21st century, we have all the modern-day conveniences that lull us into overconsumption and sedentary living. By living in America, we adopt behaviors that put our health at risk. And though we understand that lifestyle choices affect our health and well-being, we still have an extremely difficult time making changes.

Let's look at weight gain. Most people do not start life with a weight problem. By age 20, a man may weigh 160 pounds. A few years later, the weight starts to climb and may reach 170 pounds. He now adapts and accepts 170 pounds as his weight. He may go on a diet but not make the necessary lifestyle changes. Gradually his weight climbs to 180, 190, and 200 pounds. Although he may not like it and would like to weigh less, once again he adapts and accepts 200 pounds as his stable weight.

The time comes, usually around middle age, when values change, that people want to make changes in their lives but find this difficult to accomplish, illustrating the adage that "old habits die hard." Acquiring positive behaviors that will lead to better health and well-being is a long-term process and requires continual effort. Understanding why so many people are unsuccessful at changing their behaviors and are unable to live a healthy lifestyle may increase your readiness and motivation for change. Next we will examine barriers to change, what motivates people to change, behavior change theories, the transtheoretical or stages-of-change model, the process of change, techniques for change, and actions required to make permanent changes in behavior.

2.3 Values and Behavior

To understand human behavior, or why people do what they do, we need to understand values. Values are defined as the core beliefs and ideals that people have. Values govern behavior as people look to conduct themselves in a manner that is conducive to living and attaining goals consistent with their beliefs and what's important to them. A person's values reflect who they are.

Values are established through experience and learning, and their development is a lifelong process that influences all aspects of life. Personal values are first developed within family circles, schools, the media, and the culture where people grow up and live; according to what is acceptable or unacceptable, desirable or undesirable, good or bad, and rewarded or ignored/punished. Educational experiences play a key role in the establishment of values. Education is power: It provides people with knowledge to form opinions and forces them to question issues and take stands.

Values are also learned through examples and role models. People tend to emulate and adopt behaviors from people they

Activity 2.1: Exercising Control over Your Physical Activity and Nutrition Environment

Name _____ Date _____

Course _____ Section _____ Gender _____ Age _____

INSTRUCTIONS
Select the appropriate answer to each question and obtain a final score for each section. Then rate yourself according to the guidelines at the end of the lab.

I. Physical Activity

Note: Based on the definitions of *physical activity* and *exercise*, as you take this questionnaire, keep in mind that you can be physically active without exercising, but you cannot exercise without being physically active.

	NEARLY ALWAYS	OFTEN	SELDOM	NEVER
1. Do you identify daily time slots to be *physically active*?	4	3	2	1
2. Do you seek additional opportunities to be active each day (walk, cycle, park farther away, do yard work/gardening)?	4	3	2	1
3. Do you avoid labor-saving devices/activities (escalators, elevators, self-propelled lawn mowers, snow blowers, drive through windows)?	4	3	2	1
4. Does physical activity improve your health and well-being?	4	3	2	1
5. Does physical activity increase your energy level?	4	3	2	1
6. Do you seek professional and/or medical (if necessary) advice prior to starting an exercise program or when increasing the intensity, duration, and frequency of exercise?	4	3	2	1
7. Do you identify time slots to *exercise* most days of the week?	4	3	2	1
8. Do you schedule exercise during times of the day when you feel most energetic?	4	3	2	1
9. Do you have an alternative plan to be active or exercise during adverse weather conditions (walk at the mall, swim at the health club, climb stairs, skip rope, dance)?	4	3	2	1
10. Do you cross-train (participate in a variety of activities)?	4	3	2	1
11. Do you surround yourself with people who support your physical activity/exercise goals?	4	3	2	1
12. Do you let family and friends know of your physical activity/exercise interests?	4	3	2	1
13. Do you invite family and friends to exercise with you?	4	3	2	1
14. Do you seek new friendships with people who are physically active?	4	3	2	1
15. Do you select friendships with people whose fitness and skill levels are similar to yours?	4	3	2	1
16. Do you plan social activities that involve physical activity?	4	3	2	1
17. Do you plan activity/exercise when you are away from home (during business and vacation trips)?	4	3	2	1
18. When you have a desire to do so, do you take classes to learn new activity/sport skills?	4	3	2	1
19. Do you limit daily television viewing and Internet and computer game time?	4	3	2	1
20. Do you spend leisure hours being physically active?	4	3	2	1

Physical Activity Score: _____

II. Nutrition

	NEARLY ALWAYS	OFTEN	SELDOM	NEVER
1. Do you prepare a shopping list prior to going to the store?	4	3	2	1
2. Do you select food items primarily from the perimeter of the store (site of most fresh/unprocessed foods)?	4	3	2	1
3. Do you limit the unhealthy snacks you bring into the home and the workplace?	4	3	2	1
4. Do you plan your meals and is your pantry well stocked so you can easily prepare a meal without a quick trip to the store?	4	3	2	1
5. Do you help cook your meals?	4	3	2	1
6. Do you pay attention to how hungry you are before and during a meal?	4	3	2	1
7. When reaching for food, do you remind yourself that you have a choice about what and how much you eat?	4	3	2	1
8. Do you eat your meals at home?	4	3	2	1
9. Do you eat your meals at the table only?	4	3	2	1
10. Do you include whole-grain products in your diet each day (whole-grain bread/cereal/crackers/rice/pasta)?	4	3	2	1
11. Do you make a deliberate effort to include a variety of fruits and vegetables in your diet each day?	4	3	2	1
12. Do you limit your daily saturated fat and trans fat intake (red meat, whole milk, cheese, butter, hard margarines, luncheon meats, baked goods, processed foods)?	4	3	2	1
13. Do you avoid unnecessary/unhealthy snacking (at work or play, during TV viewing, at the movies or socials)?	4	3	2	1
14. Do you plan caloric allowances prior to attending social gatherings that include food and eating?	4	3	2	1
15. Do you limit alcohol consumption to two drinks a day if you are a man, one drink a day if you are a woman, or none at all if you are a woman with a family history of cancer, especially breast cancer?	4	3	2	1
16. Are you aware of strategies to decrease caloric intake when dining out (resist the server's offerings for drinks and appetizers, select a low-calorie/nutrient-dense item, drink water, resist cleaning your plate, ask for a doggie bag, share meals, request whole-wheat substitutes, get dressings on the side, avoid cream sauces, skip desserts)?	4	3	2	1
17. Do you avoid ordering larger meal sizes because you get more food for your money?	4	3	2	1
18. Do you avoid buying food when you hadn't planned to do so (gas stations, convenience stores, video rental stores)?	4	3	2	1
19. Do you fill your time with activities that will keep you away from places where you typically consume food (kitchen, coffee room, dining room)?	4	3	2	1
20. Do you know what situations trigger your desire for unnecessary snacking and overeating (vending machines, TV viewing, food ads, cookbooks, fast-food restaurants, buffet restaurants)?	4	3	2	1

Nutrition Score: _____

Environmental Control Ratings

≥71	You have good control over your environment
51–70	There is room for improvement
31–50	Your environmental control is poor
≤30	You are controlled by your environment

Total Environmental Score
(add Physical Activity and Nutrition Scores): ☐

admire, look up to, or view as heroes. Role models are most often parents, life heroes, siblings, classmates, sports figures, or people one sees on television or in movies, or reads and hears about through books or other media sources. As people look to develop values, they typically search for and emulate people of high ethical values and accomplishments that make them feel positive both about the people whose behaviors they are trying to emulate and themselves. Subsequently, the constant and habitual repetition of similar actions, behaviors, and expectations has a powerful conditioning effect on the mind and the role of the value for success in life.

Core values change throughout life based on education and the environment in which people live. Learning and gaining a belief about a particular issue is most critical in the establishment of values. For example, individuals who lead a sedentary lifestyle and never exercise lack an understanding of and don't experience the myriad benefits and vibrant quality of life obtained through fitness participation. Through a book, class, sports participation, or a friend, the person may first be exposed to exercise and an active lifestyle. The individual may then seek an environment wherein he/she can learn and actively participate in a physical activity or exercise program. The feelings of well-being and increased health, functional capacity, quality of life, and the education gained about the benefits of fitness in turn become the reward for program participation and lead to the development of the value that daily activity is vital for health and wellness. The person, often subconsciously, learns to analyze the feelings experienced through participation that lead to the development of a new value. The value now sways the person's actions to live according to what is important to achieve wellness. This feeling of "fitness" often snowballs into the adoption of other healthy behaviors that further improve the individual's state of well-being. Of utmost importance in the maintenance of core values is to live the principles involved to reap the benefits. Thus, a constant and deliberate effort is required to be in an environment that rewards the behavior(s) the individual is trying to live.

2.4 Your Brain and Your Habits

People are creatures of habit. Most of the time habits are developed based on rewards, and most people value instant rewards more than long-term rewards. A change in core values, nonetheless, often overrules instant rewards as people seek long-term gratification.

People tend to repeat actions that are pleasurable and avoid those that are unpleasant. A part of the brain known as the striatum (corpus striatum) plays a key role in habit formation. There is a biological explanation to this process. The striatum is activated by events that are rewarding, exciting, unexpected, and intense, as well as by cues from the environment that are associated with those events. The striatum then memorizes events that are pleasurable and rewarding. For example, most people love cake because its taste is much more pleasurable (immediate reward) than that of a green salad, even though the latter provides better nutrition and is conducive to weight management (long-term gratification).

The neurotransmitter dopamine is abundant in the striatum. Dopamine has many functions in the brain, including cognition, learning, behavior, motivation, and reward and punishment. As such, it plays a key role in habit formation. Any activity that links an action to a reward involves dopamine. Following repeated pairings with a reward, the behavior becomes a conditioned response that is now hardwired in the brain. Eventually, environmental cues lead the striatum to automatically elicit behaviors. These behaviors, now "ingrained" in the brain, often sabotage the desire for willful change.

There are steps you can take to change unwanted behaviors ingrained in the brain. First, recognize that there are biological processes that lead to behavioral habits. Next, a change in values, whether through education or environmental cues (relationships, surroundings, incentives, rewards) is of utmost importance.

As you are adopting a new behavior, repetition is critical. The more you repeat a new behavior under similar circumstances, the more likely you will develop the required circuitry in the striatum to make it a habit. For example, exercising at the same time of day helps develop the exercise habit. In due time, when you fail to exercise, the striatum will let you know that that specific time of the day is exercise time.

You must also consciously prepare to eliminate bad habits, such as not eating while watching television. Better yet, exercise while viewing television! Finally, realize that exces-

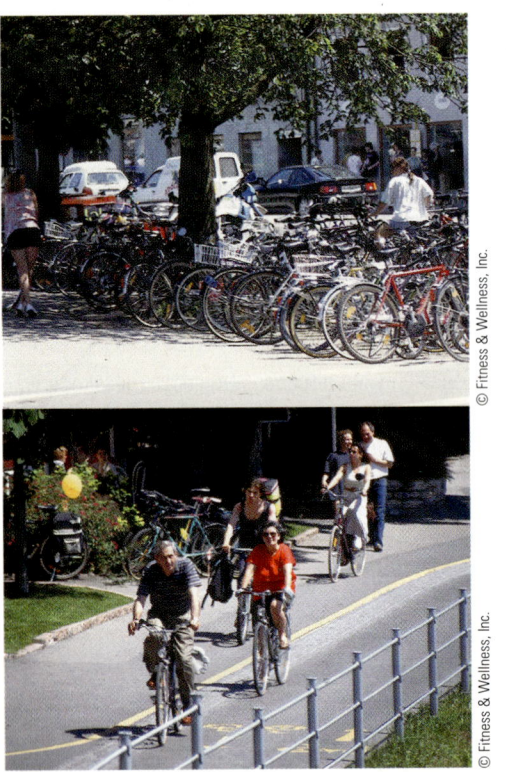

Bicycles are the preferred mode of transportation for local residents in Salzburg, Austria.

sive stress (distress; see Chapter 12) often triggers old bad habits. For example, an argument with a roommate may lead to excessive TV viewing while eating unhealthy calorie-dense foods. You must prepare for an adequate response in these situations. If you made a mistake and did not adequately respond to that specific situation, chalk it up to experience, use it as a learning tool, and next time come back with the proper response.

2.5 Barriers to Change

In spite of the best intentions, people make unhealthy choices daily. The most common reasons are:

1. Lack of core values. Most people recognize the benefits of a healthy lifestyle but are unwilling or unable to trade convenience (sedentary lifestyle, unhealthy eating, substance abuse) for health or other benefits.
   Tip to initiate change. Educate yourself regarding the benefits of a healthy lifestyle and subscribe to several reputable health, fitness, and wellness newsletters (see Chapter 15). The more you read, understand, and then start living a wellness lifestyle, the more your core values will change. At this time you should also break relationships with individuals who are unwilling to change with you.
2. Procrastination. People seem to think that tomorrow, next week, or after the holiday is the best time to start change.
   Tip to initiate change. Ask yourself: Why wait until tomorrow when you can start changing today? Lack of motivation is a key factor in procrastination. (Motivation is discussed later in this chapter.)
3. Preconditioned cultural beliefs. If we accept the idea that we are a product of our environment, our cultural beliefs and our physical surroundings pose significant barriers to change. In Salzburg, Austria, people of both genders and all ages use bicycles as a primary mode of transportation. In the United States, few people other than children ride bicycles.
   Tip to initiate change. Find a like-minded partner. In the pre-Columbian era, people thought the world was flat. Few dared to sail long distances for fear that they would fall off the edge of the Earth. If your health and fitness are at stake, preconditioned cultural beliefs shouldn't keep you from making changes. Finding people who are willing to "sail" with you will help overcome this barrier.
4. Gratification. People prefer instant gratification to long-term benefits. Therefore, they will overeat (instant pleasure) instead of using self-restraint to eat moderately to prevent weight gain (long-term satisfaction). We like tanning (instant gratification) and avoid paying much attention to skin cancer (long-term consequence).
   Tip to initiate change. Think ahead and ask yourself: How did I feel the last time I engaged in this behavior? How did it affect me? Did I really feel good about myself or about the results? In retrospect, was it worth it?
5. Risk complacency. Consequences of unhealthy behaviors often don't manifest themselves until years later. People tell themselves, "If I get heart disease, I'll deal with it then. For now, let me eat, drink, and be merry."
   Tip to initiate change. Ask yourself: How long do I want to live? How do I want to live the rest of my life and what type of health do I want to have? What do I want to be able to do when I am 60, 70, or 80 years old?
6. Complexity. People think the world is too complicated, with too much to think about. If you are living the typical lifestyle, you may feel overwhelmed by everything that seems to be required to lead a healthy lifestyle, such as:
   - getting exercise
   - decreasing intake of saturated and trans fats
   - eating high-fiber meals and cutting total calories
   - controlling use of substances
   - managing stress
   - wearing seat belts
   - practicing safe sex
   - getting annual physicals, including blood tests, Pap smears, and so on
   - fostering spiritual, social, and emotional wellness

   Tip to initiate change. Take it one step at a time. Work on only one or two behaviors at a time so that the task won't seem insurmountable.
7. Indifference and helplessness. A defeatist thought process often takes over, and we may believe that the way we live won't really affect our health, that we have no control over our health, or that our destiny is all in our genes (also see discussion of locus of control, pages 53–54).
   Tip to initiate change. As much as 84 percent of the leading causes of death in the United States are preventable. Realize that only you can take control of your personal health and lifestyle habits and affect the quality of your life. Implementing many of the behavioral modification strategies and programs outlined in this book will get you started on a wellness way of life.
8. Rationalization. Even though people are not practicing healthy behaviors, they often tell themselves that they do get sufficient exercise; that their diet is fine; that they have good, solid relationships; or that they don't smoke/drink/get high enough to affect their health.
   Tip to initiate change. Learn to recognize when you're glossing over or minimizing a problem. You'll need to face the fact that you have a problem before you can commit to change. Your health and your life are at stake. Monitoring lifestyle habits through daily logs and then analyzing the results can help you change self-defeating behaviors.
9. Illusions of invincibility. At times people believe that unhealthy behaviors will not harm them. Young adults often have the attitude that "I can smoke now, and in a

few years I'll quit before it causes any damage." Unfortunately, nicotine is one of the most addictive drugs known to us, so quitting smoking is not an easy task. Health problems may arise before you quit, and the risk of lung cancer lingers for years after you quit. Another example is drinking and driving. The feeling of "I'm in control" or "I can handle it" while under the influence of alcohol is a deadly combination. Others perceive low risk when engaging in negative behaviors with people they like (for example, sex with someone you've recently met and feel attracted to) but perceive themselves at risk just by being in the same classroom with an HIV-infected person.

Tip to initiate change. No one is immune to sickness, disease, and tragedy. The younger you are when you implement a healthy lifestyle, the better are your odds to attain a long and healthy life. Thus, initiating change right now will help you enjoy the best possible quality of life for as long as you live.

When health and appearance begin to deteriorate—usually around middle age—people seek out health care professionals in search of a "magic pill" to reverse and cure the many ills they have accumulated during years of abuse and overindulgence. The sooner we implement a healthy lifestyle program, the greater the health benefits and quality of life that lie ahead.

> **Critical Thinking**
>
> What barriers to exercise do you encounter most frequently?
> • How about barriers that keep you from managing your daily caloric intake?

2.6 Self-Efficacy

At the heart of behavior modification is the concept of **self-efficacy**, or the belief in one's own ability to perform a given task. Self-efficacy exerts a powerful influence on people's behaviors and touches virtually every aspect of their lives. It determines how you feel, think, behave, motivate yourself, make choices, set goals, and pursue courses of action, as well as the effort you put into all of your tasks or activities. It also influences your vulnerability to stress and depression. Furthermore, your confidence in your coping skills determines how resilient you are in the face of adversity. Possessing high self-efficacy enhances wellness in countless ways, including your desire to learn, be productive, be fit, and be healthy.

The knowledge and skills you possess and further develop determine your goals and what you do and choose not to do. Mahatma Gandhi once stated: "If I have the belief that I can do it, I shall surely acquire the capacity to do it even if I may not have it at the beginning." Likewise, Teilhard de Chardin, a French paleontologist and philosopher, stated: "It is our duty as human beings to proceed as though the limits of our capabilities do not exist." With this type of attitude, how can you not strive to be the best that you can possibly be?

As you have already learned in this chapter, the environment has a tremendous effect on our behaviors. We can therefore increase self-efficacy by the type of environment we choose. Experts agree that four different sources affect self-efficacy (discussed next). If you understand these sources and learn from them, you can use them to improve your degree of efficacy. Subsequently, you can apply the concepts for change provided in this chapter to increase confidence in your abilities to master challenging tasks and succeed at implementing change.

Sources of Self-Efficacy The best contributors to self-efficacy are mastery experiences, or personal experiences, that one has had with successes and failures. Successful past performances greatly enhance self-efficacy: "Nothing breeds success like success." Failures, on the other hand, undermine confidence, in particular if they occur before a sense of efficacy is established.

You should structure your activities in ways that they will bring success. Don't set your goals too high or make them too difficult to achieve. Your success at a particular activity increases your confidence in being able to repeat that activity. Once strong self-efficacy is developed through successful mastery experiences, an occasional setback does not have a significant effect on one's beliefs.

Vicarious experiences provided by role models or those one admires also influence personal efficacy. This involves the thought process of your belief that you can also do it. When you observe a peer of similar capabilities master a task, you are more likely to develop a belief that you too can perform that task—"If he can do it, so can I." Here you imitate the model's skill or you follow the same approach demonstrated by your model to complete the task. You may also visualize success. Visual imagery of successful personal performance, that is, watching yourself perform the skill in your mind, also increases personal efficacy.

Although not as effective as past performances and vicarious experiences, verbal persuasion of one's capabilities to perform a task also contributes to self-efficacy. When you are

Feelings of invincibility are a strong barrier to change that can bring about life-threatening consequences.

verbally persuaded that you possess the capabilities, you will be more likely to try the task and believe that you can get it done. The opposite is also true. Negative verbal persuasion has a far greater effect in lowering efficacy than positive messages do to enhance it. If you are verbally persuaded that you lack the skills to master a task, you will tend to avoid the activity and will be more likely to give up without giving yourself a fair chance to succeed.

The least significant source of self-efficacy beliefs are physiological cues that people experience when facing a challenge. These cues in turn affect performance. For example, feeling calm, relaxed, and self-confident enhances self-efficacy. Anxiety, nervousness, perspiration, dryness of the mouth, and a rapid heart rate are cues that may adversely affect performance. You may question your competence to successfully complete the task.

2.7 Motivation and Locus of Control

The explanation given for why some people succeed and others do not is often motivation. **Motivation** is the drive that dictates human behavior. Although motivation comes from within, external factors trigger the inner desire to accomplish a given task. These external factors, then, control behavior.

When studying motivation, understanding locus of control is helpful. People who believe they have control over events in their lives are said to have an internal locus of control. People with an external **locus of control** believe that what happens to them is a result of chance or the environment and is unrelated to their behavior. People with an internal locus of control generally are healthier and have an easier time initiating and adhering to a wellness program than those who perceive that they have no control and think of themselves as powerless and vulnerable. The latter people also are at greater risk for illness. When illness does strike a person, establishing a sense of control is vital to recovery.

Few people have either a completely external or a completely internal locus of control. They fall somewhere along a continuum. The more external one's locus of control is, the greater the challenge to change and adhere to exercise and other healthy lifestyle behaviors. Fortunately, people can develop a more internal locus of control. Understanding that most events in life are not determined genetically or environmentally helps people pursue goals and gain control over their lives. Three impediments, however, can keep people from taking action: lack of competence, confidence, and motivation.[20]

1. Problems of competence. Lacking the skills to perform a task leads to reduced competence. If your friends play basketball regularly but you don't know how to play, you might be inclined not to participate. The solution to this problem of competence is to master the skills you require to participate. Most people are not born with all-inclusive natural abilities, including playing sports.

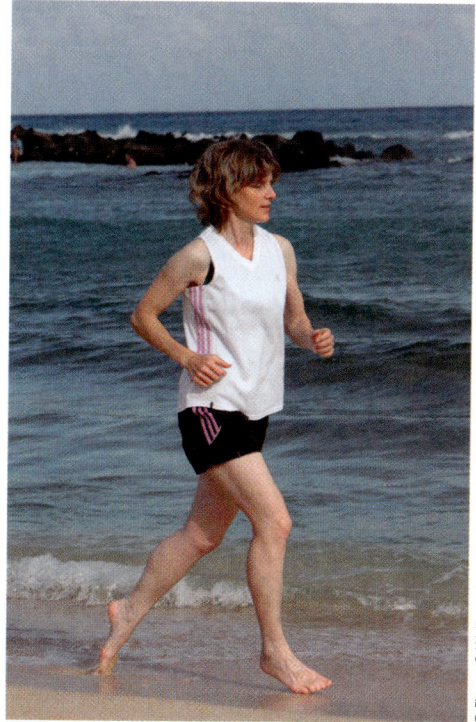

The higher quality of life experienced by people who are physically fit is hard to explain to someone who has never achieved good fitness.

Another alternative is to select an activity in which you are skilled. It may not be basketball, but it well could be aerobics. Don't be afraid to try new activities. Similarly, if your body weight is a problem, you could learn to cook healthy, low-calorie meals. Try different recipes until you find foods that you like.

2. Problems of confidence. Problems with confidence arise when you have the skill but don't believe you can get it done. Fear and feelings of inadequacy often interfere with the ability to perform the task. You shouldn't talk yourself out of something until you have given it a fair try. If you have the skills, the sky is the limit. Initially, try to visualize yourself doing the task and getting it done. Repeat this several times, then actually try it. You will surprise yourself.

Sometimes, lack of confidence arises when the task seems insurmountable. In these situations, dividing a goal into smaller, more realistic objectives helps to accomplish the task. You might know how to swim but may need to train for several weeks to swim a continuous mile. Set up your training program so that you swim a little farther each day until

> **Self-efficacy** One's belief in the ability to perform a given task.
>
> **Motivation** The desire and will to do something.
>
> **Locus of control** A concept examining the extent to which a person believes he or she can influence the external environment.

you are able to swim the entire mile. If you don't meet your objective on a given day, try it again; reevaluate; cut back a little; and, most important, don't give up.

3. Problems of motivation. With problems of motivation, both the competence and the confidence are there, but individuals are unwilling to change because the reasons to change are not important to them. For example, people begin contemplating a smoking-cessation program only when the reasons for quitting outweigh the reasons for smoking. The primary causes of unwillingness to change are lack of knowledge and lack of goals. Knowledge often determines goals, and goals determine motivation. How badly you want something dictates how hard you'll work at it.

Many people are unaware of the magnitude of benefits of a wellness program. When it comes to a healthy lifestyle, however, you may not get a second chance. A stroke, a heart attack, or cancer can have irreparable or fatal consequences. Greater understanding of what leads to disease can help initiate change. Joy, however, is a greater motivator than fear. Even fear of dying often doesn't instigate change.

Two years following coronary bypass surgery (heart disease), most patients' denial returns, and surveys show that they have not done much to alter their unhealthy lifestyle. The motivating factor for the few who do change is the "joy of living." Rather than dwelling on the "fear of dying" and causing patients to live in emotional pain, point out the fact that change will help them feel better. They will be able to enhance their quality of life by carrying out activities of daily living without concern for a heart attack, go for a walk without chest pain, play with children, and even resume an intimate relationship.

Also, feeling physically fit is difficult to explain to people unless they have experienced it themselves. Feelings of fitness, self-esteem, confidence, health, and better quality of life cannot be conveyed to someone who is constrained by sedentary living. In a way, wellness is like reaching the top of a mountain. The quiet, the clean air, the lush vegetation, the flowing water in the river, the wildlife, and the majestic valley below are difficult to explain to someone who has spent a lifetime within city limits.

2.8 Changing Behavior

The first step in addressing behavioral change is to recognize that you indeed have a problem. The five general categories of behaviors addressed in the process of willful change are:

1. Stopping a negative behavior
2. Preventing relapse to a negative behavior
3. Developing a positive behavior
4. Strengthening a positive behavior
5. Maintaining a positive behavior

Most people do not change all at once. Thus, psychotherapy has been used successfully to help people change their behavior. But most people do not seek professional help. They usually attempt to change by themselves with limited or no knowledge of how to achieve change. In essence, the process of change moves along a continuum from being not willing to change to recognizing the need for change to taking action and implementing change.

The simplest model of change is the two-stage model of unhealthy behavior and healthy behavior. This model states that either you do it or you don't. Most people who use this model attempt self-change but end up asking themselves why they're unsuccessful. They just can't do it (exercise, perhaps, or quit smoking). Their intent to change may be good, but to accomplish it, they need knowledge about how to achieve change.

Behavior Change Theories For most people, changing chronic/unhealthy behaviors to stable/healthy behaviors is challenging. The "do it or don't do it" approach seldom works when attempting to implement lifestyle changes. Thus, several theories or models have been developed over the years. Among the most accepted are learning theories, the problem-solving model, social cognitive theory, the relapse prevention model, humanistic theory of change, and the transtheoretical model.

Learning Theories
Learning theories maintain that most behaviors are learned and maintained under complex schedules of reinforcement and anticipated outcomes. The process involved in learning a new behavior requires modifying many small behaviors that shape the new pattern behavior. For example, a previously inactive individual who wishes to accumulate 10,000 steps per day may have to gradually increase the number of steps daily, park farther away from the office and stores, decrease television and Internet use, take stairs instead of elevators and escalators, and avoid the car and telephone when running errands that are only short distances away. The outcomes are better health and body weight management and feelings of well-being.

Problem-Solving Model
The **problem-solving model** proposes that many behaviors are the result of making decisions as we seek to change the problem behavior. The process of change requires conscious attention, the setting of goals, and a design for a specific plan of action. For instance, to quit smoking cigarettes, one has to understand the reasons for smoking, know under what conditions each cigarette is smoked, decide that one will quit, select a date to do so, and then draw up a plan of action to reach the goal. (A complete smoking-cessation program is outlined in Chapter 13.)

Social Cognitive Theory
In **social cognitive theory**, behavior change is influenced by the environment, self-efficacy, and characteristics of the behavior itself. You can increase self-efficacy by educating yourself about the behavior, developing the skills to master the behavior, performing smaller mastery experiences successfully, and receiving verbal reinforcement and vicarious expe-

riences. If you desire to lose weight, for example, you need to learn the principles of proper weight management, associate with people who are also losing weight or who have lost weight, eat less, shop and cook wisely, be more active, set small weight-loss goals of one to two pounds per week, praise yourself for your accomplishments, and visualize losing the weight as others you admire have done.

Relapse Prevention Model

In the **relapse prevention model**, people are taught to anticipate high-risk situations and develop action plans to prevent **lapses** and **relapses**. Examples of factors that disrupt behavior change include negative physiological or psychological states (stress, illness), social pressure, lack of support, limited coping skills, change in work conditions, and lack of motivation. For example, if the weather turns bad for your evening walk, you can choose to walk around an indoor track (or at the mall), do water aerobics, swim, or play racquetball.

Humanistic Theory of Change

Humanists believe in the basic goodness of humanity and respect for mankind. At the core of the theory is the belief that people are unique in the development of personal goals—with the ultimate goal being self-actualization. Self-actualized people are independent, are creative, set their own goals, and accept themselves. Humanists also propose that people are motivated by a hierarchy of needs that include approval, recognition, achievement, and the fulfillment of each person's potential. In this hierarchy, each need requires fulfillment before the next need becomes relevant. The present is the most important time for any person rather than the past or the future. For instance, a person will not exercise unless he or she has had something to eat within a reasonable amount of time. Similarly, a person who uses cigarette smoking to maintain weight will not give up smoking unless proper weight management is accomplished by other means (healthy eating habits and increased physical activity). The challenge, then, is to identify basic needs at the core of the hierarchy (acceptance, independence, recognition) before other healthy behaviors (exercise, stress management, altruism) are considered.

Transtheoretical Model

The **transtheoretical model**, developed by psychologists James Prochaska, John Norcross, and Carlo DiClemente, is based on the theory that change is a gradual process that involves several stages.[21] The model is used most frequently to change health-related behaviors such as physical inactivity, smoking, poor nutrition, weight problems, stress, and alcohol abuse.

An individual goes through five stages in the process of willful change. The stages describe underlying processes that people go through to change problem behaviors and replace them with healthy behaviors. A sixth stage (termination/adoption) was subsequently added to this model. The six stages of change are precontemplation, contemplation, preparation, action, maintenance, and termination/adoption (see Figure 2.2).

After years of study, researchers indicate that applying specific behavioral-change processes during each stage of the model increases the success rate for change. (The specific processes for each stage are shown in Table 2.1.) Understanding each stage of this model will help you determine where you are in relation to your personal healthy lifestyle behaviors. It also will help you identify processes to make successful changes. The discussion in the remainder of the chapter focuses on the transtheoretical model, with the other models integrated as applicable with each stage of change.

1. **Precontemplation.** Individuals in the **precontemplation stage** are not considering change or do not want to change a given behavior. They typically deny having a problem and have no intention of changing in the immediate future. These people are usually unaware or underaware of the problem. Other people around them, including family, friends, health care practitioners, and coworkers, however, identify the problem clearly. Precontemplators do not care about the problem behavior and may even avoid information and materials that address the issue. They tend to avoid free screenings and workshops that might help identify and change the problem, even if they receive financial compensation for at-

> **Learning theories** Behavioral modification perspective stating that most behaviors are learned and maintained under complex schedules of reinforcement and anticipated outcomes.
>
> **Problem-solving model** Behavioral modification model proposing that many behaviors are the result of making decisions as the individual seeks to solve the problem behavior.
>
> **Social cognitive theory** Behavioral modification model holding that behavior change is influenced by the environment, self-efficacy, and characteristics of the behavior itself.
>
> **Relapse prevention model** Behavioral modification model based on the principle that high-risk situations can be anticipated through the development of strategies to prevent lapses and relapses.
>
> **Lapse** (v.) To slip or fall back temporarily into unhealthy behavior(s); (n.) short-term failure to maintain healthy behaviors.
>
> **Relapse** (v.) To slip or fall back into unhealthy behavior(s) over a longer time; (n.) longer-term failure to maintain healthy behaviors.
>
> **Transtheoretical model** Behavioral modification model proposing that change is accomplished through a series of progressive stages in keeping with a person's readiness to change.
>
> **Precontemplation stage** Stage of change in the transtheoretical model in which an individual is unwilling to change behavior.

Figure 2.2 Stages of change model.

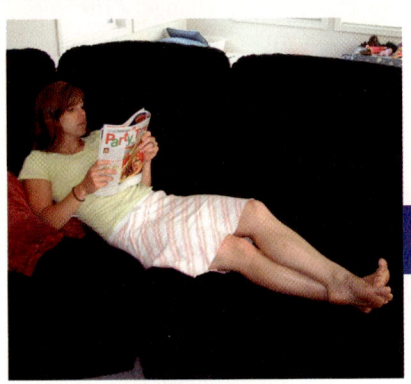
Precontemplation
Do not wish to change

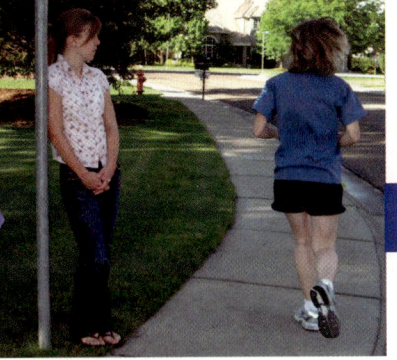
Contemplation
Contemplating change over next 6 months

Preparation
Looking to change in the next month

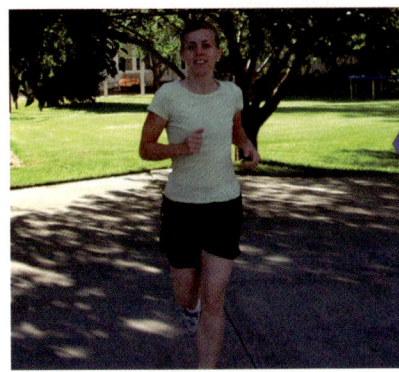
Termination/Adoption
Change has been maintained for more than 5 years

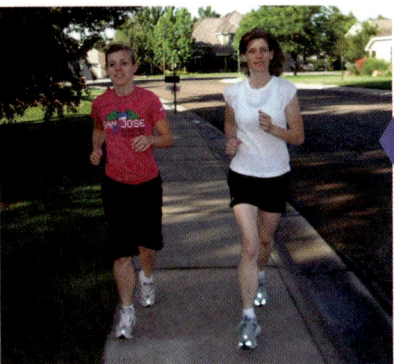
Maintenance
Maintaining change for 5 years

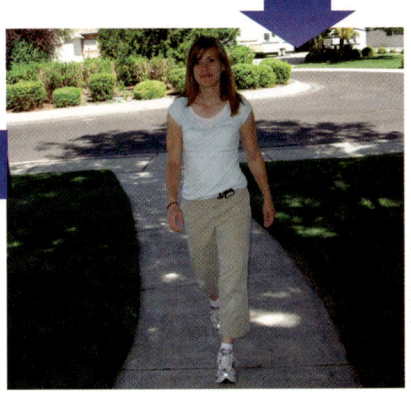
Action
Implementing change for 6 months

Table 2.1 Applicable Processes of Change During Each Stage of Change

Precontemplation	Contemplation	Preparation	Action	Maintenance	Termination/Adoption
Consciousness-raising	Consciousness-raising	Consciousness-raising			
Social liberation	Social liberation	Social liberation	Social liberation		
	Self-analysis	Self-analysis			
	Emotional arousal	Emotional arousal			
	Positive outlook	Positive outlook	Positive outlook		
		Commitment	Commitment	Commitment	Commitment
		Behavior analysis	Behavior analysis		
		Goal setting	Goal setting	Goal setting	
		Self-reevaluation	Self-reevaluation	Self-reevaluation	
			Countering	Countering	
			Monitoring	Monitoring	Monitoring
			Environment control	Environment control	Environment control
			Helping relationships	Helping relationships	Helping relationships
			Rewards	Rewards	Rewards

SOURCE: Adapted from J. O. Prochaska, J. C. Norcross, and C. C. DiClemente, *Changing for Good* (New York: William Morrow, 1994); and W. W. K. Hoeger and S. A. Hoeger, *Principles and Labs for Fitness & Wellness* (Belmont, CA: Wadsworth/Thomson Learning, 2004).

tending. Often they actively resist change and seem resigned to accepting the unhealthy behavior as their "fate."

Precontemplators are the most difficult people to inspire toward behavioral change. Many think that change isn't even a possibility. At this stage, knowledge is power. Educating them about the problem behavior is critical to help them start contemplating the process of change. The challenge is to find ways to help them realize that they are ultimately responsible for the consequences of their behavior. Typically, they initiate change only when their values change or people they respect or job requirements pressure them to do so.

2. **Contemplation.** In the **contemplation stage**, individuals acknowledge that they have a problem and begin to think seriously about overcoming it. Although they are not quite ready for change, they are weighing the pros and cons of changing. Core values are starting to change. Even though they may remain in this stage for years, in their minds they are planning to take some action within the next six months. Education and peer support remain valuable during this stage. In Activity 2.2, you will be able to list under the processes of change self-defeating and constructive habits (pros and cons) that work against and for you when attempting to accomplish that specific behavior.

3. **Preparation.** In the **preparation stage,** individuals are seriously considering change and planning to change a behavior within the next month. They are taking initial steps for change and may even try the new behavior for a short while, such as stopping smoking for a day or exercising a few times during the month. During this stage, people define a general goal for behavioral change (for example, to quit smoking by the last day of the month) and write specific actions (objectives or strategies) to accomplish this goal. The discussion on goal setting later in this chapter will help you write SMART goals and specific actions to reach your goal. Continued peer and environmental support is helpful during the preparation stage.

A key concept to keep in mind during the preparation stage is that in addition to being prepared to address the behavioral change or goal you are attempting to reach, you must prepare to address the specific actions (supportive behaviors) required to reach that goal (Figure 2.3). For example, you may be willing to give weight loss a try, but are you prepared to start eating less, eating out less often, eating less calorie-dense foods, shopping and cooking wisely, exercising more, watching television less, and becoming much more active? Achieving goals generally requires changing these supportive behaviors, and you must be prepared to do so.

4. **Action.** The **action stage** requires the greatest commitment of time and energy. Here, the individual is actively doing things to change or modify the problem behavior or to adopt a new, healthy behavior. The action stage requires that the person follow the specific guidelines set

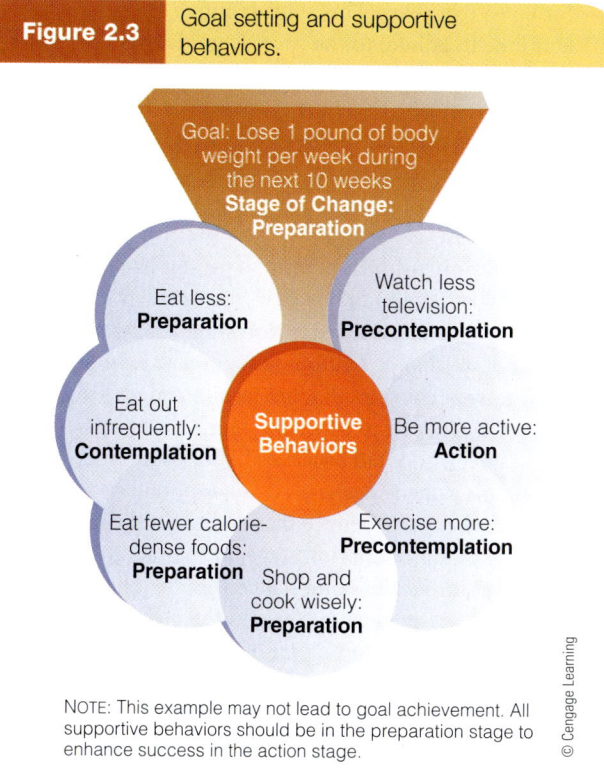

Figure 2.3 Goal setting and supportive behaviors.

NOTE: This example may not lead to goal achievement. All supportive behaviors should be in the preparation stage to enhance success in the action stage.

forth for that behavior. For example, a person has actually stopped smoking completely, is exercising aerobically three times a week according to exercise prescription guidelines, or is maintaining a healthy diet.

Relapse is common during this stage, and the individual may regress to a previous stage. If unsuccessful, a person should reevaluate his or her readiness to change supportive behaviors as required to reach the overall goal. Problem solving that includes identifying barriers to change and specific actions (strategies) to overcome supportive behaviors is useful during relapse. Once people are able to maintain the action stage for six consecutive months, they move into the maintenance stage.

5. **Maintenance.** During the **maintenance stage,** the person continues the new behavior

> **Contemplation stage** Stage of change in the transtheoretical model in which the individual is considering changing behavior within the next six months.
>
> **Preparation stage** Stage of change in the transtheoretical model in which the individual is getting ready to make a change within the next month.
>
> **Action stage** Stage of change in the transtheoretical model in which the individual is actively changing a negative behavior or adopting a new, healthy behavior.
>
> **Maintenance stage** Stage of change in the transtheoretical model in which the individual maintains behavioral change for up to five years.

for up to five years. This stage requires the person to continue to adhere to the specific guidelines that govern the behavior (such as complete smoking cessation, exercising aerobically three times a week, or practicing proper stress management techniques). At this time, the person works to reinforce the gains made through the various stages of change and strives to prevent lapses and relapses.

6. **Termination/Adoption.** Once a person has maintained a behavior more than five years, he or she is said to be in the **termination or adoption stage** and exits from the cycle of change without fear of relapse. In the case of negative behaviors that are terminated, the stage of change is referred to as termination. If a positive behavior has been adopted successfully for more than five years, this stage is designated as adoption.

Many experts believe that once an individual enters the termination/adoption stage, former addictions, problems, or lack of compliance with healthy behaviors no longer presents an obstacle in the quest for wellness. The change has become part of one's lifestyle. This phase is the ultimate goal for all people searching for a healthier lifestyle.

For addictive behaviors such as alcoholism and hard drug use, however, some health care practitioners believe that the individual never enters the termination stage. Chemical dependency is so strong that most former alcoholics and hard-drug users must make a lifetime effort to prevent relapse. Similarly, some behavioral scientists suggest that the adoption stage might not be applicable to health behaviors such as exercise and weight control because the likelihood of relapse is always high.

Use the guidelines provided in Activity 2.2 to determine where you stand in respect to behaviors you want to change or new ones you wish to adopt. As you follow the guidelines, you will realize that you might be at different stages for different behaviors. For instance, you might be in the preparation stage for aerobic exercise and smoking cessation, in the action stage for strength training, but only in the contemplation stage for a healthy diet. Realizing where you are with respect to different behaviors will help you design a better action plan for a healthy lifestyle.

Relapse

After the precontemplation stage, relapse may occur at any level of the model. Even individuals in the maintenance and termination/adoption stages may regress to any of the first three stages of the model (Figure 2.4). Relapse, however, does not mean failure. Failure comes only to those who give up and don't use prior experiences as a building block for future success. The chances of moving back up to a higher stage of the model are far better for someone who has previously made it into one of those stages.

2.9 The Process of Change

Using the same plan for everyone who wishes to change a behavior will not work. With exercise, for instance, we provide different prescriptions to people of varying fitness levels (Chapter 6). The same prescription would not provide optimal results for a person who has been inactive for 20 years, compared with one who already walks regularly 3 times each week. This principle also holds true for individuals who are attempting to change their behaviors.

Timing is also important in the process of willful change. People respond more effectively to selected **processes of change** in keeping with the stage of change they have reached at any given time. Thus, applying appropriate processes at each stage of change enhances the likelihood of changing behavior permanently. The following description of 14 of the most common processes of change will help you develop a personal plan for change. The respective stages of change in which each process works best are summarized in Table 2.1.

Consciousness-Raising The first step in a **behavior modification** program is consciousness-raising. This step involves obtaining information about the problem so that you can make a better decision about the problem behavior. For example, the problem could be physical inactivity. Learning about the benefits of exercise or the difference in benefits between physical activity and exercise (Chapter 1) can help you decide the type of fitness program (health or high fitness) that you want to pursue. Possibly, you don't even know that a certain behavior is a problem, such as being unaware of saturated and total fat content in many fast-food items. Consciousness-raising may continue from the precontemplation stage through the preparation stage.

Social Liberation Social liberation stresses external alternatives that make you aware of problem behaviors and make you begin to contemplate change. Examples of social liberation include pedestrian-only traffic areas, nonsmoking areas, health-oriented cafeterias and restaurants, advocacy groups, civic organizations, policy interventions, and self-help groups. Social liberation often provides opportunities to

Figure 2.4 Model of progression and relapse.

get involved, stir up emotions, and enhance self-esteem—helping you gain confidence in your ability to change.

Self-Analysis The next process in modifying behavior is developing a decisive desire to do so, called self-analysis. If you have no interest in changing a behavior, you won't do it. You will remain a precontemplator or a contemplator. A person who has no intention of quitting smoking will not quit, regardless of what anyone may say or how strong the evidence in favor of quitting may be. In your self-analysis, you may want to prepare a list of reasons for continuing or discontinuing the behavior. When the reasons for changing outweigh the reasons for not changing, you are ready for the next stage—either the contemplation stage or the preparation stage.

Emotional Arousal In emotional arousal, a person experiences and expresses feelings about the problem and its solutions. Also referred to as "dramatic release," this process often involves deep emotional experiences. Watching a loved one die from lung cancer caused by cigarette smoking may be all that is needed to make a person quit smoking. As in other examples, emotional arousal might be prompted by a dramatization of the consequences of drug use and abuse, a film about a person undergoing open-heart surgery, or a book illustrating damage to body systems as a result of unhealthy behaviors.

Positive Outlook Having a positive outlook means taking an optimistic approach from the beginning and believing in yourself. Following the guidelines in this chapter will help you design a plan so that you can work toward change and remain enthused about your progress. Also, you may become motivated by looking at the outcome—how much healthier you will be, how much better you will look, or how far you will be able to jog.

Commitment Upon making a decision to change, you accept the responsibility to change and believe in your ability to do so. During the commitment process, you engage in preparation and may draw up a specific plan of action. Write down your goals and, preferably, share them with others. In essence, you are signing a behavioral contract for change. You will be more likely to adhere to your program if others know you are committed to change.

Behavior Analysis How you determine the frequency, circumstances, and consequences of the behavior to be altered or implemented is known as behavior analysis. If the desired outcome is to consume less trans and saturated fats, you first must find out what foods in your diet are high in these fats, when you eat them, and when you don't eat them—all part of the preparation stage. Knowing when you don't eat them points to circumstances under which you exert control over your diet, which will help as you set goals.

Goals Goals motivate change in behavior. The stronger the goal or desire, the more motivated you'll be either to change unwanted behaviors or to implement new, healthy behaviors. The discussion on goal setting (beginning on page 61) will help you write goals and prepare an action plan to achieve them. This will aid with behavior modification.

Self-Reevaluation During the process of self-reevaluation, individuals analyze their feelings about a problem behavior. The pros and cons or advantages and disadvantages of a certain behavior can be reevaluated at this time. For example, you may decide that strength training will help you get stronger and tone up, but implementing this change will require you to stop watching an hour of TV three times per week. If you presently have a weight problem and are unable to lift certain objects around the house, you may feel good about weight loss and enhanced physical capacity as a result of a strength-training program. You also might visualize what it would be like if you were successful at changing.

Countering The process whereby you substitute healthy behaviors for a problem behavior, known as countering, is a critical part of the action and maintenance stages of changing behaviors. You need to replace unhealthy behaviors with new, healthy ones. You can use exercise to combat sedentary living, smoking, stress, or overeating. Or you may use exercise, diet, yard work, volunteer work, or reading to prevent overeating and achieve recommended body weight.

Monitoring During the action and maintenance stages, continuous behavior monitoring increases awareness of the desired outcome. Sometimes this process of monitoring is sufficient in itself to cause change. For example, keeping track of daily food intake reveals sources of excessive and/or unhealthy fats in the diet. This can help you gradually cut down and eliminate unhealthy, fatty foods. If the goal is to increase daily intake of fruit and vegetables, keeping track of the number of servings consumed each day raises awareness and may help increase intake.

Environment Control In environment control, the person restructures the physical surroundings to avoid problem behaviors and decrease temptations. If you don't buy alcohol, you can't drink any. If you shop on a full stomach, you can reduce impulse buying of junk food.

Similarly, you can create an environment in which exceptions become the norm,

> **Termination/adoption stage** Stage of change in the transtheoretical model in which the individual has eliminated an undesirable behavior or maintained a positive behavior for more than five years.
>
> **Processes of change** Actions that help you achieve change in behavior.
>
> **Behavior modification** The process of permanently changing negative behaviors to positive behaviors that will lead to better health and well-being.

Countering: Substituting healthy behaviors for problem behaviors facilitates change.

and then the norm can flourish. Instead of bringing home cookies for snacks, bring fruit. Place notes to yourself on the refrigerator and pantry to avoid unnecessary snacking. Put baby carrots or sugarless gum where you used to put cigarettes. Post notes around the house to remind you of your exercise time. Leave exercise shoes and clothing by the door so they are visible as you walk into your home. Put an electric timer on the TV so it will shut off automatically at 7:00 p.m.

All of these tactics will be helpful throughout the action, maintenance, and termination/adoption stages.

Helping Relationships Surrounding yourself with people who will work toward a common goal with you or those who care about you and will encourage you along the way—helping relationships—will be supportive during the action, maintenance, and termination/adoption stages.

Attempting to quit smoking, for instance, is easier when a person is around others who are trying to quit as well. The person also could get help from friends who have quit smoking already. Losing weight is difficult if meal planning and cooking are shared with roommates who enjoy foods that are high in fat and sugar. This situation can be even worse if a roommate also has a weight problem but does not wish to lose weight.

Peer support is a strong incentive for behavioral change. Thus, the individual should avoid people who will not be supportive and associate with those who will. Friends who have no desire to quit smoking or to lose weight, or whatever behavior a person is trying to change, may tempt one to smoke or overeat and encourage relapse into unwanted behaviors.

In some cases, people who have achieved the same goal already may not be supportive either. For instance, someone may say, "I can do six consecutive miles." Your response should be, "I'm proud that I can jog three consecutive miles."

Rewards People tend to repeat behaviors that are rewarded and to disregard those that are not rewarded or are punished. Rewarding oneself or being rewarded by others is a powerful tool during the process of change in all stages. If you have successfully cut down your caloric intake during the week, reward yourself by going to a movie or buying a new

Behavior Modification Planning

Steps for Successful Behavior Modification

1. Acknowledge that you have a problem.
2. Describe the behavior to change (increase physical activity, stop overeating, quit smoking).
3. List advantages and disadvantages of changing the specified behavior.
4. Decide positively that you will change.
5. Identify your stage of change.
6. Set a realistic goal (SMART goal), completion date, and sign a behavioral contract.
7. Define your behavioral change plan: List processes of change, techniques of change, and actions that will help you reach your goal.
8. Implement the behavior change plan.
9. Monitor your progress toward the desired goal.
10. Periodically evaluate and reassess your goal.
11. Reward yourself when you achieve your goal.
12. Maintain the successful change for good.

Try It

In your Online Journal or class notebook, record your answers to the following questions: Have you consciously attempted to incorporate a healthy behavior into or eliminate a negative behavior from your lifestyle? If so, what steps did you follow, and what helped you achieve your goal?

Rewarding oneself when a goal is achieved, such as scheduling a weekend getaway, is a powerful tool during the process of change.

pair of shoes. Do not reinforce yourself with destructive behaviors such as eating a high-fat/calorie-dense dinner. If you fail to change a desired behavior (or to implement a new one), you may want to put off buying those new shoes you had planned for that week. When a positive behavior becomes habitual, give yourself an even better reward. Treat yourself to a weekend away from home or buy a new bicycle.

> **Critical Thinking**
>
> Your friend John is a 20-year-old student who is not physically active. Exercise has never been a part of his life, and it has not been a priority in his family. He has decided to start a jogging and strength-training course in two weeks. • Can you identify his current stage of change and list processes and techniques of change that will help him maintain a regular exercise behavior?

2.10 Techniques of Change

Not to be confused with the processes of change, you can apply any number of **techniques of change** within each process to help you through it (Table 2.2). For example, following dinner, people with a weight problem often can't resist continuous snacking during the rest of the evening until it is time to retire for the night. In the process of countering, for example, you can use various techniques to avoid unnecessary snacking. Examples include going for a walk, flossing and brushing your teeth immediately after dinner, going for a drive, playing the piano, going to a show, or going to bed earlier.

As you develop a behavior modification plan, you need to identify specific techniques that may work for you within each process of change. A list of techniques for each process is provided in Table 2.2. This is only a sample list; dozens of other techniques could be used as well. For example, a discussion of behavior modification and adhering to a weight management program starts on page 147; getting started and adhering to a lifetime exercise program is presented on page 305; stress management techniques are provided in Chapter 12; and tips to help stop smoking on pages 455–465. Some of these techniques also can be used with more than one process. Visualization, for example, is helpful in emotional arousal and self-reevaluation.

Now that you are familiar with the stages of change in the process of behavior modification, use Figure 2.5 and Activity 2.2 to identify two problem behaviors in your life. In this activity, you will be asked to determine your stage of change for two behaviors according to six standard statements. Based on your selection, determine the stage of change classification according to the ratings provided in Table 2.3. Next, develop a behavior modification plan according to the processes and techniques for change that you have learned in this chapter. (Similar exercises to identify stages of change for other fitness and wellness behaviors are provided in activities for subsequent chapters.)

2.11 Goal Setting and Evaluation

To initiate change, **goals** are essential, as goals motivate behavioral change. Whatever you decide to accomplish, setting goals will provide the road map to help make your dreams a reality. Setting goals, however, is not as simple as it looks. Setting goals is more than just deciding what you want to do. A vague statement such as "I will lose weight" is not sufficient to help you achieve this goal.

SMART Goals Only a well-conceived action plan will help you attain goals. Determining what you want to accomplish is the starting point, but to reach your goal you need to write **SMART goals** (Figure 2.6). These goals are **S**pecific, **M**easurable, **A**cceptable, **R**ealistic, and **T**ime specific. In Activity 2.3, you have an opportunity to set SMART goals for two behaviors that you wish to change or adopt.

1. **Specific.** When writing goals, state exactly and in a positive manner what you would like to accomplish. For example, if you are overweight at 150 pounds and at 27 percent body fat, to simply state, "I will lose weight" is not a specific goal. Instead, rewrite your goal to state, "I will reduce my body fat to 20 percent (137 pounds) in 12 weeks."
Write down your goals. An unwritten goal is simply a wish. A writ-

> **Techniques of change** Methods or procedures used during each process of change.
>
> **Goals** The ultimate aims toward which effort is directed.
>
> **SMART (goals)** An acronym used in reference to specific, measurable, attainable, realistic, and time-specific goals.

Table 2.2 Sample Techniques for Use with Process of Change

Process	Techniques
Consciousness-Raising	Become aware that there is a problem, read educational materials about the problem behavior or about people who have overcome this same problem, find out about the benefits of changing the behavior, watch an instructional program on television, visit a therapist, talk and listen to others, ask questions, take a class.
Social Liberation	Seek out advocacy groups (Overeaters Anonymous, Alcoholics Anonymous), join a health club, buy a bike, join a neighborhood walking group, work in nonsmoking areas.
Self-Analysis	Question yourself on the problem behavior, express your feelings about it, become aware that there is a problem, analyze your values, list advantages and disadvantages of continuing (smoking) or not implementing a behavior (exercise), take a fitness test, do a nutrient analysis.
Emotional Arousal	Practice mental imagery of yourself going through the process of change, visualize yourself overcoming the problem behavior, do some role-playing in overcoming the behavior or practicing a new one, watch dramatizations (a movie) of the consequences or benefits of your actions, visit an auto salvage yard or a drug rehabilitation center.
Positive Outlook	Believe in yourself, know that you are capable, know that you are special, draw from previous personal successes.
Commitment	Just do it, set New Year's resolutions, sign a behavioral contract, set start and completion dates, tell others about your goals, work on your action plan.
Behavior Analysis	Prepare logs of circumstances that trigger or prevent a given behavior and look for patterns that prompt the behavior or cause you to relapse.
Goal Setting	Write goals and actions; design a specific action plan.
Self-Reevaluation	Determine accomplishments and evaluate progress, rewrite goals and actions, list pros and cons, weigh sacrifices (can't eat out with others) versus benefits (weight loss), visualize continued change, think before you act, learn from mistakes, and prepare new action plans accordingly.
Countering	Seek out alternatives: stay busy, walk (don't drive), read a book (instead of snacking), attend alcohol-free social events, carry your own groceries, mow your yard, dance (don't eat), go to a movie (instead of smoking), practice stress management.
Monitoring	Use exercise logs (days exercised, sets and resistance used in strength training), keep journals, conduct nutrient analyses, count grams of fat, count number of consecutive days without smoking, list days and type of relaxation technique(s) used.
Environment Control	Rearrange your home (no TVs, ashtrays, large-sized cups), get rid of unhealthy items (cigarettes, junk food, alcohol), then avoid unhealthy places (bars, happy hour), avoid relationships that encourage problem behaviors, use reminders to control problem behaviors or encourage positive ones (post notes indicating "don't snack after dinner" or "lift weights at 8:00 p.m."). Frequent healthy environments (a clean park, a health club, restaurants with low-fat/low-calorie/nutrient-dense menus, friends with goals similar to yours).
Helping Relationships	Associate with people who have and want to overcome the same problem, form or join self-help groups, join community programs specifically designed to deal with your problem.
Rewards	Go to a movie, buy a new outfit or shoes, buy a new bike, go on a weekend getaway, reassess your fitness level, use positive self-talk ("good job," "that felt good," "I did it," "I knew I'd make it," "I'm good at this").

© Cengage Learning

Table 2.3 Stage of Change Classification

Selected Statements (see Figure 2.5 and Activity 2.2)	Classification
1	Precontemplation
2	Contemplation
3	Preparation
4	Action
5	Maintenance
6	Termination/Adoption

© Cengage Learning

ten goal, in essence, becomes a contract with yourself. Show this goal to a friend or an instructor, and have him or her witness the contract you have made with yourself by signing alongside your signature.

Once you have identified and written down a specific goal, write the specific **actions** that will help you reach that goal. These actions are necessary steps. For example, a goal might be to achieve recommended body weight. Several specific actions could be to:

a. lose an average of one pound (or one fat percentage point) per week
b. monitor body weight before breakfast every morning
c. assess body composition at three-week intervals
d. limit fat intake to less than 25 percent of total daily caloric intake
e. eliminate all pastries from the diet during this time
f. walk/jog in the proper target zone for 60 minutes, 6 times a week

2. **Measurable.** Whenever possible, goals and actions should be measurable. For example, "I will lose weight"

Figure 2.5 Stage of change and behavior modification outline.

Please indicate which response most accurately describes your current [_____] behavior (in the blank space identify the behavior: smoking, physical activity, stress, nutrition, weight control). Next, select the statement below (select only one) that best represents your current behavior pattern. To select the most appropriate statement, fill in the blank for one of the first three statements if your current behavior is a problem behavior. (For example, you may say, "I currently smoke, and I do *not* intend to change in the foreseeable future," or "I currently *do not exercise,* but I am contemplating changing in the next 6 months.") If you have already started to make changes, fill in the blank in one of the last three statements. (In this case, you may say: "I currently *eat a low-fat diet,* but I have done so only within the past 6 months," or "I currently *practice adequate stress management techniques,* and I have done so for more than 6 months.") As you can see, you may use this form to identify your stage of change for any type of health-related behavior.

1. I currently [_____], and I do not intend to change in the foreseeable future.
2. I currently [_____], but I am contemplating changing in the next 6 months.
3. I currently [_____] regularly, but I intend to change in the next month.
4. I currently [_____], but I have done so only within the past 6 months.
5. I currently [_____], and I have done so for more than 6 months.
6. I currently [_____], and I have done so for more than 5 years.

---

is not measurable, but "to reduce body fat to 20 percent" is measurable. Also note that all of the sample-specific actions (a) through (f) for "Specific" in the previous point are measurable. For instance, you can figure out easily whether you are losing a pound or a percentage point per week; you can conduct a nutrient analysis to assess your average fat intake; or you can monitor your weekly exercise sessions to make sure you are meeting this specific objective.

3. **Acceptable.** Goals that you set for yourself are more motivational than goals that someone else sets for you. These goals will motivate and challenge you and should be consistent with your other goals. As you set an acceptable goal, ask yourself: Do I have the time, commitment, and necessary skills to accomplish this goal? If not, you need to restate your goal so that it is acceptable to you.

When successful completion of a goal involves others, such as an athletic team or an organization, an acceptable goal must be compatible with those of the other people involved. If a team's practice schedule is set Monday through Friday from 4:00 to 6:00 p.m., it is unacceptable for you to train only three times per week or at a different time of the day.

Acceptable goals also embrace positive thoughts. Visualize and believe in your success. As difficult as some tasks may seem, where there's a will, there's a way. A plan of action, prepared according to the guidelines in this chapter, will help you achieve your goals.

4. **Realistic.** Goals should be within reach. On the one hand, if you currently weigh 190 pounds and your target weight is 140 pounds, setting a goal to lose 50 pounds in a month would be unsound, if not impossible. Such a goal does not allow you to implement adequate behavior modification techniques or ensure weight maintenance at the target weight. Unattainable goals only set you up for failure, discouragement, and loss of interest. On the other hand, do not write goals that are too easy to achieve and do not challenge you. If a goal is too easy, you may lose interest and stop working toward it.

You can write both short-term and long-term goals. If the long-term goal is to attain recommended body weight and you are 53 pounds overweight, you might set

Figure 2.6 SMART goals.

Actions (for behavioral change) Steps required to reach a goal.

Activity 2.2: Behavior Modification Plan

Name _____ Date _____
Course _____ Section _____ Gender _____ Age _____

I. Stages of Change Instructions

Please indicate which response most accurately describes your current _____ and _____ behaviors (in the blank spaces identify the behaviors: smoking, physical activity, stress, nutrition, weight control). Next, select the statement below (select only one) that best represents your current behavior pattern for each. To select the most appropriate statement, fill in the blank for one of the first three statements if your current behavior is a problem behavior. For example, you may say:

"I currently smoke, and I do not intend to change in the foreseeable future" or

"I currently do not exercise, but I am contemplating changing in the next 6 months."

If you have already started to make changes, fill in the blank in one of the last three statements. In this case you may say:

"I currently eat a low-fat diet, but I have only done so within the last 6 months" or

"I currently practice adequate stress management techniques, and I have done so for over 6 months."

You may use this form to identify your stage of change for any health-related behavior. After identifying two problem behaviors, look up your stage of change for each one using Table 2.3 (on page 62).

Behavior #1. Fill in only one blank.

☐ 1. I currently _____, and do not intend to change in the foreseeable future.
☐ 2. I currently _____, but I am contemplating changing in the next 6 months.
☐ 3. I currently _____ regularly, but I intend to change in the next month.
☐ 4. I currently _____, but I have only done so within the last 6 months.
☐ 5. I currently _____, and I have done so for over 6 months.
☐ 6. I currently _____, and I have done so for over 5 years.

Stage of change: _____ (see Table 2.3 on page 62).

Behavior #2. Fill in only one blank.

☐ 1. I currently _____, and do not intend to change in the foreseeable future.
☐ 2. I currently _____, but I am contemplating changing in the next 6 months.
☐ 3. I currently _____ regularly, but I intend to change in the next month.
☐ 4. I currently _____, but I have only done so within the last 6 months.
☐ 5. I currently _____, and I have done so for over 6 months.
☐ 6. I currently _____, and I have done so for over 5 years.

Stage of change: _____ (see Table 2.3 on page 62).

II. Processes of Change

According to your stage of change for the two behaviors you have identified, list the processes of change that apply to each behavior (see Table 2.1 on page 56).

Behavior #1: _____

_____

Behavior #2: _____

_____

III. Techniques for Change

List a minimum of three techniques that you will use with each process of change (see Table 2.2 on page 62).

Behavior #1: _____

_____

List:	Self-Destructive Behaviors	Constructive Behaviors
	_____	_____
	_____	_____
	_____	_____
	_____	_____

Behavior #2: _____

_____

List:	Self-Destructive Behaviors	Constructive Behaviors
	_____	_____
	_____	_____
	_____	_____
	_____	_____

Today's date: _____ Completion date: _____ Signature: _____

Activity 2.3: Setting SMART Goals

Name _____ Date _____
Course _____ Section _____ Gender _____ Age _____

In Activity 2.2 you identified two behaviors that you wish to change. Using SMART goal guidelines, write goals and actions that will provide a road map for behavioral change. In the spaces provided in this lab, indicate how your stated goals meet each one of the SMART goal guidelines.

I. SMART Goals

Goal 1:
_____
_____

Indicate what makes your goal specific.
_____
_____

How is your goal measurable?
_____
_____
_____

Why is this an acceptable goal?
_____
_____
_____

State why you consider this goal realistic.
_____
_____

How is this goal time-specific?
_____
_____
_____

Goal 2: _____

_____

Indicate what makes your goal specific.

_____

_____

How is your goal measurable?

_____

_____

Why is this an acceptable goal?

_____

_____

State why you consider this goal realistic.

_____

_____

How is this goal time-specific?

_____

_____

II. Specific Actions
Write a minimum of five specific actions that will help you reach your two SMART goals.

Goal 1: _____

Actions:

1. _____
2. _____
3. _____
4. _____
5. _____

Goal 2: _____

Actions:

1. _____
2. _____
3. _____
4. _____
5. _____

a short-term goal of losing 10 pounds and write specific actions to accomplish this goal. Then the immediate task will not seem as overwhelming and will be easier.

At times, problems arise even with realistic goals. Try to anticipate potential difficulties as much as possible, and plan for ways to deal with them. If your goal is to jog for 30 minutes on 6 consecutive days, what are the alternatives if the weather turns bad? Possible solutions are to jog in the rain, find an indoor track, jog at a different time of day when the weather is better, or participate in a different aerobic activity such as stationary cycling, swimming, Zumba, or step aerobics.

Monitoring your progress as you move toward a goal also reinforces behavior. Keeping an exercise log or doing a body composition assessment periodically enables you to determine your progress at any given time.

5. **Time specific.** A goal should always have a specific date set for completion. The earlier example to reach 20 percent body fat in 12 weeks is time specific. The chosen date should be realistic but not too distant in the future. Allow yourself enough time to achieve the goal, but not too much time, as this could affect your performance. With a deadline, a task is much easier to work toward.

Goal Evaluation

In addition to the SMART guidelines provided, you should conduct periodic evaluations of your goals. Reevaluations are vital to success. You may find that after you have fully committed and put all your effort into a goal, that goal may be unreachable. If so, reassess the goal.

Recognize that you will face obstacles and you will not always meet your goals. Use your setbacks and learn from them. Rewrite your goal and create a plan that will help you get around self-defeating behaviors in the future. Once you achieve a goal, set a new one to improve on or maintain what you have achieved. Goals keep you motivated.

ASSESS YOUR BEHAVIOR

CENGAGEbrain To access course materials, including companion resources, please visit www.cengagebrain.com.

1. What are your feelings about the science of behavior modification and how its principles may help you on your journey to health and wellness?
2. Can you accept the fact that for various healthy lifestyle factors (for example, regular exercise, healthy eating, not smoking, stress management, prevention of sexually transmitted infections) you are either in the precontemplation or contemplation stage of change? As such, are you willing to learn what is required to change and actually eliminate unhealthy behaviors and adopt healthy lifestyle behaviors?
3. Are you now in the action phase (or a later phase) for exercise and healthy eating? If not, what barriers keep you from doing so?

ASSESS YOUR KNOWLEDGE

Evaluate how well you understand the concepts presented in this chapter using the chapter-specific quizzing available in the online materials at www.cengagebrain.com.

1. Most of the behaviors that people adopt in life are
   a. a product of their environment.
   b. learned early in childhood.
   c. learned from parents.
   d. genetically determined.
   e. the result of peer pressure.

2. Instant gratification is
   a. a barrier to change.
   b. a factor that motivates change.
   c. one of the six stages of change.
   d. the end result of successful change.
   e. a technique in the process of change.

3. The desire and will to do something is referred to as
   a. invincibility.
   b. confidence.
   c. competence.
   d. external locus of control.
   e. motivation.

4. People who believe they have control over events in their lives
   a. tend to rationalize their negative actions.
   b. exhibit problems of competence.
   c. often feel helpless over illness and disease.
   d. have an internal locus of control.
   e. often engage in risky lifestyle behaviors.

5. A person who is unwilling to change a negative behavior because the reasons for change are not important enough is said to have problems of
   a. competence.
   b. conduct.
   c. motivation.
   d. confidence.
   e. risk complacency.

6. Which of the following is a stage of change in the transtheoretical model?
   a. recognition
   b. motivation
   c. relapse
   d. preparation
   e. goal setting

7. A precontemplator is a person who
   a. has no desire to change a behavior.
   b. is looking to make a change in the next 6 months.
   c. is preparing for change in the next 30 days.
   d. willingly adopts healthy behaviors.
   e. is talking to a therapist to overcome a problem behavior.

8. An individual who is trying to stop smoking and has not smoked for three months is in the
   a. maintenance stage.
   b. action stage.
   c. termination stage.
   d. adoption stage.
   e. evaluation stage.

9. The process of change in which an individual obtains information to make a better decision about a problem behavior is known as
   a. behavior analysis.
   b. self-reevaluation.
   c. commitment.
   d. positive outlook.
   e. consciousness-raising.

10. A goal is effective when it is
    a. specific.
    b. measurable.
    c. realistic.
    d. time specific.
    e. all of the above.

Correct answers can be found at the back of the book.

Nutrition for Wellness

3

Healthy nutrition significantly enhances health and quality of life: Preparing most meals at home is one of the surest ways to eat healthier and enjoy a longer, more productive, and better life. If you feel that you don't have time to cook, or don't care to cook, sooner or later you will have to make time to treat and care for illness and disease.

Objectives

- **Define** nutrition and describe its relationship to health and well-being.
- **Learn** to use the U.S. Department of Agriculture MyPlate guidelines for healthier eating.
- **Describe** the functions of the nutrients—carbohydrates, fiber, fats, proteins, vitamins, minerals, and water—in the human body.
- **Define** the various energy production mechanisms of the human body.
- **Be able** to conduct a comprehensive nutrient analysis and implement changes to meet the Dietary Reference Intakes (DRIs).
- **Identify** myths and fallacies regarding nutrition.
- **Become** aware of guidelines for nutrient supplementation.
- **Learn** the *Dietary Guidelines for Americans 2010*.
- **Analyze** your diet and plan for healthy nutrition.

CENGAGEbrain.com

Visit www.cengagebrain.com to access course materials and companion resources for this text, including quiz questions designed to check your understanding of the chapter contents. See the preface on page ix for more information.

What is gluten sensitivity?

Gluten sensitivity falls under an umbrella of adverse effects on the body caused by gluten, a protein found in wheat, barley, rye, malts, and triticale. Gluten is also used as an additive for flavoring and stabilizing food or as a thickening agent.

About one percent of Americans suffer from celiac disease, an autoimmune disorder in genetically predisposed people of all ages that damages the lining of the small intestine and the ability to absorb nutrients. The disease is caused by a reaction to gluten, leading to an inflammatory reaction that induces a series of symptoms, including vomiting, severe abdominal pain, diarrhea, and fatigue. A gluten-free diet is the accepted treatment for individuals with celiac disease.

Many people test negative for celiac disease but appear to be gluten sensitive. They indicate that they feel better when they eliminate gluten from the diet. A gluten-free diet, however, is not completely free of gluten; rather, it contains a low, harmless level. Switching to a healthy diet often helps gluten-sensitive individuals because processed and junk foods tend to have high amounts of gluten. Some gluten in the diet may not affect these people much.

Should I worry about sugar in my diet?

Until recently, the most significant health concerns regarding excessive sugar intake included increased caloric intake, weight gain, obesity, tooth decay, and lower nutrient intake ("empty" or "discretionary" calories with no nutritional benefit whatsoever). A 24-year study of almost 90,000 women published in the *American Journal of Clinical Nutrition,* however, indicated that consumption of one or two sugar-sweetened beverages per day increased coronary heart disease risk by 23 or 35 percent, respectively. Regular soft drink consumers have about an 80-percent greater risk for developing type 2 diabetes. Excessive body weight increases the risk for metabolic syndrome and heart disease. Excessive added sugar in the diet also raises blood fats known as triglycerides, which, along with cholesterol, clog up the arteries. People who consume a sugar-heavy diet run a greater risk for pancreatic cancer. At present, there is no evidence that sugar directly causes other types of cancer, hyperactivity, or abnormal behavior. Other data indicate that individuals who drink more than five sugary soft drinks per week have reduced bone density in the hips and more than double joint-cushioning cartilage loss in the knees.

You do not have to eliminate all sugar from your diet. The latest data released in late 2010 indicate that the typical American consumes about 475 daily calories from added sugar, the equivalent of 30 teaspoons per day. Most people simply cannot afford all those extra daily empty calories. People should strive for a "nutrient-rich" diet—that is, a high nutrient-to-calorie ratio. The American Heart Association recommends no more than six and nine daily teaspoons of added sugar for women and men, respectively. Data also indicate that liquid calories (soft drinks) do not result in less food consumption during a meal. Adults who drink one or more sodas per day are 27 percent more likely to be overweight or obese.

Unfortunately, food labels do not differentiate between natural and added sugars, making it difficult to determine the quantity added to foods and drinks. Natural sugars in food (fructose and lactose) are acceptable because these foods contain many other healthful substances. Among others, sugars listed on food labels include ordinary table sugar (sucrose), raw sugar, cane sugar, brown sugar, invert sugar, high-fructose corn syrup (HFCS), corn syrup, corn sweetener, glucose, dextrose, fructose, lactose, maltose, maltodextrin, molasses, honey, agave syrup, maple syrup, malt syrup, fruit juice concentrate, and sorghum.

The American Diabetic Association indicates that soft drinks and sweetened drinks are the biggest source of sugar in the diet, accounting for 38 percent of all added sugar intake (each 12-ounce can of soft drink contains about 10 teaspoons of sugar). Soda consumption in the United States has increased by 500 percent over the past 50 years. The soda industry generates about 47 gallons of soft drink for each American. Other drinks that are loaded with sugar include fruit drinks, iced teas, sports drinks, and energy drinks. Plain sugar, candy, and desserts account for another 34 percent of the added sugar intake.

Currently, energy drinks are a major health concern in the United States. Besides sugar, the caffeine content in these drinks can be five times (250 to 500 mg) what's in a cup of coffee (40 to 90 mg). Five deaths have been attributed to these energy drinks, most likely due to an irregular heartbeat caused by the excess caffeine.

Many researchers have expressed particular concern over HFCS, a liquid sweetener made from cornstarch but greatly enhanced with fructose. HFCS is used in many products, including soft drinks, candies, baked goods, and breakfast cereals. HFCS is thought to be a major contributor to obesity, cardiovascular disease, diabetes, and possibly high blood pressure, liver and kidney disease, and systemic inflammation.

Only athletes who participate in vigorous-intensity exercise for longer than 60 minutes at a time can benefit from sports drinks as an additional source of energy. Sports drinks contain between 70 and 100 calories (four to six teaspoons of added sugar) per 12 ounces. Most individuals who participate in 30 to 60 minutes of physical activity/exercise for health/fitness purposes do not need and will not benefit from sports drinks. For proper weight management and healthy living, moderation is a sound principle regarding added sugar consumption.

Fish is known to be heart healthy, but should we have concerns about mercury toxicity?

Fish and shellfish contain high-quality protein, omega-3 fatty acids, and other essential nutrients. Fish is lower in saturated fat and cholesterol than meat or poultry. Data indicate that eating as little as six ounces of fatty fish per week can reduce the risk of premature death from heart disease by one-third and overall death rates by about one-sixth. Fish also appears to have anti-inflammatory properties that can help treat chronic inflammatory kidney disease, osteoarthritis, rheumatoid arthritis, Crohn's disease, and autoimmune disorders like asthma and lupus. Thus, fish is one of the healthiest foods we can consume.

Potential contaminants in fish, and in particular mercury, have created concerns among some people. Mercury cannot be removed from food. As it accumulates in the body, it harms the brain and nervous system. Mercury is a naturally occurring trace mineral that can be released into the air from industrial pollution. As mercury falls into streams and oceans, it accumulates in the aquatic food chain. Larger fish accumulate larger amounts of mercury because they eat medium- and small-size fish. Of particular concern are shark, swordfish, king mackerel, pike, bass, and tilefish, which have higher levels. Farm-raised salmon also have slightly higher levels of polychlorinated biphenyls (PCBs), which the U.S. Environmental Protection Agency lists as a "probable human carcinogen."

The American Heart Association recommends consuming fish twice a week. The risk for adverse effects from eating fish is extremely low and primarily theoretical in nature. For most people, eating two servings (up to six ounces) of fish per week poses no health threat. Pregnant and nursing women and young children, however, should avoid mercury in fish. The best recommendation is to balance the risks against the benefits. If you are still concerned, consume no more than 12 ounces per week of a variety of fish and shellfish that are lower in mercury, including canned light tuna, wild salmon, shrimp, pollock, catfish, and scallops. And check local advisories about the safety of fish caught by family and friends in local streams, rivers, lakes, and coastal areas. Many preventive medicine experts now believe that fish is most likely the single most important food an individual can consume for good health.

What do the terms "glycemic index" and "glycemic load" mean?

The glycemic index (GI) provides a numeric value that measures the blood glucose (sugar) response following ingestion of individual carbohydrate foods. Carbohydrates that are quickly absorbed and cause a rapid rise in blood glucose are said to have a high GI. Those that break down slowly and gradually release glucose into the blood have a low GI. Consumption of high glycemic foods in combination with some fat and protein, nonetheless, brings down the average index. The glycemic load (GL) is calculated by multiplying the GI of a particular food by its carbohydrate content in grams and dividing by 100. The usefulness of the glycemic load is based on the theory that a high-glycemic-index food eaten in small quantities provides a similar effect in blood sugar rise as a consumption of a larger quantity of a low-glycemic food. Research also indicates that a low-GL diet significantly reduces inflammatory conditions that lead to chronic diseases in the human body. The most accurate source of the GI and GL of 750 foods has been published in the *Journal of Clinical Nutrition*. Additional information on the GI is also provided in Chapter 5, pages 155-158.

What is the difference between antioxidants and phytonutrients?

Antioxidants, comprising vitamins, minerals, and phytonutrients, help prevent damage to cells from highly reactive and unstable molecules known as oxygen free radicals (see page 105). Antioxidants are found both in plant and animal foods, whereas phytonutrients (also known as phytochemicals) are found in plant foods only, including fruits, vegetables, beans, nuts, and seeds. Thousands of these bioactive compounds found in plants offer an array of health benefits ranging from cardiovascular disease and cancer prevention to vision health. The actions of phytonutrients go beyond those of most antioxidants. In particular, they appear to have powerful anti-cancer properties. For example, at almost every stage of cancer, phytonutrients can block, disrupt, slow, or even reverse the process. In terms of heart disease, they may reduce inflammation, inhibit blood clots, or prevent the oxidation of low-density lipoprotein cholesterol. People should consume ample amounts of plant-based foods to obtain a healthy supply of antioxidants, including a wide array of phytonutrients.

Real Life Story | Kwame's Experience

Through high school and my first couple years of college, I was in the habit of eating fast food every day. I was usually in a hurry, so going through a drive-through and getting a burger or chicken nuggets was the easiest solution. I pretty much never ate vegetables. I just didn't care for them. The only vegetable I liked was fresh corn the way my mom makes it—with lots of butter. My eating habits caused me to put on some weight over the years, but I still thought I looked okay. It wasn't until I took a Fitness and Wellness class and did a 3-day analysis of my diet that I realized how bad my eating habits really were. Some days I got more than double the amount of saturated fat and sodium that I should be having! I realized that if I went on eating this way, it would catch up with me eventually, and might even take years off my life. So I decided to try to improve my eating habits. I cut way down on the trips to fast food restaurants. It was really hard, because I drive by so many of them, and as soon as I see the sign, I start craving the foods. Sometimes I can almost smell the French fries cooking! At first it took a lot of willpower, but once I got in the habit of driving past without stopping, it got easier and I stopped thinking about it so much. I started making meals for myself, or else buying ready-made meals that were healthier, even including salads! I started out being willing to eat only a couple of vegetables, but gradually tried more, and actually started to like a lot of them. Now I usually get even more than five servings a day of fruits and vegetables. Since changing my eating habits, I have lost some weight, and I also have more energy. Eating right can still be a challenge, especially when I get stressed and am pressed for time. But I believe that my health is worth the effort.

PERSONAL PROFILE: Personal Nutrition Habits

I. Are you aware of the average daily caloric intake and macronutrient content of your diet? ___Yes ___ No If you answered "yes," please indicate your average daily caloric intake: ___ calories and your daily percentage of total calories for CHO ___%, fat ___%, and protein ___%.

II. According to nutritional guidelines, the daily average caloric intake should be distributed so that ___ to ___% of the calories come from carbohydrates, ___ to ___% from fat, and ___ to ___% from protein.

III. Nutrient supplements are encouraged for most people to achieve a balanced diet ___ True ___ False

IV. Current dietary guidelines for Americans encourage people to balance calories with physical activity to sustain healthy weight and focus on consuming nutrient-dense foods and beverages. ___ True ___ False

V. As a "pediatric disease," osteoporosis can be prevented early in life by making sure that the diet has sufficient calcium and by participating in weight-bearing activities. ___ True ___ False

Proper **nutrition** is essential to overall health and wellness. Good nutrition means that a person's diet supplies all the essential nutrients for healthy body functioning, including normal tissue growth, repair, and maintenance. The diet should also provide enough **substrates** to produce the energy necessary for work, physical activity, and relaxation.

Nutrients should be obtained from a wide variety of sources. Figure 3.1 shows U.S. Department of Agriculture (USDA) MyPlate nutrition guidelines and recommended daily food amounts according to various caloric requirements. To lower the risk for chronic disease, an effective wellness program must incorporate healthy eating guidelines. These guidelines will be discussed throughout this chapter and in later chapters.

Too much or too little of any nutrient can precipitate serious health problems. The typical U.S. diet is too high in calories, sugar, saturated fat, trans fat, and sodium, and not high enough in whole grains, fruits, and vegetables—factors that undermine good health. On a given day, nearly half of the people in the

> **Nutrition** Science that studies the relationship of foods to optimal health and performance.
>
> **Substrates** Substances acted on by an enzyme (e.g., carbohydrates, fats).
>
> **Nutrients** Substances found in food that provide energy, regulate metabolism, and help with growth and repair of body tissues.

Figure 3.1 MyPlate: Steps to a Healthier You.

Switch to fat-free or low-fat (1%) milk.

Make half your plate fruits and vegetables.

Make at least half your grains whole grains.

Choose fish and lean or low-fat meat and poultry.

ChooseMyPlate.gov

VEGETABLES	FRUITS	GRAINS	PROTEIN	DAIRY
Any vegetable or 100% vegetable juice counts as a member of the Vegetable Group. Vegetables may be raw or cooked; fresh, frozen, canned, or dried/dehydrated; and may be whole, cut-up, or mashed. Vegetables are organized into 5 subgroups, based on their nutrient content: dark green vegetables, red and orange vegetables, beans and peas, starchy vegetables, and other vegetables.	Any fruit or 100% fruit juice counts as part of the Fruit Group. Fruits may be fresh, canned, frozen, or dried, and may be whole, cut-up, or pureed.	Any food made from wheat, rice, oats, cornmeal, barley, or another cereal grain is a grain product. Bread, pasta, oatmeal, breakfast cereals, tortillas, and grits are examples of grain products. Grains are divided into 2 subgroups: whole grains and refined grains.	All foods made from meat, poultry, seafood, beans, and peas, eggs, processed soy products, nuts, and seeds are considered part of the Protein Foods Group (beans and peas are also part of the Vegetable Group). Select at least 8 ounces of cooked seafood per week. Meat and poultry choices should be lean or low-fat. Young children need less, depending on their age and calories needs. The advice to consume seafood does not apply to vegetarians. Vegetarian options in the Protein Foods Group include beans and peas, processed soy products, and nuts and seeds.	All fluid milk products and many foods made from milk are considered part of this food group. Most Dairy Group choices should be fat-free or low-fat. Foods made from milk that retain their calcium content are part of the group. Foods made from milk that have little to no calcium, such as cream cheese, cream, and butter, are not. Calcium-fortified soymilk (soy beverage) is also part of the Dairy Group.

Recommended Daily Amounts

Women	Vegetables	Fruits	Grains	Protein	Dairy
19–30 years old	2½ cups	2 cups	6 oz. equivalents	5½ oz. equivalents	3 cups
31–50 years old	2½ cups	1½ cups	6 oz. equivalents	5 oz. equivalents	3 cups
51+ years old	2 cups	1½ cups	5 oz. equivalents	5 oz. equivalents	3 cups
Men					
19–30 years old	3 cups	2 cups	8 oz. equivalents	6½ oz. equivalents	3 cups
31–50 years old	3 cups	2 cups	7 oz. equivalents	6 oz. equivalents	3 cups
51+ years old	2½ cups	2 cups	6 oz. equivalents	6½ oz. equivalents	3 cups

Source: http://www.choosemyplate.gov/. Additional information can be obtained on this site, including an online individualized MyPlate eating plan (Plan a Healthy Menu option on the site) based on your age, gender, weight, height, and activity level.

United States eat no fruit and almost a fourth eat no vegetables.

Food availability is not a problem. The problem is overconsumption of the wrong foods. Diseases of dietary excess and imbalance are among the leading causes of death in many developed countries throughout the world, including the United States.

Diet and nutrition often play a crucial role in the development and progression of chronic diseases. A diet high in saturated fat, trans fat, and cholesterol increases the risk for diseases of the cardiovascular system, including atherosclerosis, coronary heart disease (CHD), and strokes. In sodium-sensitive individuals, high salt intake has been linked to high blood pressure. Up to 50 percent of all cancers may be diet related. Obesity, diabetes, and osteoporosis also have been associated with faulty nutrition.

3.1 Nutrients

The essential nutrients that the human body requires are carbohydrates, fat, protein, vitamins, minerals, and water. The first three are called "fuel nutrients" because they are the only substances that the body uses to supply the energy (commonly measured in calories) needed for work and normal body functions. The three others—vitamins, minerals, and water—are regulatory nutrients. They have no caloric value but are still necessary for a person to function normally and maintain good health. Many nutritionists add to this list a seventh nutrient: fiber. This nutrient is vital for good health. Recommended amounts seem to provide protection against several diseases, including cardiovascular disease and some cancers.

Carbohydrates, fats, proteins, and water are termed macronutrients because we need them in proportionately large amounts daily. Vitamins and minerals are required in only small amounts—grams, milligrams, and micrograms instead of, say, ounces—and nutritionists refer to them as micronutrients.

Depending on the amount of nutrients and calories they contain, foods can be classified by their **nutrient density**. Foods that contain few or a moderate number of calories but are packed with nutrients are said to have high nutrient density. Foods that have a lot of calories but few nutrients are of low nutrient density and are commonly called "junk food."

A **calorie** is the unit of measure indicating the energy value of food to the person who consumes it. It also is used to express the amount of energy a person expends in physical activity. Technically, a kilocalorie (kcal), or large calorie, is the amount of heat necessary to raise the temperature of one kilogram of water by one degree centigrade. For simplicity, people call it a calorie rather than a kcal. For example, if the caloric value of a food is 100 calories (i.e., 100 kcal), the energy in this food would raise the temperature of 100 kilograms of water by one degree centigrade. Similarly, walking one mile would burn about 100 calories (again, 100 kcal).

Carbohydrates Carbohydrates constitute the major source of calories that the body uses to provide energy for work, to maintain cells, and generate heat. They are necessary for brain, muscle, and nervous system function and help regulate fat and metabolize protein. Each gram of carbohydrates provides the human body with four calories. The major sources of carbohydrates are breads, cereals, fruits, vegetables, and milk and other dairy products. Carbohydrates are classified into **simple carbohydrates** and complex carbohydrates (Figure 3.2).

Simple Carbohydrates

Often called "sugars," simple carbohydrates have little nutritive value. Examples are candy, soda, and cakes. Simple carbohydrates are divided into monosaccharides and disaccharides. These carbohydrates—whose names end in "ose"—often take the place of more nutritive foods in the diet.

Monosaccharides. The simplest sugars are **monosaccharides**. The three most common monosaccharides are glucose, fructose, and galactose.

1. Glucose is a natural sugar found in food and also produced in the body from other simple and complex carbohydrates. It is used as a source of energy, or it may be stored in the muscles and liver in the form of glycogen (a long chain of glucose molecules hooked together). Excess glucose in the blood is converted to fat and stored in **adipose tissue**.
2. Fructose, or fruit sugar, occurs naturally in fruits and honey and is converted to glucose in the body.
3. Galactose is produced from milk sugar in the mammary glands of lactating animals and is converted to glucose in the body.

Disaccharides. The three major **disaccharides** are:

1. Sucrose or table sugar (glucose + fructose)
2. Lactose (glucose + galactose)
3. Maltose (glucose + glucose)

Figure 3.2 Major types of carbohydrates.

Simple carbohydrates

Monosaccharides	Disaccharides
Glucose	Sucrose (glucose+fructose)
Fructose	Lactose (glucose+galactose)
Galactose	Maltose (glucose+glucose)

Complex carbohydrates

Polysaccharides	Fiber
Starches	Cellulose
Dextrins	Hemicellulose
Glycogen	Pectins
	Gums
	Mucilages

© Cengage Learning

These disaccharides are broken down in the body, and the resulting simple sugars (monosaccharides) are used as indicated earlier.

Complex Carbohydrates

Complex carbohydrates are also called polysaccharides. Anywhere from about ten to thousands of monosaccharide molecules can unite to form a single polysaccharide. Examples of complex carbohydrates are starches, dextrins, and **glycogen**.

1. Starch is the storage form of glucose in plants that is needed to promote their earliest growth. Starch is commonly found in grains, seeds, corn, nuts, roots, potatoes, and legumes. In a healthful diet, grains, the richest source of starch, should supply most of the body's energy. Once eaten, starch is converted to glucose for the body's own energy use.
2. Dextrins are formed from the breakdown of large starch molecules exposed to dry heat, such as in baking bread or producing cold cereals. These complex carbohydrates of plant origin provide many valuable nutrients and can be an excellent source of fiber.
3. Glycogen is the animal polysaccharide synthesized from glucose and is found in only tiny amounts in meats. In essence, we manufacture it; we don't consume it. Glycogen constitutes the body's reservoir of glucose. Thousands of glucose molecules are linked, to be stored as glycogen in the liver and muscle. When a surge of energy is needed, enzymes in the muscle and the liver break down glycogen and thereby make glucose readily available for energy transformation. (This process is discussed under "Nutrition for Athletes," starting on page 113.)

Fiber

Fiber is a form of complex carbohydrate. A high-fiber diet gives a person a feeling of fullness without adding too many calories to the diet. **Dietary fiber** is present mainly in plant leaves, skins, roots, and seeds. Processing and refining foods removes almost all of their natural fiber. In our diet, the main sources of fiber are whole-grain cereals and breads, fruits, vegetables, and legumes.

Fiber is important in the diet because it decreases the risk for disease, in particular cardiovascular disease. Increased fiber intake may lower the risk for CHD, because saturated fats and trans fats often take the place of fiber in the diet, increasing the absorption and formation of cholesterol. Other health disorders that have been tied to low intake of fiber are infections, respiratory diseases, constipation, diverticulitis, hemorrhoids, gallbladder disease, and obesity. Recent 2011 data showed that individuals who eat the most dietary fiber have a 22 percent lower mortality rate from any cause as compared to those who eat the least amount of fiber.[1]

The recommended fiber intake for adults of age 50 years and younger is 25 grams per day for women and 38 grams for men. As a result of decreased food consumption in people older than 50 years of age, an intake of 21 and 30 grams of fiber per day, respectively, is recommended.[2] Most people in the United States eat only 15 grams of fiber per day, putting them at increased risk for disease.

A person can increase fiber intake by eating more fruits, vegetables, legumes, whole grains, and whole-grain cereals. Research provides evidence that increasing fiber intake to 30 grams

> **Nutrient density** A measure of the amount of nutrients and calories in various foods.
>
> **Calorie** The amount of heat necessary to raise the temperature of one gram of water one degree centigrade; used to measure the energy value of food and cost (energy expenditure) of physical activity.
>
> **Carbohydrates** A classification of a dietary nutrient containing carbon, hydrogen, and oxygen; the major source of energy for the human body.
>
> **Simple carbohydrates** Formed by simple or double sugar units with little nutritive value; divided into monosaccharides and disaccharides.
>
> **Monosaccharides** The simplest carbohydrates (sugars), formed by five- or six-carbon skeletons. The three most common monosaccharides are glucose, fructose, and galactose.
>
> **Adipose tissue** Fat cells in the body.
>
> **Disaccharides** Simple carbohydrates formed by two monosaccharide units linked together, one of which is glucose. The major disaccharides are sucrose, lactose, and maltose.
>
> **Complex carbohydrates** Carbohydrates formed by three or more simple sugar molecules linked together; also referred to as polysaccharides.
>
> **Glycogen** Form in which glucose is stored in the body.
>
> **Dietary fiber** A complex carbohydrate in plant foods that is not digested but is essential to digestion.

High-fiber foods are essential in a healthy diet.

per day leads to a significant reduction in heart attacks, cancer of the colon, breast cancer, diabetes, and diverticulitis. Table 3.1 provides the fiber content of selected foods. A practical guideline to obtain your fiber intake is to eat at least five (preferably nine) daily servings of fruits and vegetables and three servings of whole-grain foods (whole-grain bread, cereal, and rice). Think of your servings of these food items as servings of absolute goodness to your taste and health.

Fiber is typically classified according to its solubility in water:

1. Soluble fiber dissolves in water and forms a gel-like substance that encloses food particles. This property allows soluble fiber to bind and excrete fats from the body. This type of fiber has been shown to lower blood cholesterol and blood sugar levels. Soluble fiber is found primarily in oats, fruits, barley, legumes, and psyllium (an ancient Indian grain added to some breakfast cereals).

2. Insoluble fiber is not easily dissolved in water, and the body cannot digest it. This type of fiber is important because it binds water, causing a softer and bulkier stool that increases **peristalsis**, the involuntary muscle contractions of intestinal walls that force the stool through the intestines and enable quicker excretion of food residues. Speeding the passage of food residues through the intestines seems to lower the risk for colon cancer, mainly because it reduces the amount of time that cancer-causing agents are in contact with the intestinal wall. Insoluble fiber is also thought to bind with carcinogens (cancer-producing substances), and more water in the stool may dilute the cancer-causing agents, lessening their potency. Sources of insoluble fiber include wheat, cereals, vegetables, and skins of fruits.

The most common types of fiber are:

1. Cellulose: water-insoluble fiber found in plant cell walls
2. Hemicellulose: water-insoluble fiber found in cereal fibers
3. Pectins: water-soluble fiber found in vegetables and fruits
4. Gums and mucilages: water-soluble fiber also found in small amounts in foods of plant origin

Surprisingly, excessive fiber intake can be detrimental to health. It can produce loss of calcium, phosphorus, and iron, to say nothing of gastrointestinal discomfort. If your fiber intake is less than the recommended amount, increase your intake gradually over several weeks to avoid gastrointestinal disturbances. While increasing your fiber intake, be sure to drink more water to avoid constipation and even dehydration. Excellent complex carbohydrate choices include quinoa (one of the best whole grains you can eat, also high in protein—a complete protein), beans, and sweet potatoes.

Fats (Lipids) The human body uses **fats** as a source of energy. Also called lipids, fats are the most concentrated energy source, with each gram of fat supplying nine calories to

Table 3.1 Dietary Fiber Content of Selected Foods

Food	Serving Size	Dietary Fiber (gr)
Almonds, shelled	¼ cup	3.9
Apple	1 medium	3.7
Banana	1 small	1.2
Beans (red kidney)	½ cup	8.2
Blackberries	½ cup	4.9
Beets, red, canned (cooked)	½ cup	1.4
Brazil nuts	1 oz	2.5
Broccoli (cooked)	½ cup	3.3
Brown rice (cooked)	½ cup	1.7
Carrots (cooked)	½ cup	3.3
Cauliflower (cooked)	½ cup	5.0
Cereal		
All Bran	1 oz	8.5
Cheerios	1 oz	1.1
Cornflakes	1 oz	0.5
Fruit and Fibre	1 oz	4.0
Fruit Wheats	1 oz	2.0
Just Right	1 oz	2.0
Wheaties	1 oz	2.0
Corn (cooked)	½ cup	2.2
Eggplant (cooked)	½ cup	3.0
Lettuce (chopped)	½ cup	0.5
Orange	1 medium	4.3
Parsnips (cooked)	½ cup	2.1
Pear	1 medium	4.5
Peas (cooked)	½ cup	4.4
Popcorn (plain)	1 cup	1.2
Potato (baked)	1 medium	4.9
Strawberries	½ cup	1.6
Summer squash (cooked)	½ cup	1.6
Watermelon	1 cup	0.1

© Cengage Learning

Figure 3.3 Major types of fats (lipids).

Simple fats
Monoglyceride (glyceride+one fatty acid*)
Diglyceride (glyceride+two fatty acids)
Triglyceride (glyceride+three fatty acids)

Compound fats
Phospholipids
Glucolipids
Lipoproteins

Derived fats
Sterols (cholesterol)

*Fatty acids can be saturated or unsaturated

© Cengage Learning

Behavior Modification Planning

Tips to Increase Fiber in Your Diet

I PLAN TO / **I DID IT**

- ❏ ❏ Eat more vegetables, either raw or steamed
- ❏ ❏ Eat salads daily that include a wide variety of vegetables
- ❏ ❏ Eat more fruit, including the skin
- ❏ ❏ Choose whole-wheat and whole-grain products
- ❏ ❏ Choose breakfast cereals with more than 3 grams of fiber per serving
- ❏ ❏ Sprinkle a teaspoon or two of unprocessed bran or 100 percent bran cereal on your favorite breakfast cereal
- ❏ ❏ Add high-fiber cereals to casseroles and desserts
- ❏ ❏ Add beans to soups, salads, and stews
- ❏ ❏ Add vegetables to sandwiches: sprouts, green and red pepper strips, diced carrots, sliced cucumbers, red cabbage, onions
- ❏ ❏ Add vegetables to spaghetti: broccoli, cauliflower, sliced carrots, mushrooms
- ❏ ❏ Experiment with unfamiliar fruits and vegetables—collards, kale, broccoflower, asparagus, papaya, mango, kiwi, starfruit
- ❏ ❏ Blend fruit juice with small pieces of fruit and crushed ice
- ❏ ❏ When increasing fiber in your diet, drink plenty of fluids

Try It

Do you know your average daily fiber intake? If you do not know, keep a three-day record of daily fiber intake. How do you fare against the recommended guidelines? If your intake is low, how can you change your diet to increase your daily fiber intake?

---

the body (in contrast to four for carbohydrates). Fats are a part of the human cell structure. Deposits of fat cells are used as stored energy and as an insulator to preserve body heat. They absorb shock; supply essential fatty acids; and carry the fat-soluble vitamins A, D, E, and K. Fats can be classified into three main groups: simple, compound, and derived (Figure 3.3). The most familiar sources of fat are whole milk and other dairy products, meats, and meat alternatives such as eggs and nuts.

Simple Fats

A simple fat consists of a glyceride molecule linked to one, two, or three units of fatty acids. Depending on the number of fatty acids attached, simple fats are divided into monoglycerides (one fatty acid), diglycerides (two fatty acids), and triglycerides (three fatty acids). More than 90 percent of the weight of fat in foods and more than 95 percent of the stored fat in the human body are in the form of triglycerides.

The length of the carbon atom chain and the amount of hydrogen saturation (i.e., the number of hydrogen molecules attached to the carbon chain) in fatty acids vary. Based on the extent of saturation, fatty acids are said to be saturated or unsaturated. Unsaturated fatty acids are classified further into monounsaturated and polyunsaturated fatty acids. Saturated fatty acids are mainly of animal origin, and unsaturated fats are found mostly in plant products.

Saturated Fats. In saturated fatty acids (or "saturated fats"), the carbon atoms are fully saturated with hydrogen atoms; only single bonds link the carbon atoms on the chain (Figure 3.4). Foods high in saturated fatty acids are meats, animal fat, lard, whole milk, cream, butter, cheese, ice cream, hydrogenated oils (hydrogenation saturates fat with hydrogens, also known as trans fats), coconut oil, and palm oils. Saturated fats typically do not melt at room temperature. Coconut and palm oils are exceptions. In general, saturated fats raise the blood cholesterol level. The data on coconut and palm oils are controversial, as some research indicates that these oils may be neutral in terms of their effects on cholesterol.

Although saturated fats raise the "bad" low-density lipoprotein (LDL) cholesterol (in particular the less-damaging larger LDL particles) and daily intake should be limited, data indicate that people who replace saturated fat in the diet with refined carbohydrates such as white bread and pasta and low-fat sweetened baked goods, are at greater risk because the latter tend to decrease the "good" high-density lipoprotein (HDL) cholesterol and increase triglycerides (blood fats) and the more dangerous smaller LDL particles.[3] Individuals who replace saturated fats with polyunsaturated fats (see discussion that follows) derive significant health benefits. A more thorough discussion on this topic is provided in Chapter 10 (page 349).

Unsaturated Fats. In unsaturated fatty acids (or "unsaturated fats"), double bonds form be-

> **Peristalsis** Involuntary muscle contractions of intestinal walls that facilitate excretion of wastes.
>
> **Fats** A classification of nutrients containing carbon, hydrogen, some oxygen, and sometimes other chemical elements.

Figure 3.4 Chemical structure of saturated and unsaturated fats.

Saturated fatty acid

```
     H   H   H   H   H   OH
     |   |   |   |   |   |
G* - C - C - C - C - C - C = O
     |   |   |   |   |
     H   H   H   H   H
```

Monounsaturated fatty acid

```
     H   H   H   H   H   OH
     |   |   |   |   |   |
G* - C - C - C = C - C - C = O
     |   |           |
     H   H           H
                ↑
            Double Bond
```

Polyunsaturated fatty acid

```
     H   H   H   H   H   H   H   H   OH
     |   |   |   |   |   |   |   |   |
G* - C - C - C - C = C - C = C - C - C = O
     |   |   |           |           |
     H   H   H           H           H
                    ↑       ↑
                   Double Bonds
```

*Glyceride component

© Cengage Learning

tween unsaturated carbons. These healthy fatty acids include monounsaturated and polyunsaturated fats, which are usually liquid at room temperature. Other shorter fatty acid chains also tend to be liquid at room temperature. Unsaturated fats help lower blood cholesterol. When unsaturated fats replace saturated fats in the diet, the former stimulate the liver to clear cholesterol from the blood.

In monounsaturated fatty acids (MUFA), only one double bond is found along the chain. Monounsaturated fatty acids are found in olive, canola, peanut, and sesame oils. They are also found in avocados, peanuts, and cashews.

Olive oil is considered the healthiest oil because of the nutrients it contains. Extra virgin olive oil contains antioxidants, polyphenols, and omega-3 fatty acids, all of which promote cardiovascular health, improved cognitive function, and a healthier immune system. Olive oil may even help prevent or reverse type 2 diabetes because it helps the body produce adiponectin, a hormone that aids with blood sugar regulation. Olive oil also has anti-inflammatory properties that protect against chronic diseases.

Extra virgin olive oil is produced from the first pressing of the olives and as such holds the most nutrients. Virgin olive oil is derived from the second pressing. Juices collected from subsequent pressings are then used to manufacture light and pure olive oils.

Canola oil is also extremely healthy. Its composition is the closest to the optimum requirements of fatty acids by the human body, and it contains a nearly ideal mix of unsaturated fatty acids that promote cardiac health. The omega-3s in canola oil also counteract fibrinogen, a compound in the blood that has been linked to thrombosis (clot formation in the blood vessels) and inflammation.

Extra virgin and virgin olive oils retain the flavor of the olives to a greater extent, thus they are best used to make tasty dish toppings and salad dressings, but may not be the most ideal for cooking or baking. Because olive oil is more expensive than canola oil, you can use canola oil for cooking, and reserve olive oil for toppings, dips, and dressings.

Polyunsaturated fatty acids (PUFA) contain two or more double bonds between unsaturated carbon atoms along the chain. Corn, cottonseed, safflower, walnut, sunflower, and soybean oils are high in polyunsaturated fatty acids and are also found in fish, almonds, and pecans.

Trans Fatty Acids. Hydrogen often is added to monounsaturated and polyunsaturated fats to increase shelf life and to solidify them so that they are more spreadable. During this process, called "partial hydrogenation," the position of hydrogen atoms may be changed along the carbon chain, transforming the fat into a **trans fatty acid**. Some margarine, spreads, shortening, pastries, nut butters, crackers, cookies, frozen breakfast foods, dairy products, snacks and chips, cake mixes, meats, processed foods, and fast foods contain trans fatty acids.

Trans fatty acids are not essential and provide no known health benefit. In truth, health-conscious people minimize their intake of these types of fats because diets high in trans fatty acids increase LDL cholesterol and decrease HDL cholesterol, increase rigidity of the coronary arteries, and contribute to the formation of blood clots that may lead to heart attacks and strokes.

Paying attention to food labels is important, because the words "partially hydrogenated" and "trans fatty acids" indicate that the product carries a health risk just as high as or higher than that of saturated fat. The U.S. Food and Drug Administration (FDA) requires that food labels list trans fatty acids so that consumers can make healthier choices.

Polyunsaturated Omega Fatty Acids. Omega fatty acids have been named based on where the first double bond appears in the carbon chain—starting from the end of the chain; hence, the term "omega" from the end of the Greek alphabet. Accordingly, omega fats are classified as omega-3, omega-6, and omega-9. **Omega-3 fatty acids** and **omega-6 fatty acids** have gained considerable attention in recent years. These fatty acids are essential to human health and cannot be manufactured by the body, they have to be consumed in the diet. Omega-9 fatty acids are defined as nonessential because the body can synthesize them from other foods we eat, and we don't have to depend on direct dietary sources to obtain them.

Maintaining a balance between omega-3 and omega-6 fatty acids appears to be important for good health. Excessive intake of omega-6 fatty acids may contribute to inflammation (a risk factor for heart disease—see Chapter 10, page 358), cancer, asthma, arthritis, and depression. A ratio of four to one (4:1) omega-6 to omega-3 fatty acids is often recommended to maintain and improve health.

Most critical in the diet are omega-3 fatty acids, which provide substantial health benefits. Omega-3 fatty acids tend to decrease cholesterol, triglycerides, inflammation, blood clots, abnormal heart rhythms, and high blood pressure. They also decrease the risk for heart attack, abnormal heart rhythms, stroke, Alzheimer's disease, dementia, macular degeneration, and joint degeneration.

Unfortunately, only 25 percent of the U.S. population consumes the recommended amount (approximately 500 mg) of omega eicosapentaenoic acid (EPA) and docosahexaenoic acid (DHA) on any given day. These are two of the three major types of omega-3 fatty acids, along with alpha-linolenic acid (ALA). The evidence is strongest for EPA and DHA as being cardioprotective. Once consumed, the body converts ALA to EPA and then to DHA, but the process is not very efficient. It is best to increase consumption of EPA and DHA to obtain the greatest health benefit.

Individuals at risk for heart disease are encouraged to get an average of .5 to 1.8 grams (500 to 1,800 mg) of EPA and DHA per day.[4] These fatty acids protect against irregular heartbeat and blood clots, reduce triglycerides and blood pressure, and defend against inflammation.[5]

Fish—especially fresh or frozen salmon, mackerel, herring, tuna, and rainbow trout—are high in EPA and DHA. Table 3.2 presents a listing of total EPA plus DHA content of selected species of fish. Canned fish is best when packed in water. In oil-packed fish, the oil mixes with some of the natural fat in fish. When the oil is drained, some of the omega-3 fatty acids are lost as well. Good sources of omega-3 ALA include flaxseeds, canola oil, walnuts, wheat germ, and green leafy vegetables.

Table 3.2 Omega-3 Fatty Acid Content (EPA + DHA) per 100 Grams (3.5 oz) of Fish

Type of Fish	Total EPA + DHA
Anchovy	1.4 gr
Bluefish	1.2 gr
Halibut	0.4 gr
Herring	1.7 gr
Mackerel	2.4 gr
Sardine	1.4 gr
Salmon, Atlantic	1.0 gr
Salmon, Chinook	1.9 gr
Salmon, Coho	1.2 gr
Salmon, Pink	1.0 gr
Salmon, Sockeye	1.3 gr
Shrimp	0.3 gr
Trout, Rainbow	0.6 gr
Trout, Lake	1.6 gr
Tuna, light (water canned)	0.3 gr
Tuna, white (Albacore)	0.8 gr

© Cengage Learning

The oil in flaxseeds is high in ALA and has been shown to reduce abnormal heart rhythm and prevent blood clots. Flaxseeds are also high in fiber and plant chemicals known as lignans. Studies are being conducted to investigate the potential cancer-fighting ability of lignans. In one report, the addition of a daily ounce (three to four tablespoons) of ground flaxseeds to the diet seemed to lead to a decrease in the onset of tumors, preventing their formation and even leading to their shrinkage.[6] Excessive flaxseed in the diet is not recommended. High doses actually may be detrimental to health. Pregnant and lactating women, especially, should not consume large amounts of flaxseed.

Because flaxseeds have a hard outer shell, they should be ground to obtain the nutrients; whole seeds will pass through the body undigested. Grinding the seeds just before use best preserves flavor and nutrients. Pre-ground seeds should be kept sealed and refrigerated. Ground flaxseeds can be mixed with salad dressings, salads, wheat flour, pancakes, muffins, cereals, rice, cottage cheese, and yogurt. Flaxseed oil also may be used, but the oil has little or no fiber and lignans and must be kept refrigerated because it spoils quickly. The oil cannot be used for cooking either, because it scorches easily.

Most of the polyunsaturated fatty acid consumption in the United States comes from omega-6. Once viewed as healthy fats, excessive intake may be detrimental to health. Omega-6 fatty acids include linoleic acid (LA), gamma-linolenic acid (GLA), and arachidonic acid (AA). The typical American diet contains 10 to 20 times more omega-6 than omega-3 fatty acids. Most omega-6 fatty acids come in the form of LA from vegetable oils, the primary oil ingredient added to most processed foods, including salad dressing. LA-rich oils include corn, soybean, sunflower, safflower, and cottonseed oils.

Although more research is required, the imbalance between omega-3 and omega-6 fatty acids is thought to be responsible for the increased rate of inflammatory conditions seen in the United States today. Furthermore, in terms of heart health, while omega-6 fatty acids lower the "bad" LDL cholesterol, they also lower the "good" HDL cholesterol; thus its overall effect on cardiac health is neutral. To decrease your intake of LA, watch for corn, soybean, sunflower, and cottonseed oils in salad dressings, mayonnaise, and margarine.

The best source of omega-3 APA and DHA, the fatty acids that provide the most health benefits, is fish. Data suggest that the amount of fish oil obtained by eating two servings of fish weekly lessens the risk for CHD and may contribute to brain, joint, and vision health. A word of caution:

Trans fatty acid Solidified fat formed by adding hydrogen to monounsaturated and polyunsaturated fats to increase shelf life.

Omega-3 fatty acids Polyunsaturated fatty acids found primarily in cold-water seafood, flaxseed, and flaxseed oil; thought to lower blood cholesterol and triglycerides.

Omega-6 fatty acids Polyunsaturated fatty acids found primarily in corn and sunflower oils and most oils in processed foods.

People who have diabetes or a history of hemorrhaging or strokes, are on aspirin or blood-thinning therapy, or are presurgical patients should not consume fish oil except under a physician's instruction.

Omega-9 fatty acids are from a family of polyunsaturated fats generally found in vegetable oils (canola, olive, peanut, safflower, and sunflower oils), but are also found in avocados, olives, and nuts (almonds, cashews, macadamias, peanuts, pecans, pistachios, and walnuts). These fatty acids are uniquely high in monounsaturated fat, low in saturated fat, and contain zero trans fat. Omega-9 fatty acids are protective against metabolic syndrome and cardiovascular disease as they have been shown to increase HDL cholesterol and decrease LDL cholesterol.

Compound Fats

Compound fats are a combination of simple fats and other chemicals. Examples are:

1. Phospholipids: similar to triglycerides, except that choline (or another compound) and phosphoric acid take the place of one of the fatty acid units
2. Glucolipids: a combination of carbohydrates, fatty acids, and nitrogen
3. Lipoproteins: water-soluble aggregates of protein and triglycerides, phospholipids, or cholesterol

Lipoproteins (a combination of lipids and proteins) are especially important because they transport fats in the blood. The major forms of lipoproteins are HDL, LDL, and very-low-density lipoprotein (VLDL). Lipoproteins play a large role in developing or in preventing heart disease. High HDL ("good" cholesterol) levels have been associated with lower risk for CHD, whereas high levels of LDL ("bad" cholesterol) levels have been linked to increased risk for CHD. HDL is more than 50 percent protein and contains little cholesterol. LDL is approximately 25 percent protein and nearly 50 percent cholesterol. VLDL contains about 50 percent triglycerides, only about 10 percent protein, and 20 percent cholesterol.

Derived Fats

Derived fats combine simple and compound fats. **Sterols** are an example. Although sterols contain no fatty acids, they are considered lipids because they do not dissolve in water. The sterol mentioned most often is cholesterol, which is found in many foods or can be manufactured in the body—primarily from saturated fats, trans fats, and refined carbohydrates.

In the 1980s and 1990s, people were concerned with overall fat intake. As a result, they cut back on fats and started to overconsume refined carbohydrates. Nowadays, people understand that healthy unsaturated fats and caloric balance are essential to good health. The latter is important because overconsumption of even healthy fats leads to weight gain. Keep in mind that as you add something healthy to your diet, you need to remove an equal amount of calories from a different food item, preferably a less healthy item.

Proteins Proteins are the main substances the body uses to build and repair tissues such as muscles, blood, internal organs, skin, hair, nails, and bones. They form a part of hormone, antibody, and enzyme molecules. **Enzymes** play a key role in all of the body's processes. Because proteins form all enzymes, this nutrient is necessary for normal functioning. Proteins also help maintain the normal balance of body fluids.

Proteins can be used as a source of energy, too, but only if sufficient carbohydrates are not available. Each gram of protein yields four calories of energy (the same as carbohydrates). The main sources of protein are meats and meat alternatives, milk, and other dairy products. Excess proteins may be converted to glucose or fat, or even excreted in the urine.

The human body uses 20 **amino acids** to form various types of protein. Amino acids contain nitrogen, carbon, hydrogen, and oxygen. Of the 20 amino acids, 9 are called essential amino acids because the body cannot produce them. The other 11, termed nonessential amino acids, can be manufactured in the body if food proteins in the diet provide enough nitrogen (see Table 3.3). For the body to function normally, all amino acids shown in Table 3.3 must be present in the diet.

Proteins that contain all the essential amino acids, known as "complete" or "higher-quality" proteins, are usually of animal origin. If one or more of the essential amino acids are missing, the proteins are termed incomplete or lower-quality proteins. The essential amino acid that is missing in an incomplete protein is called the limiting amino acid. All plant products, including grains, fruits, vegetables, beans, nuts, and seeds, are incomplete proteins. The only exceptions of complete proteins found in plant products are soy and quinoa (a grain-like crop grown for its edible seed).

Individuals have to take in enough protein to ensure nitrogen for adequate production of all amino acids. On a vegetarian diet, consumption of a variety of food sources is required so that the diet supplies all the essential amino acids within a meal or a given day. When different foods are consumed, the limiting amino acid in one food can be obtained from another food source. This principle is referred to as complementing

Table 3.3 Amino Acids

Essential Amino Acids*	Nonessential Amino Acids
Histidine	Alanine
Isoleucine	Arginine
Leucine	Asparagine
Lysine	Aspartic acid
Methionine	Cysteine
Phenylalanine	Glutamic acid
Threonine	Glutamine
Tryptophan	Glycine
Valine	Proline
	Serine
	Tyrosine

*NOTE: Must be provided in the diet because the body cannot manufacture them.

© Cengage Learning

proteins. For example, consumption of grains and legumes complement each other. Legumes and nuts also complement each other. Nuts and grains, however, are not complementary proteins. Soy and quinoa, can also be used to complement the limiting amino acids in grains, legumes, nuts, and seeds.

Protein deficiency is not a problem in the typical U.S. diet. Two glasses of skim milk combined with about four ounces of poultry or fish meet the daily protein requirement. High intake of protein foods from animal sources, however, can be a concern because they are often high in fat, saturated fat, and cholesterol, which can lead to cardiovascular disease and cancer.

Importance of Adequate Daily Protein Intake

The role of protein in the American diet, nonetheless, is gaining relevance as *adequate protein intake with each meal* is crucial for satiety and weight management and to help build, repair, and maintain lean tissue. The latter has even greater relevance for people who are physically active. Loss of lean tissue with sedentary living, aging, exhaustive exercise training, and while dieting (negative caloric balance) without proper energy and protein intake is inevitable. Loss of lean tissue is never desirable because of the decrease in functional physical capacity (the ability to perform ordinary and unusual tasks of daily living), as well as in the resting metabolic rate.

As an individual, you can prevent or even completely reverse such a loss. The recommendation is that we distribute our protein intake in equal parts throughout the day. To do so, determine your daily intake in grams (see Table 3.4) and divide by three (meals per day). For example, if you weigh 141 pounds (64 kg) and you are physically active, your total protein intake should be between 64 and 77 grams per day (64 × 1.0 and 64 × 1.2 or the equivalent of 256 to 308 calories derived from protein each day—each gram of protein supplies the body with 4 calories) or 21 to 26 grams of protein per meal.

Limiting Red Meat Consumption

Several recent research articles provide strong evidence that excessive red meat consumption increases the risk of premature death, primarily from heart disease, stroke, some cancers, and type 2 diabetes. Consumption of both unprocessed red meat (beef, pork, and lamb) and processed red meat (cold cuts, ham, bacon, bologna, sausage, hot dogs) leads to this outcome.

Researchers believe that it is not just the saturated fat and cholesterol that are the culprits. L-carnitine, a compound abundant in red meat feeds intestinal bacteria. These bacteria digest *L-carnitine* and turn it into a compound called trimethylamine-N-oxide (TMAO) that is believed to cause atherosclerosis (obstruction of the arteries). Red-meat eaters also have a higher incidence of pancreatic, prostate, and esophageal cancers. Nitrites, chemical compounds used to cure (preserve) meats, are believed to increase the risk. Processed meats labeled as "no nitrite added," most likely are not nitrite-free because nitrite and nitrate (which the body can convert to nitrite) occur naturally in meats.

Eating less red meat also protects the environment by requiring less cattle feed and water, decreasing the production of methane gas and solid waste by the animals, reducing the requirement of nitrous oxide used in fertilizers to grow the feed, and leading to less deforestation to make pasture and farmland.

The most compelling evidence comes from a 2012 study of more than 120,000 people at the Harvard School of Public Health showing a 30 percent increased risk of premature death among people who eat the most red meat as compared to those who eat the least (about a half a serving per day).[7] In the study, three ounces of unprocessed red meat were considered as one serving, but only one ounce of processed red meat was viewed as a serving. The mortality rate was highest among processed red-meat eaters. Eating just 1 serving per day increased the risk between 13 percent (unprocessed) and 20 percent (processed).

The data also indicated that replacing one serving a day of red meat with fish, poultry, nuts, beans, low-fat dairy, or whole grains decreased the chances of premature death in the range of 7 percent to 19 percent. The researchers concluded that *"The message we want to communicate is it would be great if you could reduce your intake of red meat consumption to half a serving a day or two to three servings a week, and severely limit processed red meat intake."*

As mentioned earlier, a well-balanced diet contains a variety of foods from all five basic food groups, including a wise selection of foods from animal sources (see also "Balancing the Diet" in this chapter). Based on current nutrition data, meat (particularly red meat or excessive poultry and fish) should be replaced by grains, legumes, vegetables, and fruits as main courses. Meats should be used more for flavoring than for volume. Daily consumption of beef, poultry, or fish

Table 3.4 Recommended Daily Protein Intake

Activity Level	Grams/kg of Body Weight
Sedentary	0.8 g/kg
Physically active	1.0–1.2 g/kg
Athlete	1.2–2.0 g/kg
Weight gain/loss	1.5–2.0 g/kg

SOURCE: Adapted from H. H. Fink, A. E. Mikesky, and L. A. Burgoon, *Practical Applications in Sports Nutrition*. Jones & Bartlet Learning, 2012.

Lipoproteins Lipids covered by proteins, these transport fats in the blood. Types are LDL, HDL, and VLDL.

Sterols Derived fats, of which cholesterol is the best-known example.

Proteins A classification of nutrients consisting of complex organic compounds containing nitrogen and formed by combinations of amino acids; the main substances used in the body to build and repair tissues.

Enzymes Catalysts that facilitate chemical reactions in the body.

Amino acids Chemical compounds that contain nitrogen, carbon, hydrogen, and oxygen; the basic building blocks the body uses to build different types of protein.

should be limited to three ounces (smaller than a deck of cards) or less.

Vitamins

Vitamins are necessary for normal bodily metabolism, growth, and development. Vitamins are classified into two types based on their solubility:

1. Fat soluble (A, D, E, and K)
2. Water soluble (B complex and C)

The body does not manufacture most vitamins, so they can be obtained only through a well-balanced diet. To decrease loss of vitamins during cooking, natural foods should be microwaved or steamed rather than boiled in water that is thrown out later.

A few exceptions, such as vitamins A, D, and K, are formed in the body. Vitamin A is produced from beta-carotene, found mainly in yellow foods such as carrots, pumpkin, and sweet potatoes. Vitamin D is found in certain foods and is created when ultraviolet light from the sun transforms 7-dehydrocholesterol, a compound in human skin. Vitamin K is created in the body by intestinal bacteria. The major functions of vitamins are outlined in Table 3.5.

Vitamins C, E, and beta-carotene also function as antioxidants, which are thought to play a key role in preventing chronic diseases. (The specific functions of these antioxidant nutrients and of the mineral selenium, also an antioxidant, are discussed under "Antioxidants," page 105.)

Table 3.5 Major Functions of Vitamins

Nutrient	Good Sources	Major Functions	Deficiency Symptoms
Vitamin A	Milk, cheese, eggs, liver, yellow and dark green fruits and vegetables	Required for healthy bones, teeth, skin, gums, and hair; maintenance of inner mucous membranes, thereby increasing resistance to infection; adequate vision in dim light.	Night blindness; decreased growth; decreased resistance to infection; rough, dry skin
Vitamin D	Fortified milk, cod liver oil, salmon, tuna, egg yolk	Necessary for bones and teeth; needed for calcium and phosphorus absorption.	Rickets (bone softening), fractures, muscle spasms
Vitamin E	Vegetable oils, yellow and green leafy vegetables, margarine, wheat germ, whole-grain breads and cereals	Related to oxidation and normal muscle and red blood cell chemistry.	Leg cramps, red blood cell breakdown
Vitamin K	Green leafy vegetables, cauliflower, cabbage, eggs, peas, potatoes	Essential for normal blood clotting.	Hemorrhaging
Vitamin B_1 (Thiamin)	Whole-grain or enriched bread, lean meats and poultry, fish, liver, pork, poultry, organ meats, legumes, nuts, dried yeast	Assists in proper use of carbohydrates, normal functioning of nervous system, maintaining good appetite.	Loss of appetite, nausea, confusion, cardiac abnormalities, muscle spasms
Vitamin B_2 (Riboflavin)	Eggs, milk, leafy green vegetables, whole grains, lean meats, dried beans and peas	Contributes to energy release from carbohydrates, fats, and proteins; needed for normal growth and development, good vision, and healthy skin.	Cracking of the corners of the mouth, inflammation of the skin, impaired vision
Vitamin B_6 (Pyridoxine)	Vegetables, meats, whole grain cereals, soybeans, peanuts, potatoes	Necessary for protein and fatty acids metabolism and for normal red blood cell formation.	Depression, irritability, muscle spasms, nausea
Vitamin B_{12}	Meat, poultry, fish, liver, organ meats, eggs, shellfish, milk, cheese	Required for normal growth, red blood cell formation, nervous system and digestive tract functioning.	Impaired balance, weakness, drop in red blood cell count
Niacin	Liver and organ meats, meat, fish, poultry, whole grains, enriched breads, nuts, green leafy vegetables, and dried beans and peas	Contributes to energy release from carbohydrates, fats, and proteins; normal growth and development; and formation of hormones and nerve-regulating substances.	Confusion, depression, weakness, weight loss
Biotin	Liver, kidney, eggs, yeast, legumes, milk, nuts, dark green vegetables	Essential for carbohydrate metabolism and fatty acid synthesis.	Inflamed skin, muscle pain, depression, weight loss
Folic Acid	Leafy green vegetables, organ meats, whole grains and cereals, dried beans	Needed for cell growth and reproduction and for red blood cell formation.	Decreased resistance to infection
Pantothenic Acid	All natural foods, especially liver, kidney, eggs, nuts, yeast, milk, dried peas and beans, green leafy vegetables	Related to carbohydrate and fat metabolism.	Depression, low blood sugar, leg cramps, nausea, headaches
Vitamin C (Ascorbic acid)	Fruits, vegetables	Helps protect against infection; required for formation of collagenous tissue, normal blood vessels, teeth, and bones.	Slow-healing wounds, loose teeth, hemorrhaging, rough scaly skin, irritability

Minerals Approximately 25 minerals have important roles in body functioning. **Minerals** are inorganic substances contained in all cells, especially those in hard parts of the body (bones, nails, teeth). Minerals are crucial to maintaining water balance and the acid–base balance. They are essential components of respiratory pigments, enzymes, and enzyme systems, and they regulate muscular and nervous tissue impulses, blood clotting, and normal heart rhythm. The four minerals mentioned most often are calcium, iron, sodium, and selenium. Calcium deficiency may result in osteoporosis, and low iron intake can induce iron-deficiency anemia (see page 117). High sodium intake may contribute to high blood pressure. Selenium seems to be important in preventing certain types of cancer. Specific functions of some of the most important minerals are given in Table 3.6.

Water The most important nutrient is **water**, as it is involved in almost every vital body process: in digesting and absorbing food, in producing energy, in the circulatory process, in regulating body heat, in removing waste products, in building and rebuilding cells, and in transporting other nutrients. In men, about 61 percent of total body weight is water. The proportion of body weight in women is 56 percent (Figure 3.5). The difference is due primarily to the higher amount of muscle mass in men.

Almost all foods contain water, but it is found primarily in liquid foods, fruits, and vegetables. People obtain about 80 percent of the daily water needs from beverages and the remaining 20 percent from foods. Although for decades the recommendation was to consume at least eight cups of water per day, a panel of scientists at the Institute of Medicine of the National Academy of Sciences (NAS) indicated that people are getting enough water from the liquids (milk, juices, sodas, coffee) and the moisture content of solid foods. Most Americans and Canadians remain well hydrated simply by using thirst as their guide. Caffeine-containing drinks also are acceptable as a water source because data indicate that people who regularly consume such beverages do not have more 24-hour urine output than those who don't.

An exception to not waiting for the thirst signal to replenish water loss is when an individual exercises in the heat, or does so for an extended time (see Chapter 9, page 321). Water lost under these conditions must be replenished regularly. If you wait for the thirst signal, you may have lost too much water already. At two percent of body

> **Vitamins** Organic nutrients essential for normal metabolism, growth, and development of the body.
>
> **Minerals** Inorganic nutrients essential for normal body functions; found in the body and in food.
>
> **Water** The most important classification of essential body nutrients, involved in almost every vital body process.

Table 3.6 Major Functions of Minerals

Nutrient	Good Sources	Major Functions	Deficiency Symptoms
Calcium	Milk, yogurt, cheese, green leafy vegetables, dried beans, sardines, salmon	Required for strong teeth and bone formation; maintenance of good muscle tone, heartbeat, and nerve function.	Bone pain and fractures, periodontal disease, muscle cramps
Copper	Seafood, meats, beans, nuts, whole grains	Helps with iron absorption and hemoglobin formation; required to synthesize the enzyme cytochrome oxidase.	Anemia (although deficiency is rare in humans)
Iron	Organ meats, lean meats, seafood, eggs, dried peas and beans, nuts, whole and enriched grains, green leafy vegetables	Major component of hemoglobin; aids in energy utilization.	Nutritional anemia, overall weakness
Phosphorus	Meats, fish, milk, eggs, dried beans and peas, whole grains, processed foods	Required for bone and teeth formation and for energy release regulation.	Bone pain and fracture, weight loss, weakness
Zinc	Milk, meat, seafood, whole grains, nuts, eggs, dried beans	Essential component of hormones, insulin, and enzymes; used in normal growth and development.	Loss of appetite, slow-healing wounds, skin problems
Magnesium	Green leafy vegetables, whole grains, nuts, soybeans, seafood, legumes	Needed for bone growth and maintenance, carbohydrate and protein utilization, nerve function, temperature regulation.	Irregular heartbeat, weakness, muscle spasms, sleeplessness
Sodium	Table salt, processed foods, meat	Needed for body fluid regulation, transmission of nerve impulses, heart action.	Rarely seen
Potassium	Legumes, whole grains, bananas, orange juice, dried fruits, potatoes	Required for heart action, bone formation and maintenance, regulation of energy release, acid–base regulation.	Irregular heartbeat, nausea, weakness
Selenium	Seafood, meat, whole grains	Component of enzymes; functions in close association with vitamin E.	Muscle pain, possible deterioration of heart muscle, possible hair loss and nail loss

© Cengage Learning

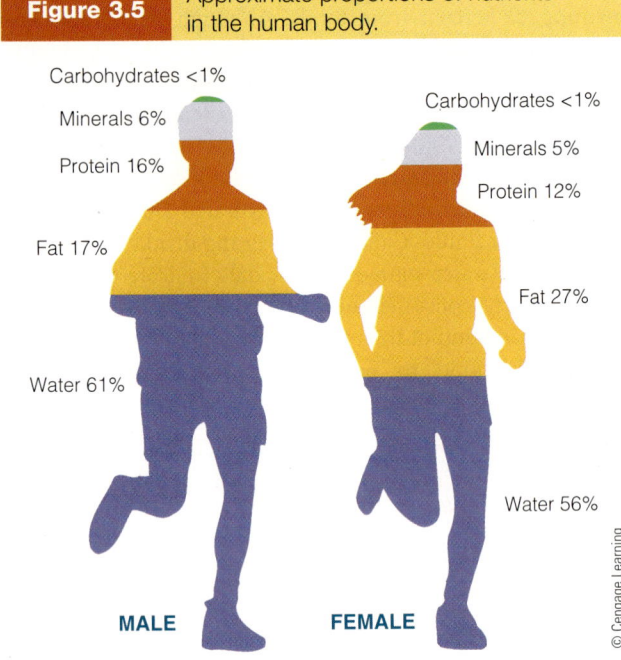

Figure 3.5 Approximate proportions of nutrients in the human body.

weight lost, a person is dehydrated. At five percent, one may become dizzy and disoriented, have trouble with cognitive skills and heart function, and even lose consciousness.

3.2 Balancing the Diet

One of the fundamental ways to enjoy good health and live life to its fullest is through a well-balanced diet. Several guidelines have been published to help you accomplish this. As illustrated in Table 3.7, the most recent recommended guidelines by the NAS state that daily caloric intake should be distributed so that 45 to 65 percent of total calories come from carbohydrates (mostly complex carbohydrates and less than 25 percent from sugar), 20 to 35 percent from fat, and 10 to 35 percent from protein.[8] The recommended ranges allow for flexibility in planning diets according to individual health and physical activity needs.

In addition to the macronutrients, the diet must include all of the essential vitamins, minerals, and water. The source of fat calories is also critical. The National Cholesterol Education Program recommends that, of total calories, saturated fat should constitute less than 7 percent, polyunsaturated fat up to 10 percent, and monounsaturated fat up to 20 percent. Rating a particular diet accurately is difficult without a complete nutrient analysis. You have an opportunity to perform this analysis in Activity 3.1.

The NAS guidelines vary slightly from those previously issued by major national health organizations, which recommend 50 to 60 percent of total calories from carbohydrates, less than 30 percent from fat, and about 15 percent from protein. These percentages are within the ranges recommended by the NAS. The most drastic difference appears in the NAS-allowed range of fat intake, up to 35 percent of total calories. This higher percentage, however, was included to accommodate individuals with metabolic syndrome (see Chapter 10, page 360), who have an abnormal insulin response to carbohydrates and may need additional fat in the diet. For all other individuals, daily fat intake should not exceed 30 percent of total caloric intake.

The NAS recommendations will be effective only if people consistently replace saturated and trans fatty acids with unsaturated fatty acids. The latter will require changes in the typical "unhealthy" American diet, which is generally high in red meat, whole dairy products, and fast foods—all of which are high in saturated and/or trans fatty acids.

Diets in most developed countries changed significantly in the early 20th century. Today, people eat more calories and fat, fewer carbohydrates, and about the same amount of protein. People also weigh more than they did in 1900, an indication that we are eating more calories and are not as physically active as our forebears.

Surveys indicate that on average people now eat out one meal per day compared to only two per week in the 1970s. Not only do Americans eat more when they eat out, but they also eat far fewer healthy foods than at home. Among the most popular foods ordered at restaurants and fast-food places today are French fries, hamburgers, and pizza. About one-fifth of all restaurant meals are purchased at drive-throughs, with almost one-half of young people and a third of baby boomers indicating that they eat full meals in the car. In contrast, whenever possible, healthy eating implies consuming primarily whole, fresh, or locally grown food items made with few ingredients and minimal processing and packaging.

Nutrition Standards Nutritionists use a variety of nutrient standards, the most widely known of which is **Recommended Dietary Allowance (RDA)**. Others are the **Dietary Reference Intakes (DRI)** and the **Daily Values (DV)** on food labels. Each standard has a different purpose and utilization in dietary planning and assessment.

Table 3.7 The American Diet: Current and Recommended Carbohydrate, Fat, and Protein Intake Expressed as a Percentage of Total Calories

	Current Percentage	Recommended Percentage*
Carbohydrates:	50%	45–65%
Simple	26%	Less than 25%
Complex	24%	20–40%
Fat:	34%	20–30%**
Monounsaturated:	11%	Up to 20%
Polyunsaturated:	10%	Up to 10%
Saturated:	13%	Less than 7%
Protein:	16%	10–35%

*SOURCE: Adapted from the National Academy of Sciences, Institute of Medicine. *Dietary Reference Intakes for Energy, Carbohydrates, Fiber, Fat, Protein and Amino Acids (macronutrients).* Washington D.C.: National Academy Press, 2002.

**Less than 30% is recommended by most major national health organizations. Up to 35% is allowed for individuals with metabolic syndrome who may need additional fat in the diet.

Dietary Reference Intakes

To help people meet dietary guidelines, the NAS developed the DRIs for healthy people in the United States and Canada. The DRIs are based on a review of the most current research on nutrient needs of healthy people. The DRI reports are written by the Food and Nutrition Board of the Institute of Medicine in cooperation with scientists from Canada.

The DRI encompass four types of reference values—including the RDA—for planning and assessing diets and for establishing adequate amounts and maximum safe nutrient intakes in the diet. The other three reference values are **Estimated Average Requirement (EAR)**, **Adequate Intakes (AI)**, and **Tolerable Upper Intake Levels (UL)**. The type of reference value used for a given nutrient and a specific age/gender group is determined according to available scientific information and the intended use of the dietary standard.

Nutrients for which a daily DRI has been set are given in Table 3.8.

Estimated Average Requirement. The EAR is the amount of a nutrient that is estimated to meet the nutrient requirement of half the healthy people in specific age and gender groups. At this nutrient intake level, the nutritional requirements of 50 percent of the people are not met. For example, looking at 300 healthy women at age 26, the EAR would meet the nutritional requirement for only half of these women.

Recommended Dietary Allowance. The RDA is the daily amount of a nutrient that is considered adequate to meet the known nutrient needs of nearly all healthy people in the United States. A committee of the Food and Nutrition Board of the NAS determines RDAs of nutrients. Because the committee must decide what level of intake to recommend for everybody, the RDA is set well above the EAR and covers about 98 percent of the population. Stated another way, the RDA recommendation for any nutrient is well above almost everyone's actual requirement. The RDA could be considered a goal for adequate intake. The process for determining the RDA depends on being able to set an EAR, because RDAs are determined statistically from the EAR values. If an EAR cannot be set, no RDA can be established.

Adequate Intake. When data are insufficient or inadequate to set an EAR, an AI value is determined instead of the RDA. A group or groups of healthy people derive the AI value from approximations of observed nutrient intakes. The AI value for children and adults is expected to meet or exceed the nutritional requirements of a corresponding healthy population.

Tolerable Upper Intake Level. The UL establishes the highest level of nutrient intake that seems to be safe for most healthy people, beyond which exists an increased risk for adverse effects. As intakes increase above the UL, so does the risk for adverse effects. Established UL values are presented in Table 3.9.

Daily Values

The DVs are reference values for nutrients and food components listed on food-packaging labels. The DVs include measures of fat, saturated fat, and carbohydrates (as a percent of total calories); cholesterol, sodium, and potassium (in milligrams); and fiber and protein (in grams). The DVs for total fat, saturated fat, and carbohydrates are expressed as percentages for a 2,000-calorie diet and therefore may require adjustments depending on an individual's daily **estimated energy requirement (EER)** in calories. For example, for a 2,000-calorie diet (the EER), the recommended carbohydrate intake is about 300 grams (about 60 percent

> **Recommended Dietary Allowance (RDA)** The daily amount of a nutrient (statistically determined from the EARs) that is considered adequate to meet the known nutrient needs of almost 98 percent of all healthy people in the United States.
>
> **Dietary Reference Intakes (DRI)** A general term that describes four types of nutrient standards that establish adequate amounts and maximum safe nutrient intakes in the diet: Estimated Average Requirements (EAR), Recommended Dietary Allowances (RDA), Adequate Intakes (AI), and Tolerable Upper Intake Levels (UL).
>
> **Daily Values (DV)** Reference values for nutrients and food components used in food labels.
>
> **Estimated Average Requirement (EAR)** The amount of a nutrient that meets the dietary needs of half the people.
>
> **Adequate Intake (AI)** The recommended amount of a nutrient intake when sufficient evidence is not available to calculate the EAR and subsequent RDA.
>
> **Tolerable Upper Intake Level (UL)** The highest level of nutrient intake that seems safe for most healthy people, beyond which exists an increased risk of adverse effects.
>
> **Estimated Energy Requirement (EER)** The average dietary energy (caloric) intake that is predicted to maintain energy balance in a healthy adult of defined age, gender, weight, height, and level of physical activity, consistent with good health.

The typical American diet is too high in calories and unhealthy fats.

Table 3.8 Dietary Reference Intakes (DRIs): Recommended Dietary Allowances (RDA) and Adequate Intakes (AI) for Selected Nutrients

	Recommended Dietary Allowances (RDA)															Adequate Intakes (AI)			
	Thiamin (mg)	Riboflavin (mg)	Niacin (mg NE)	Vitamin B$_6$ (mg)	Folate (µg)	Vitamin B$_{12}$ (µg)	Phosphorus (mg)	Magnesium (mg)	Vitamin A (µg)	Vitamin C (mg)	Vitamin D (µg)	Vitamin E (mg)	Selenium (mcg)	Iron (mg)	Calcium (mg)	Fluoride (mg)	Pantothenic acid (mg)	Biotin (mg)	Choline (mg)
Males																			
14–18	1.2	1.3	16	1.3	400	2.4	1,250	410	900	75	15	15	55	11	1,300	3	5.0	25	550
19–30	1.2	1.3	16	1.3	400	2.4	700	400	900	90	15	15	55	8	1,000	4	5.0	30	550
31–50	1.2	1.3	16	1.3	400	2.4	700	420	900	90	15	15	55	8	1,000	4	5.0	30	550
51–70	1.2	1.3	16	1.7	400	2.4	700	420	900	90	15	15	55	8	1,000	4	5.0	30	550
>70	1.2	1.3	16	1.7	400	2.4	700	420	900	90	20	15	55	8	1,200	4	5.0	30	550
Females																			
14–18	1.0	1.0	14	1.2	400	2.4	1,250	360	700	65	15	15	55	15	1,300	3	5.0	25	400
19–30	1.1	1.1	14	1.3	400	2.4	700	310	700	75	15	15	55	18	1,000	3	5.0	30	425
31–50	1.1	1.1	14	1.3	400	2.4	700	320	700	75	15	15	55	18	1,000	3	5.0	30	425
51–70	1.1	1.1	14	1.5	400	2.4	700	320	700	75	15	15	55	8	1,200	3	5.0	30	425
>70	1.1	1.1	14	1.5	400	2.4	700	320	700	75	20	15	55	8	1,200	3	5.0	30	425
Pregnant (19–30)	1.4	1.4	18	1.9	600	2.6	*	+40	770	85	15	15	60	27	1,000	3	6.0	30	450
Lactating (19–30)	1.4	1.6	17	2.0	500	2.8	*	*	1,300	120	15	19	70	9	1,000	3	7.0	35	550

*Values for these nutrients do not change with pregnancy or lactation. Use the value listed for women of comparable age.

SOURCE: Reprinted with permission from "Dietary Reference Intakes: Recommended Dietary Allowances and Adequate Intakes, Elements," and "Dietary Reference Intakes for Calcium and Vitamin D," 2011 by the National Academy of Sciences, Courtesy of the National Academics Press, Washington D.C.

Table 3.9 Tolerable Upper Intake Levels (UL) of Selected Nutrients for Adults (19–70 years)

Nutrient	UL per Day
Calcium	2.5 gr
Phosphorus	4.0 gr*
Magnesium	350 mg
Vitamin D	50 mcg
Fluoride	10 mg
Niacin	35 mg
Iron	45 mg
Vitamin B$_6$	100 mg
Folate	1,000 mcg
Choline	3.5 gr
Vitamin A	3,000 mcg
Vitamin C	2,000 mg
Vitamin E	1,000 mg
Selenium	400 mcg

*3.5 gr per day for pregnant women.

SOURCE: Adapted from the National Academy of Sciences, Institute of Medicine. Dietary Reference Intakes for Tolerable Upper Intake Levels, Vitamins. Washington D.C. National Academy Press, 2011.

of the EER), and the recommendation for fat is 65 grams (about 30 percent of EER). The vitamin, mineral, and protein DV were adapted from the RDA. The DV also are not as specific for age and gender groups as are the DRI. Both the DRI and the DV apply to only healthy adults. They are not intended for people who are ill, who may require additional nutrients. Figure 3.6 shows a food label with U.S. Recommended Daily Values.

Critical Thinking

What do the nutrition standards mean to you? • How much of a challenge would it be to apply those standards in your daily life?

Nutrient Analysis The first step in evaluating your diet is to conduct a nutrient analysis. This can be quite educational, because most people do not realize how harmful and nonnutritious many common foods are. The top sources of

Figure 3.6 Food label with U.S. Recommended Daily Values.

1 Better by Design
How to recognize the new food labels
The new food labels feature a revamped nutrition panel titled "Nutrition Facts," with nutrient listings that reflect current health concerns. Now you'll be able to find information on fat, fiber, and other food components fundamental to lowering your risk of cancer and other chronic diseases. Listings for nutrients like thiamin and riboflavin will no longer be required because Americans generally eat enough of them these days.

2 Size Up the Situation
All serving sizes are created equal
Now you can compare similar products and know that their serving sizes are basically identical. So when you realize how much fat is packed into that carton of double-dutch-chocolate-caramel-chew ice cream you're eyeing, you might opt for low-fat frozen yogurt instead. Serving sizes will also be standardized, so manufacturers can't make nutrition claims for unrealistically small portions. That means a chocolate cake, for example, must be divided into 8 servings sized to satisfy the average person—not 16 servings sized to satisfy the average munchkin.

3 Look Before You Leap
Use the Daily Values
You will find the Daily Values on the bottom half of the "Nutrition Facts" panel. Some represent maximum levels of nutrients that should be consumed each day for a healthful diet (as with fat), while others refer to minimum levels that can be exceeded (as with carbohydrates). They are based on both a 2,000 and 2,500 calorie diet. Your own needs may be more or less, but these figures give you a point from which to compare. For example, the sample label indicates that someone with a 2,000 calorie diet should eat no more than 65 grams of fat per day. This is based on a diet getting 30 percent of calories as fat. If you normally eat less calories or want to eat less than 30 percent of calories as fat, your daily fat consumption will be lower.

4 Rate It Right
Scan the % Daily Values
The % Daily Values make judging the nutritional quality of a food a snap. For instance, you can look at the % Daily Value column and find that a food has 25 percent of the Daily Value for fiber. This means the product will give you a substantial portion of the recommended amount of fiber for the day. You can also use this column to compare nutrients in similar products. The % Daily Values are based on a 2,000 calorie diet.

5 Trust Adjectives
Descriptors have legal definitions
Terms like "low," "high," and "free" have long been used on food labels. What these words actually mean, however, could vary. Thanks to the new labeling laws, such descriptions must now meet legal definitions. For example, you may be shopping for foods high in vitamin A, which has been linked to lower risk of certain cancers. Under the new label laws, a food described as "high" in a particular nutrient must contain 20 percent or more of the Daily Value for that nutrient. So if the bottle of juice you're thinking of buying says "high in vitamin A," you can now feel confident that it really is a good source of the vitamin.

6 Read Health Claims with Confidence
The nutrient link to disease prevention
You can also expect to see food packages with health claims linking certain nutrients to reduced risk of cancer and other diseases. The federal government has approved three health claims dealing with cancer prevention: a low-fat diet may reduce your risk for cancer; high-fiber foods may reduce your risk for cancer; and fruits and vegetables may reduce your risk for cancer. A food may not make such a health claim for one nutrient if it contains other nutrients that undermine its health benefits. A high-fiber, but high-fat, jelly doughnut cannot carry a health claim!

Reprinted with permission from the American Institute for Cancer Research.

An apple a day will not keep the doctor away if most meals are high in calories, saturated fat, and trans fat content.

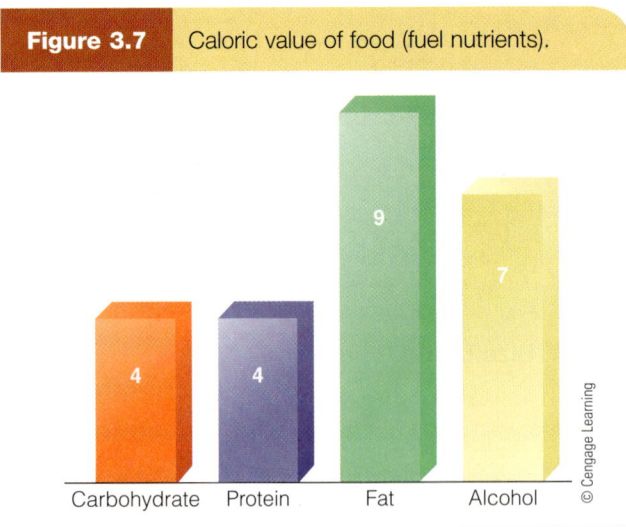

Figure 3.7 Caloric value of food (fuel nutrients).

calories in the American diet are soft drinks, sweet rolls, pastries, doughnuts, cakes, hamburgers, cheeseburgers, meatloaf, pizza, potato and corn chips, and buttered popcorn, all of which are low in essential nutrients and high in fat and/or sugar and calories.

Most nutrient analyses cover calories, carbohydrates, fats, cholesterol, and sodium, as well as eight essential nutrients: protein, calcium, iron, vitamin A, thiamin, riboflavin, niacin, and vitamin C. If the diet has enough of these eight nutrients, the foods consumed in natural form to provide these nutrients typically contain all the other nutrients the human body needs.

To do your own nutrient analysis, keep a three-day record of everything you eat using Activity 3.1 (make additional copies of this form as needed). At the end of each day, look up the nutrient content for those foods in the list of Nutritive Values of Selected Foods (in Appendix A). Record this information on the form in Activity 3.1. If you do not find a food in Appendix A, the information may be on the food container itself.

When you have recorded the nutritive values for each day, add up each column and write the totals at the bottom of the chart. After the third day, fill in your totals in Activity 3.2 and compute an average for the three days. To rate your diet, compare your figures with those in the RDA (see Table 3.8). The results will give a good indication of areas of strength and deficiency in your current diet.

Some of the most revealing information learned in a nutrient analysis is the source of fat and saturated fat intake in the diet. The average daily fat consumption in the U.S. diet is about 34 percent of the total caloric intake, much of it from saturated fats, which increases the risk for chronic diseases such as cardiovascular disease, cancer, diabetes, and obesity. Although fat provides a smaller percentage of our total daily caloric intake compared with two decades ago (37 percent), the decrease in percentage is simply because Americans now eat more calories than 20 years ago (335 additional daily calories for women and 170 for men).

As illustrated in Figure 3.7, one gram of carbohydrate or protein supplies the body with four calories, and fat provides nine calories per gram consumed (alcohol yields seven calories per gram). Therefore, looking at only the total grams consumed for each type of food can be misleading.

For example, a person who eats 160 grams of carbohydrates, 100 grams of fat, and 70 grams of protein has a total intake of 330 grams of food. This indicates that 30 percent of the total grams of food is in the form of fat (100 grams of fat ÷ 330 grams of total food = 0.30; .30 × 100 = 30 percent)—and, in reality, almost half of that diet is in the form of fat calories.

In the sample diet, 640 calories are derived from carbohydrates (160 grams × 4 calories per gram), 280 calories from protein (70 grams × 4 calories per gram), and 900 calories from fat (100 grams × 9 calories per gram), for a total of 1,820 calories. If 900 calories are derived from fat, almost half of the total caloric intake is in the form of fat (900 ÷ 1,820 × 100 = 49.5 percent).

Each gram of fat provides nine calories—more than twice the calories of a gram of carbohydrate or protein. When figuring out the percentage of fat calories of individual foods, you may find Figure 3.8 to be a useful guideline. Multiply the total fat grams by nine and divide by the total calories in that particular food (per serving). Then multiply that number by 100 to get the percentage. For example, the food label in Figure 3.8 lists a total of 120 calories and five grams of fat, and the equation below it shows the fat content to be 38 percent of total calories. This simple guideline can help you decrease the fat in your diet.

The fat content of selected foods, given in grams and as a percent of total calories, is presented in Figure 3.9. The percentage of fat is further subdivided into saturated, monounsaturated, polyunsaturated, and other fatty acids.

Behavior Modification Planning

Caloric and Fat Content of Selected Fast Food Items

Item	Calories	Total Fat (grams)	Saturated Fat (grams)	Percent Fat Calories
Burgers				
McDonald's Big Mac	590	34	11	52
McDonald's Big N' Tasty with Cheese	590	37	12	56
McDonald's Quarter Pounder with Cheese	530	30	13	51
Burger King Whopper	760	46	15	54
Burger King Bacon Double Cheeseburger	580	34	18	53
Burger King BK Smokehouse Cheddar Griller	720	48	19	60
Burger King Whopper with Cheese	850	53	22	56
Burger King Double Whopper	1,060	69	27	59
Burger King Double Whopper with Cheese	1,150	76	33	59
Wendy's Baconator	830	51	22	55
Sandwiches				
Arby's Regular Roast Beef	350	16	6	41
Arby's Super Roast Beef	470	23	7	44
Arby's Roast Chicken Club	520	28	7	48
Arby's Market Fresh Roast Beef & Swiss	810	42	13	47
McDonald's Crispy Chicken	430	21	8	43
McDonald's Filet-O-Fish	470	26	5	50
McDonald's Chicken McGrill	400	17	3	38
Wendy's Chicken Club	470	19	4	36
Wendy's Breast Fillet	430	16	3	34
Wendy's Grilled Chicken	300	7	2	21
Burger King Specialty Chicken	560	28	6	45
Subway Veggie Delight*	226	3	1	12
Subway Turkey Breast	281	5	2	16
Subway Sweet Onion Chicken Teriyaki	374	5	2	12
Subway Steak & Cheese	390	14	5	32
Subway Cold Cut Trio	440	21	7	43
Subway Tuna	450	22	6	44
Mexican				
Taco Bell Crunchy Taco	170	10	4	53
Taco Bell Taco Supreme	220	14	6	57
Taco Bell Soft Chicken Taco	190	7	3	33
Taco Bell Bean Burrito	370	12	4	29
Taco Bell Fiesta Steak Burrito	370	12	4	29
Taco Bell Grilled Steak Soft Taco	290	17	4	53
Taco Bell Double Decker Taco	340	14	5	37
French Fries				
Wendy's, biggie (5½ oz)	440	19	7	39
McDonald's, large (6 oz)	540	26	9	43
Burger King, large (5½ oz)	500	25	13	45
Shakes				
Wendy's Frosty, medium (16 oz)	440	11	7	23
McDonald's McFlurry, small (12 oz)	610	22	14	32
Burger King, Old Fashioned Ice Cream Shake, medium (22 oz)	760	41	29	49
Hash Browns				
McDonald's Hash Browns (2 oz)	130	8	4	55
Burger King, Hash Browns, small (2½ oz)	230	15	9	59

*6-inch sandwich with no mayo

Try It

Using the information in the table, record in your Online Journal or class notebook ways you can restructure fast-food consumption to decrease caloric value and fat and saturated fat content in your diet.

SOURCE: Adapted from *Restaurant Confidential* Copyright © 2002 by the Center for Science in the Public Interest. Used by permission of Workman Publishing Co., Inc., New York. All rights reserved.

Figure 3.8 Computation for fat content in food.

Nutrition Facts
Serving Size 1 cup (240 ml)
Servings Per Container 4

Amount Per Serving	
Calories 120	Calories from Fat 45
	% Daily Value*
Total Fat 5g	8%
Saturated Fat 3g	15%
Trans Fat 0g	0%
Cholesterol 20mg	7%
Sodium 120mg	5%
Total Carbohydrate 12g	4%
Dietary Fiber 0g	0%
Sugars 12g	
Protein 8g	

| Vitamin A | 10% | • | Vitamin C | 4% |
| Calcium | 30% | • | Iron | 0% |

* Percent Daily Values are based on a 2,000 calorie diet. Your daily values may be higher or lower depending on your calorie needs:

		Calories	2,000	2,500
Total Fat	Less than		65g	80g
Sat Fat	Less than		20g	25g
Cholesterol	Less than		300mg	300mg
Sodium	Less than		2,300mg	2,300mg
Total Carbohydrate			300g	375g
Fiber			25g	30g

Calories per gram:
Fat 9 • Carbohydrate 4 • Protein 4

Percent fat calories = (grams of fat × 9) ÷ calories per serving × 100

5 grams of fat × 9 calories per grams of fat = 45 calories from fat

45 calories from fat ÷ 120 calories per serving × 100 = 38% fat

3.3 Achieving a Balanced Diet

Anyone who has completed a nutrient analysis and has given careful attention to Tables 3.3 (vitamins) and 3.4 (minerals) probably will realize that a well-balanced diet entails eating a variety of nutrient-dense foods and monitoring total daily caloric intake. The MyPlate healthy food plan in Figure 3.1 (page 75) contains five major food groups. The food groups are fruits, vegetables, grains, protein, and dairy. A Healthy Eating Plate, based on the MyPlate guidelines, was subsequently developed by the Harvard School of Public Health to offer specific recommendations for healthier food choices within the various food groups (Figure 3.10).

For most meals, three quarters of the plate should be taken up by fruits, vegetables, and grains, as they provide the nutritional base for a healthy diet. When increasing the intake of these food groups, it is important to decrease the intake of low-nutrient foods to effectively balance caloric intake with energy needs. These foods should be complemented with low-fat milk/dairy products and small amounts of lean sources of protein.

In addition to providing nutrients crucial to health, fruits and vegetables are the sole source of **phytonutrients** ("phyto" comes from the Greek word for plant). These compounds show promising results in the fight against cancer and heart disease. More than 4,000 phytonutrients have been identified. The main function of phytonutrients in plants is to protect them from sunlight. In humans, phytonutrients seem to have a powerful ability to block the formation of cancerous tumors. Their actions are so diverse that at almost every stage of cancer, phytonutrients have the ability to block, disrupt, slow, or even reverse the process. In terms of heart disease, they may reduce inflammation, inhibit blood clots, or prevent the oxidation of LDL cholesterol.

The consistent message is to eat a diet with ample fruits and vegetables. The daily recommended amount of fruits and vegetables has absolutely no substitute. Science has not yet found a way to allow people to eat a poor diet, pop a few pills, and derive the same benefits.

Whole grains are a major source of fiber as well as other nutrients. Whole grains contain the entire grain kernel (the bran, germ, and endosperm). Examples include whole-wheat flour, whole cornmeal, oatmeal, cracked wheat (bulgur), and brown rice. Refined grains have been milled—a process that removes the bran and germ. The process also removes fiber, iron, and many B vitamins. Refined grains include white flour, white bread, white rice, and degermed cornmeal. Refined grains are often enriched to add back B vitamins and iron. Fiber, however, is not added back.

Milk and milk products (select low-fat or nonfat) can decrease the risk of low bone mass (osteoporosis) throughout life. Besides calcium, other nutrients from milk are potassium, vitamin D, and protein.

Foods in the protein group consist of poultry, fish, eggs, nuts, legumes, and seeds. Nutrients in this group include protein, B vitamins, vitamin E, iron, zinc, and magnesium. Choose low-fat or lean meats and poultry and bake, grill, or broil them at low temperature (to prevent the formation of advanced glycation end products; see page 102). Most Americans eat sufficient food in this group but need to choose leaner foods and a greater variety of fish, dry beans, nuts, and seeds. In terms of meat, poultry, and fish, the recommendation is to consume about three ounces and not to exceed six ounces daily. All visible fat and skin should be trimmed off meats and poultry before cooking.

Oils are fats that come from different plants and fish and are liquid at room temperature. Choose carefully and avoid oils that have trans fats (check the food la-

> **Phytonutrients** Compounds thought to prevent and fight cancer; found in large quantities in fruits and vegetables.

Activity 3.1: Daily Nutrient Intake

Date:

Foods	Amount	Calories	Protein (g)	Fat (total g)	Sat. Fat (g)	Cho- lesterol (mg)	Carbo- hydrates (g)	Dietary Fiber (g)	Calcium (mg)	Iron (mg)	Sodium (mg)	Vit. E (mg)	Folate (mcg)	Vit. C (mg)	Selenium (mcg)
Totals															

Activity 3.2: Analysis of Daily Nutrient Intake

Name: _____

Day	Calories	Protein (g)	Fat (g)	Sat. Fat (g)	Cho-lesterol (mg)	Carbo-hydrates (g)	Dietary Fiber (g)	Calcium (mg)	Iron (mg)	Sodium (mg)	Vit. E (mg)	Folate (mcg)	Vit. C (mg)	Selenium (mcg)
One														
Two														
Three														
Totals														
Average[a]														
Percentages[b]														
Recommended Dietary Allowances*														
Men														
14–18 yrs.	See below[c]	See below[d]	20–30%[e]	7%	<300	45–65%	38	1,300	12	2,300	15	400	75	55
19–30 yrs.			20–30%[e]	7%	<300	45–65%	38	1,000	10	2,300	15	400	90	55
31–50 yrs.			20–30%[e]	7%	<300	45–65%	38	1,000	10	2,300	15	400	90	55
51+ yrs.			20–30%[e]	7%	<300	45–65%	30	1,000	10	2,300	15	400	90	55
Women														
14–18 yrs.			20–30%[e]	7%	<300	45–65%	25	1,300	15	2,300	15	400	65	55
19–30 yrs.			20–30%[e]	7%	<300	45–65%	25	1,000	15	2,300	15	400	75	55
31–50 yrs.			20–30%[e]	7%	<300	45–65%	25	1,000	15	2,300	15	400	75	55
51+ yrs.			20–30%[e]	7%	<300	45–65%	21	1,200	15	2,300	15	400	75	55
Pregnant			20–30%[e]	7%	<300	45–65%	25	1,200	30	2,300	15	600	85	60
Lactating			20–30%[e]	7%	<300	45–65%	25	1,200	15	2,300	15	500	120	70

[a] Divide totals by 3 or number of days assessed.
[b] Percentages: Protein and carbohydrates = multiply average by 4, divide by average calories, and multiply by 100.
Fat and saturated fat = multiply average by 9, divide by average calories, and multiply by 100.
[c] Use Table 5.5 (page 176) for all categories.
[d] Protein intake should be between .8 and 2.0 grams per kilogram of body weight (see Table 3.4 page 83). Pregnant women should consume an additional 15 grams of daily protein, and lactating women should have an extra 20 grams.
[e] Up to 35% is allowed for individuals who suffer from metabolic syndrome.
*Based on recommendations by nutrition experts.
*Adapted from *Recommended Dietary Allowances*, 10th Edition, and the Dietary Reference Intakes series, National Academy of Sciences 1989, 1997, 1998, 2000, 2001. Washington, DC.

Figure 3.9 Fat content of selected foods.

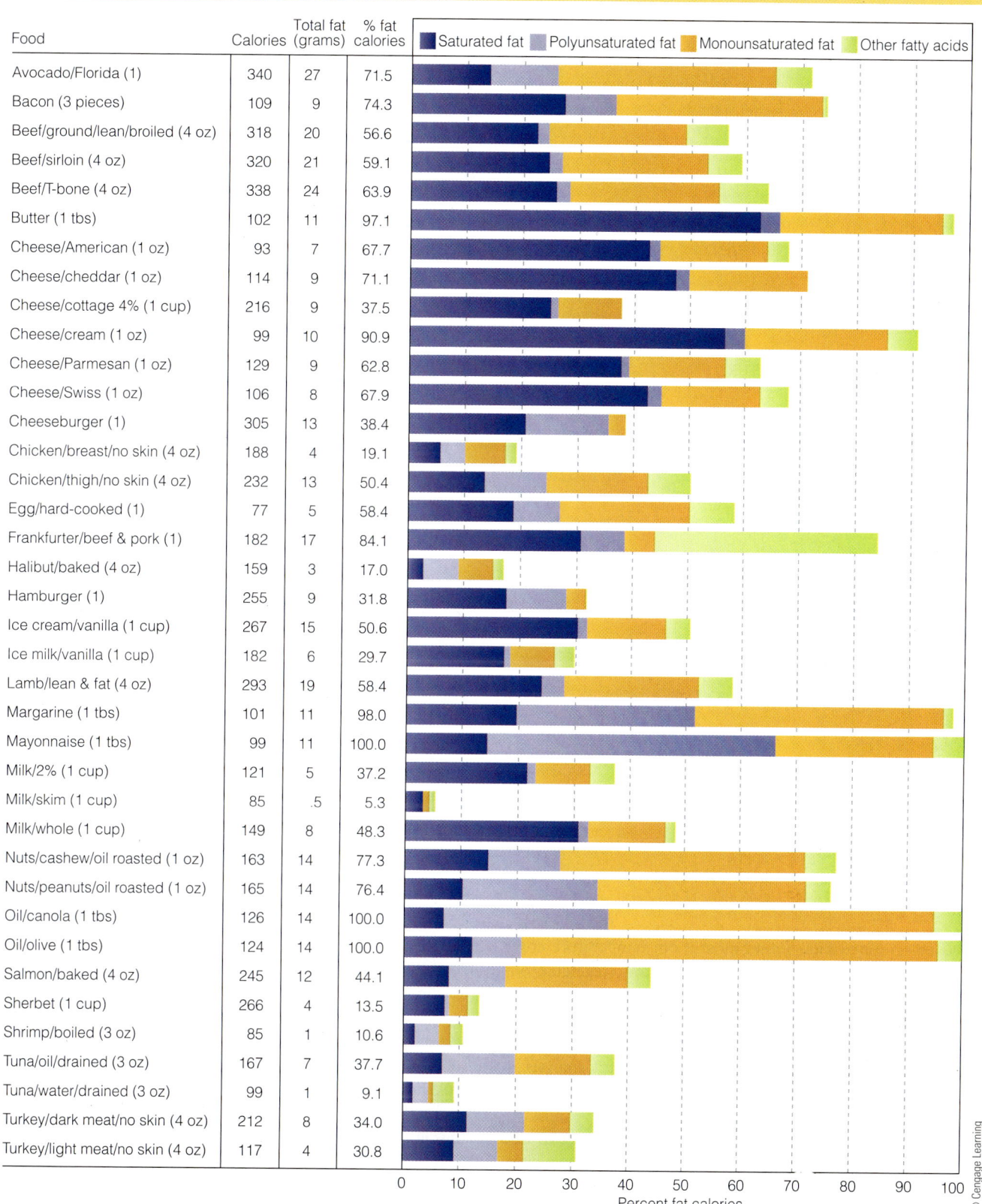

Food	Calories	Total fat (grams)	% fat calories
Avocado/Florida (1)	340	27	71.5
Bacon (3 pieces)	109	9	74.3
Beef/ground/lean/broiled (4 oz)	318	20	56.6
Beef/sirloin (4 oz)	320	21	59.1
Beef/T-bone (4 oz)	338	24	63.9
Butter (1 tbs)	102	11	97.1
Cheese/American (1 oz)	93	7	67.7
Cheese/cheddar (1 oz)	114	9	71.1
Cheese/cottage 4% (1 cup)	216	9	37.5
Cheese/cream (1 oz)	99	10	90.9
Cheese/Parmesan (1 oz)	129	9	62.8
Cheese/Swiss (1 oz)	106	8	67.9
Cheeseburger (1)	305	13	38.4
Chicken/breast/no skin (4 oz)	188	4	19.1
Chicken/thigh/no skin (4 oz)	232	13	50.4
Egg/hard-cooked (1)	77	5	58.4
Frankfurter/beef & pork (1)	182	17	84.1
Halibut/baked (4 oz)	159	3	17.0
Hamburger (1)	255	9	31.8
Ice cream/vanilla (1 cup)	267	15	50.6
Ice milk/vanilla (1 cup)	182	6	29.7
Lamb/lean & fat (4 oz)	293	19	58.4
Margarine (1 tbs)	101	11	98.0
Mayonnaise (1 tbs)	99	11	100.0
Milk/2% (1 cup)	121	5	37.2
Milk/skim (1 cup)	85	.5	5.3
Milk/whole (1 cup)	149	8	48.3
Nuts/cashew/oil roasted (1 oz)	163	14	77.3
Nuts/peanuts/oil roasted (1 oz)	165	14	76.4
Oil/canola (1 tbs)	126	14	100.0
Oil/olive (1 tbs)	124	14	100.0
Salmon/baked (4 oz)	245	12	44.1
Sherbet (1 cup)	266	4	13.5
Shrimp/boiled (3 oz)	85	1	10.6
Tuna/oil/drained (3 oz)	167	7	37.7
Tuna/water/drained (3 oz)	99	1	9.1
Turkey/dark meat/no skin (4 oz)	212	8	34.0
Turkey/light meat/no skin (4 oz)	117	4	30.8

Percent fat calories

Behavior Modification Planning

"Super" Foods

The following "super" foods that fight disease and promote health should be included often in the diet.

I PLAN TO / I DID IT

- ❏ ❏ Acai berries
- ❏ ❏ Avocados
- ❏ ❏ Bananas
- ❏ ❏ Barley
- ❏ ❏ Beans
- ❏ ❏ Beets
- ❏ ❏ Blueberries
- ❏ ❏ Broccoli
- ❏ ❏ Butternut squash
- ❏ ❏ Carrots
- ❏ ❏ Goji berries
- ❏ ❏ Grapes
- ❏ ❏ Kale
- ❏ ❏ Kiwifruit
- ❏ ❏ Flaxseeds
- ❏ ❏ Lentils
- ❏ ❏ Nuts (Brazil, walnuts)
- ❏ ❏ Salmon (wild)
- ❏ ❏ Soy
- ❏ ❏ Oats and oatmeal
- ❏ ❏ Olives and olive oil
- ❏ ❏ Onions
- ❏ ❏ Oranges
- ❏ ❏ Peppers
- ❏ ❏ Pomegranates
- ❏ ❏ Quinoa
- ❏ ❏ Strawberries
- ❏ ❏ Spinach
- ❏ ❏ Sweet potatoes
- ❏ ❏ Tea (green, black, red)
- ❏ ❏ Tomatoes
- ❏ ❏ Walnuts
- ❏ ❏ Watermelon
- ❏ ❏ Yogurt

Try It

Using the above list, make a list of which super foods you can add to your diet and when you can eat them (snacks/meals). List meals that you can add these foods to.

© Cengage Learning

---

bel) or saturated fats. Solid fats at room temperature come from animal sources or can be made from vegetable oils through the process of hydrogenation.

As an aid to balancing your diet, the form in Activity 3.3 enables you to record your daily food intake. This record is much easier to keep than the complete dietary analysis in Activities 3.1 and 3.2. Make one copy for each day you wish to record.

To start the activity, go to www.choosemyplate.gov/ and establish your personal Daily Food Plan based on your age, gender, height, weight, and physical activity level. To do so, select the 'SuperTracker & Other Tools' tab and choose 'Daily Food Plans.' Now click on 'Daily Food Plan' at the beginning of the text under 'Daily Food Plans and Worksheets.' You may also go directly to www.choosemyplate.gov/myplate/index.aspx. Now fill in your personal information and record it on the form provided in Activity 3.2. Next, whenever you have something to eat, record the food and the amount eaten according to the MyPlate standard amounts (ounce, cup, or teaspoon—Figure 3.1). Do this immediately after each meal so you will be able to keep track of your actual food intake more easily. At the end of the day, evaluate your diet by checking whether you ate the minimum required amounts for each food group. If you meet the minimum required servings at the end of each day and your caloric intake is in balance with the recommended amount, you are taking good steps to a healthier you.

Choosing Healthy Foods Once you have completed the nutrient analysis and the healthy diet plan (Activities 3.1 and 3.2), you may conduct a self-evaluation of your current nutritional habits. In Activity 3.4, you can also assess your

Figure 3.10 Healthy Eating Plate.

current stage of change regarding healthy nutrition and list strategies to help you improve your diet.

Initially, developing healthy eating habits requires a conscious effort to select nutritious foods (see box on page 100).

You can restructure your meals so that whole grains and vegetables constitute the major portion of the meal; meats or fish are on the side and added primarily for flavoring; fruits are used for desserts; and low-fat or nonfat milk products are used.

You must learn the nutritive value of typical foods that you eat. You can do so by reading food labels and looking up the nutritive values using listings such as that provided in Appendix A or by using computer software available for such purposes.

Although not a major concern, be aware that in a few cases there is label misinformation. Whether it is a simple mistake or outright deception is difficult to determine because there is little testing of food products and limited risks (penalties) if label misrepresentation occurs. The FDA simply does not have adequate staffing to regularly check food labels.

A limited number of organizations are trying to help. For example, the Florida Department of Agriculture and Consumer Services has found a 10 percent violation rate in food products tested. As a consumer, you may never know which products are mislabeled, although in a few cases you may be able to discern the truth by yourself. If a product claims to be low in calories and fat but tastes "too good to be true," that may indeed be the case. For example, an independent analysis of Rising Dough Bakery cookies found that the oatmeal cranberry cookie (the size of a compact disk) had more than twice as many calories as those listed on the label.

In most cases, when monitoring caloric intake, doing your own food preparation using healthy cooking methods is a better option than eating out or purchasing processed

Activity 3.3: MyPlate Record Form

Name: _____

Course: _____ Section: _____ Gender: _____ Date: _____ Age: _____

No.	Food*	Calories	Fat (gr)	Grains (oz.)	Vegetables (cups)	Fruits (cups)	Dairy (cups)	Protein Foods (oz.)	Oils (tsp.)
				\multicolumn{6}{c	}{Food Groups — Daily Goals (see Figure 3.1)}
1									
2									
3									
4									
5									
6									
7									
8									
9									
10									
11									
12									
13									
14									
15									
16									
17									
18									
19									
20									
21									
22									
23									
24									
25									
26									
27									
28									
29									
30									
Totals									
Recommended Amount: Obtain online at www.choosemyplate.gov based on age, gender, weight, height, and activity level (see page 75 for a complete explanation)			**						
Deficiencies/Excesses									

*See "List of Nutritive Value of Selected Foods" in Appendix A.
**Multiply the recommended amount of calories by .30 (30%) and divide by 9 to obtain the daily recommended amount of grams of fat.

© Cengage Learning

Activity 3.4: Nutrition Behavior Modification Plan

Name _____ Date _____

Course _____ Section _____ Gender _____ Age _____

Nutrition Stage of Change
Using Figure 2.5 (page 63) and Table 2.3 (page 62) identify your current stage of change for nutrition (healthy diet):

[   ]

What I Learned and What I Can Do to Improve My Nutrition:
Based on the nutrient analysis and your healthy diet plan, explain what these experiences have taught you, and list specific changes and strategies that you can use to improve your present nutrition habits. Use an extra blank sheet of paper as needed.

Briefly state what you learned from the online MyPlate experience at www.choosemyplate.gov/: _____

_____

_____

_____

_____

_____

Specific changes I plan to make: _____

_____

_____

_____

_____

_____

Strategies I will use: _____

_____

_____

_____

_____

_____

_____

Current number of daily steps: [   ]   Category (Use Table 1.2, page 12): _____

Behavior Modification Planning

Selecting Nutritious Foods

To select nutritious foods:

I PLAN TO / I DID IT

☐ ☐ 1. Given the choice between whole foods and refined, processed foods, choose the former (apples rather than apple pie, potatoes rather than potato chips). No nutrients have been refined out of the whole foods, and they contain less fat, salt, and sugar.

☐ ☐ 2. Choose the leaner cuts of meat. Select fish or poultry often, beef seldom. Ask for broiled, not fried, to control your fat intake.

☐ ☐ 3. Use both raw and cooked vegetables and fruits. Raw foods offer more fiber and vitamins, such as folate and thiamin, that are destroyed by cooking. Cooking foods frees other vitamins and minerals for absorption.

☐ ☐ 4. Include milk, milk products, or other calcium sources for the calcium you need. Use low-fat or nonfat items to reduce fat and calories.

☐ ☐ 5. Learn to use margarine, butter, and oils sparingly. A little gives flavor, a lot overloads you with fat and calories.

☐ ☐ 6. Vary your choices. Eat broccoli today, carrots tomorrow, and corn the next day. Eat Chinese today, Italian tomorrow, and broiled fish with brown rice and steamed vegetables the third day.

☐ ☐ 7. Load your plate with vegetables and unrefined starchy foods. A small portion of meat or cheese is all you need for protein.

☐ ☐ 8. When choosing breads and cereals, choose the whole-grain varieties.

To select nutritious fast foods:

☐ ☐ 9. Choose the broiled sandwich with lettuce, tomatoes, and other goodies—and hold the mayo—rather than the fish or chicken patties coated with breadcrumbs and cooked in fat.

☐ ☐ 10. Select a salad—and use more plain vegetables than those mixed with oily or mayonnaise-based dressings.

☐ ☐ 11. Order chili with more beans than meat. Choose a soft bean burrito over tacos with fried shells.

☐ ☐ 12. Drink low-fat milk rather than a cola beverage.

When choosing from a vending machine:

☐ ☐ 13. Choose cracker sandwiches over chips and pork rinds (virtually pure fat). Choose peanuts, pretzels, and popcorn over cookies and candy.

☐ ☐ 14. Choose milk and juices over cola beverages.

Try It

Based on what you have learned, list strategies you can use to increase food variety, enhance the nutritive value of your diet, and decrease fat and caloric content in your meals.

Adapted from W. W. K. Hoeger, L. W. Turner, & B. Q. Hafen. *Wellness: Guidelines for a Healthy Lifestyle* (Wadsworth Thomson Learning, 2007).

---

foods. Healthy eating requires proper meal planning and adequate coping strategies when confronted with situations that encourage unhealthy eating and overindulgence. Additional information on these topics is provided in the weight management chapter (Chapter 5).

Vegetarianism About 7.5 million people in the United States are vegetarians and another 23 million people follow a vegetarian-inclined diet. **Vegetarians** rely primarily on foods from the bread, cereal, rice, pasta, and fruit and vegetable groups and avoid most foods from animal sources in the dairy and protein groups. The five basic types of vegetarians are as follows:

1. **Vegans** eat no animal products at all.
2. **Ovovegetarians** allow eggs in the diet.
3. **Lactovegetarians** allow foods from the milk group.
4. **Ovolactovegetarians** include egg and milk products in the diet.
5. **Semivegetarians** do not eat red meat, but do include fish and poultry in addition to milk products and eggs in their diet.

Vegetarian diets can be healthful and consistent with the Dietary Guidelines for Americans and can meet the DRIs for nutrients. Vegetarians who do not select their food combinations properly, however, can develop nutritional deficiencies of protein, vitamins, minerals, and even calories. Even greater attention should be paid when planning vegetarian diets for infants and children. Unless carefully planned, a strict plant-based diet will prevent proper growth and development.

3.4 Nutrient Concerns

In some vegetarian diets, protein deficiency can be a concern. Vegans in particular must be careful to eat foods that provide a balanced distribution of essential amino acids, such as grain products and legumes. Strict vegans also need a supplement of vitamin B_{12}. This vitamin is not found in plant foods; its only source is animal foods. Deficiency of this vitamin can lead to anemia and nerve damage.

The key to a healthful vegetarian diet is to eat foods that possess complementary proteins, because most plant-based products lack one or more essential amino acids in adequate amounts. For example, both grains and legumes are good protein sources, but neither provides all the essential amino acids. Grains and cereals are low in the amino acid lysine, and legumes lack methionine. Foods from these two groups—such as combinations of tortillas and beans, rice and beans, rice and soybeans, or wheat bread and peanuts—complement each other and provide all required protein nutrients. Complementing protein foods include grains with legumes; legumes with nuts and seeds; or soy and quinoa with grains, legumes, or nuts and seeds. These complementary proteins may be consumed over the course of one day, but it is best if they are consumed during the same meal (also see discussion under Proteins on pages 82-83).

Other nutrients likely to be deficient in vegetarian diets—and ways to compensate—are as follows:

- Vitamin D can be obtained from moderate exposure to the sun or by taking a supplement.
- Riboflavin can be found in green leafy vegetables, whole grains, and legumes.
- Calcium can be obtained from fortified soybean milk or fortified orange juice, calcium-rich tofu, and selected cereals. A calcium supplement is also an option.
- Iron can be found in whole grains, dried fruits and nuts, and legumes. To enhance iron absorption, a good source of vitamin C should be consumed with these foods. (Calcium and iron are the most difficult nutrients to consume in sufficient amounts in a strict vegan diet.)
- Zinc can be obtained from whole grains, wheat germ, beans, nuts, and seeds.

MyPlate also can be used as a guide for vegetarians. The key is food variety. Most vegetarians today eat dairy products and eggs. They can replace meat with legumes, nuts, seeds, eggs, and meat substitutes (tofu, tempeh, soy milk, and commercial meat replacers such as veggie burgers and soy hot dogs). For additional MyPlate healthy eating tips for vegetarians and how to get enough of the previously mentioned nutrients, go to www.choosemyplate.gov/. Those who are interested in vegetarian diets are encouraged to consult additional resources, because special vegetarian diet planning cannot be covered adequately in a few paragraphs.

Nuts

Consumption of nuts, commonly used in vegetarian diets, has received considerable attention in recent years. Although nuts are 70 to 90 percent fat, most of this is healthy unsaturated fats. Nuts are known to be nutrient powerhouses. They are an excellent source of vitamin E and magnesium, and provide selenium, folate, vitamin K, beta-carotene, phosphorus, copper, potassium, zinc, and many phytonutrients. And research indicates that people who eat nuts several times a week have a lower incidence of heart disease, and eating nuts aids blood pressure and blood glucose control.

The research indicates that people who eat nuts several times a week have a lower incidence of heart disease. Eating two to three ounces (about one-half cup) of almonds, walnuts, or peanuts a day may decrease high LDL cholesterol by about seven percent. Nuts can even enhance the cholesterol-lowering effects of the Mediterranean diet. Other data indicate that consumption of one daily serving of mixed nuts decreases oxidized LDL cholesterol concentrations. LDL cholesterol causes even greater damage when it is oxidized, inflaming the arteries, promoting atherosclerosis, and increasing the risk of a heart attack and stroke. Furthermore, studies have shown that nut consumption is associated with lower concentrations of other circulating inflammatory molecules. Daily substitution

Most fruits and vegetables contain large amounts of cancer-preventing phytonutrients.

> **Vegetarians** Individuals whose diet is of vegetable or plant origin.
>
> **Vegans** Vegetarians who eat no animal products at all.
>
> **Ovovegetarians** Vegetarians who allow eggs in their diet.
>
> **Lactovegetarians** Vegetarians who eat foods from the milk group.
>
> **Ovolactovegetarians** Vegetarians who include eggs and milk products in their diet.
>
> **Semivegetarians** Vegetarians who include milk products, eggs, and fish and poultry in the diet.

of 200 grams of carbohydrates with 22 ounces of nuts also helps control blood glucose in type 2 diabetics.

Heart-health benefits are attributed not only to the unsaturated fats but also to other nutrients found in nuts, including vitamin E and folic acid. And nuts are also packed with additional B vitamins, calcium, copper, potassium, magnesium, fiber, and phytonutrients. Many of these nutrients are cancer- and cardio-protective, help lower homocysteine levels, and act as antioxidants (discussed in "Antioxidants," page 105, and "Folate," page 108).

Nuts do have a drawback: They are high in calories. A handful of nuts provide as many calories as a piece of cake, so nuts should be avoided as a snack. Excessive weight gain is a risk factor for cardiovascular disease. Nuts are recommended for use in place of high-protein foods such as meats, bacon, and eggs or as part of a meal in fruit or vegetable salads, homemade bread, pancakes, casseroles, yogurt, and oatmeal. Peanut butter is also healthier than cheese or some cold cuts in sandwiches.

Soy Products

The popularity of soy foods, including use in vegetarian diets, is attributed primarily to Asian research that points to less heart disease and fewer hormone-related cancers in people who regularly consume soy foods. A benefit of eating soy is that it replaces unhealthy animal products high in saturated fat. Soy is rich in plant protein, unsaturated fat, and fiber, and some soy is high in calcium.

The benefits of soy lie in its high protein content and plant chemicals, known as isoflavones, that act as antioxidants and are thought to protect against estrogen-related cancers (breast, ovarian, and endometrial). The compound genistein, one of many phytonutrients in soy, may reduce the risk for breast cancer, and soy consumption also may lower the risk for prostate cancer. Limited animal studies have suggested an actual increase in breast cancer risk. Human studies are still inconclusive but tend to favor a slight protective effect in premenopausal women.

Until more data become available, the University of California Wellness Letter has issued the following recommendations[9]:

1. Do not exceed three servings of soy per day (a serving constitutes half a cup of tofu, edamame, or tempeh; one-fourth cup of roasted soy nuts; or one cup of soy yogurt or soy milk).
2. Limit soy intake to just a few servings per week if you now have or have had breast cancer.
3. Avoid soy supplements, as they may contain higher levels of isoflavones than those found in soy foods. Individuals with a history of breast cancer and women who are pregnant or lactating should especially avoid them altogether.

Probiotics

Yogurt is rated in the "super-foods" category because, in addition to being a good source of calcium, potassium, riboflavin, and protein, it contains **probiotics**. The latter are friendly "for life" microbes that are thought to rebalance the naturally present intestinal bacteria. These microorganisms help break down foods and are thought to prevent disease-causing organisms from settling in. Although low-fat or nonfat yogurt is an excellent choice, you should not consume yogurt expecting miraculous medical benefits. Probiotics have been found to offer protection against gastrointestinal infections and boost immune activity. Additional research, nonetheless, is needed to further investigate probiotic benefits.

Yogurts are cultured with *Lactobacillus bulgaricus* and *Streptococcus thermophilus* probiotics. When selecting yogurt, preferably look for low-fat or nonfat products that also contain L-acidophilus, Bifidus, and the prebiotic (substances on which probiotics feed) inulin. The latter, a soluble fiber, appears to enhance calcium absorption. Avoid yogurt with added fruit jam, sugar, and candy. Most yogurts have lots of added sugar and limited fruit. Thus, it is best to buy plain yogurt and add fresh fruit.

Advanced Glycation End Products

A new area of research in nutrition has to do with **advanced glycation end products (AGEs)**, compounds that have been implicated in aging, adverse effects, and chronic diseases by increasing oxidation and inflammation. AGEs are thought to contribute to the development of atherosclerosis, heart disease, diabetes and diabetes-related complications, kidney disease, osteoarthritis, rheumatoid arthritis, and Alzheimer's disease among others. These compounds are produced when glucose combines with proteins, lipids, and other ingredients in foods.

AGEs are found primarily in foods cooked in dry heat, at high temperatures, in processed foods, and in foods high in fat content. Broiling, grilling, and frying create the highest levels of AGEs, whereas braising, steaming, stewing, roasting, boiling, and poaching decrease the levels. French-fried potatoes have about eight times the amount of AGEs compared with the same amount in a baked potato. Fast-food restaurants take advantage of the flavor-enhancing effects of AGEs by adding these toxic compounds to their foods to increase the foods' appeal to the consumer. The take-home message to the consumer here is once again moderation. You do not have to completely eliminate grilling, frying, and fast foods, but common sense is vital to maintain good health.

The following guidelines can help you decrease AGEs in your diet:

1. Limit cooking meats at high temperatures.
2. Avoid high-fat foods (whole-milk products and meats).
3. Increase intake of fruits, vegetables, grains, fish, and low-fat milk products.
4. Choose unprocessed rather than processed foods by cooking fresh foods from scratch.
5. Eat at home most of the time and avoid prepackaged and fast foods as much as possible.
6. Avoid browning. (The process of browning sugars and proteins on food surfaces increases the formation of AGEs.)

Figure 3.11 Mediterranean Diet Pyramid.

SOURCE: © 2009 Oldways Preservation and Exchange Trust. www.oldwayspt.org. Reprinted with permission.

Diets from Other Cultures Increasingly, Americans are eating foods reflecting the ethnic composition of people from other countries. Learning how to wisely select from the wide range of options is the task of those who seek a healthy diet.

Mediterranean Diet

The **Mediterranean diet** receives much attention because people in that region have notably lower rates of diet-linked diseases and a longer life expectancy. The diet features olive oil, grains (whole, not refined), legumes, vegetables, fruits, and, in moderation, fish, red wine, nuts, and dairy products. Although it is a semivegetarian diet, up to 40 percent of the total daily caloric intake may come from fat—mostly monounsaturated fat from olive oil. Moderate intake of red wine is included with meals. The dietary plan also encourages regular physical activity (Figure 3.11).

More than a "diet," the Mediterranean diet is a dietary pattern that has existed for centuries. According to the largest and most comprehensive **observational study** on this dietary pattern, the health benefits and decreased mortality are not linked to any specific component of the diet (such as olive oil or red wine) but are achieved through the interaction of all the components of the pattern.[10] Those who adhere most closely to the dietary pattern have a lower incidence of heart disease (33 percent) and deaths from cancer (24 percent). A subsequent study published in 2013, the first randomized **clinical study** on the diet, was terminated early because individuals on a Mediterranean diet had an almost 30 percent decreased risk of heart disease.[11] The Mediterranean diet has also been linked to lower risk for metabolic syndrome and stroke, improved brain health and cognitive function, and lower risk for Alzheimer's disease. Although most people in the United States focus on the olive oil component of the diet, olive oil is used mainly as a means to increase consumption of vegetables because vegetables sautéed in oil taste better than steamed vegetables.

Ethnic Diets

As people migrate, they take their dietary practices with them. Many ethnic diets are healthier than the typical American diet because they emphasize consumption of complex carbohydrates and limit fat intake. The predominant minority ethnic groups in the United States are African American, Hispanic American, and Asian American. Unfortunately, the generally healthier ethnic diets quickly become Americanized when these groups adapt to the United States. Often, they cut back on vegetables and add meats and salt to the diet in conformity with the American consumer.

Ethnic dishes can be prepared at home. They are easy to make and much healthier when one uses the typical (original) variety of vegetables, corn, rice, spices, and condiments. Ethnic health recommendations also encourage daily physical activity and suggest no more than two alcoholic drinks per day. Three typical ethnic diets are as follows:

- The African American diet ("soul food") is

> **Probiotics** Healthy microbes (bacteria) that help break down foods and prevent disease-causing organisms from settling in the intestines.
>
> **Advanced glycation end products (AGEs)** Derivatives of glucose-protein and glucose-lipid interactions that are linked to aging and chronic diseases.
>
> **Mediterranean diet** Typical diet of people around the Mediterranean region, focusing on olive oil, red wine, fish, grains, legumes, vegetables, and fruits, with limited amounts of red meat, fish, milk, and cheese.
>
> **Observational study** A research study in which the investigator does not intervene to make changes but only observes the outcomes based on a particular lifestyle pattern.
>
> **Clinical study** A research study in which the investigator intervenes (makes certain changes or uses certain interventions or programs) to prevent or treat a disease.

based on the regional cuisine of the American South. Soul food includes yams, black-eyed peas, okra, and peanuts. The latter have been combined with American foods such as corn products and pork. Today, most people think of soul food as meat, fried chicken, sweet potatoes, and chitterlings.
- Hispanic foods in the United States arrived with the conquistadores and evolved through combinations with other ethnic diets and local foods available in Latin America. For example, Cuban cuisine combined Spanish, Chinese, and native foods; Puerto Rican cuisine developed from Spanish, African, and native products; and Mexican diets evolved from Spanish and native foods. Prominent in all of these diets were corn, beans, squash, chili peppers, avocados, papayas, and fish. The colonists later added rice and citrus foods. Today, the Hispanic diet incorporates a wide variety of foods, including red meat and cheese, but the staple still consists of rice, corn, and beans.
- Asian American diets are characteristically rich in vegetables and use minimal meat and fat. The Okinawan diet in Japan, where some of the healthiest and oldest people in the world live, is high in fresh (versus pickled) vegetables, high in fiber, and low in fat and salt. Chinese cuisine includes more than 200 vegetables, and fat-free sauces and seasoning are used to enhance flavor. The Chinese diet varies by region in China. The lowest in fat is that of southern China, with most meals containing fish, seafood, and stir-fried vegetables. Chinese food in American restaurants contains a much higher percentage of fat and protein than traditional Chinese cuisine.

Table 3.10 provides a list of healthier foods to choose from when dining at selected ethnic restaurants. Additionally, you can consult the box on page 104 for strategies that you can use for healthy dining out.

All healthy diets have similar characteristics: They are high in fruits, vegetables, and grains and low in fat and satu-

Behavior Modification Planning

Strategies for Healthier Restaurant Eating

On average, Americans eat out six times per week. Research indicates that when dining out, most people consume too many calories and too much fat. Such practice is contributing to the growing obesity epidemic and chronic conditions afflicting most Americans in the 21st century. The following are strategies that you can implement to eat healthier when dining out.

I PLAN TO / I DID IT

☐ ☐ Plan ahead. Decide before you get to the restaurant that you will select a healthy meal. Then stick to your decision. If you are unfamiliar with the menu, you may be able to access the menu at the restaurant's Web site beforehand or you can obtain valuable nutrition information at HealthyDiningFinder.com. This Web site is maintained by registered dietitians and provides information on many restaurant chains located in your area.

☐ ☐ Be aware of calories in drinks. You can gulp down several hundred extra calories through drinks alone. Restaurants and beverage industries are eager to get your money, and servers wouldn't mind a larger tip by having you consume additional items on the menu. Water, sparkling soda water, or unsweetened teas are good choices. If you do munch on food freebies or appetizers (or make a meal out of them), have your server box up half or the entire meal for you to take home. If you box up an entire meal, you now have two additional meals that you can consume at home; that is because most restaurant meals can be split into two meals.

☐ ☐ Request a half-size or a child's portion. If you are unable to do so, split the meal with your dining partner or box up half the meal before you start to eat.

☐ ☐ Inquire about ingredients and cooking methods. Don't be afraid to ask for healthy substitutes. For example, you may request that meat be sautéed instead of deep fried or that canola or olive oil be used instead of other oil choices. You can also request a baked potato or brown rice instead of French fries or white rice. Ask for dressing, butter, or sour cream on the side. Request whole-wheat bread for sandwiches. Furthermore, avoid high-fat foods or ingredients such as creamy or cheese sauces, butter, oils, and fatty/fried/crispy meats. When in doubt, ask the server for additional information. If the server can't answer your questions, select a different meal.

Try It

Implement as many of these strategies every time you dine out. Take pride in your healthy choices. Your long-term health and well-being are at stake. You will feel much better about yourself following a healthy meal than you would otherwise.

© Cengage Learning

Table 3.10 Ethnic Eating Guide

	Choose Often	Choose Less Often
Chinese	Beef with broccoli Chinese greens Steamed rice, brown or white Steamed beef with pea pods Stir-fry dishes Teriyaki beef or chicken Wonton soup	Crispy duck Egg rolls Fried rice Kung pao chicken (fried) Peking duck Pork spareribs
Japanese	Chiri nabe (fish stew) Grilled scallops Sushi, sashimi (raw fish) Teriyaki Yakitori (grilled chicken)	Tempura (fried chicken, shrimp, or vegetables) Tonkatsu (fried pork)
Italian	Cioppino (seafood stew) Minestrone (vegetarian soup) Pasta with marinara sauce Pasta primavera (pasta with vegetables) Steamed clams	Antipasto Cannelloni, ravioli Fettuccini alfredo Garlic bread White clam sauce
Mexican	Beans and rice Black bean/vegetable soup Burritos, bean Chili Enchiladas, bean Fajitas Gazpacho Taco salad Tamales Tortillas, steamed	Chili rellenos Chimichangas Enchiladas, beef or cheese Flautas Guacamole Nachos Quesadillas Tostadas Sour cream (as topping)
Middle Eastern	Tandoori chicken Curry (yogurt-based) Rice pilaf Lentil soup Shish kebab	Falafel
French	Poached salmon Spinach salad Consommé Salad niçoise	Beef Wellington Escargot French onion soup Sauces in general
Soul Food	Baked chicken Baked fish Roasted pork (not smothered or "etouffe") Sautéed okra Baked sweet potato	Fried chicken Fried fish Smothered pork tenderloin Okra in gumbo Sweet potato casserole or pie
Greek	Gyros Pita Lentil soup	Baklava Moussaka

SOURCE: Adapted from P. A. Floyd, S. E. Mimms, and C. Yelding-Howard. *Personal Health: Perspectives & Lifestyles* (Belmont, CA: Wadsworth/Thomson Learning, 1998).

rated fat. Healthy diets also use low-fat or fat-free dairy products, and they emphasize portion control—essential in a healthy diet plan.

Many people now think that if a food item is labeled "low fat" or "fat free," they can consume it in large quantities. "Low fat" or "fat free" does not imply "calorie free." Many people who consume low-fat diets eat more (and thus increase their caloric intake), which in the long term leads to obesity and its associated health problems.

3.5 Nutrient Supplementation

Approximately half of all adults in the United States take daily nutrient **supplements**. Nutrient requirements for the body normally can be met by consuming as few as 1,500 calories per day, as long as the diet contains the recommended amounts of food from the different food groups. Still, many people consider it necessary to take vitamin supplements.

It's true that the body cannot retain water-soluble vitamins as long as fat-soluble vitamins. The body excretes excessive intakes readily, although it can retain small amounts for weeks or months in various organs and tissues. Fat-soluble vitamins, by contrast, are stored in fatty tissue. Therefore, daily intake of these vitamins is not as crucial.

People should not take **megadoses** of vitamins and minerals. For some nutrients, a dose of five times the RDA taken over several months may create problems. For other nutrients, it may not pose a threat to human health. Vitamin and mineral doses should not exceed the UL (with the possible exception of vitamin D; see page 107). For nutrients that do not have an established UL, one day's dose should be no more than three times the RDA.

Iron deficiency (determined through blood testing) is more common in women than men. Iron supplementation is frequently recommended for women who have a heavy menstrual flow. Pregnant and lactating women also may require supplements. The average pregnant woman who eats an adequate amount of a variety of foods should take a low dose of iron supplement daily. Women who are pregnant with more than one baby may need additional supplements. Folate supplements also are encouraged prior to and during pregnancy to prevent certain birth defects (see the following discussions of antioxidants and folate). In the previously listed instances, individuals should take supplements under a physician's supervision.

Adults older than the age of 60 may need to supplement with a daily multivitamin. Aging may decrease the body's ability to absorb and utilize certain nutrients. Nutrient deficiencies in older adults include vitamins C, D, B_6, B_{12}, folate, and the minerals calcium, zinc, and magnesium. Iron needs, however, decrease with age; thus a supplement with lower levels of iron is recommended.

Other people who may benefit from supplementation are those

> **Supplements** Tablets, pills, capsules, liquids, or powders that contain vitamins, minerals, antioxidants, amino acids, herbs, or fiber that individuals take to increase their intake of these nutrients.
>
> **Megadoses** For most vitamins, 10 times the RDA or more; for vitamin A, 5 times the RDA.

with nutrient deficiencies, alcoholics and street-drug users who do not have a balanced diet, smokers, vegans (strict vegetarians), individuals on low-calorie diets (fewer than 1,500 calories per day), and people with disease-related disorders or who are taking medications that interfere with proper nutrient absorption.

Although supplements may help a small group of individuals, most supplements do not provide benefits to healthy people who eat a balanced diet. Supplements do not seem to prevent chronic diseases or help people run faster, jump higher, relieve stress, improve sexual prowess, cure a common cold, or boost energy levels.

Antioxidants Much research and discussion are taking place regarding the effectiveness of **antioxidants** in thwarting several chronic diseases. Although foods probably contain more than 4,000 antioxidants, the four most studied antioxidants are vitamins E, C, beta-carotene (a precursor to vitamin A), and the mineral selenium (technically not an antioxidant but a component of antioxidant enzymes).

Oxygen is used during metabolism to change carbohydrates and fats into energy. During this process, oxygen is transformed into stable forms of water and carbon dioxide. A small amount of oxygen, however, ends up in an unstable form, referred to as **oxygen free radicals**. A free radical molecule has a normal proton nucleus with a single unpaired electron. Having only one electron makes the free radical extremely reactive, and it looks constantly to pair its electron with one from another molecule. When a free radical steals a second electron from another molecule, that other molecule in turn becomes a free radical. This chain reaction goes on until two free radicals meet to form a stable molecule.

Free radicals attack and damage proteins and lipids—in particular, cell membranes and DNA. This damage is thought to contribute to the development of conditions such as cardiovascular disease, cancer, emphysema, cataracts, Parkinson's disease, and premature aging. Solar radiation, cigarette smoke, air pollution, radiation, some drugs, injury, infection, chemicals (such as pesticides), and other environmental factors also seem to encourage the formation of free radicals. Antioxidants are thought to offer protection by absorbing free radicals before they can cause damage and also by interrupting the sequence of reactions once damage has begun, thwarting certain chronic diseases (Figure 3.12).

The body's own defense systems typically neutralize free radicals so they don't cause any damage. When free radicals are produced faster than the body can neutralize them, they can damage the cells. Research, however, indicates that the body's antioxidant defense system improves as fitness improves.[12] That is, physically fit people have greater protection against free radicals.

Antioxidants are found abundantly in food, especially in fruits and vegetables. Unfortunately, most Americans do not eat the minimum recommended amounts of fruits and vegetables.

Antioxidants work best in the prevention and progression of disease, but they cannot repair damage that has already occurred or cure people who have disease. The benefits are obtained primarily from food sources themselves, and controversy surrounds the benefits of antioxidants taken in supplement form.

For years people believed that taking antioxidant supplements could further prevent free radical damage, but adding to the controversy, a report published in the *Journal of the American Medical Association* indicated that antioxidant supplements actually increase the risk of death.[13] Vitamin E, beta-carotene, and vitamin A increased the risk for mortality by 4 percent, 7 percent, and 16 percent, respectively. Vitamin C had no effect on mortality, while selenium decreased risk by 9 percent. Some researchers, however, have questioned the design and conclusions of this report. More research is definitely required to settle the controversy.

Vitamin E

The RDA for vitamin E is 15 mg or 22 **IU (international units)**. Although no evidence indicates that vitamin E supplementation less than the upper limit of 1,000 mg per day is harmful, little or no clinical research supports any health benefits. Vitamin E is found primarily in oil-rich seeds and vegetable oils. Foods high in vitamin E include almonds, hazelnuts, peanuts, canola oil, safflower oil, cottonseed oil, kale, sunflower seeds, shrimp, wheat germ, sweet potato, avocado, and tomato sauce. You should incorporate some of these foods regularly in the diet to obtain the RDA.

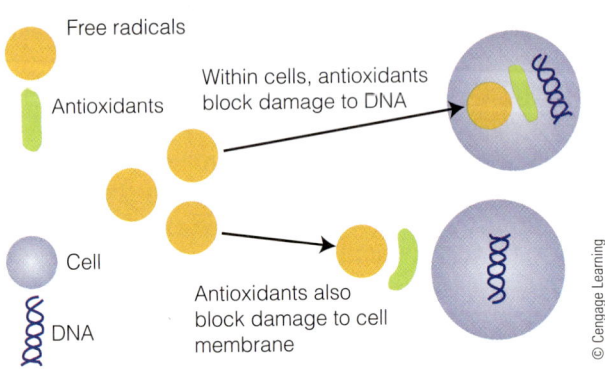

Figure 3.12 Antioxidant protection: blocking and absorbing oxygen free radicals to prevent chronic disease.

Vitamin C

Studies have shown that vitamin C may offer benefits against heart disease, cancer, and cataracts. People who consume the recommended amounts of daily fruits and vegetables, nonetheless, need no supplementation because they obtain their daily vitamin C requirements through the diet alone.

Vitamin C is water soluble, and the body eliminates it in about 12 hours. For best results, consume food rich in vitamin C twice a day. High intake of a vitamin C supplement, above 500 mg per day, is not recommended. The body absorbs very little vitamin C beyond the first 200 mg per serving or dose. Foods high in vitamin C include oranges and other citrus fruit, kiwi fruit, cantaloupe, guava, bell peppers, strawberries, broccoli, kale, cauliflower, and tomatoes.

Beta-Carotene

Obtaining the daily recommended dose of beta-carotene (20,000 IU) from food sources rather than supplements is preferable. Clinical trials have found that beta-carotene supplements do not offer protection against heart disease or cancer or provide any other health benefits. Therefore, the recommendation is to "skip the pill and eat the carrot." One medium raw carrot contains about 20,000 IU of beta-carotene. Other foods high in beta-carotene include sweet potatoes, pumpkin, cantaloupe, squash, kale, broccoli, tomatoes, peaches, apricots, mangoes, papaya, turnip greens, and spinach.

Selenium

Early research on individuals who took 200 micrograms (mcg) of selenium daily indicates that it decreased the risk for prostate, colorectal, and lung cancers by about 50 percent and may have decreased the risk for cancers of the breast, liver, and digestive tract. More recent research, however, has failed to confirm such benefits, and experts recommend caution with selenium supplements. One report indicated that men and women taking 200 mcg per day for eight years were almost three times more likely to suffer from diabetes than those taking a placebo.[14]

At present, the best recommendation available is not to exceed a daily supplement that contains more than 100 mcg of selenium. Based on the current body of research, 100 to 200 mcg of selenium per day seems to provide the necessary amount of antioxidant for this nutrient. Although the UL for selenium has been set at 400 mcg, a person has no reason to take more than 200 mcg daily. Too much selenium can damage cells rather than protect them.

One Brazil nut that you crack yourself provides about 100 mcg of selenium. Shelled nuts found in supermarkets average only about 20 mcg each. Other foods high in selenium include red snapper, salmon, cod, tuna, noodles, whole grains, and meats.

Multivitamins

Although much interest has been generated in the previously mentioned individual supplements, the American people still prefer multivitamins as supplements. At present, several large-scale, well-designed studies have provided no evidence that multivitamins decrease the risk for either cardiovascular disease or cancer. The most convincing data came in a 2009 study on more than 161,000 postmenopausal women taking multivitamin pills.[15] The results showed no benefits in terms of cardiovascular, cancer, or premature mortality risk reduction in women taking a multivitamin complex for an average of eight years compared with those who did not. A panel of experts from the National Institutes of Health (NIH) has indicated that there aren't enough data to support the use of multivitamins.

If you take a multivitamin for general health reasons, it doesn't grant you a license to eat carelessly. Multivitamins are not magic pills. They don't provide energy, fiber, or phytonutrients. People who eat a healthy diet, with ample amounts of fruits, vegetables, and grains, have a low risk of cardiovascular disease and cancer compared with people with deficient diets who take a multivitamin complex.

Vitamin D

Vitamin D is attracting a lot of attention because research suggests that the vitamin possesses anticancer properties, especially against breast, colon, and prostate cancers and possibly lung and digestive cancers. It also decreases inflammation, fighting cardiovascular disease, periodontal disease, and atherosclerosis. Furthermore, vitamin D strengthens the immune system, controls blood pressure, helps maintain muscle strength, decreases the risk for arthritis and dementia, prevents birth defects, and may help deter diabetes and fight depression. It is also necessary for absorption of calcium, a nutrient critical for building and maintaining bones to prevent osteoporosis and for dental health.

The theory that vitamin D protects against cancer is based on studies showing that people who live farther north (who have less sun exposure during the winter months) have a higher incidence of cancer. Furthermore, people diagnosed with breast, colon, or prostate cancer during the summer months, when vitamin D production by the body is at its highest, are 30 percent less likely to die from cancer, even 10 years following the initial diagnosis. Researchers think that vitamin D level at the time of cancer onset affects survival rates.

Technically, vitamin D is a prohormone. Its metabolic product, calcitriol, is a secosteroid hormone that influences more than 2,000 genes affecting health and well-being. During the winter months, most people in the United States living north of a 35-degree latitude (above the states of Georgia and Texas) and in Canada are not getting enough vitamin D. The body uses ultraviolet

> **Antioxidants** Compounds such as vitamins C and E, beta-carotene, and selenium that prevent oxygen from combining with other substances in the body to form harmful compounds.
>
> **Oxygen free radicals** Substances formed during metabolism that attack and damage proteins and lipids, in particular the cell membrane and DNA, leading to diseases such as heart disease, cancer, and emphysema.
>
> **International unit (IU)** Measure of nutrients in foods.

Table 3.11 Good Sources of Vitamin D

Food	Amount	IU*
Multivitamins (most brands)	Daily dose	400
Salmon	3.5 oz	360
Mackerel	3.5 oz	345
Sardines (oil/drained)	3.5 oz	250
Shrimp	3.5 oz	200
Orange juice (D-fortified)	8 oz	100
Milk (any type/D-fortified)	8 oz	100
Margarine (D-fortified)	1 tbsp	60
Yogurt (D-fortified)	6–8 oz	60
Cereal (D-fortified)	¾–1 c	40
Egg	1	20

*IU = International units
© Cengage Learning

B (UVB) rays to generate vitamin D. UVB rays are shorter than ultraviolet A rays, so they penetrate the atmosphere at higher angles. During the winter season, the sun is too far south for the UVB rays to get through.

In 2010, the Institute of Medicine of the NAS increased the DRI of vitamin D to 600 IU (15 mcg) for children and adults up to 70 years of age. Older adults should get 800 IU (20 mcg) per day. Vitamin D experts had hoped for higher levels, considering amounts to be too low for most individuals, especially during the winter months. Preliminary evidence suggests that people should get between 1,000 and 2,000 IU (25 to 50 mcg) of vitamin D per day.[16] For now, the UL has been set at 2,000 IU (50 mcg).

The most accurate test to measure how much vitamin D is in the body is the 25-hydroxyvitamin D test. Blood levels should remain between 50 and 80 ng/mL all year long. To increase your levels, the Vitamin D Council recommends that all adults supplement their diets with 5,000 IU of vitamin D daily for three months and then take a 25-hydroxyvitamin D test.[17] You may then adjust your supplement dosage based on your test results, daily sun exposure, and the season of the year.

Depending on skin tone and sun intensity, about 15 minutes of unprotected sun exposure (without sunscreen) of the face, arms, hands, and lower legs during peak daylight hours (10:00 a.m. and 4:00 p.m.—when your shadow is shorter than your actual height) generates between 2,000 and 5,000 IU of vitamin D. Thus, it makes no sense that the UL is set at 2,000 when the human body manufactures more than that in just 15 minutes of unprotected sun exposure. The UL of 2,000 IU will most likely be revised in the next update of the DRI.

Good sources of vitamin D in the diet include salmon, mackerel, tuna, and sardines. Fortified milk, yogurt, orange juice, margarines, and cereals are also good sources. To obtain up to 2,000 IU per day from food sources alone, however, is difficult (see Table 3.11). Thus, daily safe sun exposure and supplementation (especially during the winter months) are highly recommended.

The best source of vitamin D is sunshine. UVB rays lead to the production on the surface of the skin of inactive oil-soluble vitamin D3. The inactive form is then transformed by the liver, and subsequently the kidneys, into the active form of vitamin D. Sun-generated vitamin D is better than that obtained from foods or supplements.

Vitamin D_3 generated on the surface of the skin, however, doesn't immediately penetrate into the blood. It takes up to 48 hours to absorb most of the vitamin. Because it is an oil-soluble compound, experts recommend that you avoid using soap following safe sun exposure, as it would wash off most of the vitamin. You may use soap for your armpits, groin area, and feet, but avoid using soap on the newly sun-exposed skin.

Excessive sun exposure can lead to skin damage and skin cancer. It is best to strive for daily *safe sun* exposure, that is, 10 to 20 minutes (based on skin tone and sun intensity) of unprotected sun exposure during peak hours of the day a few times a week. Generating too much vitamin D from the sun is impossible because the body generates only what it needs. If you have sensitive skin, you may start with five minutes and progressively increase sun exposure by one minute per day. If your skin turns a slight pink, following exposure, you have overdone it and need to cut back on the time that you are out in the sun.

People at the highest risk for low vitamin D levels are older adults, those with dark skin (they make less vitamin D), and individuals who spend most of their time indoors and get little sun exposure. Over a span of 6 to 7 years, individuals 65 and older with low blood levels of vitamin D are two-and-a-half times more likely to die in that time frame than those with high levels, 2 studies have found. People with darker skin also need 5 to 10 times the sun exposure of lighter-skinned people to generate the same amount of vitamin D. The skin's dark pigment reduces the ability of the body to synthesize vitamin D from the sun by up to 95 percent.

In the United States and Canada, most of the population does not make vitamin D from the sun during the winter months when UVB rays do not get through, most people's time is spent indoors, and extra clothing is worn to protect against the cold. According to the National Health and Nutrition Examination Survey published in 2011, 41.6 percent of the U.S. population doesn't have a 25-hydroxyvitamin D level of even 20 ng/mL. The highest deficiency rate is seen in Blacks and Hispanics, with 82.1 percent and 69.2 percent deficiency rates respectively. During periods of limited sun exposure, you should consider a daily vitamin D_3 supplement of up to 2,000 IU per day. (Some vitamins contain vitamin D_2, which is a less potent form of the vitamin.)

Folate

Although it is not an antioxidant, 400 mcg of **folate** (a B vitamin) is recommended for all premenopausal women. Folate helps prevent some birth defects and seems to offer protection against colon and cervical cancers. Women who might become pregnant should plan to take a folate supplement, because studies have shown that folate before and during pregnancy can prevent serious birth defects (in particular spina bifida). Some of these defects occur during the first few days and weeks of pregnancy. Adequate folate intake can also prevent congenital heart defects, early miscarriages, and premature birth. Thus, women who may become pregnant need to have adequate folate levels before conception and throughout pregnancy.

Some evidence also indicates that adequate intake of folate along with vitamins B_6 and B_{12} prevents heart attacks by reducing homocysteine levels in the blood (see Chapter 10). High concentrations of homocysteine accelerate the process of plaque formation (atherosclerosis) in the arteries. Five servings of fruits and vegetables per day usually meet the needs for these nutrients. Almost 9 of 10 adults in the United States do not obtain the recommended 400 mcg of folate per day and less than 8 percent eat the recommended daily servings of fruits and vegetables.

With the possible exception of women of childbearing age, obtaining your daily folate RDA from natural foods is preferable to getting it from supplements. The UL for folate has been set at 1,000 mcg/day. Recent evidence suggests that exceeding 1,000 mcg through a combination of diet and supplements may actually fuel the progression of precancerous growths and cancer.[18] A daily multivitamin or a serving of a highly fortified cereal each provides 400 mcg of folate. In combination with a supplement, one can easily exceed the UL of 1,000 mcg/day. To date, no data have linked folate obtained from natural foods to increased cancer risk. On the contrary, natural foods have been found to have a cancer-protective effect.

Benefits of Foods In its latest position statement on nutrient supplements, the American Dietetic Association stated, "The best nutrition-based strategy for promoting optimal health and reducing the risk of chronic disease is to wisely choose a wide variety of foods. Additional nutrients from supplements can help some people meet their nutrient needs as specified by science-based nutrition standards such as the Dietary Reference Intakes."[19]

Fruits and vegetables are the richest sources of antioxidants and phytonutrients. For example, researchers at the U.S. Department of Agriculture (USDA) compared the antioxidant effects of vitamins C and E with those of various common fruits and vegetables. The results indicated that three-fourths of a cup of cooked kale (which contains only 11 IU of vitamin E and 76 mg of vitamin C) neutralized as many free radicals as did approximately 800 IU of vitamin E or 600 mg of vitamin C. A list of top antioxidant foods is presented in Table 3.12.

Many people who eat unhealthily think that they need supplementation to balance their diets. This is a fallacy about nutrition. The problem here is not necessarily a lack of vitamins and minerals but, rather, a diet too high in calories, saturated fat, trans fats, and sodium. Vitamin, mineral, and fiber supplements do not supply all of the nutrients and other beneficial substances present in food and needed for good health.

Wholesome foods contain vitamins, minerals, carbohydrates, fiber, proteins, fats, and phytonutrients, along with other substances not yet discovered. Researchers do not know whether the protective effects are caused by the antioxidants alone, by a combination of antioxidants with other nutrients or by some other nutrients in food that have not been investigated yet. Many nutrients work in **synergy**, enhancing chemical processes in the body.

Supplementation will not offset poor eating habits. Pills are no substitute for common sense. If you think your diet is not balanced, you first need to conduct a nutrient analysis (see Activities 3.1 and 3.2, pages 93-95) to determine which nutrients you lack in sufficient amounts. Eat more of them, as well as foods that are high in antioxidants and phytonutrients. Following a nutrient assessment, a **registered dietitian** can help you decide what supplement(s), if any, might be necessary.

Furthermore, the American Heart Association does not recommend antioxidant supplements either, until more definite research is available. If you take any supplements in pill form, however, look for products that meet the disintegration standards of the U.S. Pharmacopoeia (USP) on the bottle. The USP standard suggests that the supplement should completely dissolve in 45 minutes or less. Supplements that do not dissolve, of course, cannot get into the bloodstream.

> **Critical Thinking**
>
> Do you take supplements? • If so, for what purposes are you taking them—and do you think you could restructure your diet so that you could do without them?

Functional Foods Functional foods are foods or food ingredients that offer specific health benefits beyond those supplied by the traditional nutrients they contain. Many functional foods come in their natural forms. A tomato, for example, is a

Table 3.12 Top Antioxidant Foods

Food
Red beans
Wild blueberries
Red kidney beans
Pinto beans
Blueberries
Cranberries
Artichokes
Blackberries
Kale
Prunes
Raspberries

SOURCE: U.S. Department of Agriculture.

> **Folate** One of the B vitamins.
>
> **Synergy** A reaction in which the result is greater than the sum of its two parts.
>
> **Registered dietitian (RD)** A person with a college degree in dietetics who meets all certification and continuing education requirements of the American Dietetic Association or Dietitians of Canada.
>
> **Functional foods** Foods or food ingredients containing physiologically active substances that provide specific health benefits beyond those supplied by basic nutrition.

Behavior Modification Planning

Guidelines for a Healthy Diet

I PLAN TO / I DID IT

- ☐ ☐ Use portion control by keeping them small to moderate.
- ☐ ☐ Base your diet on a large variety of foods and focus on high-fiber foods.
- ☐ ☐ Consume ample amounts of green, yellow, red, blue/purple, and orange fruits and vegetables.
- ☐ ☐ Eat more whole grains, foods high in complex carbohydrates, including at least three one-ounce servings of whole-grain foods per day. Limit refined carbohydrates.
- ☐ ☐ Obtain most of your vitamins and minerals from food sources.
- ☐ ☐ Eat foods rich in vitamin D.
- ☐ ☐ Maintain adequate daily calcium intake from food sources and consider a supplement with vitamin D_3.
- ☐ ☐ Consume protein in moderation.
- ☐ ☐ Limit meat consumption to three to six ounces per day.
- ☐ ☐ Emphasize healthy unsaturated fats and limit trans fat and saturated fat intake, and excessive total fat intake.
- ☐ ☐ Limit cholesterol consumption to less than 300 mg per day.
- ☐ ☐ Limit sodium intake to 2,300 mg per day.
- ☐ ☐ Limit sugar intake.
- ☐ ☐ Limit liquid calories, especially those with added sugar.
- ☐ ☐ If you drink alcohol, do so in moderation (one daily drink for women and two for men).
- ☐ ☐ Obtain most vitamins and minerals from food sources. If deficient, consider taking a daily multivitamin (preferably one that includes vitamin D_3).

Try It

Carefully analyze these guidelines and note the areas where you can improve your diet. Work on one guideline each week until you are able to adhere to all of the guidelines.

© Cengage Learning

---

functional food because it contains the phytonutrient lycopene, thought to reduce the risk for prostate cancer. Other examples of functional foods are kale, broccoli, blueberries, red grapes, and green tea.

The term "functional food," however, has been used primarily as a marketing tool by the food industry to attract consumers. Unlike **fortified foods**, which have been modified to help prevent nutrient deficiencies, functional foods are created by the food industry by the addition of ingredients aimed at treating or preventing symptoms or disease. In functional foods, the added ingredient(s) is typically not found in the food item in its natural form but is added to allow manufacturers to make appealing health claims.

In most cases, only one extra ingredient is added (a vitamin, mineral, phytonutrient, or herb). An example is calcium added to orange juice to make the claim that this brand offers protection against osteoporosis. Food manufacturers now offer cholesterol-lowering margarines (enhanced with plant stanol), cancer-protective ketchup (fortified with lycopene), memory-boosting candy (with ginkgo added), calcium-fortified chips, and corn chips containing kava kava (to enhance relaxation).

The use of some functional foods, however, may undermine good nutrition. Margarines still may contain saturated fats or partially hydrogenated oils. Regularly consuming ketchup on top of large orders of fries adds many calories and fat to the diet. Sweets are also high in calories and sugar. Chips are high in calories, salt, and fat. In all of these cases, the consumer would be better off taking the specific ingredient in a supplement form rather than consuming the functional food with its extra calories, sugar, salt, and/or fat.

Functional foods can provide added benefits if used in conjunction with a healthful diet. You may use nutrient-dense functional foods in your overall wellness plan as an adjunct to health-promoting strategies and treatments.

Organic Foods Concerns over food safety have led many people to turn to organic foods. Currently, there's no solid evidence that organic food is more nutritious than conventional food, but pesticide residues in organic foods are substantially lower than conventionally grown foods. Health risks from pesticide exposure from foods are relatively small for healthy adults. The health benefits of produce far outweigh the risks. Children, older adults, pregnant and lactating women, and people with weak immune systems, however, may be vulnerable to some types of pesticides.

Organic foods, including crops, meat, poultry, eggs, and dairy products, are produced under strict government regulations. Organic crops have to be grown without the use of

Behavior Modification Planning

Minimizing the Risk of Food Contamination and Pesticide Residues

Most food is safe to eat, but there is no 100 percent guarantee that all produce is free of contamination.

I PLAN TO / **I DID IT**

- ☐ ☐ Wash your hands thoroughly before and after touching raw produce.
- ☐ ☐ Do not place raw fruits and vegetables next to uncooked meat, poultry, or fish.
- ☐ ☐ Trim all visible fat from meat and remove the skin from poultry and fish prior to cooking (pesticides concentrate in animal fat).
- ☐ ☐ Use a scrub brush to wash fresh produce under running water. Pay particular attention to crevices in the produce. Washing fresh produce reduces pesticide levels but does not completely eliminate them. Eat a variety of foods to decrease exposure to any given pesticide.
- ☐ ☐ Select produce that is free of dirt and does not have holes or cuts or other signs of spoilage.
- ☐ ☐ Discard the outermost leaves of leafy vegetables such as lettuce and cabbage.
- ☐ ☐ Cut your own fruits and vegetables instead of getting them precut. Wash all produce thoroughly before cutting, even melons and avocados. Cutting into potentially contaminated (unwashed) inedible rinds of fruit can contaminate the inside of the fruit. Always use a knife to remove orange peels instead of biting into them. Peel waxed fruits and vegetables, and other produce as necessary (cucumbers, carrots, peaches, apples).
- ☐ ☐ Store produce in the refrigerator in clean containers or clean plastic bags (previously used bags that are not kept cold can grow harmful bacteria).
- ☐ ☐ For some produce, consider buying certified organic foods. Look for the "USDA Organic" seal. According to data from the Environmental Working Group, a nonprofit consumer activist organization, conventional produce with the most pesticide residue include peaches, apples, sweet bell peppers, celery, nectarines, strawberries, cherries, grapes, lettuce, imported grapes, pears, spinach, and potatoes. Among the least contaminated are onions, avocados, sweet corn, pineapples, mangoes, sweet peas, asparagus, kiwifruit, bananas, cabbage, broccoli, and eggplant (list of foods downloaded from www.foodnews.org).

Try It

Lifestyle behavior patterns are difficult to change. These recommendations can minimize your risk of food contamination and ingestion of pesticide residues. Make a copy of the recommendations and determine how many of these suggestions you are able to include in daily life over the course of the next seven days.

---

conventional pesticides, artificial fertilizers, human waste, or sewage sludge, and have been processed without ionizing radiation or food additives. Harmful microbes in manure must also be destroyed prior to use, and genetically modified organisms may not be used. Organic livestock are raised under certain grazing conditions, using organic feed, and without the use of antibiotics and growth hormones.

Organic foods can just as easily be contaminated with bacteria, pathogens, and heavy metals that pose major health risks. The soil itself may become contaminated, or if the produce comes in contact with feces of grazing cattle, wild animals/birds, farm workers, or any other source, potentially harmful microorganisms can contaminate the produce. Recent *Escherichia coli*–contaminated spinach, sold nationwide, was grown in a field that was in transition from conventional crops to an organic field. The best safeguard to protect yourself is to follow the food safety guidelines provided on this page.

Genetically Modified Crops In a genetically modified organism (GMO), the DNA (or basic genetic material) is manipulated to obtain certain results. This is done by inserting genes with desirable traits from one plant, animal, or microorganism into another one to either introduce new traits or enhance existing traits.

Crops are genetically modified to make them better resist disease and extreme environmental conditions (such as heat and frost), require fewer fertilizers and pesticides, last longer, and improve their nutrient content and taste. GMOs could help save billions of dollars by producing more crops and helping to feed the hungry in developing countries around the world.

> **Fortified foods** Foods that have been modified by the addition or increase of nutrients that either were not present or were present in insignificant amounts with the intent of preventing nutrient deficiencies.

Concern over the safety of **genetically modified (GM) foods** has led to heated public debates in Europe and, to a lesser extent, in the United States. The concern is that genetic modifications create "transgenic" organisms that have not previously existed and that have potentially unpredictable effects on the environment and on humans. Also, there is some concern that GM foods may cause illness or allergies in humans and that cross-pollination may destroy other plants or create "superweeds" with herbicide-resistant genes. Some researchers believe that GM crops have increased usage of harmful herbicides, causing an overall negative impact on the environment.

Genetically modified crops were first introduced into the United States in 1996. This technology is moving forward so rapidly that the USDA already has approved more than 50 GM crops. Today, about 40 percent of U.S. cropland produced GM foods. Now, more than 80 percent of our soybeans, 73 percent of cotton, 50 percent of canola, and 40 percent of corn come from GM crops.

Avoiding GM foods is difficult because more than 75 percent of processed foods on the market today contain GMOs. Americans have been consuming GM foods for almost two decades now with no apparent detrimental health consequences. If people do not wish to consume GM foods, organic foods are an option because organic trade organizations do not certify foods with genetic modifications. Produce bought at the local farmers' market also may be an option, because small farmers are less likely to use this technology.

At this point, no evidence indicates that GM foods are harmful—but no compelling evidence guarantees that they are safe, either. Many questions remain, and much research is required in this field. As a consumer, you will have to continue educating yourself as more evidence becomes available in the next few years.

3.6 Energy Substrates for Physical Activity

The two main fuels that supply energy for physical activity are glucose (sugar) and fat (fatty acids). The body uses amino acids, derived from proteins, as an energy substrate when glucose is low, such as during fasting, prolonged aerobic exercise, or a low-carbohydrate diet.

Glucose is derived from foods that are high in carbohydrates, such as breads, cereals, grains, pasta, beans, fruits, vegetables, and sweets in general. Glucose is stored as glycogen in muscles and the liver. Fatty acids (discussed on pages 79-80) are the product of the breakdown of fats. Unlike glucose, an almost unlimited supply of fatty acids, stored as fat in the body, can be used during exercise.

3.7 Energy (ATP) Production

The energy derived from food is not used directly by the cells. It is first transformed into **adenosine triphosphate (ATP)**. The subsequent breakdown of this compound provides the energy used by all energy-requiring processes of the body (Figure 3.13).

ATP must be recycled continually to sustain life and work. ATP can be resynthesized in three ways:

1. ATP-CP system. The body stores small amounts of ATP and creatine phosphate (CP). These stores are used during all-out activities such as sprinting, long jumping, and weight lifting. The amount of stored ATP provides energy for just one or two seconds. During brief all-out efforts, ATP is resynthesized from CP, another high-energy phosphate compound. This is the ATP-CP, or phosphagen, system. Depending on the amount of physical training, the concentration of CP stored in cells is sufficient to allow maximum exertion for up to 10 seconds. Once the CP stores are depleted, the person is forced to slow down or rest to allow ATP to form through anaerobic and aerobic pathways.

2. Anaerobic or lactic acid system. During maximal-intensity exercise that is sustained for 10 to 180 seconds, ATP is replenished primarily from the breakdown of glucose through a series of chemical reactions that do not require oxygen (hence "anaerobic"). In the process, though, **lactic acid** is produced. As lactic acid accumulates, it leads to muscle fatigue.

   Because of the accumulation of lactic acid with high-intensity exercise, the formation of ATP during anaerobic activities is limited to about three minutes. A recovery period of several minutes then is necessary to allow for the removal of lactic acid. Formation of ATP through the anaerobic system requires glucose (carbohydrates).

3. Aerobic system. The production of energy during slow-sustained exercise is derived primarily through aerobic metabolism. Glucose (carbohydrates), fatty acids (fat), and oxygen (hence "aerobic") are required to form ATP

Figure 3.13 Contributions of the energy formation mechanisms during various forms of physical activity.

using this process; and under steady-state exercise conditions, lactic acid accumulation is minimal or nonexistent.

Because oxygen is required, a person's capacity to utilize oxygen is crucial for successful athletic performance in aerobic events. The higher one's maximal oxygen uptake (VO_{2max}) (see pages 201-202), the greater is one's capacity to generate ATP through the aerobic system—and the better is one's athletic performance in long-distance events. From the previous discussion, it becomes evident that for optimal performance, both recreational and highly competitive athletes make the required nutrients a part of their diet.

3.8 Nutrition for Athletes

During resting conditions, fat supplies about two-thirds of the energy to sustain the body's vital processes. During exercise, the body uses both glucose (glycogen) and fat in combination to supply the energy demands. The proportion of fat to glucose changes with the intensity of exercise. When a person is exercising below 60 percent of his or her maximal work capacity (VO_{2max}), fat is used as the primary energy substrate. As the intensity of exercise increases, so does the percentage of glucose utilization—up to 100 percent during maximal work that can be sustained for only 2 to 3 minutes.

In general, athletes do not require special supplementation or any other special type of diet. Unless the diet is deficient in basic nutrients, no special secret or magic diet will help people perform better or develop faster as a result of what they eat. As long as they eat a balanced diet—that is, based on a large variety of nutrients from all basic food groups—athletes do not require additional supplements. Even in strength training and bodybuilding, protein in excess of 20 percent of total daily caloric intake is not necessary. The recommended daily protein intake ranges from 0.8 gram per kilogram of body weight for sedentary people to 2.0 grams per kilogram for extremely active individuals (Table 3.4).

The main difference between a sensible diet for a sedentary person and a sensible diet for a highly active individual is the total number of calories required daily and the amount of carbohydrate intake needed during prolonged physical activity. People in training consume more calories because of their greater energy expenditure—which is required as a result of intense physical training.

Carbohydrate Loading

On a regular diet, the body is able to store between 1,500 and 2,000 calories in the form of glycogen. About 75 percent of this glycogen is stored in muscle tissue. This amount, however, can be increased greatly through **carbohydrate loading**.

A regular diet should be altered during several days of heavy aerobic training or when a person is going to participate in a long-distance event of more than 90 minutes (e.g., marathon, triathlon, road cycling). For events shorter than 90 minutes, carbohydrate loading does not seem to enhance performance.

During prolonged exercise, glycogen is broken down into glucose, which then is readily available to the muscles for energy production. In comparison with fat, glucose frequently is referred to as the "high-octane fuel," because it provides about six percent more energy per unit of oxygen consumed.

Heavy training over several consecutive days leads to depletion of glycogen faster than it can be replaced through the diet. Glycogen depletion with heavy training is common in athletes. Signs of depletion include chronic fatigue, difficulty in maintaining accustomed exercise intensity, and lower performance.

On consecutive days of exhaustive physical training (this means several hours daily), a carbohydrate-rich diet—70 percent of total daily caloric intake or eight grams of carbohydrate per kilogram (2.2 pounds) of body weight—is recommended. This diet often restores glycogen levels in 24 hours. Along with the high-carbohydrate diet, a day of rest often is needed to allow the muscles to recover from glycogen depletion following days of intense training. For people who exercise less than an hour a day, a 60-percent carbohydrate diet, or 6 grams of carbohydrate per kilogram of body weight, is enough to replenish glycogen stores.

Following an exhaustive workout, eating a combination of carbohydrates and protein (such as a tuna sandwich) within 30 minutes of exercise seems to speed up glycogen storage even more. Protein intake increases insulin activity, thereby enhancing glycogen replenishment. A 70 percent carbohydrate intake then should be maintained throughout the rest of the day.

By following a special diet and exercise regimen five days before a long-distance event, highly (aerobically) trained individuals are capable of storing two to three times the amount of glycogen found in the average person. Athletic performance may be enhanced for long-distance events of more than 90 minutes by eating a regular balanced diet (50 to 60 percent carbohydrates), along with intensive physical training on the fifth and fourth days before the event, followed by a diet high in carbohydrates (about 70 percent) and a gradual decrease in training intensity over the last 3 days before the event.

The amount of glycogen stored as a result of a carbohydrate-rich diet does not seem to be affected by the proportion of complex and simple carbohydrates. The intake of simple carbohydrates (sugars) can be raised while on a 70 percent carbohydrate diet, as long as it doesn't exceed 25 per-

> **Genetically modified (GM) foods** Foods whose basic genetic material (DNA) is manipulated by inserting genes with desirable traits from one plant, animal, or microorganism into another one either to introduce new traits or to enhance existing ones.
>
> **Adenosine triphosphate (ATP)** A high-energy chemical compound that the body uses for immediate energy.
>
> **Lactic acid** End product of anaerobic glycolysis (metabolism).
>
> **Carbohydrate loading** Increasing intake of carbohydrates during heavy aerobic training or prior to aerobic endurance events that last longer than 90 minutes.

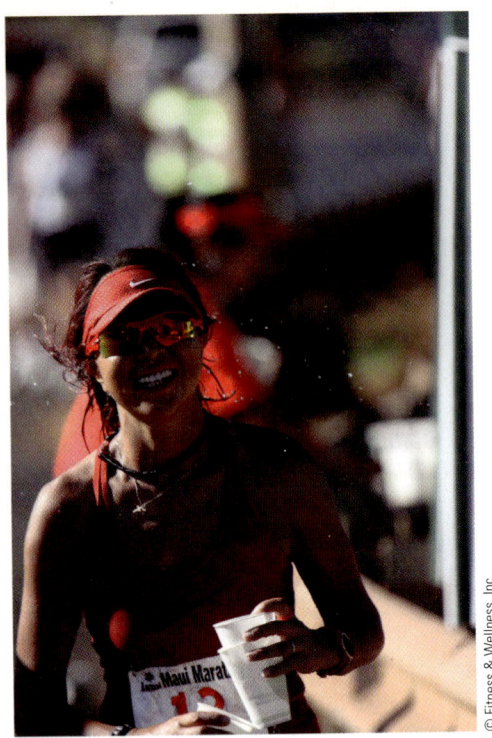

Fluid and carbohydrate replenishment during exercise is essential when participating in long-distance aerobic endurance events, such as a marathon or a triathlon.

cent of the total calories. Complex carbohydrates provide more nutrients and fiber, making them a better choice for a healthier diet.

On the day of the long-distance event, carbohydrates are still the recommended choice of substrate. As a general rule, athletes should consume one gram of carbohydrate for each kilogram (2.2 pounds) of body weight one hour prior to exercise (i.e., if you weigh 160 pounds, you should consume 160 ÷ 2.2 = 72 grams). If the pre-event meal is eaten earlier, the amount of carbohydrate can be increased to two, three, or four grams per kilogram of weight two, three, or four hours, respectively, before exercise.

During the long-distance event, researchers recommend that the athlete consume 30 to 60 grams of carbohydrates (120 to 240 calories) every hour. This is best accomplished by drinking 8 ounces of a 6- to 8-percent carbohydrate sports drink every 15 minutes (check labels to ensure proper carbohydrate concentration). This also lessens the chance of dehydration during exercise, which hinders performance and endangers health. The percentage of the carbohydrate drink is determined by dividing the amount of carbohydrate (in grams) by the amount of fluid (in milliliters) and then multiplying by 100. For example, 18 grams of carbohydrate in 240 milliliters (8 ounces) of fluid yields a drink that is 7.5 percent (18 ÷ 240 × 100) carbohydrate.

Hyponatremia In some cases, athletes participating in long- or ultra-long-distance races may suffer from **hyponatremia**, or low sodium concentration in the blood. The longer the race, the greater the risk of hyponatremia. This condition occurs as lost sweat, which contains salt and water, is replaced by only water (no salt) during a very long-distance race. Although the athlete is overhydrated, blood sodium is diluted and hyponatremia occurs. Typical symptoms are similar to those of heat illness and include fatigue, weakness, disorientation, muscle cramps, bloating, nausea, dizziness, confusion, slurred speech, fainting, and even seizures and coma in severe cases.

Based on estimates, about 30 percent of the participants in the Hawaii Ironman Triathlon suffer from hyponatremia. The condition, however, is rare in the everyday exerciser. To help prevent hyponatremia, athletes should ingest extra sodium prior to the event and then adequately monitor fluid intake during the race to prevent overhydration. Sports drinks that contain sodium (ingest about one gram of sodium per hour) should be used during the race to replace **electrolytes** lost in sweat and to prevent blood sodium dilution.

Creatine Supplementation Creatine is an organic compound obtained in the diet primarily from meat and fish. In the human body, creatine combines with inorganic phosphate and forms **creatine phosphate (CP)**, a high-energy compound. CP then is used to resynthesize ATP during short bursts of all-out physical activity. Individuals on a normal mixed diet consume an average of one gram of creatine per day. Each day, one additional gram is synthesized from various amino acids. One pound of meat or fish provides approximately two grams of creatine.

Creatine supplementation is popular among individuals who want to increase muscle mass and improve athletic performance. Creatine monohydrate—a white, tasteless powder that is mixed with fluids prior to ingestion—is the form most popular among people who use the supplement. Supplementation can result in an approximate 20 percent increase in the amount of creatine that is stored in muscles. Most of this creatine binds to phosphate to form CP, and 30 to 40 percent remains as free creatine in the muscle. Increased creatine storage is believed to enable individuals to train more intensely—thereby building more muscle mass and enhancing performance in all-out activities of very short duration (less than 30 seconds).

Creatine supplementation has two phases: the loading phase and the maintenance phase. During the loading phase, the person consumes between 20 and 25 grams (one teaspoonful is about 5 grams) of creatine per day for 5 to 6 days, divided into 4 or 5 dosages of five grams each throughout the day (this amount represents the equivalent of consuming 10 or more pounds of meat per day). Research also suggests that the amount of creatine stored in muscle is enhanced by taking creatine in combination with a high-carbohydrate food. Once the loading phase is complete, taking 2 grams per day seems to be sufficient to maintain the increased muscle stores.

To date, no serious side effects have been documented in people who take up to 25 grams of creatine per day for 5 days. Stomach distress and cramping have been reported only in rare instances. The two grams taken per day during the maintenance phase is just slightly above the average intake in our daily diet. Long-term effects of creatine supplementation on health, however, have not been established.

A frequently documented result following five to six days of creatine loading is an increase of two to three pounds in body weight. This increase appears to be related to the increased water retention necessary to maintain the additional creatine stored in muscles. Some data, however, suggest that the increase in stored water and CP stimulates protein synthesis, leading to an increase in lean body mass.

The benefits of elevated creatine stores may be limited to high-intensity/short-duration activities such as sprinting, strength training (weight lifting), and sprint cycling. Supplementation is most beneficial during exercise training itself, rather than as an aid to enhance athletic performance a few days before competition.

Enhanced creatine stores do not benefit athletes competing in aerobic endurance events, because CP is not used in energy production for long-distance events. Actually, the additional weight can be detrimental in long-distance running and swimming events, because the athlete must expend more energy to carry the extra weight during competition.

3.9 Bone Health and Osteoporosis

Osteoporosis, literally meaning "porous bones," is a condition in which bones lack the minerals required to keep them strong. In osteoporosis, bones—primarily of the hip, wrist, and spine—become so weak and brittle that they fracture readily. The process begins slowly in the third and fourth decades of life. Women are especially susceptible after menopause because of the accompanying loss of **estrogen**, which increases the rate at which bone mass is broken down.

According to the National Osteoporosis Foundation, 10 million Americans (8 million women and 2 million men) already have the disease and another 34 million have low bone density, placing them at increased risk for osteoporosis and bone fractures. About 30 percent of postmenopausal women have osteoporosis, but only about 2 percent are actually diagnosed and treated for this condition.

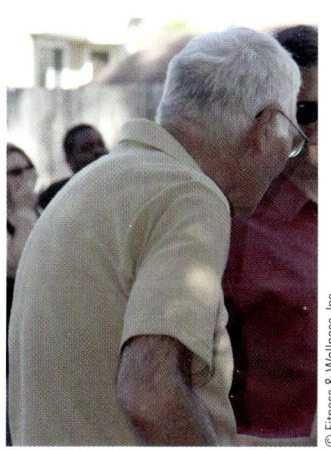

Osteoporosis is a leading cause of serious morbidity and functional loss in the elderly.

Osteoporosis is the leading cause of serious morbidity and functional loss in the elderly population. One of every two women and up to one in four men over age 50 will have an osteoporotic-related fracture at some point in their lives. The chances of a postmenopausal woman developing osteoporosis are much greater than her chances of developing breast cancer or incurring a heart attack or stroke. Up to 20 percent of people who have a hip fracture die within a year because of complications related to the fracture. As alarming as these figures are, they do not convey the pain and loss of quality of life in people who suffer the crippling effects of osteoporotic fractures.

Although osteoporosis is viewed primarily as a woman's disease, more than 30 percent of all men will be affected by age 75. About 100,000 of the yearly 300,000 hip fractures in the United States occur in men.

Despite the strong genetic component, osteoporosis is preventable. Maximizing bone density at a young age and subsequently decreasing the rate of bone loss later in life are critical factors in preventing osteoporosis.

Normal hormone levels prior to menopause and adequate calcium intake and physical activity throughout life cannot be overemphasized. These factors are all crucial in preventing osteoporosis. The absence of any one of these three factors leads to bone loss for which the other two factors never completely compensate. Smoking and excessive use of alcohol and corticosteroid drugs also accelerate the rate of bone loss in women and men alike. And osteoporosis is more common in whites, Asians, and people with small frames. Figure 3.14 depicts these variables.

Bone health begins at a young age. Some experts have called osteoporosis a "pediatric disease." Bone density can be promoted early in life by making sure the diet has sufficient calcium and participating in weight-bearing activities. Adequate calcium intake in women and men alike is also associated with a reduced risk for colon cancer. The RDA for calcium is between 1,000 and 1,300 mg per day (see Table 3.13).

> **Hyponatremia** A low sodium concentration in the blood caused by overhydration with water.
>
> **Electrolytes** Substances that become ions in solution and are critical for proper muscle and neuron activation (include sodium, potassium, chloride, calcium, magnesium, phosphate, and bicarbonate among others).
>
> **Creatine** An organic compound derived from meat, fish, and amino acids that combines with inorganic phosphate to form creatine phosphate.
>
> **Creatine phosphate (CP)** A high-energy compound that the cells use to resynthesize ATP during all-out activities of very short duration.
>
> **Osteoporosis** A condition of softening, deterioration, or loss of bone mineral density that leads to disability, bone fractures, and even death from medical complications.
>
> **Estrogen** Female sex hormone essential for bone formation and conservation of bone density.

Figure 3.14 Threats to bone health (osteoporosis).

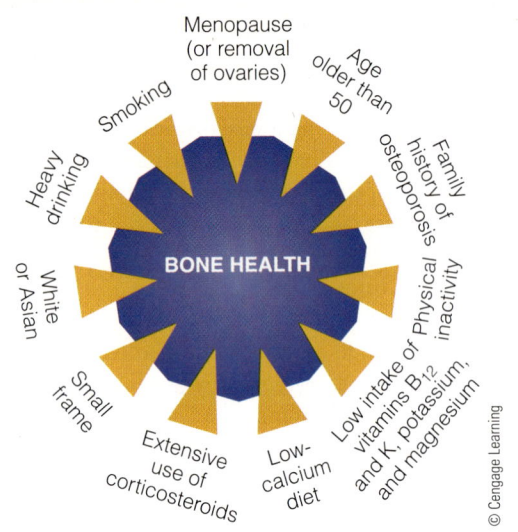

Table 3.14 Low-Fat Calcium-Rich Foods

Food	Amount	Calcium (mg)	Calories
Beans, red kidney, cooked	1 cup	70	218
Beet, greens, cooked	½ cup	82	19
Bok choy (Chinese cabbage)	1 cup	158	20
Broccoli, cooked, drained	1 cup	72	44
Burrito, bean (no cheese)	1	57	225
Cottage cheese, 2% low-fat	½ cup	78	103
Ice milk (vanilla)	½ cup	102	100
Instant Breakfast, nonfat milk	1 cup	407	216
Kale, cooked, drained	1 cup	94	36
Milk, nonfat, powdered	1 tbsp	52	15
Milk, skim	1 cup	296	88
Oatmeal, instant, fortified, plain	½ cup	109	70
Okra, cooked, drained	½ cup	74	23
Orange juice, fortified	1 cup	300	110
Soy milk, fortified, fat free	1 cup	400	110
Spinach, raw	1 cup	56	12
Turnip greens, cooked	1 cup	197	29
Tofu (some types)	½ cup	138	76
Yogurt, fruit	1 cup	372	250
Yogurt, low-fat, plain	1 cup	448	155

© Cengage Learning

To obtain your daily calcium requirement, get as much calcium as possible from calcium-rich foods, including calcium-fortified foods. If you don't get enough, you need to make a conscious and deliberate effort to reach the RDA. Calcium supplements are no longer recommended because they may cause more harm than good; including a higher risk of heart attack, kidney stones in both men and women, and possibly increased risk of prostate cancer in men. Calcium obtained from food, has not been linked to these negative health risks. Supplements are only warranted in extreme cases, when dietary intake from food absolutely does not supply the need.

Table 3.14 provides a list of selected foods and their calcium content. Along with having an adequate calcium intake, taking a minimum of 400 to 800 IU of vitamin D daily is recommended for optimal calcium absorption (for overall health benefits, 1,000 to 2,000 IU of vitamin D is preferable). Close to half of people older than 50 are also vitamin D deficient. Without vitamin D, it is practically impossible for the body to absorb sufficient calcium to protect the bones.

Protein is also necessary for the continuous rebuilding of bones. Excessive protein, however, is detrimental to bone health because it makes the blood more acidic. To neutralize the acid, calcium is taken from the bones and released into the bloodstream. The more protein we eat, the higher the calcium content in the urine (i.e., the more calcium excreted). This might be the reason that countries with a high protein intake, including the United States, also have the highest rates of osteoporosis. Individuals should aim to achieve the RDA for protein nonetheless, because people who consume too little protein (less than 35 grams per day) lose more bone mass than those who eat too much (more than 100 grams per day).

Vitamin B_{12} may also be a key nutrient in the prevention of osteoporosis. Several reports have shown an association between low vitamin B_{12} and lower bone mineral density in both men and women. Vitamin B_{12} is found primarily in dairy products, meats, poultry, fish, and some fortified cereals. Other nutrients vital for bone health are potassium (also neutralizes acid), vitamin K (works with bone-building proteins), and magnesium (also keeps bone from becoming too brittle).

Soft drinks and alcoholic beverages also can contribute to a loss in bone density if consumed in large quantities. Although they may not cause the damage directly, they often take the place of dairy products in the diet.

Exercise plays a key role in preventing osteoporosis by decreasing the rate of bone loss following the onset of menopause. Active people are able to maintain bone density much more effectively than their inactive counterparts. A combina-

Table 3.13 Recommended Daily Calcium Intake

Age	Amount (mg)
9–18	1,300
19–50	1,000
51–70 Men	1,000
51–70 Women	1,200
>70	1,200

Pregnant and lactating women should follow the recommendation for their respective age group.

© Cengage Learning

tion of weight-bearing exercises, such as walking or jogging and weight training, is especially helpful.

The benefits of exercise go beyond maintaining bone density. Exercise strengthens muscles, ligaments, and tendons—all of which provide support to the bones (skeleton). Exercise also improves balance and coordination, which can help prevent falls and injuries.

People who are active have higher bone mineral density than inactive people do. Similar to other benefits of participating in exercise, there is no such thing as "bone in the bank." To have good bone health, people need to participate in a regular lifetime exercise program.

Prevailing research also tells us that estrogen is the most important factor in preventing bone loss. Lumbar bone density in women who have always had regular menstrual cycles exceeds that of women with a history of **oligomenorrhea** and **amenorrhea** interspersed with regular cycles. Furthermore, the lumbar density of these two groups of women is higher than that of women who have never had regular menstrual cycles.

For instance, athletes with amenorrhea (who have lower estrogen levels) have lower bone mineral density than even nonathletes with normal estrogen levels. Studies have shown that amenorrheic athletes at age 25 have the bones of women older than 50. It has become clear that sedentary women with normal estrogen levels have better bone mineral density than active amenorrheic athletes. Many experts believe the best predictor of bone mineral content is the history of menstrual regularity.

As a baseline, women age 65 and older should have a bone density test to establish the risk for osteoporosis. Younger women who are at risk for osteoporosis should discuss a bone density test with their physician at menopause. The test also can be used to monitor changes in bone mass over time and to predict the risk of future fractures. The bone density test is a painless scan requiring only a small amount of radiation to determine bone mass of the spine, hip, wrist, heel, or fingers. The amount of radiation is so low that technicians administering the test can sit next to the person receiving it. The procedure often takes less than 15 minutes.

Various therapy modalities available to prevent and/or treat osteoporosis should be discussed with a physician. If you have osteoporosis, lifestyle changes may be required, and you may also need medication to prevent future fractures. A calcium-rich diet, adequate vitamin D, daily exercise, and drug therapy are all treatment options.

New medical treatments have been developed and continue to evolve to prevent and treat bone loss. The newer medications can be classified into two categories: antiresorptive and anabolic. Antiresorptive medications slow bone loss, but the body still makes new bone at the same rate, so bone density may increase. The drugs that fall into this category include bisphosphonates, calcitonin, denosumab, estrogen agonists/antagonists (also referred to as selective estrogen receptor modulators, or SERMs), and menopausal hormone therapy (MHT). Anabolic medications increase the rate of bone formation. The only FDA approved drug in this category is teriparatide, a form of parathyroid hormone.

Menopausal hormone therapy (MHT) may be the most effective treatment to relieve acute (short-term) symptoms of menopause, such as hot flashes, mood swings, sleep difficulties, and vaginal dryness. Due to potential health risks, experts recommend that women on MHT use the lowest dose that still provides benefits and use it for the shortest time needed. Regardless of the treatment modality, women should always work with a physician to determine the best course of action.

3.10 Iron Deficiency

Iron is a key element of **hemoglobin** in blood. The RDA for iron for adult women is between 15 and 18 mg per day (8 to 11 mg for men). Inadequate iron intake is often seen in children, teenagers, women of childbearing age, and endurance athletes. If iron absorption does not compensate for losses or if dietary intake is low, iron deficiency develops. As many as half of American women have an iron deficiency. Over time, excessive depletion of iron stores in the body leads to iron-deficiency anemia, a condition in which the concentration of hemoglobin in the red blood cells is lower than it should be.

Physically active individuals, in particular women, have a greater than average need for iron. Heavy training creates a demand for iron that is higher than the recommended intake because small amounts of iron are lost through sweat, urine, and stools. Mechanical trauma, caused by the pounding of the feet on the pavement during extensive jogging, may also lead to destruction of iron-containing red blood cells.

A large percentage of female endurance athletes are reported to have iron deficiency. The blood ferritin levels of women who participate in intense physical training should be checked frequently.

The rates of iron absorption and iron loss vary from person to person. In most cases, though, people can get enough iron by eating more iron-rich foods such as beans, peas, green leafy vegetables, enriched grain products, egg yolk, fish, and lean meats. Although organ meats, such as liver, are especially good sources, they also are high in cholesterol. A list of foods high in iron is given in Table 3.15.

If you are iron-deficient, be aware that calcium interferes with iron absorption. Thus, try not to include dietary sources of calcium with your main iron-rich meal. The intake of these two minerals should be separated as much as possible. This is particularly critical in young menstruating women who need the iron and calcium can be detrimental with the absorption of iron.

Oligomenorrhea Irregular menstrual cycles.

Amenorrhea Cessation of regular menstrual flow.

Hemoglobin Protein–iron compound in red blood cells that transports oxygen in the blood.

Table 3.15 Iron-Rich Foods

Food	Amount	Iron (mg)	Calories	% Calories From Fat
Beans, red kidney, cooked	1 cup	3.2	218	4
Beef, ground lean (21% fat)	3 oz	2.1	237	57
Beef, sirloin, lean only	3 oz	2.9	171	36
Beef, liver, fried	3 oz	5.3	184	33
Beet, greens, cooked	½ cup	1.4	19	—
Broccoli, cooked, drained	1 cup	1.3	44	—
Burrito, bean (no cheese)	1	2.3	225	28
Egg, hard-cooked	1	.7	77	58
Farina (Cream of Wheat), cooked	½ cup	5.2	65	—
Instant Breakfast, nonfat milk	1 cup	4.8	216	4
Peas, frozen, cooked, drained	½ cup	1.3	62	—
Shrimp, boiled	3 oz	2.7	87	10
Spinach, raw	1 cup	1.5	12	—
Vegetables, mixed, cooked	1 cup	1.5	108	—

© Cengage Learning

3.11 2010 Dietary Guidelines for Americans

The secretaries of the Department of Health and Human Services (DHHS) and the USDA appoint an expert Dietary Guidelines advisory committee every five years to issue a report and make recommendations concerning dietary guidelines for Americans. The guidelines should be used as a goal to help people achieve a healthier life.

The *2010 Dietary Guidelines for Americans* are intended for healthy people two years and older. Due to the dramatic increase in obesity, eating and physical activity patterns that are focused on consuming fewer calories, making informed food choices, and being physically active are emphasized to help people attain and maintain a healthy weight, reduce their risk of chronic disease, and promote overall health. The improved recommendations give individuals the necessary information to make thoughtful choices of healthier foods in the right portions and to complement those choices with physical activity. Two key concepts are emphasized in the 2010 guidelines:

- Balance calories with physical activity to sustain a healthy weight.
- Focus on consuming nutrient-dense foods and beverages. This includes a greater consumption of certain foods and nutrients such as fruits, vegetables, whole grains, fat-free and low-fat dairy products, and seafood; and decreased consumption of foods with sodium (salt), saturated fats, trans fats, cholesterol, added sugars, and refined grains.

The 2010 dietary guidelines include 20 key recommendations for the general population and 9 additional key recommendations for specific population groups.[20] The recommendations are intended to help people choose an overall healthy diet.

Additional information on the following guidelines is posted at www.dietaryguidelines.gov.

Balancing Calories to Manage Weight

1. Prevent and/or reduce overweight and obesity through improved eating and physical activity behaviors.
2. Control total calorie intake to manage body weight. For people who are overweight or obese, this will mean consuming fewer calories from foods and beverages.

Specific Nutrition Recommendations in the 2010 Dietary Guidelines for Americans

Increase consumption of
- Fruits and vegetables
- Whole grains
- Low-fat dairy products
- A variety of lean protein choices
- Seafood
- Healthy fats
- Foods high in fiber, calcium, potassium, and vitamin D

Decrease intake of
- Saturated fat
- Trans fats
- Dietary cholesterol
- Sodium
- Refined grains
- Alcohol

3. Increase physical activity and reduce time spent in sedentary behaviors.
4. Maintain appropriate calorie balance during each stage of life—childhood, adolescence, adulthood, pregnancy and breastfeeding, and older age.
5. Reduce daily sodium intake to less than 2,300 milligrams (mg) and further reduce intake to 1,500 mg among persons who are 51 and older and those of any age who are African American or have hypertension, diabetes, or chronic kidney disease. The 1,500 mg recommendation applies to about half of the U.S. population, including children, and the majority of adults.
6. Consume less than 10 percent of calories from saturated fatty acids by replacing them with monounsaturated and polyunsaturated fatty acids.
7. Consume less than 300 mg per day of dietary cholesterol.
8. Keep trans fatty acid consumption as low as possible by limiting foods that contain synthetic sources of trans fats, such as partially hydrogenated oils, and by limiting other solid fats.
9. Reduce the intake of calories from solid fats and added sugars.
10. Limit the consumption of foods that contain refined grains, especially refined grain foods that contain solid fats, added sugars, and sodium.
11. If alcohol is consumed, it should be consumed in moderation—up to one drink per day for women and two drinks per day for men—and only by adults of legal drinking age.

Foods and Nutrients to Increase Individuals should meet the following recommendations as part of a healthy eating pattern while staying within their calorie needs.

12. Increase vegetable and fruit intake.
13. Eat a variety of vegetables, especially dark-green and red and orange vegetables and beans and peas.
14. Consume at least half of all grains as whole grains. Increase whole-grain intake by replacing refined grains with whole grains.
15. Increase intake of fat-free or low-fat milk and milk products, such as milk, yogurt, cheese, or fortified soy beverages.
16. Choose a variety of protein foods, which include seafood, lean meat and poultry, eggs, beans and peas, soy products, and unsalted nuts and seeds.
17. Increase the amount and variety of seafood consumed by choosing seafood in place of some meat and poultry.
18. Replace protein foods that are higher in solid fats with choices that are lower in solid fats and calories and/or are sources of oils.
19. Use oils to replace solid fats where possible.
20. Choose foods that provide more potassium, dietary fiber, calcium, and vitamin D, which are nutrients of concern in American diets. These foods include vegetables, fruits, whole grains, and milk and milk products.

Recommendations for Specific Population Groups

Women Capable of Becoming Pregnant

1. Choose foods that supply heme iron, which is more readily absorbed by the body, additional iron sources, and enhancers of iron absorption such as vitamin C–rich foods.
2. Consume 400 micrograms (mcg) per day of synthetic folic acid (from fortified foods and/or supplements) in addition to food forms of folate from a varied diet.

Pregnant or Breastfeeding Women

1. Consume 8 to 12 ounces of seafood per week from a variety of seafood types.
2. Due to their high methyl mercury content, limit white (albacore) tuna to six ounces per week and do not eat the following four types of fish: tilefish, shark, swordfish, and king mackerel.
3. If pregnant, take an iron supplement, as recommended by an obstetrician or other health care provider.

For Individuals 50 Years and Older

1. Consume foods fortified with vitamin B12, such as fortified cereals, or dietary supplements.

Building Healthy Eating Patterns

1. Select an eating pattern that meets nutrient needs over time at an appropriate calorie level.
2. Account for all foods and beverages consumed and assess how they fit within a total healthy eating pattern.
3. Follow food safety recommendations when preparing and eating foods to reduce the risk of food-borne illnesses.

Additional information on these guidelines is posted at www.DietaryGuidelines.gov/.

3.12 Proper Nutrition: A Lifetime Prescription for Healthy Living

The three factors that do the most for health, longevity, and quality of life are proper nutrition, a sound exercise program, and quitting (or never starting) smoking. Achieving and maintaining a balanced diet is not as difficult as most people think. If everyone were more educated about their own nutrition habits and the nutrition habits of their children, the current magnitude of nutrition-related health problems would be much smaller. Although treatment of obesity is important, we should place far greater emphasis on preventing obesity in youth and adults in the first place.

Children tend to eat the way their parents do. If parents adopt a healthy diet, children most likely will follow. The difficult part for most people is to retrain themselves—to closely examine the eating habits they learned from their parents—to follow a lifetime healthy nutrition plan that includes lots of grains, legumes, fruits, vegetables, and low-fat dairy products, with moderate use of animal protein, junk food, sodium, and alcohol.

> **Critical Thinking**
>
> What factors in your life and the environment have contributed to your current dietary habits? • Do you need to make changes? • What may prevent you from doing so?

In spite of the ample scientific evidence linking poor dietary habits to early disease and mortality rates, many people remain precontemplators: They are not willing to change their eating patterns. Even when faced with obesity, elevated blood lipids, hypertension, and other nutrition-related conditions, people do not change. The motivating factor to change one's eating habits seems to be a major health breakdown, such as a heart attack, a stroke, or cancer—by which time the damage has been done already. In many cases it is irreversible and, for some, fatal.

An ounce of prevention is worth a pound of cure. The sooner you implement the dietary guidelines presented in this chapter, the better your chances of preventing chronic diseases and reaching a higher state of wellness.

ASSESS YOUR BEHAVIOR

CENGAGEbrain To access course materials, including companion resources, please visit www.cengagebrain.com.

1. Are whole grains, fruits, and vegetables the staples of your diet?
2. Are you meeting your personal MyPlate recommendations for daily fruits, vegetables, grains, protein, and dairy?
3. Will the information presented in this chapter change in any manner the way you eat?
4. Are there dietary changes that you need to implement to meet energy, nutrition, and disease risk-reduction guidelines and improve health and wellness? If so, list these changes and indicate what you will do to make it happen.

ASSESS YOUR KNOWLEDGE

Evaluate how well you understand the concepts presented in this chapter using the chapter-specific quizzing available in the online materials at www.cengagebrain.com.

1. The science of nutrition studies the relationship of
   a. vitamins and minerals to health.
   b. foods to optimal health and performance.
   c. carbohydrates, fats, and proteins to the development and maintenance of good health.
   d. the macronutrients and micronutrients to physical performance.
   e. kilocalories to calories in food items.

2. Faulty nutrition often plays a crucial role in the development and progression of which disease?
   a. cardiovascular disease
   b. cancer
   c. osteoporosis
   d. diabetes
   e. All are correct choices.

3. According to MyPlate, daily vegetable consumption is measured in
   a. servings.
   b. ounces.
   c. cups.
   d. calories.
   e. all of the above.

4. The recommended amount of fiber intake for adults 50 years and younger is
   a. 10 grams per day for women and 12 grams for men.
   b. 21 grams per day for women and 30 grams for men.
   c. 28 grams per day for women and 35 grams for men.
   d. 25 grams per day for women and 38 grams for men.
   e. 45 grams per day for women and 50 grams for men.

5. Unhealthy fats include
   a. unsaturated fatty acids.
   b. monounsaturated fats.
   c. polyunsaturated fatty acids.
   d. saturated fats.
   e. all of the above.

6. The daily recommended carbohydrate intake is
   a. 45 to 65 percent of the total calories.
   b. 10 to 35 percent of the total calories.
   c. 20 to 35 percent of the total calories.
   d. 60 to 75 percent of the total calories.
   e. 35 to 50 percent of the total calories.

7. The amount of a nutrient that is estimated to meet the nutrient requirement of half the healthy people in specific age and gender groups is known as the
   a. estimated average requirement.
   b. recommended dietary allowance.
   c. daily values.
   d. adequate intake.
   e. dietary reference intake.

8. The percent fat intake for an individual who on a given day consumes 2,385 calories with 106 grams of fat is
   a. 44 percent of total calories.
   b. 17.7 percent of total calories.
   c. 40 percent of total calories.
   d. 31 percent of total calories.
   e. 22.5 percent of total calories.

9. Carbohydrate loading is beneficial for
   a. endurance athletes.
   b. people with diabetes.
   c. strength athletes.
   d. sprinters.
   e. All of the above are correct.

10. Osteoporosis is
    a. crippling disease.
    b. more prevalent in women.
    c. more prevalent in people who were calcium deficient at a young age.
    d. linked to heavy drinking and smoking.
    e. All are correct choices.

Correct answers can be found at the back of the book.

Body Composition

4

Achieving recommended body weight improves health parameters, but most importantly, it improves quality of life by allowing you to pursue tasks of daily living, along with leisure and recreational activities, without functional limitations. You will also rejoice in the way you feel if you follow a healthy diet, remain physically active, and maintain a lifetime exercise program.

Objectives

- **Define** body composition and understand its relationship to assessment of recommended body weight.
- **Explain** the difference between essential fat and storage fat.
- **Describe** various techniques used to assess body composition.
- **Be able** to assess body composition using skinfold thickness and girth measurements.
- **Understand** the importance of body mass index (BMI), waist circumference, and waste-to-height ratio in the assessment of risk for disease.
- **Be able** to determine recommended weight according to recommended percent body fat values and BMI.
- **Learn** how to measure body composition.
- **Assess** your risks for potential disease.

CENGAGEbrain.com

Visit **www.cengagebrain.com** to access course materials and companion resources for this text, including quiz questions designed to check your understanding of the chapter contents. See the preface on page ix for more information.

FAQ

What constitutes ideal body weight?

There is no such thing as "ideal" body weight. Health/fitness professionals prefer to use the terms "recommended" or "healthy" body weight. Let's examine the question in more detail. For instance, 25 percent body fat is the recommended health fitness standard for a 40-year-old man. For the average "apparently healthy" individual, this body fat percentage does not constitute a threat to good health. Due to genetic and lifestyle conditions, however, if a person this same age at 25 percent body fat is prediabetic, prehypertensive, and with abnormal blood lipids (cholesterol and triglycerides—see Chapter 10), weight (fat) loss and a lower percent body fat may be recommended. Thus, what will work as recommended weight for most individuals may not be the best standard for individuals with disease risk factors. The current recommended or healthy weight standards (based on percent body fat or BMI) are established at the point where there appears to be a lower incidence for overweight-related conditions for most people. Individual differences have to be taken into consideration when making a final recommendation, especially in people with risk factors or a personal and family history of chronic conditions.

How accurate are body composition assessments?

Most of the techniques to determine body composition require proper training on the part of the technician administering the test (skinfolds, hydrostatic weighing, DXA, Bod Pod) and, in the case of hydrostatic weighing, proper performance on the part of the person being tested. As detailed in this chapter, body composition assessment is not a precise science. Some of the procedures are more accurate than others. Before undergoing body composition testing, make sure that you understand the accuracy of the technique (see standard error of estimates [SEEs] included under the description of each technique); and even more important, inquire about the training and experience of the person administering the test. We often encounter individuals who have been tested elsewhere by any number of assessments, particularly skinfolds, who come to our laboratory in disbelief (and rightfully so) because of the results that were given to them. To obtain the best possible results, look for trained and experienced technicians.

Is there a future trend in body composition assessment?

Results of research data indicate that the area of the body where people store fat is more critical than how much is stored. Individuals with a higher amount of intra-abdominal or abdominal visceral fat (located around internal organs), as opposed to primarily abdominal fat stored beneath the skin (subcutaneous fat), are at greater risk for disease. Thus, to increase disease risk evaluation, future body composition tests will be designed to get a clearer view of where the abdominal fat lies.

Additionally, although not a body composition assessment, body mass index (BMI) guidelines to detect thinness and excessive fatness (see BMI section on page 130) will most likely change based on age, gender, and physical activity patterns. BMIs of 25 or greater are not accurate predictors of excessive fatness in younger people and in athletic populations. Furthermore, because of differences in essential fat between men and women, the same standard may not apply for men and women alike.

Real Life Story | Shondra's Experience

I was surprised at my results of the body composition assessments that we did in our lab. The BMI calculation told me I was at a healthy weight (about 24). But when we did the skinfold test, I found out that I was almost 29 percent body fat, which is considered overweight. I talked about it with my instructor, and I told her that for the first two years after starting college I had yo-yo dieted. I would eat a lot less, lose weight, and then get sick of dieting, eat what I wanted, and gain it all back, plus more. Also, I hated to exercise, so I didn't do anything other than just walking from class to class. My instructor said she felt that my higher percent body fat might be due to my weight loss history. Each time I dieted, I probably lost lean body mass along with fat, and then when I gained weight back, I mainly gained fat, so over time my percent body fat went up. The good news is that over the course of the year, I became much more active and even started doing some basic strength training. Even though I didn't lose any weight, my percent body fat went down to 23 percent, which is a lot healthier.

PERSONAL PROFILE: Personal Body Composition Profile

Please answer the following questions to the best of your ability. If you cannot answer all of them at this time, you will be able to do so as you work through the chapter contents.

I. Do you understand the concept of body composition and its relationship to recommended body weight, proper weight management, and good health? Yes ___ No ___

II. Current values
Body weight: ___ lb
Percent body fat is: ___ %
Classification: ___
Lean body mass: ___ lb

Body Mass Index (BMI): Disease risk: ___
Classification: ___
Waist Circumference (WC): Disease risk: ___
Classification: ___

III. Goals for the end of the term:
Body weight: ___ lb
Percent body fat: ___ %
BMI: ___ WC: ___

IV. Can you relate to Shondra's experience, and what can you do in your life to avoid the same pitfalls?

To understand the concept of **body composition**, we must recognize that the human body consists of fat and nonfat components. The fat component is called fat mass or **percent body fat**. The nonfat component is termed **lean body mass**.

To determine **recommended body weight**, we need to find out what percent of total body weight is fat and what amount is lean tissue—in other words, assess body composition. Body composition should be assessed by a well-trained technician who understands the procedure being used.

Once the fat percentage is known, recommended body weight can be calculated from recommended body fat. Recommended body weight, also called "healthy weight," implies the absence of any medical condition that would improve with weight loss and a fat distribution pattern that is not associated with higher risk for illness.

Formerly, people relied on simple height/weight charts to determine their recommended body weight, but these tables can be highly inaccurate and fail to identify critical fat values associated with higher risk for disease. Standard height/weight tables, first published in 1912, were based on average weights (including shoes and clothing) for men and women who obtained life insurance policies between 1888 and 1905—a notably unrepresentative population. The recommended body weight on these tables was obtained according to gender, height, and frame size. Because no scientific guidelines were given to determine frame size, most people chose their frame size based on the column in which the weight came closest to their own!

The best way to determine whether people are truly **overweight** or falsely at recommended body weight is through assessment of body composition. **Obesity** is an excess of body fat. If body weight is the only criterion, an individual might easily appear to be overweight according to height/weight charts, yet not have too much body fat. Typical examples are football players, body builders, weight lifters, and other athletes with large muscle size. Some athletes who appear to be 20 or 30 pounds overweight really have little body fat.

The importance of body composition was clearly demonstrated when a young man who weighed about 225 pounds applied to join a city police force but was turned down without having been granted an interview. The reason? He was "too fat." When this young man's body composition was assessed at a preventive medicine clinic, it was determined that only 5 percent of his total body weight was in the form of fat—considerably less than the recommended standard. In the words of the director of the clinic, "The only way this fellow could come down to the chart's target weight would have been through surgical removal of a large amount of his muscle tissue."

At the other end of the spectrum, some people who weigh very little (and may be viewed as skinny or underweight) actually can be classified as overweight because of their high body fat content. People who weigh as little as 120 pounds but are more than 30 percent fat (about one-third of their total body weight) are not rare. These cases are found more readily in the sedentary population and among people who are always dieting. Physical inactivity and a constant negative caloric balance both lead to a loss in lean body mass (see Chapter 5).

Body composition The fat and nonfat components of the human body; important in assessing recommended body weight.

Percent body fat Proportional amount of fat in the body based on the person's total weight; includes both essential fat and storage fat; also termed fat mass.

Lean body mass Body weight without body fat.

Recommended body weight Body weight at which there seems to be no harm to human health; healthy weight.

Overweight An excess amount of weight against a given standard, such as height or recommended percent body fat.

Obesity An excessive accumulation of body fat, usually at least 30 percent greater than recommended body weight.

These examples illustrate that body weight alone clearly does not tell the whole story.

4.1 Essential and Storage Fat

Total fat in the human body is classified into two types: **essential fat** and **storage fat**. Essential fat is needed for normal physiological function. Without it, human health and physical performance deteriorate. This type of fat is found within tissues such as muscles, nerve cells, bone marrow, intestines, heart, liver, and lungs. Essential fat constitutes about 3 percent of the total weight in men and 12 percent in women (see Figure 4.1). The percentage is higher in women because it includes sex-specific fat, such as that found in the breast tissue, the uterus, and other sex-related fat deposits.

Storage fat is the fat stored in adipose tissue, mostly just beneath the skin (subcutaneous fat) and around major organs in the body. This fat serves three basic functions:

1. As an insulator to retain body heat
2. As energy substrate for metabolism
3. As padding against physical trauma to the body

The amount of storage fat does not differ between men and women, except that men tend to store fat around the waist and women around the hips and thighs.

4.2 Techniques to Assess Body Composition

Body composition can be estimated through the several procedures described in the following pages. Each procedure includes a standard error of estimate (SEE), a measure of the accuracy of the prediction made through the regression equation for that specific technique. For example, if the SEE for a given technique is 3.0 and the individual tests at a fat percentage of 18.0, the actual fat percentage may range from 15 to 21 percent.

Dual Energy X-ray Absorptiometry Dual energy x-ray absorptiometry (DXA) is a method to assess body composition that is used most frequently in research and by medical facilities. A radiographic technique, DXA uses very low-dose beams of x-ray energy (hundreds of times lower than a typical body x-ray) to measure total body fat mass, fat distribution pattern (see "Waist Circumference" on page 133), and bone density. Bone density is measured to assess the risk for osteoporosis. The procedure itself is simple and takes less than 15 minutes to administer. Many exercise scientists consider DXA to be the standard technique to assess body composition. The SEE for this technique is ±1.8 percent.

Due to costs, DXA is not readily available to most fitness participants. Thus, other methods to estimate body composition are used. The most common of these are:

1. Hydrostatic or underwater weighing
2. Air displacement
3. Skinfold thickness
4. Girth measurements
5. Bioelectrical impedance

Because these procedures yield estimates of body fat, each technique may yield slightly different values. Therefore, when assessing changes in body composition, be sure to use the same technique for pre- and post-test comparisons.

The most accurate technique presently available in fitness laboratories is still hydrostatic weighing. Other techniques to assess body composition are available, but the equipment is costly and not easily accessible to the general population. In addition to percentages of lean tissue and body fat, some of these methods also provide information on total body water and bone mass. These techniques include air displacement, magnetic resonance imaging (MRI), computed tomography (CT), and total body electrical conductivity (TOBEC). In terms of predicting percent body fat, these techniques are not more accurate than hydrostatic weighing.

Figure 4.1 Typical body composition of an adult man and woman.

Male: 43% Muscle, 3% Essential fat, 14% Bone, 15% Storage fat, 25% Other tissues

Female: 36% Muscle, 12% Essential fat, 15% Bone, 12% Storage fat, 25% Other tissues

The dual energy x-ray absorptiometry (DXA) technique to assess body composition and bone density.

Hydrostatic Weighing For decades, **hydrostatic weighing** has been the most common technique used in determining body composition in exercise physiology laboratories. In essence, a person's "regular" weight is compared with a weight taken underwater. Because fat is more buoyant than lean tissue, comparing the two weights can determine a person's percent of fat. Almost all other indirect techniques to assess body composition have been validated against hydrostatic weighing. The procedure requires a considerable amount of time, skill, space, and equipment and must be administered by a well-trained technician. The SEE for hydrostatic weighing is ±2.5 percent.

This technique has several drawbacks. First, because each individual assessment can take as long as 30 minutes, hydrostatic weighing is not feasible when testing a lot of people. Furthermore, the person's residual lung volume (amount of air left in the lungs following complete forceful exhalation) should be measured before testing. If residual volume cannot be measured, as is the case in some laboratories and health/fitness centers, it is estimated using the predicting equations, which may decrease the accuracy of hydrostatic weighing. Also, the requirement of being completely underwater makes hydrostatic weighing difficult to administer to **aquaphobic** people. For accurate results, the individual must be able to perform the test properly.

For each underwater weighing trial, the person has to (a) force out all of the air in the lungs, (b) lean forward and completely submerge underwater for about 5 to 10 seconds (long enough to get the underwater weight), and (c) remain as calm as possible (chair movement makes reading the scale difficult). This procedure is repeated 8 to 10 times.

Forcing all of the air out of the lungs is not easy for everyone but is important to obtain an accurate reading. Leaving additional air (beyond residual volume) in the lungs makes a person more buoyant. Because fat is less dense than water, overweight individuals weigh less in water. Additional air in the lungs makes a person lighter in water, yielding a false, higher body fat percentage.

Bod Pod, used for assessment of body composition.

Hydrostatic or underwater weighing technique.

Air Displacement Air displacement (also known as air displacement plethysmography) is a newer technique to assess body composition that holds considerable promise. With this method, an individual sits inside a small chamber, commercially known as the **Bod Pod**. Computerized pressure sensors determine the amount of air displaced by the person inside the

> **Essential fat** Minimal amount of body fat needed for normal physiological functions; constitutes about 3 percent of total weight in men and 12 percent in women.
>
> **Storage fat** Body fat in excess of essential fat; stored in adipose tissue.
>
> **Dual energy x-ray absorptiometry (DXA)** Method to assess body composition that uses very low-dose beams of x-ray energy to measure total body fat mass, fat distribution pattern, and bone density.
>
> **Hydrostatic weighing** Underwater technique to assess body composition; considered the most accurate of the body composition assessment techniques.
>
> **Aquaphobic** Having a fear of water.
>
> **Air displacement** Technique to assess body composition by calculating the body volume from the air replaced by an individual sitting inside a small chamber.
>
> **Bod Pod** Commercial name of the equipment used to assess body composition through the air displacement technique.

Various types of calipers used to assess skinfold thickness.

Skinfold thickness technique.

chamber. Body volume is calculated by subtracting the air volume with the person inside the chamber from the volume of the empty chamber. The amount of air in the person's lungs also is taken into consideration when determining actual body volume. Body density and percent body fat then are calculated from the obtained body volume. The procedure to assess body composition according to air displacement takes only about 15 minutes. Initial research showed that this technique compared favorably with hydrostatic weighing, and it is less cumbersome to administer. The published SEE for air displacement compared with hydrostatic weighing was approximately ±2.2 percent; however, the SEE may actually be higher. Recent research has determined that percent body fat is about 5 percentage points higher with air displacement than with hydrostatic weighing.[1] The strong positive correlations found between the two techniques resulted from air displacement consistently overestimating percent body fat. The researchers concluded that further technical work is required to make air displacement an acceptable technique to determine body composition. Other investigators also found this method to overestimate percent body fat.[2] Furthermore, research is required to determine its accuracy among different age groups, ethnic backgrounds, and athletic populations. At present, the Bod Pod is not readily available in most fitness centers and exercise laboratories.

Skinfold Thickness

Because of the cost, time, and complexity of hydrostatic weighing and the expense of Bod Pod equipment, most health and fitness programs use **anthropometric measurement** techniques. These techniques, primarily skinfold thickness and girth measurements, allow quick, simple, and inexpensive estimates of body composition.

Assessing body composition using **skinfold thickness** is based on the principle that the amount of **subcutaneous fat** is proportional to total body fat. Valid and reliable measurements of this tissue give a good indication of percent body fat. The SEE for skinfold analysis is ±3.5 percent.

The skinfold test is done with the aid of pressure calipers. Several techniques requiring measurement of three to seven sites have been developed. The following three-site procedure is the most commonly used technique. The sites measured are as follows (also see Figure 4.2):

Women: triceps, suprailium, and thigh skinfolds
Men: chest, abdomen, and thigh
All measurements should be taken on the right side of the body.

With the skinfold technique, training is necessary to obtain accurate measurements. In addition, different technicians may produce slightly different measurements of the same person. Therefore, the same technician should take pre- and post-test measurements.

Measurements should be done at the same time of the day—preferably in the morning—because changes in water hydration from activity and exercise can affect skinfold girth. The procedure is given in Figure 4.2. If skinfold calipers are available, you may assess your percent body fat with the help of your instructor or an experienced technician (also see Activity 4.1). Then locate the percent fat estimates in Table 4.1, 4.2, or 4.3, as appropriate.

Girth Measurements

Another method that is frequently used to estimate body fat is to measure circumferences, or **girth measurements**, at various body sites. This technique requires only a standard measuring tape. The limitation is that it may not be valid for athletic individuals (men or women) who participate actively in strenuous physical activity or for people who can be classified visually as thin or obese. The SEE for girth measurements is approximately ±4 percent.

The required procedure for girth measurements is given in Figure 4.3; conversion factors are in Tables 4.4 and 4.5. Measurements for women are the upper arm, hip, and wrist; for men, the waist and wrist.

Chapter 4 Body Composition

Figure 4.2 Procedure and anatomical landmarks for skinfold measurements.

Skinfold Measurement

1. Select the proper anatomical sites. For men, use chest, abdomen, and thigh skinfolds. For women, use triceps, suprailium, and thigh skinfolds. Take all measurements on the right side of the body with the person standing.

2. Measure each site by grasping a double thickness of skin firmly with the thumb and forefinger, pulling the fold slightly away from the muscular tissue. Hold the caliper perpendicular to the fold and take the measurement 1/2" below the finger hold. Measure each site three times and read the values to the nearest .1 to .5 mm. Record the average of the two closest readings as the final value for that site. Take the readings without delay to avoid excessive compression of the skinfold. Release and refold the skinfold between readings.

3. When doing pre- and post-assessments, conduct the measurement at the same time of day. The best time is early in the morning to avoid water hydration changes resulting from activity or exercise.

4. Obtain percent fat by adding the skinfold measurements from all three sites and looking up the respective values in Tables 4.1, 4.2, or 4.3.

For example, if the skinfold measurements for an 18-year-old female are (a) triceps = 16, (b) suprailium = 4, and (c) thigh = 30 (total = 50), the percent body fat is 20.6%.

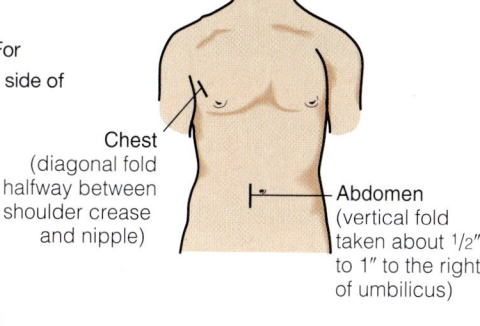

Chest (diagonal fold halfway between shoulder crease and nipple)

Abdomen (vertical fold taken about 1/2" to 1" to the right of umbilicus)

Triceps (vertical fold on back of upper arm, halfway between shoulder and elbow)

Suprailium (diagonal fold above crest of ilium, on the side of the hip)

Thigh (vertical fold on front of thigh, midway between knee and hip)

Bioelectrical Impedance

The **bioelectrical impedance** technique is much simpler to administer, but its accuracy is questionable. In this technique, sensors are applied to the skin and a weak (totally painless) electrical current is run through the body to measure its electrical resistance, which is then used to estimate body fat, lean body mass, and body water.

The technique is based on the principle that fat tissue is a less efficient conductor of electrical current than is lean tissue. The easier the conductance is, the leaner the individual. Specialized equipment or simple body weight scales with sensors on the surface can be used to perform this procedure.

The accuracy of equations used to estimate percent body fat with this technique is questionable. A single equation cannot be used for everyone, but rather valid and accurate equations to estimate body fat for the specific population (age, gender, and ethnicity) being tested are required. Several factors can affect the results, including hydration and body temperature. Following all manufacturers' instructions will ensure the most accurate result, but even then percent body fat may be off—typically on the higher end, by as much as 10 percentage points (or even more on some scales).

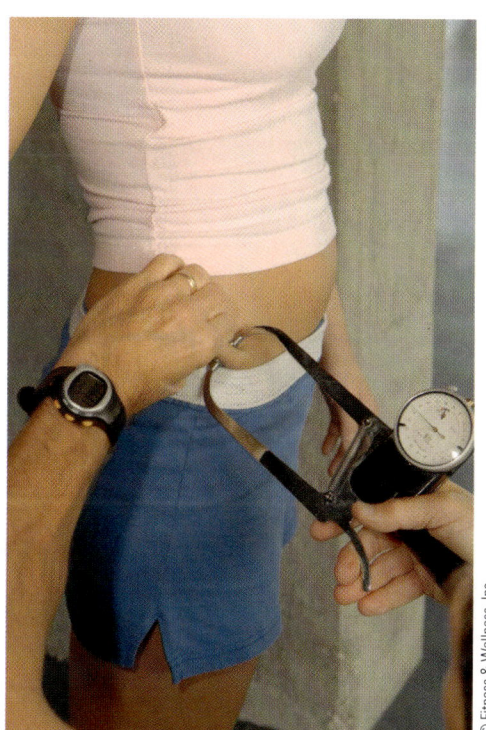

Suprailium skinfold assessment.

Anthropometric measurement Techniques to measure body girths at different sites.

Skinfold thickness Technique to assess body composition by measuring a double thickness of skin at specific body sites.

Subcutaneous fat Deposits of fat directly under the skin.

Girth measurements Technique to assess body composition by measuring circumferences at specific body sites.

Bioelectrical impedance Technique to assess body composition by running a weak electrical current through the body.

Table 4.1 Skinfold Thickness Technique: Percent Fat Estimates for Women Calculated from Triceps, Suprailium, and Thigh

Sum of 3 Skinfolds	Age at Last Birthday								
	22 or Under	23 to 27	28 to 32	33 to 37	38 to 42	43 to 47	48 to 52	53 to 57	58 and Over
23–25	9.7	9.9	10.2	10.4	10.7	10.9	11.2	11.4	11.7
26–28	11.0	11.2	11.5	11.7	12.0	12.3	12.5	12.7	13.0
29–31	12.3	12.5	12.8	13.0	13.3	13.5	13.8	14.0	14.3
32–34	13.6	13.8	14.0	14.3	14.5	14.8	15.0	15.3	15.5
35–37	14.8	15.0	15.3	15.5	15.8	16.0	16.3	16.5	16.8
38–40	16.0	16.3	16.5	16.7	17.0	17.2	17.5	17.7	18.0
41–43	17.2	17.4	17.7	17.9	18.2	18.4	18.7	18.9	19.2
44–46	18.3	18.6	18.8	19.1	19.3	19.6	19.8	20.1	20.3
47–49	19.5	19.7	20.0	20.2	20.5	20.7	21.0	21.2	21.5
50–52	20.6	20.8	21.1	21.3	21.6	21.8	22.1	22.3	22.6
53–55	21.7	21.9	22.1	22.4	22.6	22.9	23.1	23.4	23.6
56–58	22.7	23.0	23.2	23.4	23.7	23.9	24.2	24.4	24.7
59–61	23.7	24.0	24.2	24.5	24.7	25.0	25.2	25.5	25.7
62–64	24.7	25.0	25.2	25.5	25.7	26.0	26.2	26.4	26.7
65–67	25.7	25.9	26.2	26.4	26.7	26.9	27.2	27.4	27.7
68–70	26.6	26.9	27.1	27.4	27.6	27.9	28.1	28.4	28.6
71–73	27.5	27.8	28.0	28.3	28.5	28.8	29.0	29.3	29.5
74–76	28.4	28.7	28.9	29.2	29.4	29.7	29.9	30.2	30.4
77–79	29.3	29.5	29.8	30.0	30.3	30.5	30.8	31.0	31.3
80–82	30.1	30.4	30.6	30.9	31.1	31.4	31.6	31.9	32.1
83–85	30.9	31.2	31.4	31.7	31.9	32.2	32.4	32.7	32.9
86–88	31.7	32.0	32.2	32.5	32.7	32.9	33.2	33.4	33.7
89–91	32.5	32.7	33.0	33.2	33.5	33.7	33.9	34.2	34.4
92–94	33.2	33.4	33.7	33.9	34.2	34.4	34.7	34.9	35.2
95–97	33.9	34.1	34.4	34.6	34.9	35.1	35.4	35.6	35.9
98–100	34.6	34.8	35.1	35.3	35.5	35.8	36.0	36.3	36.5
101–103	35.2	35.4	35.7	35.9	36.2	36.4	36.7	36.9	37.2
104–106	35.8	36.1	36.3	36.6	36.8	37.1	37.3	37.5	37.8
107–109	36.4	36.7	36.9	37.1	37.4	37.6	37.9	38.1	38.4
110–112	37.0	37.2	37.5	37.7	38.0	38.2	38.5	38.7	38.9
113–115	37.5	37.8	38.0	38.2	38.5	38.7	39.0	39.2	39.5
116–118	38.0	38.3	38.5	38.8	39.0	39.3	39.5	39.7	40.0
119–121	38.5	38.7	39.0	39.2	39.5	39.7	40.0	40.2	40.5
122–124	39.0	39.2	39.4	39.7	39.9	40.2	40.4	40.7	40.9
125–127	39.4	39.6	39.9	40.1	40.4	40.6	40.9	41.1	41.4
128–130	39.8	40.0	40.3	40.5	40.8	41.0	41.3	41.5	41.8

Body density is calculated based on the generalized equation for predicting body density of women developed by A. S. Jackson, M. L. Pollock, and A. Ward and published in *Medicine and Science in Sports and Exercise* 12 (1980): 175–182. Percent body fat is determined from the calculated body density using the Siri formula.

© Cengage Learning

Body Mass Index The most common technique to determine thinness and excessive fatness is the **body mass index (BMI)**. BMI incorporates height and weight to estimate critical fat values at which the risk for disease increases.

BMI is calculated by either (1) dividing the weight in kilograms by the square of the height in meters or (2) multiplying body weight in pounds by 705 and dividing this figure by the square of the height in inches. For example, the BMI for an individual who weighs 172 pounds (78 kg) and is 67 inches (1.7 m) tall would be 27: [78 ÷ (1.7)^2] or [172 × 705 ÷ (67)^2]. You also can look up your BMI in Table 4.6 according to your height and weight.

Because of its simplicity and measurement consistency across populations, BMI is the most widely used method to determine overweight and obesity. Due to the various limitations of previously mentioned body composition techniques—including cost, availability to the general population, lack of consistency among technicians and laboratories, inconsistent

Table 4.2 Skinfold Thickness Technique: Percent Fat Estimates for Men Younger Than 40 Calculated from Chest, Abdomen, and Thigh

Sum of 3 Skinfolds	Age at Last Birthday							
	19 or Under	20 to 22	23 to 25	26 to 28	29 to 31	32 to 34	35 to 37	38 to 40
8–10	.9	1.3	1.6	2.0	2.3	2.7	3.0	3.3
11–13	1.9	2.3	2.6	3.0	3.3	3.7	4.0	4.3
14–16	2.9	3.3	3.6	3.9	4.3	4.6	5.0	5.3
17–19	3.9	4.2	4.6	4.9	5.3	5.6	6.0	6.3
20–22	4.8	5.2	5.5	5.9	6.2	6.6	6.9	7.3
23–25	5.8	6.2	6.5	6.8	7.2	7.5	7.9	8.2
26–28	6.8	7.1	7.5	7.8	8.1	8.5	8.8	9.2
29–31	7.7	8.0	8.4	8.7	9.1	9.4	9.8	10.1
32–34	8.6	9.0	9.3	9.7	10.0	10.4	10.7	11.1
35–37	9.5	9.9	10.2	10.6	10.9	11.3	11.6	12.0
38–40	10.5	10.8	11.2	11.5	11.8	12.2	12.5	12.9
41–43	11.4	11.7	12.1	12.4	12.7	13.1	13.4	13.8
44–46	12.2	12.6	12.9	13.3	13.6	14.0	14.3	14.7
47–49	13.1	13.5	13.8	14.2	14.5	14.9	15.2	15.5
50–52	14.0	14.3	14.7	15.0	15.4	15.7	16.1	16.4
53–55	14.8	15.2	15.5	15.9	16.2	16.6	16.9	17.3
56–58	15.7	16.0	16.4	16.7	17.1	17.4	17.8	18.1
59–61	16.5	16.9	17.2	17.6	17.9	18.3	18.6	19.0
62–64	17.4	17.7	18.1	18.4	18.8	19.1	19.4	19.8
65–67	18.2	18.5	18.9	19.2	19.6	19.9	20.3	20.6
68–70	19.0	19.3	19.7	20.0	20.4	20.7	21.1	21.4
71–73	19.8	20.1	20.5	20.8	21.2	21.5	21.9	22.2
74–76	20.6	20.9	21.3	21.6	22.0	22.2	22.7	23.0
77–79	21.4	21.7	22.1	22.4	22.8	23.1	23.4	23.8
80–82	22.1	22.5	22.8	23.2	23.5	23.9	24.2	24.6
83–85	22.9	23.2	23.6	23.9	24.3	24.6	25.0	25.3
86–88	23.6	24.0	24.3	24.7	25.0	25.4	25.7	26.1
89–91	24.4	24.7	25.1	25.4	25.8	26.1	26.5	26.8
92–94	25.1	25.5	25.8	26.2	26.5	26.9	27.2	27.5
95–97	25.8	26.2	26.5	26.9	27.2	27.6	27.9	28.3
98–100	26.6	26.9	27.3	27.6	27.9	28.3	28.6	29.0
101–103	27.3	27.6	28.0	28.3	28.6	29.0	29.3	29.7
104–106	27.9	28.3	28.6	29.0	29.3	29.7	30.0	30.4
107–109	28.6	29.0	29.3	29.7	30.0	30.4	30.7	31.1
110–112	29.3	29.6	30.0	30.3	30.7	31.0	31.4	31.7
113–115	30.0	30.3	30.7	31.0	31.3	31.7	32.0	32.4
116–118	30.6	31.0	31.3	31.6	32.0	32.3	32.7	33.0
119–121	31.3	31.6	32.0	32.3	32.6	33.0	33.3	33.7
122–124	31.9	32.2	32.6	32.9	33.3	33.6	34.0	34.3
125–127	32.5	32.9	33.2	33.5	33.9	34.2	34.6	34.9
128–130	33.1	33.5	33.8	34.2	34.5	34.9	35.2	35.5

Body density is calculated based on the generalized equation for predicting body density of men developed by A. S. Jackson, M. L. Pollock, and A. Ward and published in *Medicine and Science in Sports and Exercise* 40 (1978): 497–504. Percent body fat is determined from the calculated body density using the Siri formula.

© Cengage Learning

results between techniques, and standard error of measurement of the procedures—BMI is used almost exclusively to determine health risks and mortality rates associated with excessive body weight.

Scientific evidence indicates that the risk for disease starts to

> **Body mass index (BMI)** Technique to determine thinness and excessive fatness that incorporates height and weight to estimate critical fat values at which the risk for disease increases.

Table 4.3 Skinfold Thickness Technique: Percent Fat Estimates for Men Older Than 40 Calculated from Chest, Abdomen, and Thigh

Sum of 3 Skinfolds	Age at Last Birthday							
	41 to 43	44 to 46	47 to 49	50 to 52	53 to 55	56 to 58	59 to 61	62 and Over
8–10	3.7	4.0	4.4	4.7	5.1	5.4	5.8	6.1
11–13	4.7	5.0	5.4	5.7	6.1	6.4	6.8	7.1
14–16	5.7	6.0	6.4	6.7	7.1	7.4	7.8	8.1
17–19	6.7	7.0	7.4	7.7	8.1	8.4	8.7	9.1
20–22	7.6	8.0	8.3	8.7	9.0	9.4	9.7	10.1
23–25	8.6	8.9	9.3	9.6	10.0	10.3	10.7	11.0
26–28	9.5	9.9	10.2	10.6	10.9	11.3	11.6	12.0
29–31	10.5	10.8	11.2	11.5	11.9	12.2	12.6	12.9
32–34	11.4	11.8	12.1	12.4	12.8	13.1	13.5	13.8
35–37	12.3	12.7	13.0	13.4	13.7	14.1	14.4	14.8
38–40	13.2	13.6	13.9	14.3	14.6	15.0	15.3	15.7
41–43	14.1	14.5	14.8	15.2	15.5	15.9	16.2	16.6
44–46	15.0	15.4	15.7	16.1	16.4	16.8	17.1	17.5
47–49	15.9	16.2	16.6	16.9	17.3	17.6	18.0	18.3
50–52	16.8	17.1	17.5	17.8	18.2	18.5	18.8	19.2
53–55	17.6	18.0	18.3	18.7	19.0	19.4	19.7	20.1
56–58	18.5	18.8	19.2	19.5	19.9	20.2	20.6	20.9
59–61	19.3	19.7	20.0	20.4	20.7	21.0	21.4	21.7
62–64	20.1	20.5	20.8	21.2	21.5	21.9	22.2	22.6
65–67	21.0	21.3	21.7	22.0	22.4	22.7	23.0	23.4
68–70	21.8	22.1	22.5	22.8	23.2	23.5	23.9	24.2
71–73	22.6	22.9	23.3	23.6	24.0	24.3	24.7	25.0
74–76	23.4	23.7	24.1	24.4	24.8	25.1	25.4	25.8
77–79	24.1	24.5	24.8	25.2	25.5	25.9	26.2	26.6
80–82	24.9	25.3	25.6	26.0	26.3	26.6	27.0	27.3
83–85	25.7	26.0	26.4	26.7	27.1	27.4	27.8	28.1
86–88	26.4	26.8	27.1	27.5	27.8	28.2	28.5	28.9
89–91	27.2	27.5	27.9	28.2	28.6	28.9	29.2	29.6
92–94	27.9	28.2	28.6	28.9	29.3	29.6	30.0	30.3
95–97	28.6	29.0	29.3	29.7	30.0	30.4	30.7	31.1
98–100	29.3	29.7	30.0	30.4	30.7	31.1	31.4	31.8
101–103	30.0	30.4	30.7	31.1	31.4	31.8	32.1	32.5
104–106	30.7	31.1	31.4	31.8	32.1	32.5	32.8	33.2
107–109	31.4	31.8	32.1	32.4	32.8	33.1	33.5	33.8
110–112	32.1	32.4	32.8	33.1	33.5	33.8	34.2	34.5
113–115	32.7	33.1	33.4	33.8	34.1	34.5	34.8	35.2
116–118	33.4	33.7	34.1	34.4	34.8	35.1	35.5	35.8
119–121	34.0	34.4	34.7	35.1	35.4	35.8	36.1	36.5
122–124	34.7	35.0	35.4	35.7	36.1	36.4	36.7	37.1
125–127	35.3	35.6	36.0	36.3	36.7	37.0	37.4	37.7
128–130	35.9	36.2	36.6	36.9	37.3	37.6	38.0	38.5

Body density is calculated based on the generalized equation for predicting body density of men developed by A. S. Jackson and M. L. Pollock and published in the *British Journal of Nutrition* 40 (1978): 497–504. Percent body fat is determined from the calculated body density using the Siri formula.

© Cengage Learning

increase when BMI exceeds 25.[3] Although a BMI index between 18.5 and 25 is considered normal (see Tables 4.7 and 4.9), the lowest risk for chronic disease is in the 22 to 25 range.[4] Individuals are classified as overweight if their index lies between 25 and 30. A BMI greater than 30 is defined as obese, and one less than 18.5 is considered **underweight**. Scientific evidence has shown that even though the risk for premature illness and death is greater for those who are overweight, the risk is also increased for individuals who are underweight[5] (see Figure 4.4).

Figure 4.3 Procedure for body fat assessment according to girth measurements.

Girth Measurements for Women*

1. Using a regular tape measure, determine the following girth measurements in centimeters (cm):

   Upper arm: Take the measure halfway between the shoulder and the elbow.

   Hip: Measure at the point of largest circumference.

   Wrist: Take the girth in front of the bones where the wrist bends.

2. Obtain the person's age.

3. Using Table 4.4, find the subject's age and girth measurement for each site, then look up the respective constant value for each. These values will allow you to derive body density (BD) by substituting the constants in the following formula:

   $BD = A - B - C + D$

4. Using the derived body density, calculate percent body fat (%F) according to the following equation:

   $\%F = (495 \div BD) - 450$**

Example: Jane is 20 years old, and the following girth measurements were taken: biceps = 27 cm, hip = 99.5 cm, wrist = 15.4 cm

Data		Constant	
Upper arm	= 27 cm	A =	1.0813
Age	= 20	B =	.0102
Hip	= 99.5 cm	C =	.1206
Wrist	= 15.4 cm	D =	.0971

$BD = A - B - C + D$
$BD = 1.0813 - .0102 - .1206 + .0971 = 1.0476$
$\%F = (495 \div BD) - 450$
$\%F = (495 \div 1.0476) - 450 = 22.5$

Girth Measurements for Men**

1. Using a regular tape measure, determine the following girth measurements in inches (the men's measurements are taken in inches, as opposed to centimeters for women):

   Waist: Measure at the umbilicus (belly button).

   Wrist: Measure in front of the bones where the wrist bends.

2. Subtract the wrist from the waist measurement.

3. Obtain the weight of the subject in pounds.

4. Look up the percent body fat (%F) in Table 4.5 by using the difference obtained in number 2 above and the person's body weight.

Example: John weighs 160 pounds, and his waist and wrist girth measurements are 36.5 and 7.5 inches, respectively.

Waist girth = 36.5 inches
Wrist girth = 7.5 inches
Difference = 29.0 inches
Body weight = 160.0 lbs.
%F = 22

*From R. B. Lambson, "Generalized body density prediction equations for women using simple anthropometric measurements." Unpublished doctoral dissertation, Brigham Young University, Provo, UT, August 1987. Reproduced by permission.
**From W. E. Siri, *Body Composition from Fluid Spaces and Density* (Berkeley: University of California, Donner Laboratory of Medical Physics, March 19, 1956.)
***K. W. Penrouse, A. G. Nelson, and A. G. Fisher, "Generalized body composition equation for men using simple measurement techniques," *Medicine and Science in Sports and Exercise* 17, no. 2 (1985): 189.
© American College of Sports Medicine, 1985.

Compared with individuals who have a BMI between 22 and 25, people with a BMI between 25 and 30 (overweight) exhibit a mortality rate up to 25 percent higher; the rate for those with a BMI greater than 30 (obese) is 50 to 100 percent higher.[6] Table 4.7 provides disease risk categories when BMI is used as the sole criterion to identify people at risk. About one-third of the U.S. adult population has a BMI of 30 or more. Overweight and obesity trends starting in 1960 according to BMI are given in Figure 4.5. In addition, the prevalence of obesity by classification (obesity I, II, and III) is provided in Figure 4.6.

BMI is a useful screening tool in general, but its weakness is that it fails to differentiate fat from lean body mass or note where most of the fat is located (waist circumference—see discussion that follows). Using BMI, athletes with a large amount of muscle mass (such as body builders and football players) can easily fall in the moderate- or even high-risk categories.

Waist Circumference Scientific evidence suggests that the way people store fat affects their risk for disease. The total amount of body fat by itself is not the best predictor of increased risk for disease but, rather, the location of the fat. **Android obesity** is seen in individuals who tend to store fat in the trunk or abdominal area (which produces the "apple" shape). **Gynoid obesity** is seen in people who store fat primarily around the hips and thighs (which creates the "pear" shape).

Compared with people with body fat that is

> **Underweight** Extremely low body weight.
> **Android obesity** Obesity pattern seen in individuals who tend to store fat in the trunk or abdominal area.
> **Gynoid obesity** Obesity pattern seen in people who store fat primarily around the hips and thighs.

Table 4.4 Girth Measurement Technique: Conversion Constants to Calculate Body Density for Women

Upper Arm (cm)	Constant A	Age	Constant B	Hip (cm)	Constant C	Hip (cm)	Constant C	Wrist (cm)	Constant D
20.5	1.0966	17	.0086	79	.0957	114.5	.1388	13.0	.0819
21	1.0954	18	.0091	79.5	.0963	115	.1394	13.2	.0832
21.5	1.0942	19	.0096	80	.0970	115.5	.1400	13.4	.0845
22	1.0930	20	.0102	80.5	.0976	116	.1406	13.6	.0857
22.5	1.0919	21	.0107	81	.0982	116.5	.1412	13.8	.0870
23	1.0907	22	.0112	81.5	.0988	117	.1418	14.0	.0882
23.5	1.0895	23	.0117	82	.0994	117.5	.1424	14.2	.0895
24	1.0883	24	.0122	82.5	.1000	118	.1430	14.4	.0908
24.5	1.0871	25	.0127	83	.1006	118.5	.1436	14.6	.0920
25	1.0860	26	.0132	83.5	.1012	119	.1442	14.8	.0933
25.5	1.0848	27	.0137	84	.1018	119.5	.1448	15.0	.0946
26	1.0836	28	.0142	84.5	.1024	120	.1454	15.2	.0958
26.5	1.0824	29	.0147	85	.1030	120.5	.1460	15.4	.0971
27	1.0813	30	.0152	85.5	.1036	121	.1466	15.6	.0983
27.5	1.0801	31	.0157	86	.1042	121.5	.1472	15.8	.0996
28	1.0789	32	.0162	86.5	.1048	122	.1479	16.0	.1009
28.5	1.0777	33	.0168	87	.1054	122.5	.1485	16.2	.1021
29	1.0775	34	.0173	87.5	.1060	123	.1491	16.4	.1034
29.5	1.0754	35	.0178	88	.1066	123.5	.1497	16.6	.1046
30	1.0742	36	.0183	88.5	.1072	124	.1503	16.8	.1059
30.5	1.0730	37	.0188	89	.1079	124.5	.1509	17.0	.1072
31	1.0718	38	.0193	89.5	.1085	125	.1515	17.2	.1084
31.5	1.0707	39	.0198	90	.1091	125.5	.1521	17.4	.1097
32	1.0695	40	.0203	90.5	.1097	126	.1527	17.6	.1109
32.5	1.0683	41	.0208	91	.1103	126.5	.1533	17.8	.1122
33	1.0671	42	.0213	91.5	.1109	127	.1539	18.0	.1135
33.5	1.0666	43	.0218	92	.1115	127.5	.1545	18.2	.1147
34	1.0648	44	.0223	92.5	.1121	128	.1551	18.4	.1160
34.5	1.0636	45	.0228	93	.1127	128.5	.1558	18.6	.1172
35	1.0624	46	.0234	93.5	.1133	129	.1563		
35.5	1.0612	47	.0239	94	.1139	129.5	.1569		
36	1.0601	48	.0244	94.5	.1145	130	.1575		
36.5	1.0589	49	.0249	95	.1151	130.5	.1581		
37	1.0577	50	.0254	95.5	.1157	131	.1587		
37.5	1.0565	51	.0259	96	.1163	131.5	.1593		
38	1.0554	52	.0264	96.5	.1169	132	.1600		
38.5	1.0542	53	.0269	97	.1176	132.5	.1606		
39	1.0530	54	.0274	97.5	.1182	133	.1612		
39.5	1.0518	55	.0279	98	.1188	133.5	.1618		
40	1.0506	56	.0284	98.5	.1194	134	.1624		
40.5	1.0495	57	.0289	99	.1200	134.5	.1630		
41	1.0483	58	.0294	99.5	.1206	135	.1636		
41.5	1.0471	59	.0300	100	.1212	135.5	.1642		
42	1.0459	60	.0305	100.5	.1218	136	.1648		
42.5	1.0448	61	.0310	101	.1224	136.5	.1654		
43	1.0434	62	.0315	101.5	.1230	137	.1660		
43.5	1.0424	63	.0320	102	.1236	137.5	.1666		
44	1.0412	64	.0325	102.5	.1242	138	.1672		
		65	.0330	103	.1248	138.5	.1678		
		66	.0335	103.5	.1254	139	.1685		

Upper Arm (cm)	Constant A	Age	Constant B	Hip (cm)	Constant C	Hip (cm)	Constant C	Wrist (cm)	Constant D
		67	.0340	104	.1260	139.5	.1691		
		68	.0345	104.5	.1266	140	.1697		
		69	.0350	105	.1272	140.5	.1703		
		70	.0355	105.5	.1278	141	.1709		
		71	.0360	106	.1285	141.5	.1715		
		72	.0366	106.5	.1291	142	.1721		
		73	.0371	107	.1297	142.5	.1728		
		74	.0376	107.5	.1303	143	.1733		
		75	.0381	108	.1309	143.5	.1739		
				108.5	.1315	144	.1745		
				109	.1321	144.5	.1751		
				109.5	.1327	145	.1757		
				110	.1333	145.5	.1763		
				110.5	.1339	146	.1769		
				111	.1345	146.5	.1775		
				111.5	.1351	147	.1781		
				112	.1357	147.5	.1787		
				112.5	.1363	148	.1794		
				113	.1369	148.5	.1800		
				113.5	.1375	149	.1806		
				114	.1382	149.5	.1812		
						150	.1818		

© Cengage Learning

stored primarily in the hips and thighs, an increasing amount of evidence is showing that obese individuals with abdominal fat are clearly at higher risk for heart disease, hypertension, type 2 diabetes ("non–insulin-dependent" diabetes), stroke, some types of cancer, dementia, migraines, and diminished lung function. Evidence also indicates that among individuals with a lot of abdominal fat, those whose fat deposits are located around internal organs (intra-abdominal or visceral fat) rather than subcutaneously or retroperitoneally (see Figure 4.7) have an even greater risk for disease than those with fat mainly just

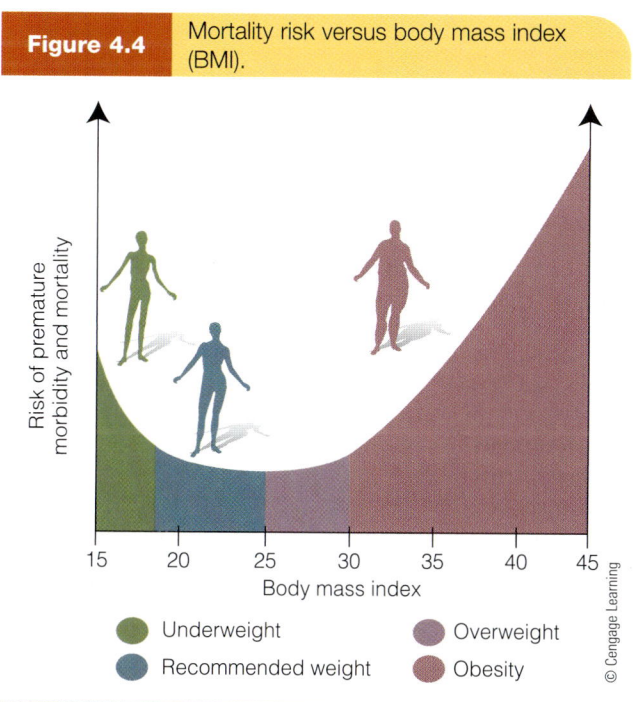

Figure 4.4 Mortality risk versus body mass index (BMI).

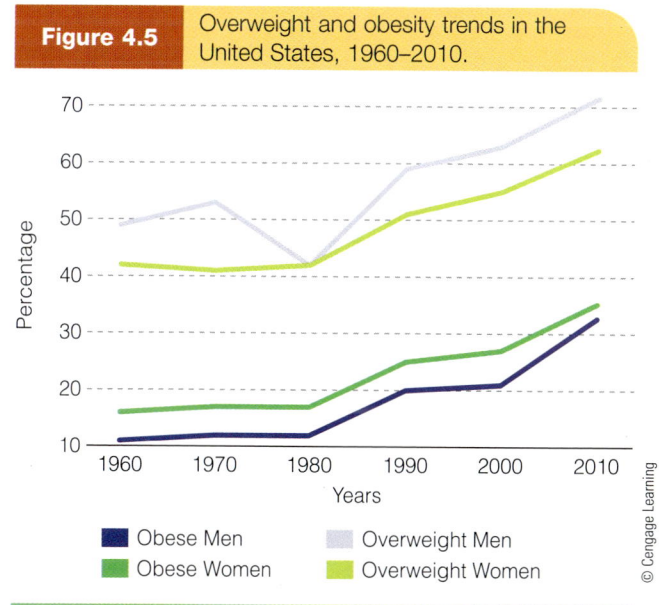

Figure 4.5 Overweight and obesity trends in the United States, 1960–2010.

SOURCE: Adapted from the National Center for Health Statistics, Centers for Disease Control and Prevention, and the *Journal of the American Medical Association*.

Table 4.5 Girth Measurement Technique: Estimated Percent Body Fat for Men

(Table content omitted due to size and complexity of numerical data.)

© Cengage Learning

Table 4.6 Determination of Body Mass Index (BMI)

Determine your BMI by looking up the number where your weight and height intersect on the table. According to the results, look up your disease risk in Tables 4.7 and 4.9.

Height	110	115	120	125	130	135	140	145	150	155	160	165	170	175	180	185	190	195	200	205	210	215	220	225	230	235	240	245	250
5'0"	21	22	23	24	25	26	27	28	29	30	31	32	33	34	35	36	37	38	39	40	41	42	43	44	45	46	47	48	49
5'1"	21	22	23	24	25	26	26	27	28	29	30	31	32	33	34	35	36	37	38	39	40	41	42	43	43	44	45	46	47
5'2"	20	21	22	23	24	25	26	27	27	28	29	30	31	32	33	34	35	36	37	37	38	39	40	41	42	43	44	45	46
5'3"	19	20	21	22	23	24	25	26	27	27	28	29	30	31	32	33	34	35	35	36	37	38	39	40	41	42	43	43	44
5'4"	19	20	21	21	22	23	24	25	26	27	27	28	29	30	31	32	33	33	34	35	36	37	38	39	39	40	41	42	43
5'5"	18	19	20	21	22	22	23	24	25	26	27	27	28	29	30	31	32	32	33	34	35	36	37	37	38	39	40	41	42
5'6"	18	19	19	20	21	22	23	23	24	25	26	27	27	28	29	30	31	31	32	33	34	35	36	36	37	38	39	40	40
5'7"	17	18	19	20	20	21	22	23	23	24	25	26	27	27	28	29	30	31	31	32	33	34	34	35	36	37	38	38	39
5'8"	17	17	18	19	20	21	21	22	23	24	24	25	26	27	27	28	29	30	30	31	32	33	33	34	35	36	36	37	38
5'9"	16	17	18	18	19	20	21	21	22	23	24	24	25	26	27	27	28	29	30	30	31	32	32	33	34	35	35	36	37
5'10"	16	16	17	18	19	19	20	21	22	22	23	24	24	25	26	27	27	28	29	29	30	31	32	32	33	34	34	35	36
5'11"	15	16	17	17	18	19	20	20	21	22	22	23	24	24	25	26	26	27	28	29	29	30	31	31	32	33	33	34	35
6'0"	15	16	16	17	18	18	19	20	20	21	22	22	23	24	24	25	26	26	27	28	28	29	30	31	31	32	33	33	34
6'1"	15	15	16	16	17	18	19	19	20	20	21	22	22	23	24	24	25	26	26	27	28	28	29	30	30	31	32	32	33
6'2"	14	15	15	16	17	17	18	19	19	20	21	21	22	23	23	24	24	25	26	26	27	28	28	29	30	30	31	31	32
6'3"	14	14	15	16	16	17	17	18	19	19	20	21	21	22	22	23	24	24	25	26	26	27	27	28	29	29	30	31	31
6'4"	13	14	15	15	16	16	17	18	18	19	19	20	21	21	22	23	23	24	24	25	26	26	27	27	28	29	29	30	30

Weight shown at top of table.

© Cengage Learning

beneath the skin (subcutaneous fat).[7] Of even greater significance, the results of a recent study that followed more than 350,000 people over almost 10 years concluded that even when body weight is viewed as "normal," individuals with a large waist circumference nearly double the risk for premature death.[8] Researchers believe that visceral fat secretes harmful inflammatory substances that contribute to chronic conditions.

Figure 4.6 Obesity prevalence by classification in U.S. Adults (>20 years of age), 2008.

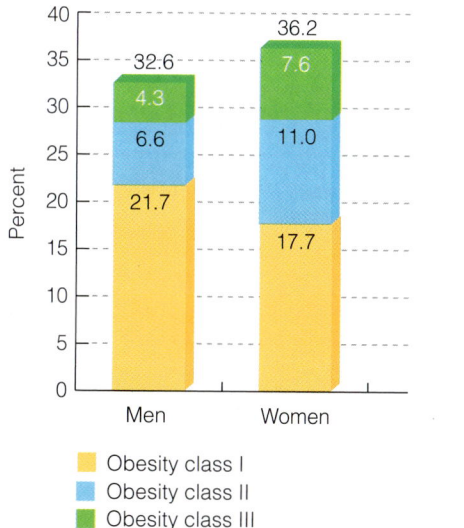

Men: 32.6 total (Obesity class I: 21.7, Obesity class II: 6.6, Obesity class III: 4.3)
Women: 36.2 total (Obesity class I: 17.7, Obesity class II: 11.0, Obesity class III: 7.6)

From Hoeger/Hoeger, Principals and Labs for Fitness and Wellness, 12E. © 2014 Cengage Learning.

Complex scanning techniques used to identify individuals at risk because of high intra-abdominal fatness are costly, so a simple **waist circumference (WC)** measure, designed by the National Heart, Lung, and Blood Institute, is used to assess this risk.[9] WC seems to predict abdominal visceral fat as accurately as the DXA technique.[10] A waist circumference of more than 40 inches in men and 35 inches in women indicates a higher risk for cardiovascular disease, hypertension, and type 2 diabetes (Table 4.8). Weight loss is encouraged when individuals exceed these measurements.

Research indicates that WC is a better predictor than BMI of the risk for disease.[11] Thus, BMI in conjunction with WC provides the best combination to identify individuals at higher risk resulting from excessive body fat. Table 4.9 provides guidelines to identify people at risk according to BMI and WC.

Waist-to-Height Ratio: "Keep your waist circumference to less than half your height."

The **waist-to-height ratio (WHtR)** is a new health risk assessment also used to ascertain the health risks of obesity. The ratio is rapidly gaining popularity in the

Waist circumference (WC) A waist girth measurement to assess potential risk for disease based on intra-abdominal fat content.

Waist-to-Height Ratio (WHtR) A waist-to-height ratio assessment equally applicable to tall and short persons used to determine potential risk for disease based on excessive body weight.

Table 4.7 Disease Risk according to Body Mass Index (BMI)

BMI	Disease Risk	Classification
<18.5	Increased	Underweight
18.5–21.99	Low	Acceptable
22.0–24.99	Very low	Acceptable
25.0–29.99	Increased	Overweight
30.0–34.99	High	Obesity I
35.0–39.99	Very high	Obesity II
≥40.0	Extremely high	Obesity III

© Cengage Learning

Table 4.8 Disease Risk according to Waist Circumference (WC)

Men	Women	Disease Risk
<35.5	32.5	Low
35.5–40.0	32.5–35.0	Moderate
>40.0	>35.0	High

© Cengage Learning

Individuals who accumulate body fat around the midsection are at greater risk for disease than those who accumulate body fat in other areas.

scientific community as research indicates that it is a better predictor of health outcomes, including multiple coronary heart disease risk factors, than BMI or WC.[12] While WC is superior to BMI, two individuals with a similar WC (e.g., 43) but of different heights, may not be at the same risk for disease; whereas, the new WHtR method discriminates between individuals of different heights.

A systematic review of the literature that included 31 research studies, including more than 300,000 adults of several ethnic groups, showed that WHtR has significantly greater discriminatory power in predicting cardiac and metabolic complications as compared to BMI and WC.[13] Another study presented at the 2013 European Congress on Obesity compared the effect of abdominal obesity on life expectancy in terms of years of life lost. The data showed that a 30-year-old man with a BMI greater than 40 has a years-of-life-lost value of 10.5 years as compared to 16.7 years using the most severe category of the WHtR. A 30-year-old woman in these same categories loses 5.3 years of life using BMI as a calculator as compared to 9.5 years using WHtR.[14]

WHtR is determined by dividing the waist circumference in inches by the height in inches. As illustrated in Figure 4.8, a ratio of .4 to .5 indicates the lowest risk for disease, whereas less than .4 or between .5 and .7 require "care" to decrease health risks, and a ratio of .7 or greater requires "action" to conform with the lowest health risk category of .4 to .5. An example of the WHtR for a person with a WC of 32 inches and a height of 68 inches (5'8") would be .47 (32 ÷ 68). The findings of many of these studies have prompted researchers to promote a public health message indicating that you should "keep your waist circumference to less than half your height." Table 4.10 below lists the various risk categories according to WHtR.

Table 4.9 Disease Risk according to Body Mass Index (BMI) and Waist Circumference (WC)

		Disease Risk Relative to Normal Weight and WC	
Classification	BMI (kg/m^2)	Men ≤40" (102 cm) Women ≤35" (88 cm)	Men >40" (102 cm) Women >35" (88 cm)
Underweight	<18.5	Increased	Low
Normal	18.5–24.9	Very low	Increased
Overweight	25.0–29.9	Increased	High
Obesity Class I	30.0–34.9	High	Very high
Obesity Class II	35.0–39.9	Very high	Very high
Obesity Class III	40.0	Extremely high	Extremely high

Adapted from Expert Panel, Executive Summary of the Clinical Guidelines on the Identification, Evaluation, and Treatment of Overweight and Obesity in Adults, *Archives of Internal Medicine* 158:1855-1867, 1998.

Table 4.10 Health Categories according to Waist-to-Height Ratio (WHtR)

Category	WHtR (Waist/Height)	Disease Risk
Take Care	<.4	Increased
Acceptable (OK)	.4–.5	Very low
Take Care	.5–.7	Increased
Take Action	>.7	Highest

© Cengage Learning 2015

4.3 Determining Recommended Body Weight

After finding out your percent body fat, you can determine your current body composition classification by consulting Table 4.11, which presents percentages of fat according to both the health fitness standard and the high physical fitness standard (see discussion in Chapter 1).

For example, the recommended health fitness fat percentage for a 20-year-old female is 28 percent or less. Although there are no clearly identified percent body fat levels at which the risk for disease definitely increases, the health fitness standard in Table 4.11 is currently the best estimate of the point at which there seems to be no harm to health.

According to Table 4.11, the high physical fitness range for this same 20-year-old woman would be between 18 and 23 percent. The high physical fitness standard does not mean that you cannot be somewhat less than this number. Many highly trained male athletes are as low as 3 percent, and some female distance runners have been measured at 6 percent body fat (which may not be healthy).

Scientists generally agree that the mortality rate is higher for obese people, and some evidence indicates that the same is true for underweight people. "Underweight" and "thin" do not necessarily mean the same thing. The body fat of a healthy thin person is near the high physical fitness standard, whereas an underweight person has extremely low body fat, even to the point of compromising the essential fat.

The 3 percent essential fat for men and 12 percent for women seem to be the lower limits for people to maintain good health. Below these percentages, normal physiological functions can be seriously impaired. Some experts point out that a little storage fat (in addition to the essential fat) is better than none at all. As a result, the health and high fitness standards for percent fat in Table 4.11 are set higher than the minimum essential fat requirements, at a point beneficial to optimal health and well-being. Finally, because lean tissue decreases with age, one extra percentage point is allowed for every additional decade of life.

> **Critical Thinking**
>
> Do you think you have a weight problem? • Do your body composition results make you feel any different about the way you perceive your current body weight and image?

Your recommended body weight is computed based on the selected health or high fitness fat percentage for your age and gender. Your decision to select a "desired" fat percentage should be based on your current percent body fat and your personal health/fitness objectives. Following are steps to compute your own recommended body weight:

1. Determine the pounds of body weight that are fat (FW) by multiplying your body weight (BW) by the current percent fat (%F) expressed in decimal form (FW = BW × %F)
2. Determine lean body mass (LBM) by subtracting the weight in fat from the total body weight (LBM = BW − FW). (Anything that is not fat must be part of the lean component.)
3. Select a desired body fat percentage (DFP) based on the health or high fitness standards given in Table 4.11.
4. Compute recommended body weight (RBW) according to the formula RBW = LBM ÷ (1.0 − DFP).

Table 4.11 Body Composition Classification according to Percent Body Fat

MEN						
Age	Underweight	Excellent	Good	Moderate	Overweight	Obese
19	<3	12.0	12.1–17.0	17.1–22.0	22.1–27.0	≥27.1
20–29	<3	13.0	13.1–18.0	18.1–23.0	23.1–28.0	≥28.1
30–39	<3	14.0	14.1–19.0	19.1–24.0	24.1–29.0	≥29.1
40–49	<3	15.0	15.1–20.0	20.1–25.0	25.1–30.0	≥30.1
50	<3	16.0	16.1–21.0	21.1–26.0	26.1–31.0	≥31.1

WOMEN						
Age	Underweight	Excellent	Good	Moderate	Overweight	Obese
≤19	<12	17.0	17.1–22.0	22.1–27.0	27.1–32.0	≥32.1
20–29	<12	18.0	18.1–23.0	23.1–28.0	28.1–33.0	≥33.1
30–39	<12	19.0	19.1–24.0	24.1–29.0	29.1–34.0	≥34.1
40–49	<12	20.0	20.1–25.0	25.1–30.0	30.1–35.0	≥35.1
≥50	<12	21.0	21.1–26.0	26.1–31.0	31.1–36.0	≥36.1

High physical fitness standard
Health fitness standard

© Cengage Learning

Figure 4.7 Visceral (VSC) fat is a greater risk factor for heart diseases, stroke, hypertension, diabetes, and cancer than subcutaneous (SBC) or retroperitoneal (RTP) fats.

As an example of these computations, a 19-year-old female who weighs 160 pounds and is 30 percent fat would like to know what her recommended body weight would be at 22 percent:

Sex: female
Age: 19
BW: 160 lbs
%F: 30% (.30 in decimal form)

1. FW = BW × %F
   FW = 160 × .30 = 48 lbs
2. LBM = BW − FW
   LBM = 160 − 48 = 112 lbs
3. DFP: 22% (.22 in decimal form)
4. RBW = LBM ÷ (1.0 − DFP)
   RBW = 112 ÷ (1.0 − .22)
   RBW = 112 ÷ .78 = 143.6 lbs

Behavior Modification Planning

Tips for Lifetime Weight Management

Maintenance of recommended body composition is one of the most significant health issues of the 21st century. If you are committed to lifetime weight management, the following strategies will help:

I PLAN TO / I DID IT

- ❑ ❑ Accumulate 60 to 90 minutes of physical activity daily.
- ❑ ❑ Exercise at a brisk aerobic pace for a minimum of 20 minutes 3 times per week.
- ❑ ❑ Strength train two to three times per week.
- ❑ ❑ Manage daily caloric intake by keeping in mind long-term benefits (recommended body weight) instead of instant gratification (overeating).
- ❑ ❑ "Junior-size" instead of "super-size."
- ❑ ❑ Regularly monitor body weight, body composition, body mass index, and waist circumference.
- ❑ ❑ Do not allow increases in body weight (percent fat) to accumulate; deal immediately with the problem through moderate reductions in caloric intake and maintenance of physical activity and exercise habits.

Try It

In your Online Journal or your class notebook, note which of these tips you are already using and which ones you can incorporate into your daily habits right away.

Figure 4.8 The Ashwell® Shape Chart (waist-to-height ratio).

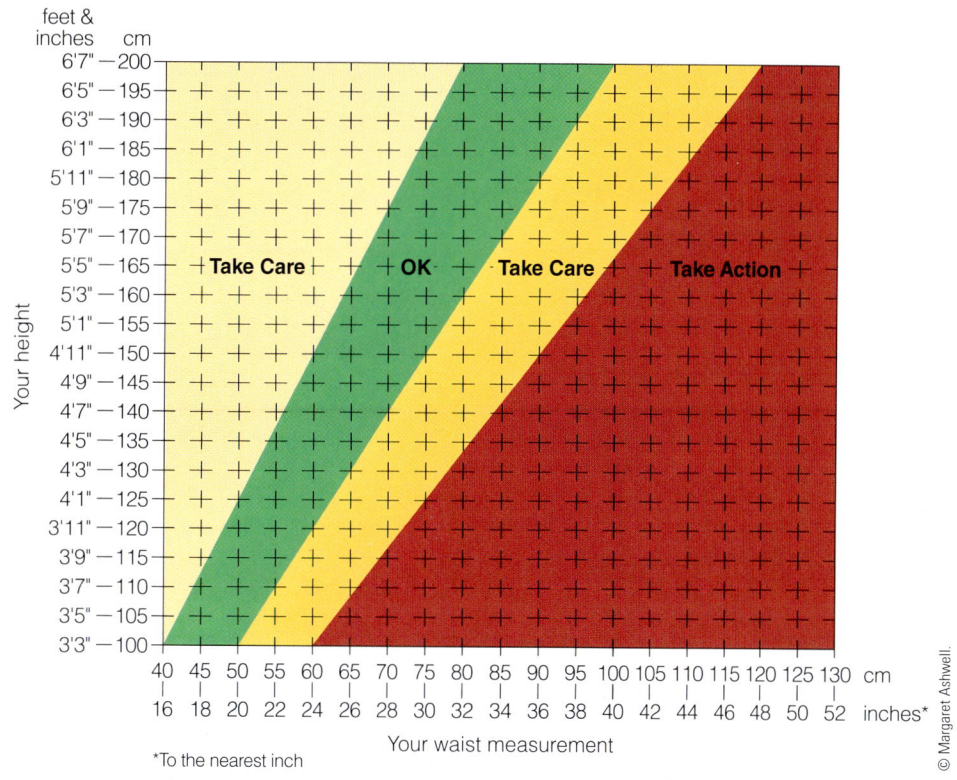

In Activity 4.1, you will have the opportunity to determine your own body composition and recommended body weight. A second column is provided in the activity for a follow-up assessment at a future date. The disease risk according to BMI and WHtR category and recommended body weight according to BMI, WC, also are determined in Activity 4.2. You can also record these results in Appendix A and set goals to accomplish by the end of the term.

Other than hydrostatic weighing, skinfold thickness seems to be the most practical and valid technique to estimate body fat, unless the person is significantly overweight and an accurate skinfold cannot be measured. If skinfold calipers are available, use this technique to assess your percent body fat. If none of these techniques is available to you, estimate your percent fat according to girth measurements (or another technique available to you). You also may wish to use several techniques and compare the results.

Critical Thinking

How do you feel about your current body weight? • What influence does society have on the way you perceive yourself in terms of your weight? • Do your body composition results make you feel any different about the way you see your current body weight and image?

Importance of Regular Body Composition Assessment Children in the United States do not start with a weight problem. Although a few struggle with weight throughout life, most are not overweight in the early years of life.

Trends indicate that adults in the United States gain one to two pounds per year. Thus, during a span of 40 years, the average American will have gained 40 to 80 pounds. Because of the typical reduction in physical activity in our society, however, the average person also loses half a pound of lean tissue each year. Therefore, this span of 40 years has produced an actual fat gain of 60 to 100 pounds accompanied by a 20-pound loss of lean body mass (Figure 4.9). These changes cannot be detected without assessing body composition periodically.

If you are on a diet/exercise program, you should repeat your percent body fat assessment and recommended weight computations about once a month. This is important because lean body mass is affected by weight-reduction programs and amount of physical activity. As lean body mass changes, so will your recommended body weight. To make valid comparisons, use the same technique for both pre- and post-program assessments. Knowing your percent body fat also is useful to identify fad diets that promote water loss and lean body mass loss, especially muscle mass.

Changes in body composition resulting from a weight control/exercise program were illustrated in a co-ed aerobic dance course taught during a six-week summer term. Students participated in a 60-minute aerobics routine four times a week. On the first and last days of class, several physiological parameters, including body composition, were assessed. Students also were given information on diet and nutrition, but they followed their own dietary program.

At the end of the six weeks, the average weight loss for the entire class was three pounds (Figure 4.10). But, because body composition was assessed, class members were surprised to find that the average fat loss was actually six pounds, accompanied by a three-pound increase in lean body mass.

When dieting, have your body composition reassessed periodically because of the effects of negative caloric balance on lean body mass. As discussed in Chapter 5, dieting does decrease lean body mass. This loss of lean body mass can be offset or eliminated by combining a sensible diet with exercise.

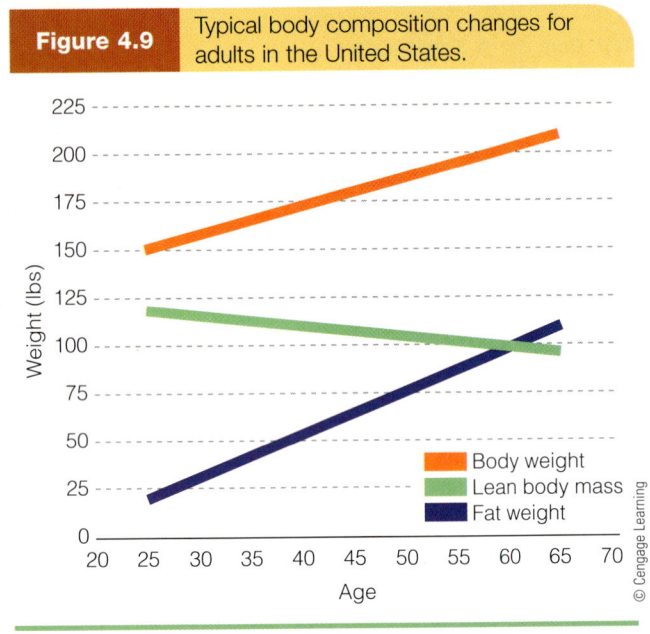

Figure 4.9 Typical body composition changes for adults in the United States.

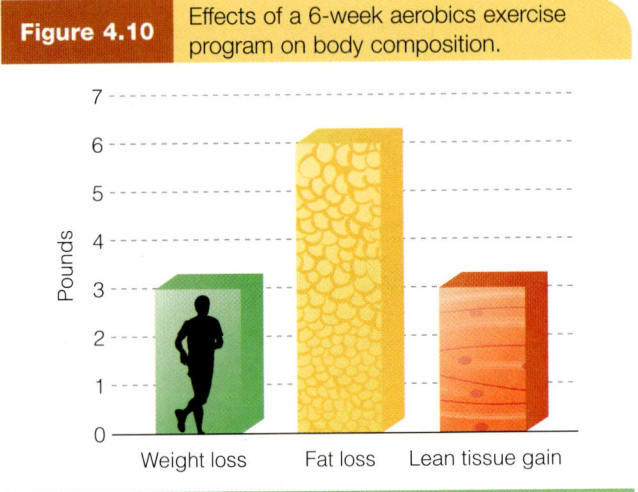

Figure 4.10 Effects of a 6-week aerobics exercise program on body composition.

Source: W. W. K. Hoeger, data collected at the University of Texas of the Permian Basin, 1985.

ASSESS YOUR BEHAVIOR

CENGAGEbrain To access course materials, including companion resources, please visit www.cengagebrain.com.

1. Do you know what your percent body fat is according to a reliable body composition assessment technique administered by a qualified technician?

2. Do you know your disease risk according to BMI and WC parameters?

3. Have you been able to maintain your body weight at a stable level during the past 12 months?

ASSESS YOUR KNOWLEDGE

Evaluate how well you understand the concepts presented in this chapter using the chapter-specific quizzing available in the online materials at www.cengagebrain.com.

1. Body composition incorporates
    a. a fat component.
    b. a nonfat component.
    c. percent body fat.
    d. lean body mass.
    e. all of the above.

2. Recommended body weight can be determined through
    a. body mass index.
    b. body composition analysis.
    c. BMI and waist circumference.
    d. waist circumference.
    e. all of the above.

3. Essential fat in women is
    a. 3 percent.
    b. 5 percent.
    c. 8 percent.
    d. 12 percent.
    e. 17 percent.

4. Which of the following is *not* a technique to assess body fat?
    a. body mass index
    b. skinfold thickness
    c. hydrostatic weighing
    d. circumference measurements
    e. air displacement

5. Which of the following sites is used to assess percent body fat according to skinfold thickness in men?
    a. suprailium
    b. chest
    c. scapular
    d. triceps
    e. All four sites are used.

6. Which variable is *not* used to assess percent body fat in women according to girth measurements?
    a. age
    b. hip
    c. wrist
    d. upper arm
    e. height

7. Waist circumference can be used to
    a. determine percent body fat.
    b. assess risk for disease.
    c. measure lean body mass.
    d. identify underweight people.
    e. All of the above are correct.

8. An acceptable BMI is between
    a. 15 and 18.49.
    b. 18.5 and 24.99.
    c. 25 and 29.99.
    d. 30 and 34.99.
    e. 35 and 39.99.

9. The health fitness percent body fat for women of various ages is in the range of
    a. 3 to 7 percent.
    b. 7 to 12 percent.
    c. 12 to 20 percent.
    d. 20 to 27 percent.
    e. 27 to 31 percent.

10. When a previously inactive individual starts an exercise program, the person may
    a. lose weight.
    b. gain weight.
    c. improve body composition.
    d. lose more fat pounds than total weight pounds.
    e. do all of the above.

Correct answers can be found at the back of the book.

Activity 4.1: Body Composition Assessment and Recommended Body Weight Determination

Name _____ Date _____

Course _____ Section _____ Gender _____ Age _____

I. Percent Body Fat according to Skinfold Thickness

Men

Chest (mm): _____
Abdomen (mm): _____
Thigh (mm): _____
Total (mm): _____
% Fat: _____

Women

Triceps (mm): _____
Suprailium (mm): _____
Thigh (mm): _____
Total (mm): _____
% Fat: _____

Follow-up

Date _____
% Fat _____ %

II. Percent Fat according to Girth Measurements (use inches for men and centimeters for women.)

Men — Waist (inches): ____ Wrist (inches): ____ Difference: ____ Body weight: ____ lbs. % Fat: ____

Women — Upperarm (cm): ____ Age: ____ Hip (cm): ____ Wrist (cm): ____

Constants: A = Upperarm ____ B = Age ____ C = Hip ____ D = Wrist ____

BD* = A − B − C + D = ____ − ____ − ____ + ____ = ____

% Fat = (495/BD) − 450 = (495/____) − 450 = ____

*BD = body density, carry the computation out to at least four decimal places.

III. Recommended Body Weight Determination

A. Body weight (BW): ____ lbs.

B. Current %F*: ____ %

C. Fat weight (FW) = BW × %F
   FW = ____ × ____ = ____ lbs.

D. Lean body mass (LBM) = BW − FW = ____ − ____ = ____ lbs.

E. Age: ____

F. Desired fat percent (DFP — see Table 4.11, page 139): ____ %

G. Recommended body weight (RBW) = LBM ÷ (1.0 − DFP*)
   RBW = ____ ÷ (1.0 − ____) = ____ lbs.

*Express percentages in decimal form (for example, 25% = .25).

Follow Up

Date: ____
A. BW: ____ lbs.
B. %F: ____ %
C. FW: ____ lbs.
D. LBM: ____ lbs.
E. Age: ____
F. DFP: ____ %
G. RBW: ____ lbs.

Chapter 4 Body Composition 145

Activity 4.2: Disease Risk Using Waist Circumference and Body Mass Index

I. Body Mass Index

Weight: [ ] lb [ ] kg
Height: [ ] in [ ] m

BMI = Weight (lb) × 705 ÷ Height (in) ÷ Height (in)

BMI = [ ] (lb) ÷ 705 ÷ [ ] (in) ÷ [ ] (in)

BMI = [ ]   Disease Risk: (use Table 4.7, page 138): [ ]

Follow-up   Date [ ]   BMI = [ ]   Disease Risk (use Table 4.7, page 138): [ ]

II. Waist Circumference

Waist (in): [ ]
Disease Risk (use Table 4.8, page 138): [ ]

Follow Up

Date: [ ]
Waist: [ ]
Disease Risk: [ ]

III. Disease Risk according to BMI and WC (use Table 4.9, page 138): [ ]

IV. Target Body Weight (TBW) according to BMI

TBW based on BMI = Desired BMI × height (in) × height (in) ÷ 705

TBW at BMI of 25 = 25 × [ ] × [ ] ÷ 705 = [ ] lbs.

TBW at BMI of 22 = 22 × [ ] × [ ] ÷ 705 = [ ] lbs.

V. Waist-to-Height Ratio (WHtR)

WHtR = [ ] (Waist, in) ÷ [ ] (Height, in) = [ ]
Health Category (use Table 4.10, page 138): [ ]

VI. Determining Body Composition Results and Goals

Briefly state your feelings about your body composition results and your recommended body weight using both percent body fat and BMI. Do you plan to reduce your percent body fat and increase your lean body mass? Write the goal(s) you want to achieve by the end of the term and indicate how you plan to achieve them.

Weight Management

5

Physical activity is the cornerstone of any sound weight management program. If you are unwilling to increase daily physical activity, you might as well not even attempt to lose weight because most likely you won't be able to keep it off.

Objectives

- **Describe** the health consequences of obesity.
- **Expose** some popular fad diets and myths and fallacies regarding weight control.
- **Describe** eating disorders and their associated medical problems and behavior patterns, and outline the need for professional help in treating these conditions.
- **Explain** the physiology of weight loss, including setpoint theory and the effects of diet on basal metabolic rate.
- **Explain** the role of a lifetime exercise program as the key to a successful weight loss and weight maintenance program.
- **Be able** to implement a physiologically sound weight reduction and weight maintenance program.
- **Describe** behavior modification techniques that help support adherence to a lifetime weight maintenance program.
- **On** your exercise log, check your progress.

CENGAGEbrain.com

Visit www.cengagebrain.com to access course materials and companion resources for this text, including quiz questions designed to check your understanding of the chapter contents. See the preface on page ix for more information.

Why can't I lose weight with exercise?

During the last few years, there has been a fair amount of media distortion stating "exercise makes a person fat," "why most of us believe that exercise makes us thinner—and why we are wrong," and "the myth about exercise: of course it's good for you, but it won't make you lose weight." There is ample scientific evidence that exercise is an important component of a successful weight loss program. The problem is that following exercise, many people eat more (particularly more junk food). They feel justified in doing so because they exercised. It is clear that weight loss is more effective when you cut back on calories (dieting), as opposed to only increasing physical activity or exercise.

When attempting to lose weight, initial lengthy exercise sessions (longer than 60 minutes) by unfit people may not be the best approach to weight loss—unless they carefully monitor daily caloric intake and avoid caloric compensation for the energy expended during exercise. In active or fit individuals, lengthy exercise sessions are not counterproductive.

Body composition changes are also more effective when dieting and exercise are combined while attempting to lose body weight. Most weight loss when dieting with exercise comes in the form of body fat and not lean body tissue, a desirable outcome. Weight loss maintenance, however, in most cases is possible only with 60 to 90 minutes of sustained daily physical activity and exercise.

If you are still not convinced that exercise is the best approach to weight management, take a look around the gym or the jogging trail. If this were the case, wouldn't those who regularly exercise be the fattest? Additional information on this subject is provided throughout this chapter, in particular in the section "The Role of Exercise Intensity and Duration in Weight Management" on page 168.

Does the time of day when calories are consumed matter in a weight loss program?

The time of day when a person eats food appears to play a part in weight reduction. When attempting to lose weight, intake should consist of a minimum of 25 percent of the total daily calories for breakfast, 50 percent for lunch, and 25 percent or less at dinner. Also, try not to eat within three hours of going to bed. This is the time of day when your metabolism is slowest. Your caloric intake is less likely to be used for energy and more likely to be stored as fat.

Are some diet plans more effective than others?

The term "diet" implies a negative caloric balance. A negative caloric balance means that you are consuming fewer calories than those required to maintain your current weight. When energy output surpasses energy intake, weight loss will occur. Popular diets differ widely in the food choices that you are allowed to have. The more limited the choices, the lower the chances to overeat, and thus you will have a lower caloric intake. And the fewer the calories that you consume, the greater the weight loss. For health reasons, to obtain the variety of nutrients the body needs, even during weight loss periods, you should not consume fewer than 1,500 calories per day (except very small individuals). These calories should be distributed over a wide range of foods, emphasizing grains, fruits, vegetables, and small amounts of low-fat animal products or fish.

Why is it so difficult to change dietary habits?

In most developed countries, there is an overabundance of food and practically an unlimited number of food choices. With unlimited supply and choices, most people do not have the willpower, stemming from their core values, to avoid overconsumption.

Our bodies were not created to go hungry or to overeat. We are uncomfortable overeating and we feel even worse when we have to go hungry. Our health values, however, are not strong enough to prevent overconsumption. The end result: weight gain. Next, we restrict calories (go on a diet), we feel hungry, and we have a difficult time adhering to the diet. Stated quite simply, going hungry is an uncomfortable and unpleasant experience.

To avoid this vicious cycle, our dietary habits (and most likely physical activity habits) must change. A question you need to ask yourself is: Do you value health and quality of life more than food overindulgence? If you do not, then the achievement and maintenance of recommended body weight and good health is a moot point. If you desire to avoid disease and increase quality of life, you have to value health more than food overconsumption. If we have spent the past 20 years tasting and "devouring" every food item in sight, it is now time to make healthy choices and consume only moderate amounts of food at a time (portion control). You do not have to taste and eat everything that is placed before your eyes. If you can make such a change in your eating habits, you may not have to worry about another diet for the rest of your life.

Real Life Story | Sam's Experience

A couple of times over the last few years, I tried to diet. It would usually start around New Year's, when I would make a resolution to lose the extra weight I was carrying. For a few weeks I would try to cut out desserts, avoid second helpings, and eat lower fat foods. At times when I would weigh myself, even if I thought I had really followed my diet well, the scale still wouldn't show any difference, which was really discouraging. Sometimes when I lost a few pounds, I would look in the mirror, but I still looked flabby. I didn't consider adding any exercise to my routine because I hate to sweat, I hate being out of breath, and I hate feeling bad because I'm not able to keep up with other, more fit people. Besides, after a long day of classes and homework, I would rather spend my free time updating Facebook, playing video games, or watching TV. But when I took a health and fitness class as a general elective, I learned about how important exercise was for proper weight management. It turns out that even if you are successful at losing weight through diet alone, you probably lose muscle along with the fat, so that even if your weight goes down, your body stays flabby. Also, your metabolism slows down, so it is easy to gain back all the weight. While taking the class, I got motivated and started exercising while also changing my diet. I started lifting weights, and walking and jogging on the treadmill at the student fitness center. I tried not to pay attention to how other people could lift more or run so much faster than me, and gradually my fitness improved. Now, several months later, my efforts have really paid off. So far I have lost more than 30 pounds. And what's more, getting regular exercise has helped me be more positive and feel stronger and more energetic. I am pretty sure that exercise is going to be a lifetime habit and that I will never want to go back to my couch potato ways.

PERSONAL PROFILE: Personal Lifetime Weight Management Program

I. Do you understand the concept of recommended body weight, and do you consider yourself to be at this weight? Yes ___ No ___

II. What type of exercise program do you consider most effective for weight management: aerobic exercise or strength training? Explain why you feel this way.

III. Have you gained weight since you started college? If so, what do you attribute this weight gain to?

IV. What can you learn from Sam's experience, and what strategies can you use to help you properly manage your body weight?

V. Do you understand the concept of long-term gratification derived through a lifetime exercise program and the required process to do so?

The current 21st century environment in which we live is rich in cues to overeat high-calorie, high-fat, sugary foods 24 hours a day, promoting weight gain and the array of chronic conditions cause by excessive weight. Essentially, the current obesogenic culture in which we live makes gaining weight the norm.

Obesity is a health hazard of epidemic proportions in most developed countries around the world. According to the World Health Organization, an estimated 35 percent of the adult population in industrialized nations is obese. Obesity has been defined as a body mass index (BMI) of 30 or higher. The obesity level is the point at which excess body fat can lead to serious health problems. The number of people who are obese and overweight in the United States has increased dramatically, a direct result of physical inactivity and poor dietary habits. The average weight of American adults between the ages of 20 and 74 has increased by 25 pounds or more since 1965, most of the weight gain has been (15 pounds) since 1990. More than one-half of all adults in the United States do not achieve the minimum recommended amount of physical activity (see Figure 1.8, page 11). In 2004, American women consumed 335 more calories daily than they had 20 years earlier, and men an additional 170 calories per day.[1]

About 68 percent of U.S. adults age 20 and older are overweight (have a BMI greater than 25), and 34 percent are obese (see Figure 5.1).[2] More than 120 million people are overweight and 30 million are obese. Between 1960 and 2002, the overall (men and women combined) prevalence of adult obesity increased from about 13 percent to 30 percent. Most of this increase occurred in the 1990s.

As illustrated in Figure 5.2, the obesity epidemic continues to escalate. Before 1990, not a single state reported an obesity rate greater than 15 percent of the state's total population (includes both adults and children). By the year 2010, not a single state had an obesity rate less than 20 percent,

| Figure 5.1 | Percentage of the adult population (20 years) that is normal weight (BMI ≥25), overweight (BMI 25–29.99), or obese (BMI ≥30) in the United States. |

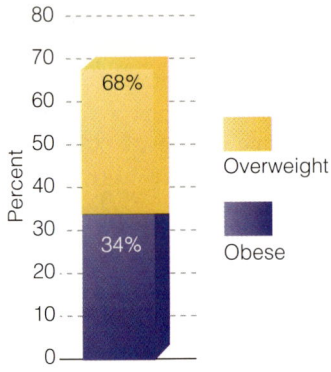

SOURCE: Centers for Disease Control and Prevention, 2012.

| Figure 5.2 | Obesity trends in the United States 1985–2010, based on BMI ≥30 or 30 pounds overweight. |

Percentages of the total number of people in the respective state who are obese.

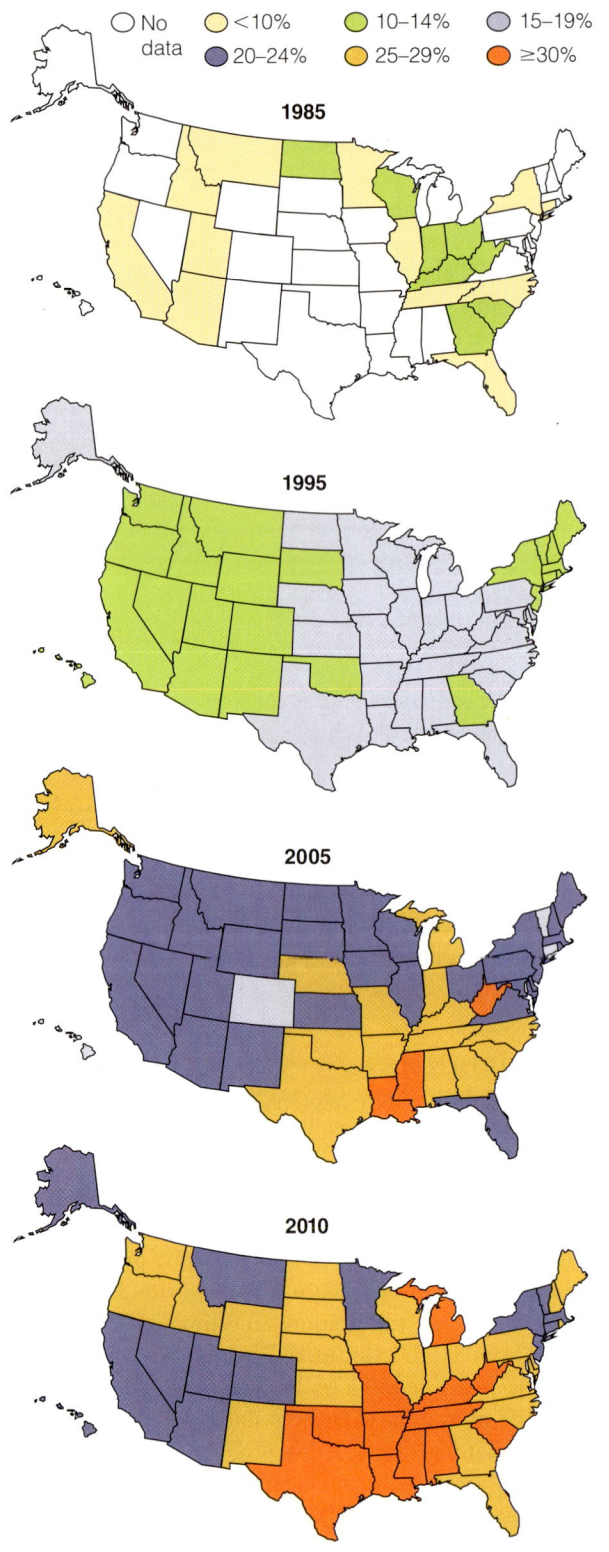

SOURCE: *Obesity Trends Among U.S. Adults Between 1985 and 2011.* (Atlanta: Centers for Disease Control and Prevention, 2013).

more than half had an obesity rate equal to or greater than 25 percent, including 12 states with a rate greater than 30 percent.

As of the end of 2012, the average man now weighs in at 196 pounds and the average woman at 156 pounds. As pointed out in Chapter 2, the human mind has a tremendous capability to adapt and accept change, even if it is detrimental to one's health. And so it is with body weight. According to a Gallup poll conducted in November 2012, men now indicate their "ideal" body weight is 185 pounds, the highest ever, and 14 pounds greater than the 1990 weight as determined by this same poll. Women indicate their "ideal" weight to be 11 pounds heavier than in 1990, at 140 pounds.

The prevalence of obesity is even higher in certain ethnic groups, especially African Americans and Hispanic Americans. Further, as the nation continues to evolve into a more mechanized and automated society (relying on escalators, elevators, remote controls, computers, e-mail, cell phones, and automatic-sensor doors), the amount of required daily physical activity continues to decrease. We are being lulled into a high-risk sedentary lifestyle.

The data in Figure 5.3 illustrate that the current obesity epidemic is not due to a change in the genetic code, as it doesn't change from one generation to the next. The data compare the obesity rates in the United States from 1988 to 1994 and with those from 2005 to 2008 and quite clearly illustrate that lifestyle changes over the last 15 to 20 years are responsible for the drastic increase in the escalating obesity rate. Furthermore, the prevalence of obesity is significantly lower among college graduates compared to those with only a high school degree or less.

More than a third of the population is on a diet at any given moment. People spend about $40 billion yearly attempting to lose weight, with more than $10 billion going to memberships in weight reduction centers and another $30 billion to diet food sales. Furthermore, the total cost attributable to treating obesity-related diseases is estimated at $117 billion per year.[3]

Excessive body weight combined with physical inactivity is the second leading cause of preventable death in the United States.[4] Furthermore, obesity is more prevalent than smoking (19 percent), poverty (14 percent), and problem drinking (6 percent).[5] Obesity and unhealthy lifestyle habits are the most critical public health problems we face in the 21st century.

Excessive body weight and obesity are associated with poor health status and are risk factors for many physical ailments, including cardiovascular disease, type 2 diabetes, and some types of cancer. Evidence indicates that health risks associated with increased body weight start at a BMI greater than 25 and are enhanced greatly at a BMI greater than 30.

The American Heart Association has identified obesity as one of the six major risk factors for coronary heart disease. Estimates also indicate that 14 percent of all cancer deaths in men and 20 percent in women are related to current overweight and obesity patterns in the United States.[6] Excessive body weight also is implicated in psychological maladjustment and a higher accidental death rate. Extremely obese people have a lower mental health–related quality of life.

Health Consequences of Excessive Body Weight

Being overweight or obese increases the risk for

- high blood pressure
- elevated blood lipids (high blood cholesterol and triglycerides)
- type 2 (non–insulin-dependent) diabetes
- insulin resistance, glucose intolerance
- coronary heart disease
- angina pectoris
- congestive heart failure
- stroke
- gallbladder disease
- gout
- osteoarthritis
- gastroesophageal reflux disease (GERD, or acid reflux)
- obstructive sleep apnea and respiratory problems
- some types of cancer (endometrial, breast, prostate, and colon)
- complications of pregnancy (gestational diabetes, gestational hypertension, preeclampsia, and complications during C-sections)
- poor female reproductive health (menstrual irregularities, infertility, irregular ovulation)
- bladder control problems (stress incontinence)
- psychological disorders (depression, eating disorders, distorted body image, discrimination, and low self-esteem)
- shortened life expectancy
- decreased quality of life

SOURCE: Centers for Disease Control and Prevention, downloaded May 30, 2013.

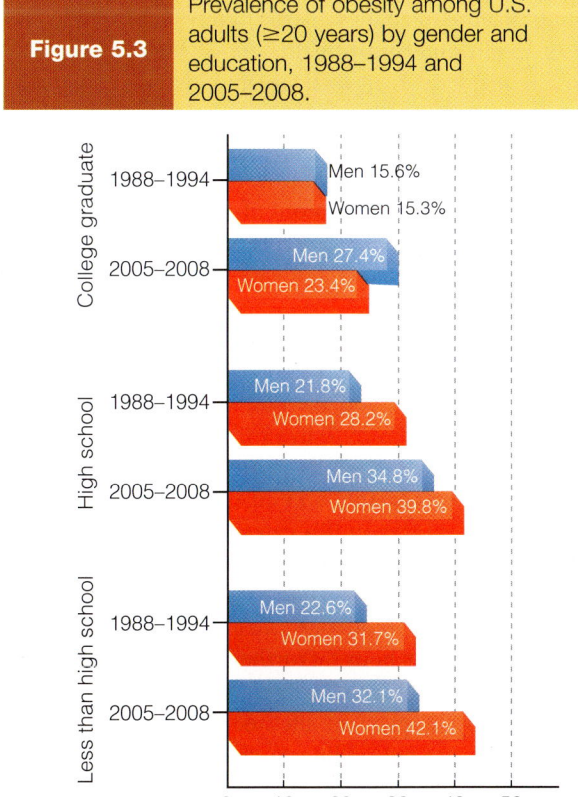

Figure 5.3 Prevalence of obesity among U.S. adults (≥20 years) by gender and education, 1988–1994 and 2005–2008.

From Hoeger/Hoeger, Principals and Labs for Fitness and Wellness, 12E. © 2014 Cengage Learning

5.1 Overweight versus Obesity

Overweight and obesity are not the same thing. Many overweight people (who weigh about 10 to 20 pounds more than the recommended weight) are not obese. Although a few pounds of excess weight may not be harmful to most people, this is not always the case. People with excessive body fat who have type 2 diabetes and other cardiovascular risk factors (elevated blood lipids, high blood pressure, physical inactivity, and poor eating habits) benefit from losing weight. People who have a few extra pounds of weight but are otherwise healthy and physically active, exercise regularly, and eat a healthy diet may not be at higher risk for early death. Such is not the case, however, with obese individuals.

Research indicates that individuals who are 30 or more pounds overweight during middle age (30 to 49 years of age) lose about 7 years of life, whereas being 10 to 30 pounds overweight decreases the lifespan by about 3 years.[7] These decreases are similar to those seen with tobacco use. Severe obesity (BMI greater than 45) at a young age, nonetheless, may cut up to 20 years off one's life.[8]

Although the loss of years of life is significant, the decreased life expectancy doesn't even begin to address the loss in quality of life and increase in illness and disability throughout the years. Even a modest reduction of 2 to 3 percent can reduce the risk for chronic diseases, including heart disease, high blood pressure, high cholesterol, and diabetes.[9]

A primary objective to achieve overall physical fitness and enhanced quality of life is to attain recommended body composition. Individuals at recommended body weight are able to participate in a wide variety of moderate to vigorous activities without functional limitations. These people have the freedom to enjoy most of life's recreational activities to their fullest potential. Excessive body weight does not afford an individual the fitness level to enjoy many lifetime activities such as basketball, soccer, racquetball, surfing, mountain cycling, or mountain climbing. Maintaining high fitness and recommended body weight gives a person a degree of independence throughout life that most people in developed nations no longer enjoy.

Scientific evidence also recognizes problems with being underweight. Although the social pressure to be thin has declined slightly in recent years, the pressure to attain model-like thinness is still with us and contributes to the gradual increase in the number of people who develop eating disorders (anorexia nervosa and bulimia, discussed under "Eating Disorders" on pages 158–161).

Extreme weight loss can lead to medical conditions such as heart damage, gastrointestinal problems, shrinkage of internal organs, abnormalities of the immune system, disorders of the reproductive system, loss of muscle tissue, damage to the nervous system, and even death. About 14 percent of people in the United States are underweight.

Critical Thinking

Do you consider yourself overweight? • If so, how long have you had a weight problem, what attempts have you made to lose weight, and what has worked best for you?

5.2 Tolerable Weight

Many people want to lose weight so they will look better. That's a worthy goal. The problem, however, is that they have a distorted image of what they would really look like if they were to reduce to what they think is their ideal weight. Hereditary factors play a big role, and only a small fraction of the population has the genes for a "perfect body."

The media have the greatest influence on people's perception of what constitutes "ideal" body weight. Most people consult fashion, fitness, and beauty magazines to determine what they should look like. The "ideal" body shapes, physiques, and proportions illustrated in these magazines are rare and are achieved mainly through airbrushing and medical reconstruction.[10] Many individuals, primarily young women, go to extremes in attempts to achieve these unrealistic figures. Failure to attain a "perfect body" may lead to eating disorders in some individuals.

When people set their own target weight, they should be realistic. Attaining the "Excellent" percent of body fat shown in Table 4.11 (page 139) is extremely difficult for some. It is even more difficult to maintain over time, unless the person makes a commitment to a vigorous lifetime exercise program and permanent dietary changes. Few people are willing to do that. The "Moderate" percent body fat category may be more realistic for many people.

The question you should ask yourself is: Am I happy with my weight? Part of enjoying a higher quality of life is being happy with yourself. If you are not, you need to either do something about it or learn to live with it.

If your percent of body fat is higher than those in the Moderate category of Table 4.11 in Chapter 4, you should try to reduce it and stay in this category for health reasons. This is the category that seems to pose no detriment to health.

If you are in the Moderate category but would like to reduce your percent of body fat further, you need to ask yourself a second question: How badly do I want it? Do I want it badly enough to implement lifetime exercise and dietary changes? If you are not willing to change, you should stop worrying about your weight and deem the Moderate category "tolerable" for you.

Obesity is a health hazard of epidemic proportions in industrialized nations.

5.3 The Weight Loss Dilemma

"Yo-yo" dieting carries as great a health risk as being overweight and remaining overweight in the first place. Epidemiological data show that frequent fluctuations in weight (up or down) markedly increase the risk for dying from cardiovascular disease. Experts theorize that the constant shrinking and growing with yo-yo dieting causes micro tears in the blood vessels that increase their susceptibility to atherosclerosis (obstruction of the arteries; see Chapter 10). Based on the findings that constant losses and regains can be hazardous to health, quick-fix diets should be replaced by a slow but permanent weight loss program (as described under "Losing Weight the Sound and Sensible Way," page 172). Individuals reap the benefits of recommended body weight when they get to that weight and stay there throughout life.

Unfortunately, only about 10 percent of all people who begin a traditional weight loss program without exercise are able to lose the desired weight. Worse, only 5 in 100 are able to keep the weight off. The body is highly resistant to permanent weight changes through caloric restrictions alone.

Traditional diets have failed because few of them incorporate permanent behavioral changes in food selection and an overall increase in physical activity and exercise as fundamental to successful weight loss and weight maintenance. When the diet stops, weight gain begins. The $40 billion diet industry tries to capitalize on the false idea that a person can lose weight quickly without considering the consequences of fast weight loss or the importance of lifetime behavioral changes to ensure proper weight loss and maintenance.

In addition, various studies indicate that most people, especially obese people, underestimate their energy intake. Those who try to lose weight but apparently fail to do so are often described as "diet resistant." One study found that while on a "diet," a group of obese individuals with a self-reported history of diet resistance underreported their average daily caloric intake by almost 50 percent (1,028 self-reported versus 2,081 actual calories) (see Figure 5.4).[11] These individuals also overestimated their amount of daily physical activity by about 25 percent (1,022 self-reported versus 771 actual calories). These differences represent an additional 1,304 calories of energy per day unaccounted for by the subjects in the study. The findings indicate that failing to lose weight often is related to misreports of actual food intake and level of physical activity.

Diet Crazes Capitalizing on hopes that the latest diet to hit the market will really work this time, fad diets continue to appeal to people of all shapes and sizes. These diets may work for a while, but their success is usually short-lived. Regarding the effectiveness of these diets, Dr. Kelly Brownell, one of the foremost researchers in the field of weight management, has stated: "When I get the latest diet fad, I imagine a trick birthday cake candle that keeps lighting up and we have to keep blowing it out." Fad diets deceive people and claim that dieters will lose weight by following all instructions. Many diets are very low in calories. Under these conditions, a lot of the weight lost is in the form of water and protein, and not fat.

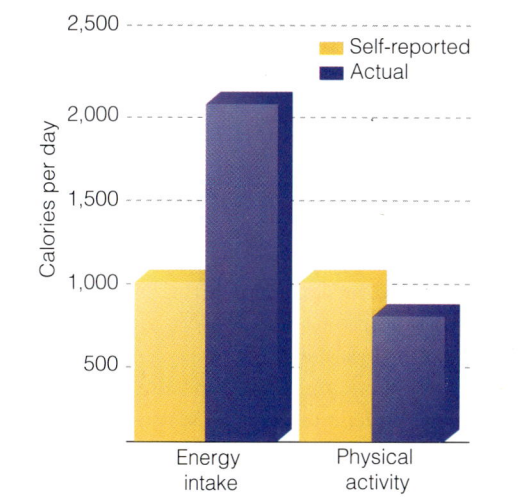

Figure 5.4 Differences between self-reported and actual daily caloric intake and exercise in obese individuals attempting to lose weight.

SOURCE: S. W. Lichtman et al., "Discrepancy Between Self-Reported and Actual Caloric Intake and Exercise in Obese Subjects," *New England Journal of Medicine* 327 (1992): 1893–1898.

On average, a 150-pound person stores about 1.3 pounds of glycogen (carbohydrate or glucose storage) in the body. This amount of glycogen is higher in aerobically trained individuals, as intense training (elite athletes) can more than double the body's capacity to store glycogen. About 80 percent of the glycogen is stored in muscles and the remaining 20 percent in the liver. Water, however, is required to store glycogen. A 2.6-to-1 water-to-glycogen ratio is necessary to store **glycogen**.[12] Thus, our 150-pound person stores about 3.4 pounds of water (1.3 × 2.6), along with the 1.3 pounds of glycogen, accounting for a total of 4.7 pounds of the person's normal body weight.

When fasting or on a crash diet (typically defined as less than 800 calories per day), glycogen storage can be completely depleted in just a few days. This loss of weight is not in the form of body fat and is typically used to promote and guarantee rapid weight loss with many fad diets on the market today. When the person resumes a normal eating plan, the body will again store its glycogen, along with the water required to do so, and there is a subsequent weight gain.

Furthermore, on a crash diet, close to half the weight loss is in lean (protein) tissue. When the

Glycogen Manner in which carbohydrates (glucose molecules) are stored in the human body, predominantly in the liver and muscles.

body uses protein instead of a combination of fats and carbohydrates as a source of energy, weight is lost as much as 10 times faster. This is because a gram of protein produces half the amount of energy that fat does. In the case of muscle protein, one-fifth of protein is mixed with four-fifths water. Therefore, each pound of muscle yields only one-tenth the amount of energy of a pound of fat. As a result, most of the weight lost is in the form of water, which on the scale, of course, looks good.

Long-term or frequent crash dieting also increases the risk of heart attacks because low calorie intake eventually leads to heart muscle (protein) loss. Limiting potassium, magnesium, and copper intake as a result of very low calorie diets may induce fatal cardiac arrhythmias. Furthermore, sodium depletion may cause a dangerous drop in blood pressure. Very low calorie diets should always be followed under a physician's supervision. Unfortunately, most crash dieters simply consult a friend rather than seek a physician's advice.

Diet books are frequently found on best-seller lists. The market is flooded with these books. Examples include *The DASH diet, The Volumetrics Eating Plan, the Ornish Diet, the Atkins Diet, the Zone Diet, the South Beach Diet, the Best Life Diet, the Abs Diet,* and *The Biggest Loser Diet*. Some of these popular diets have sound dietary principles, while others are becoming more nutritionally balanced and encourage consumption of fruits and vegetables, whole grains, some lean meat and fish, and low-fat milk and dairy products. Such plans reduce the risk for chronic diseases, including cardiovascular diseases and cancer.

While it is clear that some diets are healthier than others, strictly from a weight loss point of view, it doesn't matter what diet plan you follow, if caloric intake is lower than your caloric output, weight will come off. Dropout rates for many popular diets, however, are high because of the difficulty in long-term adherence to limited dietary plans.

Low-Carb Diets Among the most popular diets on the market in recent years were the low-carbohydrate/high-protein (LCHP) diet plans. Although they vary slightly, low-carb diets, in general, limit the intake of carbohydrate-rich foods—bread, potatoes, rice, pasta, cereals, crackers, juices, sodas, sweets (candy, cake, cookies), and even fruits and vegetables. Dieters are allowed to eat all the protein-rich foods they desire, including steak, ham, chicken, fish, bacon, eggs, nuts, cheese, tofu, high-fat salad dressings, butter, and small amounts of a few fruits and vegetables. Typically, these diets also are high in fat content. Examples of these diets are the Atkins Diet, the Zone, Protein Power, the Scarsdale Diet, the Carb Addict's Diet, the South Beach Diet, and Sugar Busters.

During digestion, carbohydrates are converted into glucose, a basic fuel used by every cell in the body. As blood glucose rises, the pancreas releases insulin. Insulin is a hormone that facilitates the entry of glucose into the cells, thereby lowering the glucose level in the bloodstream. A rapid rise in glucose also causes a rapid spike in insulin, which is followed by a rapid removal and drop in blood glucose that leaves you hungry again. A slower rise in blood glucose is desirable because the level is kept constant longer, delaying the onset of hunger. If the cells don't need the glucose for normal cell functions or to fuel physical activity, and if cellular glucose stores are already full, glucose is converted to, and stored as, body fat.

Not all carbohydrates cause a similar rise in blood glucose. The rise in glucose is based on the speed of digestion, which depends on a number of factors, including the size of the food particles. Small-particle carbohydrates break down rapidly and cause a quick, sharp rise in blood glucose. Thus, to gauge a food's effect on blood glucose, carbohydrates are classified by their **glycemic index**.

A high glycemic index signifies a food that causes a quick rise in blood glucose. At the top of the 100-point scale is glucose itself. This index is not directly related to simple and complex carbohydrates, and the glycemic values are not always what one might expect. Rather, the index is based on the actual laboratory-measured speed of absorption. Processed foods generally have a high glycemic index, whereas high-fiber foods tend to have a lower index (see Table 5.1). Other factors that affect the index are the amount of carbohydrate, fat, and protein in the food; how refined the ingredients are; and whether the food was cooked.

The body functions best when blood sugar remains at a constant level. Although this is best accomplished by consuming foods with a low glycemic index (nuts, apples, oranges, low-fat yogurt), a person does not have to eliminate all high–glycemic index foods (sugar, potatoes, bread, white rice, soda drinks) from the diet. Foods with a high glycemic index along with some protein are useful to replenish depleted glycogen stores following prolonged or exhaustive aerobic exercise. Combining high– with low–glycemic index items or with some fat and protein brings down the average index.

Regular consumption of high-glycemic foods by themselves may increase the risk for cardiovascular disease, especially in people at risk for diabetes. A person does not need to plan the diet around the index itself, as many popular diet programs indicate. The glycemic index deals with single foods eaten alone. Most people eat high-glycemic index foods in combination with other foods as part of a meal. In combination, these foods have a lower effect on blood sugar. Even people at risk for diabetes or who have the disease can eat high-glycemic foods in moderation.

Low-glycemic foods may also aid in weight loss and weight maintenance. As blood sugar levels drop between snacks and meals, hunger increases. Keeping blood sugar levels constant by including low-glycemic foods in the diet helps stave off hunger, appetite, and overeating (see Figure 5.5).

Proponents of LCHP diets claim that if a person

> **Glycemic index** A measure that is used to rate the plasma glucose response of carbohydrate-containing foods with the response produced by the same amount of carbohydrate from a standard source, usually glucose or white bread.

Popular Diets

The DASH Diet

The Dietary Approaches to Stop Hypertension (DASH) diet was originally designed as a heart-healthy diet to help lower high blood pressure. The diet plan is rich in fruits, vegetables, fat-free or low-fat milk and milk products, whole grains, fish, poultry, beans, seeds, and nuts. It also contains less sodium, fats, red meats, sweets, added sugars, and sugar-containing beverages than the typical American diet. Because it is such a healthy diet, the plan has been embraced by people seeking to lose weight. For weight-loss purposes, the recommended daily caloric intake ranges from about 1,600 to 2,200 calories. The macronutrient composition of the diet includes 50 to 60 percent carbohydrates, less than 30 percent fat, and 15 to 20 percent protein.

The Volumetrics Eating Plan

The Volumetrics diet plan focuses on maximizing the volume of food and limiting calories by emphasizing high–water content or low-fat foods (lower energy density), low-fat cooking techniques, and extensive use of vegetables. The average daily caloric intake is reduced by 500 to 1,000 calories, with a macronutrient composition of approximately 55 percent carbohydrates, less than 30 percent fat, and more than 20 percent protein.

The Best Life Diet

The initial phase of the Best Life Diet plan encourages exercise and a recommended eating schedule. The second phase requires a reduction in caloric intake through consumption of healthful foods to satisfy hunger. The plan deals extensively with emotional eating. Caloric intake averages about 1,700 calories, with maintenance of daily moderate physical activity. The diet composition is about 50 percent carbohydrates, 30 percent fat, and 20 percent protein.

Weight Watchers Diet

Dieters are given a daily point allowance in which calorie-dense foods with a higher fat content, simple carbohydrate content, or both are given more points. The points are determined using the patented Weight Watchers Point Calculator formula that looks to create an approximate 1,000-calorie per day deficit. The program encourages dieters to use points wisely by eating filling foods that keep hunger at bay, primarily foods rich in protein and fiber. The diet contains approximately 50 percent carbohydrates, 30 percent fat, and 20 percent protein.

Ornish Diet

Ornish is a very low-fat, vegetarian-type diet. Dieters are not allowed to drink alcohol or eat meat, fish, oils, sugar, or white flour. Data indicate that strict adherence to the Ornish Diet can prevent and reverse heart disease. An average daily caloric intake is about 1,500 calories, composed of approximately 75 percent carbohydrates, less than 10 percent fat, and 15 percent protein.

The Zone Diet

The Zone Diet proposes that proper macronutrient (carbohydrate/fat/protein) distribution is critical to keep blood sugar and hormones in balance and thus prevent weight gain and disease. Daily caloric allowance is about 1,100 calories for women and 1,400 for men. All meals need to provide 40 percent carbohydrate calories, 30 percent fat calories, and 30 percent protein calories.

Atkins Diet

In the LCHP Atkins Diet, practically all carbohydrates are eliminated during the first 2 weeks. Thereafter, very small amounts of carbohydrates are allowed, primarily in the form of limited fruits, vegetables, and wine. No caloric guidelines are given, but a typical daily diet plan is about 1,500 calories and is extremely high in fat (about 60 percent of calories), followed by protein (about 30 percent of calories), and limited carbohydrates (about 10 percent of calories). Dieters may not be as hungry on the Atkins Diet but may find it too restrictive for long-term adherence.

The South Beach Diet

Also an LCHP diet, the South Beach Diet is not as restrictive as the Atkins Diet. It emphasizes low-glycemic foods thought to decrease cravings for sugar and refined carbohydrates. Sugar, fruits, and grains are initially eliminated. In phase two, some high-fiber grains, fruit, and dark chocolate are permitted. No caloric guidelines are given, but a typical dietary plan provides about 1,400 calories per day, composed of 40 percent carbohydrate, 40 percent fat, and 20 percent protein calories.

The Glycemic Index Diet

The Glycemic Index Diet is based on the system of ranking carbohydrate foods according to how much each food raises the person's blood sugar level. This diet is also the basis for the Zone and South Beach diets. Dieters are encouraged to choose carbohydrate foods with a low glycemic index, such as whole fruits, vegetables, and beans. The hypothesis behind the diet is that low–glycemic index foods are absorbed more slowly,

(continued)

delaying hunger and making you less likely to overeat. Caloric intake ranges between 1,000 and 1,500 calories per day, and the diet composition is around 40 to 50 percent carbohydrates, 30 percent fat, and 30 percent protein.

The Biggest Loser Diet

Based on the popular TV show, The Biggest Loser Diet encourages small, frequent meals that emphasize filling calories from fruits, vegetables, lean protein sources, and whole grains; portion control; a food journal to monitor food intake; and an increase in daily physical activity and exercise. Caloric intake ranges from about 1,200 to 1,800 calories. The macronutrient composition of the diet is approximately 45 percent carbohydrate, 25 percent fat, and 30 percent protein calories.

The Mediterranean Diet

Although not specifically a dietary plan for weight reduction, the Mediterranean Diet (different cultures around the Mediterranean have slightly different patterns) emphasizes daily fruits, vegetables, whole grains, beans, nuts, legumes, olive oil, and flavorful herbs and spices; seafood at least twice a week; and poultry, eggs, cheese, yogurt, and red wine in moderation. Sweets and red meat are reserved for special occasions only, and physical activity is a part of the daily pattern. A calorie-restricted plan of the dietary pattern has been used to promote weight loss. Typically, the diet includes 40 to 50 percent carbohydrates, 25 to 40 percent fat, and 10 to 20 percent protein.

---

eats fewer carbohydrates and more protein, the pancreas will produce less insulin, and as insulin drops, the body will turn to its own fat deposits for energy. There is no scientific proof, however, that high levels of insulin lead to weight gain. None of the authors of these diets published any studies validating their claims. Yet, these authors base their diets on the faulty premise that high insulin leads to obesity. We know the opposite to be true: Excessive body fat causes insulin levels to rise, thereby increasing the risk for developing diabetes.

The reason for rapid weight loss in LCHP dieting is that a low carbohydrate intake forces the liver to produce glucose. The source for most of this glucose is body proteins—your lean body mass, including muscle. As indicated earlier, protein is mostly water; thus, weight is lost rapidly. When a person terminates the diet, the body rebuilds some of the protein tissue and quickly regains some weight.

Research studies indicated that individuals on an LCHP (Atkins) diet lost slightly more weight in the first few months than those on a low-fat diet.[13] The effectiveness of the diet, however, seemed to dwindle over time. In one of the studies, at 12 months into the diet, participants in the LCHP diet had regained more weight than those on the low-fat diet plan.

Years of research will be required to determine the extent to which adhering over the long term to LCHP diets increases the risk for heart disease, cancer, and kidney or bone damage. Low-carb diets are contrary to the nutrition advice of most national leading health organizations (which recommend a diet lower in saturated fat and trans fats and high in complex carbohydrates). Without fruits, vegetables, and whole grains, high-protein diets lack many vitamins, minerals, antioxidants, phytonutrients, and fiber—all dietary factors that protect against an array of ailments and diseases.

The major risk associated with long-term adherence to LCHP diets could be the increased risk for heart disease, because high-protein foods are also high in fat content (see Chapter 10). Short-term (a few weeks or months) adherence to LCHP diets does not appear to increase heart disease risk. The long-term (years) effects of these types of diet, nonetheless, have not been evaluated by scientific research (very few people would be willing to adhere to such a diet for several years). A possible long-term adverse effect of adherence to an LCHP diet is a potential increase in cancer risk. Phytonutrients found in fruits, vegetables, and whole grains protect against certain types of cancer. A low-carbohydrate intake also produces a loss of vitamin B, calcium, and potassium. Potential bone loss can accentuate the risk for osteoporosis.

Table 5.1 Glycemic Index of Selected Foods

Item	Index	Item	Index
All-Bran cereal	38	Milk, chocolate	43
Apples	40	Milk, chocolate, low-fat	34
Bagel, white	72	Milk, skim	32
Banana	56	Milk, whole	40
Bread, French	95	Jelly beans	80
Bread, wheat	73	Oatmeal	75
Bread, white	70	Oranges	48
Carrots, boiled (Australia)	41	Pasta, white	50
Carrots, boiled (Canada)	92	Pasta, wheat	32
Carrots, raw	47	Peanuts	20
Cherries	20	Peas	50
Colas	65	Pizza, cheese	60
Corn, sweet	60	Potato, baked	56–100
Corn Flakes	92	Potato, French fries	75
Doughnut	76	Potato, sweet	51
Frosted Flakes	55	Rice, white	56
Fruit cocktail	55	Sugar, table	65
Gatorade	78	Watermelon	72
Glucose	100	Yogurt, low-fat	32
Honey	58		

Figure 5.5 Effects of high- and low-glycemic carbohydrate intake on blood glucose levels.

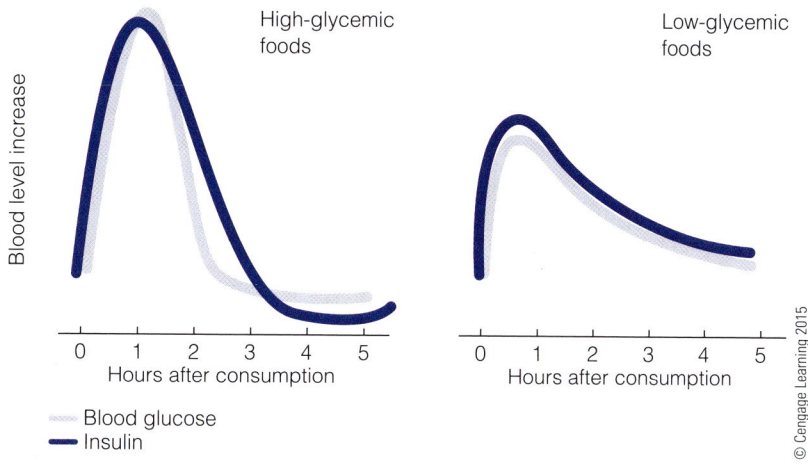

Are Low-Carb/High-Protein Diets More Effective?

Studies suggest that, at least over the short-term, low-carb/high-protein (LCHP) diets are more effective in producing weight loss than carbohydrate-based diets. The results are somewhat controversial. In LCHP diets:

- A large amount of weight loss is water and muscle protein, not body fat. Some of this weight is quickly regained when regular dietary habits are resumed.
- Few people are able to stay with LCHP diets for more than a few weeks at a time. The majority stop dieting before the targeted program completion.
- LCHP dieters are rarely found in a national weight loss registry of people who have lost 30 pounds and kept them off for a minimum of 6 years.
- Food choices are severely restricted in LCHP diets. With less variety, individuals tend to eat less (800 to 1,200 calories/day) and thus lose more weight.
- LCHP diets are fundamentally high in fat (about 60 percent fat calories) and a higher intake of saturated fat may promote heart disease, cancer, and increase the risk for osteoporosis.
- LCHP diets are not recommended for people with diabetes, high blood pressure, heart disease, or kidney disease.
- LCHP diets do not promote long-term healthy eating patterns.
- The higher protein and fat intake help control hunger pangs, thus making it easier to adhere to the diet plan.

Side effects commonly associated with LCHP diets include weakness, nausea, bad breath, constipation, irritability, lightheadedness, and fatigue. If you choose to go on an LCHP diet for longer than a few weeks, let your physician know so that he or she may monitor your blood lipids, bone density, and kidney function.

The benefit of adding extra protein to a weight loss program may be related to the hunger-suppressing effect of protein. Data suggest that protein curbs hunger more effectively than carbohydrates or fat. Dieters feel less hungry when caloric intake from protein is increased to about 30 percent of total calories and fat intake is cut to about 20 percent (while carbohydrate intake is kept constant at 50 percent of total calories). Thus, if you struggle with frequent hunger pangs, try to include lean protein with each meal. This amount of protein is the equivalent of one and a half ounces of lean meat (beef, fowl, or fish), two tablespoons of natural peanut butter, or eight ounces of plain low-fat yogurt.

The reason why many of these diets succeed is because they restrict a large number of foods. Thus, people tend to eat less food overall. With the extraordinary variety of foods available to us, it is unrealistic to think that people will adhere to these diets for very long. People eventually get tired of eating the same thing day in and day out and start eating less, leading to weight loss. If they happen to achieve the lower weight but do not make permanent dietary changes, they regain the weight quickly once they go back to their previous eating habits.

A few diets recommend exercise along with caloric restrictions—the best method for weight reduction, of course. People who adhere to these programs will succeed, so the diet has achieved its purpose. Unfortunately, if the people do not change their food selection and activity level permanently, they gain back the weight once they discontinue dieting and exercise.

> ### How to Recognize Fad Diets
>
> Fad diets have characteristics in common. These diets typically
>
> - are nutritionally unbalanced.
> - rely primarily on a single food (for example, grapefruit).
> - are based on testimonials.
> - were developed according to "confidential research."
> - are based on a "scientific breakthrough."
> - promote rapid and "painless" weight loss.
> - promise miraculous results.
> - restrict food selection.
> - are based on pseudo claims that excessive weight is related to a specific condition such as insulin resistance, combinations or timing of nutrient intake, food allergies, hormone imbalances, and certain foods (fruits, for example).
> - require the use of selected products.
> - use liquid formulas instead of foods.
> - misrepresent salespeople as individuals qualified to provide nutrition counseling.
> - fail to provide information on risks associated with weight loss and of the diet use.
> - do not involve physical activity.
> - do not encourage healthy behavioral changes.
> - are not supported by the scientific community or national health organizations.
> - fail to provide information for weight maintenance on completion of the diet phase.
>
> © Cengage Learning

If people only accepted that no magic foods will provide all of the necessary nutrients and that a person has to eat a variety of foods to be well nourished, dieters would be more successful and the diet industry would go broke. Also, let's not forget that we eat for pleasure and for health. Two of the most essential components of a wellness lifestyle are healthy eating and regular physical activity, and they provide the best weight management program available today.

5.4 Eating Disorders

Eating disorders are medical illnesses that involve crucial disturbances in eating behaviors thought to stem from some combination of environmental pressures. These disorders are characterized by an intense fear of becoming fat, which does not disappear even when the person is losing weight in extreme amounts. The three most common types of eating disorders are **anorexia nervosa**, **bulimia nervosa**, and **binge-eating disorder**. A fourth disorder, **emotional eating**, can also be listed under disordered eating.

Most people who have eating disorders are afflicted by significant family and social problems. They may lack fulfillment in many areas of their lives. The eating disorder then becomes the coping mechanism to avoid dealing with these problems. Taking control over their own body weight helps them believe that they are restoring some sense of control over their lives.

Anorexia nervosa and bulimia nervosa are common in industrialized nations where society encourages low calorie diets and thinness. The female role in society has changed rapidly, which makes women more susceptible to eating disorders. Although frequently seen in young women, eating disorders are most prevalent among individuals between the ages of 25 and 50. Surveys, nonetheless, indicate that as many as 40 percent of college-age women are struggling with an eating disorder.

Eating disorders are not limited to women. Every 1 in 10 cases occurs in men. But because men's role and body image are viewed differently in our society, these cases often go unreported.

Although genetics may play a role in the development of eating disorders, most cases are environmentally related. Individuals who have clinical depression and obsessive-compulsive behavior are more susceptible. About half of all people with eating disorders have some sort of chemical dependency (alcohol and drugs), and most of them come from families with alcohol- and drug-related problems. Of reported cases of eating disorders, a large number are individuals who are, or have been, victims of sexual molestation.

Eating disorders develop in stages. Typically, individuals who are already dealing with significant issues in life start a diet. At first they feel in control and are happy about the weight loss, even if they are not overweight. Encouraged by the prospect of weight loss and the control they can exert over their own weight, the dieting becomes extreme and often is combined with exhaustive exercise and the overuse of laxatives and diuretics.

The syndrome typically emerges following emotional issues or a stressful life event and the uncertainty about one's ability to cope efficiently. Life experiences that can trigger the syndrome might be gaining weight, starting the menstrual period, beginning college, losing a boyfriend, having poor self-esteem, being socially rejected, starting a professional career, or becoming a wife or a mother.

The eating disorder then takes on a life of its own and becomes the primary focus of attention for the individual afflicted with it. Her self-worth revolves around what the scale reads every day, her relationship with food, and her perception of how she looks each day.

Anorexia Nervosa An estimated 1 percent of the population in the United States has the eating disorder anorexia nervosa. Anorexic individuals seem to fear weight gain more than death from starvation. Furthermore, they have a distorted image of their bodies and think of themselves as being fat even when they are emaciated.

Society's unrealistic view of what constitutes recommended weight and "ideal" body image contributes to the development of eating disorders.

maintenance of body weight less than 85 percent of that expected, or failure to make expected weight gain during periods of growth, leading to body weight less than 85 percent of that expected)
- Intense fear of gaining weight or becoming fat, even though underweight
- Disturbance in the way in which one's body weight, size, or shape is perceived, undue influences of body weight or shape on self-evaluation, or denial of the seriousness of the current low body weight
- In postmenarcheal females, amenorrhea (absence of at least three consecutive menstrual cycles). (A woman is considered to have amenorrhea if her periods occur only following estrogen therapy.)

Many of the changes induced by anorexia nervosa can be reversed. Individuals with this condition can get better with professional therapy, or they sometimes turn to bulimia nervosa, or they die from the disorder. Anorexia nervosa has the highest mortality rate of all psychosomatic illnesses today—20 percent of anorexic individuals die as a result of their condition. The disorder is 100 percent curable, but treatment almost always requires professional help. The sooner it is started, the better are the chances for reversibility and cure. Therapy consists of a combination of medical and psychological techniques to restore proper nutrition, prevent medical complications, and modify the environment or events that triggered the syndrome.

Seldom can anorexia sufferers overcome the problem by themselves. They strongly deny their condition. They are able to hide it and deceive friends and relatives. Based on their behavior, many of them meet all of the characteristics of anorexia nervosa, but it goes undetected because both thinness and dieting are socially acceptable. Only a well-trained clinician is able to diagnose anorexia nervosa.

Anorexic patients commonly develop obsessive and compulsive behaviors and emphatically deny their condition. They are preoccupied with food, meal planning, and grocery shopping, and they have unusual eating habits. As they lose weight and their health begins to deteriorate, they feel weak and tired. They might realize they have a problem, but they will not stop the starvation, and refuse to consider the behavior abnormal.

Once they have lost a lot of weight and malnutrition sets in, the physical changes become more visible. Typical changes are amenorrhea (absence of menstruation), digestive problems, extreme sensitivity to cold, hair problems, fluid and electrolyte abnormalities (which may lead to an irregular heartbeat and sudden stopping of the heart), injuries to nerves and tendons, abnormalities of immune function, anemia, growth of fine body hair, mental confusion, inability to concentrate, lethargy, depression, dry skin, lower skin and body temperature, and osteoporosis.

Diagnostic criteria for anorexia nervosa are[14]:
- Refusal to maintain body weight over a minimal normal weight for age and height (weight loss leading to

Bulimia Nervosa Bulimia nervosa is more prevalent than anorexia nervosa. As many as one in five women on college campuses may be bulimic, according to some estimates. Bulimia nervosa also is more prevalent than anorexia nervosa in males, although bulimia is still much more prevalent in females.

People with bulimia usually are healthy looking, well educated, and near recommended body weight. They seem

Anorexia nervosa An eating disorder characterized by self-imposed starvation to lose and maintain very low body weight.

Bulimia nervosa An eating disorder characterized by a pattern of binge eating and purging in an attempt to lose weight and maintain low body weight.

Binge-eating disorder An eating disorder characterized by uncontrollable episodes of eating excessive amounts of food within a relatively short time.

Emotional eating The consumption of large quantities of food to suppress negative emotions.

to enjoy food and often socialize around it. In actuality, they are emotionally insecure, rely on others, and lack self-confidence and self-esteem. Recommended weight and food are important to them.

The binge–purge cycle usually occurs in stages. As a result of stressful life events or the simple compulsion to eat, bulimic individuals engage periodically in binge eating that may last an hour or longer. With some apprehension, bulimics anticipate and plan the cycle. Next they feel an urgency to begin, followed by large and uncontrollable food consumption, during which time they may eat several thousand calories (up to 10,000 calories in extreme cases). After a short period of relief and satisfaction, feelings of deep guilt and shame and intense fear of gaining weight emerge. Purging seems to be an easy answer, as the bingeing cycle can continue without fear of gaining weight.

The diagnostic criteria for bulimia nervosa follow[15]:

- Recurrent episodes of binge eating. An episode of binge eating is characterized by both of the following: (a) eating in a discrete period of time (e.g., within any two-hour period) an amount of food that is definitely more than most people would eat during a similar period and under similar circumstances; (b) a sense of lack of control over eating during the episode (a feeling that one cannot stop eating or control what or how much one is eating)
- Recurring inappropriate compensatory behaviors to prevent weight gain, such as self-induced vomiting; misuse of laxatives, diuretics, other medications, or enemas; fasting; or excessive exercise
- Occurrence of the binge eating and inappropriate compensatory behaviors both occur, on average, at least twice a week for three months
- Undue influence of body shape and weight on self-evaluation

The most typical form of purging is self-induced vomiting. Bulimics also frequently ingest strong laxatives and emetics. Near-fasting diets and strenuous bouts of exercise are common. Medical problems associated with bulimia nervosa include cardiac arrhythmias, amenorrhea, kidney and bladder damage, ulcers, colitis, tearing of the esophagus or stomach, tooth erosion, gum damage, and general muscular weakness.

Unlike anorexics, bulimia sufferers realize that their behavior is abnormal and feel shame about it. Fearing social rejection, they pursue the binge–purge cycle in secrecy and at unusual hours of the day.

Bulimia nervosa can be treated successfully when the person realizes that this destructive behavior is not the solution to life's problems. A change in attitude can prevent permanent damage or death.

Binge-Eating Disorder Binge-eating disorder is probably the most common of the three main eating disorders. About 2 percent of American adults are afflicted with binge-eating disorder in any six-month period. Although most people overeat from time to time, eating more than one should now and then does not mean the individual has a binge-eating disorder. The disorder is slightly more common in women than in men; three women for every two men have the disorder.

Binge-eating disorder is characterized by uncontrollable episodes of eating excessive amounts of food within a relatively short time. The causes of binge-eating disorder are unknown, although depression, anger, sadness, boredom, and worry can trigger an episode. Unlike bulimic sufferers, binge eaters do not purge; thus, most people with this disorder are either overweight or obese.

Typical symptoms of binge-eating disorder include:

- Eating what most people think is an unusually large amount of food
- Eating until uncomfortably full
- Eating out of control
- Eating much faster than usual during binge episodes
- Eating alone because of embarrassment of how much food one is consuming
- Feeling disgusted, depressed, or guilty after overeating

Emotional Eating In addition to physiological purposes, eating also fulfills psychological, social, and cultural purposes. We eat to sustain our daily energy requirements, but we also eat at family celebrations, national holidays, social gatherings, sporting events (as spectators), and even when we become very emotional (some people stop eating when emotional). Emotional eating involves the consumption of large quantities of food, mostly "comfort" and junk food, to suppress negative emotions. Such emotions include stress, anxiety, uncertainty, guilt, anger, pain, depression, loneliness, sadness, boredom, and foods that have a nostalgic or sentimental appeal. In such circumstances, people eat for comfort when they are at their weakest point emotionally. Comfort foods often include calorie-dense, sweet, salty, and fatty foods. Excessive emotional eating hinders proper weight management.

Some palatable foods, such as chocolate, cause the body to release small amounts of mood-elevating opiates, helping to offset negative emotions. A preference for certain foods is also present when one experiences specific feelings (loneliness, anxiety, fear). Eating helps to divert the stressor away for a while, but the distraction is only temporary. The emotions return and may be compounded by a feeling of guilt from overeating.

If you are an emotional overeater, you can always seek help from a therapist at the school's counseling center. The following list of suggestions may also help:

1. Learn to differentiate between emotional and physical hunger.
2. Avoid storing and snacking on unhealthy foods.
3. Keep healthy snacks handy.
4. Use countering techniques (going for a walk instead of reaching for the ice cream, listening to music instead of eating the candy bar).

5. Keep a "trigger log" and get to know what triggers your emotional food consumption.
6. Work it out with exercise instead of food.

Treatment   Treatment for eating disorders is available on most school campuses through the school's counseling center or health center. Local hospitals also offer treatment for these conditions. Many communities have support groups, frequently led by professional personnel and often free of charge. All information and the individual's identity are kept confidential, so the person need not fear embarrassment or repercussions when seeking professional help.

5.5 Physiology of Weight Loss

Traditional concepts related to weight control have centered on three assumptions:

1. Balancing food intake against output allows a person to achieve recommended weight.
2. All fat people simply eat too much.
3. The human body doesn't care how much (or little) fat it stores.

Although these statements contain some truth, they are open to much debate and research. We now know that the causes of obesity are complex, involving a combination of genetics, behavior, and lifestyle factors.

Energy-Balancing Equation   The principle embodied in the **energy-balancing equation** is simple: As long as caloric input equals caloric output, the person will not gain or lose weight. If caloric intake exceeds output, the person gains weight; when output exceeds input, the person loses weight. If daily energy requirements could be determined accurately, caloric intake could be balanced against output. This is not always the case, though, because genetic and lifestyle-related individual differences determine the number of calories required to maintain or lose body weight.

Table 5.3 (page 173) offers general guidelines to determine the **estimated energy requirement (EER)** in calories per day. This is an estimated figure and (as discussed under "Losing Weight the Sound and Sensible Way," page 172) serves only as a starting point from which individual adjustments have to be made.

The total daily energy requirement has three basic components (see Figure 5.6):

1. Resting metabolic rate
2. Thermic effect of food
3. Physical activity

The **resting metabolic rate (RMR)**—the energy requirement to maintain the body's vital processes in the resting state—accounts for approximately 60 to 70 percent of the total daily energy requirement. The thermic effect of food—the energy required to digest, absorb, and store food—accounts for about 5

Figure 5.6   Components of total daily energy requirement.

RMR = resting metabolic rate
TEF = thermic effect of food
PA = physical activity

to 10 percent of the total daily requirement. Physical activity accounts for 15 to 30 percent of the total daily requirement.

One pound of fat is the equivalent of 3,500 calories. If a person's EER is 2,500 calories and that person were to decrease intake by 500 calories per day, it should result in a loss of one pound of fat in seven days ($500 \times 7 = 3,500$). But research has shown—and many people have experienced—that even when dieters carefully balance caloric input against caloric output, weight loss does not always result as predicted. Furthermore, two people with similar measured caloric intake and output seldom lose weight at the same rate.

The rule of thumb is that a person needs a 3,500-calorie deficit to lose a pound of fat. This figure, however, is an oversimplification of what really happens. There are too many individual, behavior, and lifestyle variables that keep weight loss from happening at the same rate among individuals, including gender, body composition, metabolic rate, and activity level. As will be discussed in this chapter, most notably are differences in daily physical activity and the drop in basal metabolic rate as a person loses weight (that is, the body burns fewer calories as weight is lost). The 3,500-calorie rule, nonetheless, is a good guideline to work off when writing weight-loss programs.

The most common explana-

> **Energy-balancing equation**   A principle holding that as long as caloric input equals caloric output, the person will not gain or lose weight. If caloric intake exceeds output, the person gains weight; when output exceeds input, the person loses weight.
>
> **Estimated energy requirement (EER)**   The average dietary energy (caloric) intake that is predicted to maintain energy balance in a healthy adult of defined age, gender, weight, height, and level of physical activity, consistent with good health.
>
> **Resting metabolic rate (RMR)**   The energy requirement to maintain the body's vital processes in the resting state.

tion for individual differences in weight loss and weight gain has been variation in human metabolism from one person to another. We are all familiar with people who can eat "all day long" and not gain an ounce of weight, while others cannot even "dream about food" without gaining weight. Because experts did not believe that human metabolism alone could account for such extreme differences, they developed other theories that might better explain these individual variations.

In terms of physical activity, all activity or movement a person does during the course of the day counts. This principle is known as "spontaneous non-exercise activity," or "fidgeting." Such activity can easily account for several hundred calories a day, resulting in significant differences in weight management among people.

Setpoint Theory Results of research studies point toward a **weight-regulating mechanism (WRM)** in the human body that has a **setpoint** for controlling both appetite and the amount of fat stored. Setpoint is hypothesized to work like a thermostat for body fat, maintaining fairly constant body weight, because it "knows" at all times the exact amount of adipose tissue stored in the fat cells. Some people have high settings; others have low settings.

If body weight decreases (as in dieting), the setpoint senses this change and triggers the WRM to increase the person's appetite or make the body conserve energy to maintain the "set" weight. The opposite also may be true. Some people have a hard time gaining weight. In this case, the WRM decreases appetite or causes the body to waste energy to maintain the lower weight.

Every person has his or her own certain body fat percentage (as established by the setpoint) that the body attempts to maintain. The genetic instinct to survive tells the body that fat storage is vital, and therefore it sets an acceptable fat level. This level may remain somewhat constant or may climb gradually because of poor lifestyle habits.

For instance, under strict calorie reduction, the body may make extreme metabolic adjustments in an effort to maintain its setpoint for fat. The **basal metabolic rate (BMR)**, the lowest level of caloric intake necessary to sustain life, may drop dramatically when operating under a consistent negative caloric balance, and that person's weight loss may plateau for days or even weeks. A low metabolic rate compounds a person's problems in maintaining recommended body weight.

These findings were substantiated by research conducted at Rockefeller University in New York.[16] The authors showed that the body resists maintaining altered weight. Obese and lifetime nonobese individuals were used in the investigation. Following a 10 percent weight loss, the body, in an attempt to regain the lost weight, compensated by burning up to 15 percent fewer calories than expected for the new reduced weight (after accounting for the 10 percent loss). The effects were similar in the obese and nonobese participants. These results imply that after a 10 percent weight loss, a person would have to eat even less or exercise even more to compensate for the estimated 15 percent slowdown (a difference of about 200 to 300 calories).

In this same study, when the participants were allowed to increase their weight to 10 percent above their "normal" body (before weight loss) weight, the body burned 10 to 15 percent *more* calories than expected—attempting to waste energy and maintain the preset weight. This is another indication that the body is highly resistant to weight changes unless additional lifestyle changes are incorporated to ensure successful weight management. (These methods are discussed under "Losing Weight the Sound and Sensible Way," page 172.)

> **Critical Thinking**
>
> Do you see a difference in the amount of food that you are now able to eat compared with the amount that you ate in your mid- to late-teen years? • If so, to what do you attribute this difference? • What actions are you taking to account for the difference?

Dietary restriction alone will not lower the setpoint, even though the person may lose weight and fat. When the dieter goes back to the normal or even below-normal caloric intake (at which the weight may have been stable for a long time), he or she quickly regains the lost fat as the body strives to regain a comfortable fat store.

An Example

Let's use a practical illustration. A person would like to lose some body fat and assumes that his or her current stable body weight has been reached at an average daily caloric intake of 1,800 calories (no weight gain or loss occurs at this daily intake). In an attempt to lose weight rapidly, this person now goes on a **very low calorie diet** (defined as 800 calories per day or less), or, even worse, a near-fasting diet. This immediately activates the body's survival mechanism and readjusts the metabolism to a lower caloric balance. After a few weeks of dieting at the 800-calories-per-day level, the body now can maintain its normal functions at 1,300 calories per day. This new figure (1,300) represents a drop of 500 calories per day in the metabolic rate.

Having lost the desired weight, the person terminates the diet but realizes that the original intake of 1,800 calories per day will have to be lower to maintain the new lower weight. To adjust to the new lower body weight, the person restricts intake to about 1,600 calories per day. The individual is surprised to find that even at this lower daily intake (200 fewer calories), the weight comes back at a rate of one pound every one to two weeks. After the diet is over, this new lowered metabolic rate may take several months to kick back up to its normal level.

Based on this explanation, individuals clearly should not go on very low calorie diets. This will slow the RMR and also will deprive the body of basic daily nutrients required for normal function. Very low calorie diets should be used only in conjunction with dietary supplements and under proper medical supervision. Furthermore, people who use very low calorie diets are not as effective in keeping the weight off once the diet is terminated.

Chapter 5 Weight Management

Achieving and maintaining a high physical fitness percent body fat standard requires a lifetime commitment to regular physical activity and proper nutrition.

Recommendation

A daily caloric intake of approximately 1,500 calories provides the necessary nutrients if a variety of nonprocessed foods are distributed properly over the basic food groups (meeting the daily recommended amounts from each group). Of course, the individual will have to learn to select healthy foods from among 100 percent whole grains, fiber-rich fruits and vegetables, beans, lean proteins, and modest amounts of healthy oils (olive and canola), and nuts while on a calorie-restricted plan.

Under no circumstances should a person go on a diet that calls for a level of 1,200 calories or less for petite women or 1,500 calories or less for most men and women. Weight (fat) is gained over months and years, not overnight. Likewise, weight loss should be gradual, not abrupt. At 1,200 calories per day you may require a multivitamin supplement. Your health care professional should be consulted regarding such supplement.

A second way in which the setpoint may work is by keeping track of the nutrients and calories consumed daily. It is thought that the body, like a cash register, records the daily food intake, and that the brain will not feel satisfied until the calories and nutrients have been "registered."

This setpoint for calories and nutrients seems to operate even when people participate in moderate-intensity exercise. Some evidence suggests that people do not become hungrier with moderate physical activity. Therefore, people can choose to lose weight either by going hungry or by combining a sensible calorie-restricted diet with an increase in daily physical activity.

Lowering the Setpoint

The most common question regarding the setpoint is how to lower it so that the body will feel comfortable at a reduced fat percentage. The following factors seem to affect the setpoint directly by lowering the fat thermostat:

- Exercise
- A diet high in complex carbohydrates
- Nicotine
- Amphetamines

The last two are more destructive than the extra fat weight, so they are not reasonable alternatives (as far as the extra strain on the heart is concerned, smoking one pack of cigarettes per day is said to be the equivalent of carrying 50 to 75 pounds of excess body fat). A diet high in fats and refined carbohydrates, near-fasting diets, and perhaps even artificial sweeteners seem to raise the setpoint. Therefore, the only practical and sensible way to lower the setpoint and lose fat weight is a combination of exercise and a diet high in complex carbohydrates and only moderate amounts of fat.

Because of the effects of proper food management on the body's setpoint, most of the successful dieter's effort should be spent in reforming eating habits, increasing the intake of complex carbohydrates, high-fiber foods, moderate amounts of protein, and decreasing the consumption of processed foods that are high in refined carbohydrates (sugars) and fats. This change in eating habits will bring about a decrease in total daily caloric intake. Because one gram of carbohydrates provides only four calories, as opposed to nine calories per gram of fat, you could eat twice the volume of food (by weight) when substituting carbohydrates for fat. Some fat, however, is recommended in the diet—preferably polyunsaturated and monounsaturated fats. These so-called good fats do more than help protect the heart; they help delay hunger pangs.

A "diet" should not be viewed as a temporary tool to aid in weight loss but, instead, as a permanent change in eating behaviors to ensure weight management and better health. The role of increased physical activity also must be considered, because successful weight loss, maintenance, and recommended body composition are seldom attained without a moderate reduction in caloric intake combined with a regular exercise program.

> **Weight-regulating mechanism (WRM)** A feature of the hypothalamus of the brain that controls how much the body should weigh.
>
> **Setpoint** Weight control theory that the body has an established weight and strongly attempts to maintain that weight.
>
> **Basal metabolic rate (BMR)** The lowest level of oxygen consumption (and energy requirement) necessary to sustain life.
>
> **Very low calorie diet** A diet that allows an energy intake (consumption) of only 800 calories or less per day.

Behavior Modification Planning

Eating Right When on the Run

Current lifestyles often require people to be on the run. We don't seem to have time to eat right, but fortunately it doesn't have to be that way. If you are on the run, it is even more critical to make healthy choices to keep up with a challenging schedule. Look at the following food choices for eating on the run:

- Water
- Whole-grain cereal and skim milk
- Whole-grain bread and bagels
- Whole-grain bread with peanut butter
- Nonfat or low-fat yogurt
- Fresh fruits
- Frozen fresh fruit (grapes, cherries, banana slices)
- Dried fruits
- Raw vegetables (carrots, red peppers, cucumbers, radishes, cauliflower, asparagus)
- Whole-grain crackers
- Pretzels
- Whole-grain bread sticks
- Low-fat cheese sticks
- Granola bars
- Snack-size cereal boxes
- Nuts
- Trail mix
- Plain popcorn
- Vegetable soups

Try It

In your Online Journal or class notebook, plan your fast-meal menus for the upcoming week. It may require extra shopping and some food preparation (for instance, cutting vegetables to place in snack-size plastic bags). At the end of the week, evaluate how many days you had a "healthy eating on the run day." What did you learn from the experience?

5.6 Diet and Metabolism

Fat can be lost by selecting the proper foods, exercising, or restricting calories. However, when dieters try to lose weight by dietary restrictions alone, they also lose lean body mass (muscle protein, along with vital organ protein). The amount of lean body mass lost depends entirely on caloric limitation. When people go on a near-fasting diet, up to half of the weight loss is lean body mass and the other half is actual fat loss (see Figure 5.7).[17] When diet is combined with exercise, close to 100 percent of the weight loss is in the form of fat, and lean tissue actually may increase. Loss of lean body mass is never good, because it weakens the organs and muscles and slows metabolism. Large losses in lean tissue can cause disturbances in heart function and damage to other organs. Equally important is not to overindulge (binge) following a very low calorie diet, as this may cause changes in metabolic rate and electrolyte balance, which could trigger fatal cardiac arrhythmias.

Contrary to some beliefs, aging is not the main reason for the lower metabolic rate. It is not so much that metabolism slows down as that people slow down. As people age, they tend to rely more on the amenities of life (remote controls, cell phones, intercoms, single-level homes, riding lawnmowers) that lull a person into sedentary living.

Basal metabolism also is related to lean body weight. More lean tissue yields a higher metabolic rate. As a consequence of sedentary living and less physical activity, the lean component decreases and fat tissue increases. The human body requires a certain amount of oxygen per pound of lean body mass. Given that fat is considered metabolically inert from the point of view of caloric use, the lean tissue uses most of the oxygen, even at rest. As muscle and organ mass (lean body mass) decrease, so do the energy requirements at rest.

Diets with caloric intakes below 1,500 calories cannot guarantee the retention of lean body mass. Even at this intake level, some loss is inevitable unless the diet is combined with exercise. Despite the claims of many diets that they do not alter the lean component, the simple truth is that regardless of what nutrients may be added to the diet, severe caloric restrictions *always* prompt the loss of lean tissue. Sadly, many

Figure 5.7 Outcome of three forms of diet on fat loss.

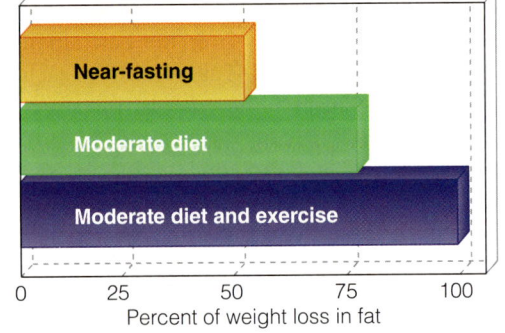

SOURCE: Adapted from R. J. Shephard, *Alive Man: The Physiology of Physical Activity* (Springfield, IL: Charles C. Thomas, 1975): 484–488.

people go on very low calorie diets constantly. Every time they do, their metabolic rate slows as more lean tissue is lost.

People in their 40s and older who weigh the same as they did when they were 20 tend to think they are at recommended body weight. During this span of 20 years or more, though, they may have dieted many times without participating in an exercise program. After they terminate each diet, they regain the weight, and much of that gain is additional body fat. Maybe at age 20 they weighed 150 pounds, of which only 15 percent was fat. Now at age 40, even though they still weigh 150 pounds, they might be 30 percent fat (see Figure 5.8). At "recommended" body weight, they wonder why they are eating very little and still having trouble staying at that weight.

5.7 Hormonal Regulation of Appetite

Ghrelin and leptin are two hormones currently being extensively researched because they appear to play a role in appetite. Ghrelin, produced primarily in the stomach, stimulates appetite: that is, the more ghrelin the body produces, the more you want to eat. Leptin, produced by fat cells, on the other hand, lets the brain know when you are full; the more leptin you produce, the less you want to eat. Similar to insulin resistance (leading to type 2 diabetes), research is beginning to show that a lack of physical activity also leads to leptin resistance, setting up a vicious cycle that leads to excessive eating. Scientists are now looking into the role these hormones play in weight gain and weight loss, as well as at the effects of sleep deprivation and exercise dose on these hormones and subsequent appetite regulation.

5.8 Sleep and Weight Management

As presented under the Healthy Lifestyle Habits box in Chapter 1 (see page 28), adequate sleep is one of the 12 key components that enhance health and extend life. New evidence shows that sleep is also important to adequate weight management. Sleep deprivation appears to be conducive to weight gain and may interfere with the body's capability to lose weight.

Current obesity and sleep deprivation data point toward a possible correlation between excessive body weight and sleep deprivation. About 68 percent of the U.S. population is overweight or obese, and according to the National Sleep Foundation, 63 percent of Americans report that they do not get eight hours of sleep per night. The question must be raised: Is there a connection? Let's examine some of the data.

One of the most recent studies examining this issue showed that individuals who get less than six hours of sleep per night have a higher average BMI (28.3) compared with those who average eight hours per night (24.5).[18] Another study on more than 68,000 women between the ages of 30 and 55 found that those who got 5 or less hours of sleep per night were 30 percent more likely to gain 30 or more pounds compared with women who got 8 hours per night.[19]

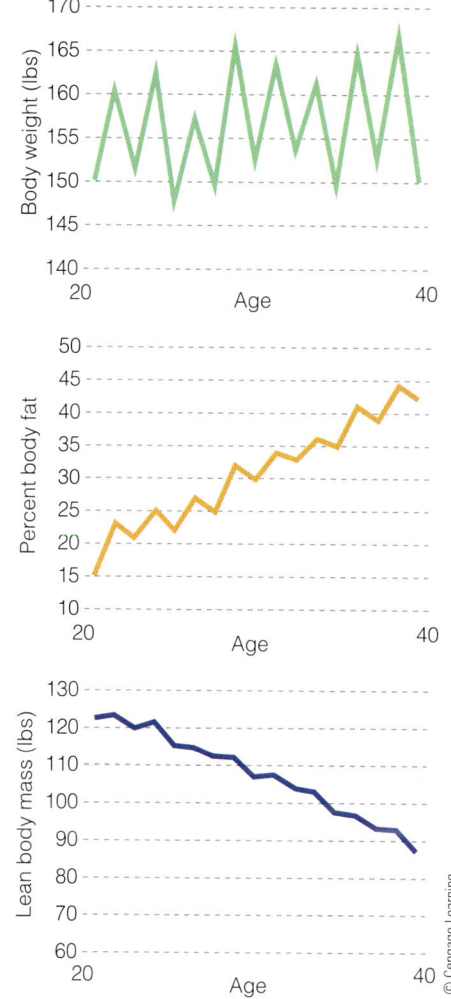

Figure 5.8 Body composition changes as a result of frequent dieting without exercise.

Researchers believe that lack of sleep disrupts normal body hormonal balances. Sleep deprivation has now been shown to elevate ghrelin levels and decrease leptin levels, potentially leading to weight gain or keeping you from losing weight.[20] Data comparing these hormone levels in five-hour versus eight-hour sleepers found that the short sleepers had a 14.9 percent increase in ghrelin levels and a 15.5-percent decrease in leptin levels. The short sleepers also had a 3.6 percent higher BMI than the regular sleepers.[21]

Based on all these studies, the data appear to indicate that sleep deprivation has a negative impact on weight loss or maintenance. Thus, an important component to a well-designed weight management program should include a good night's rest (eight hours of sleep).

5.9 Monitoring Body Weight

A most critical component to lifetime weight management is to regularly monitor your body weight. Get into the habit of weighing yourself, preferably at the same time of day and under the same conditions; for instance, in the morning just as you get out of bed. Data indicate that daily weigh-ins are associated with better weight maintenance and enhanced weight loss, while infrequent weighing leads to weight gain.

Depending on your body size, activity patterns, rehydration level, and dietary intake on any given day, your weight will fluctuate by a pound or more from one day to the next. You do not want to be obsessed with body weight that can potentially lead to an eating disorder, but monitoring your *recommended body weight* (and that is the key: *"healthy" recommended body weight*) on a regular basis allows you to make immediate adjustments in food intake and physical activity if your weight increases and stays there for several days. *Do not adapt and accept* the higher weight as your new stable weight. Understand that it is a lot easier to make sensible short-term dietary and activity changes to lose one or two pounds of weight, rather than having to make drastic long term changes to lose 10, 20, 50, or more pounds that you allowed yourself to gain over the course of several months or years. Whenever feasible, you also want to do periodic assessments of body composition using experienced technicians and valid techniques.

5.10 Exercise and Weight Management

To tilt the energy-balancing equation in your favor, you need to burn more calories through physical activity. Research indicates that exercise accentuates weight loss while on a negative caloric balance (diet) as long as you do not replenish the calories expended during exercise. The debate, however, centers on what amount of exercise is best for individuals who are trying to lose weight and those who are trying to maintain weight. The data are clear, nonetheless, that exercise is the best predictor of long-term maintenance of weight loss.[22]

Regular exercise seems to exert control over how much a person weighs. On average, the typical adult American gradually becomes overweight by gaining one to two pounds of weight per year. A one-pound weight gain represents a simple energy surplus of less than 10 calories per day (10×365 days $= 3{,}650$ calories and 1 pound of fat represents 3,500 calories). This simple surplus of less than 10 calories per day is the equivalent of less than one teaspoon of sugar. Weight gain is clearly related to a decrease in physical activity and an increase in caloric intake. Physical inactivity, however, might very well be the primary cause leading to excessive weight and obesity. The human body was meant to be physically active and *a minimal level of activity* appears to be necessary to accurately balance caloric intake to caloric expenditure. In sedentary individuals, the body seems to lose control over this fine energy balance.

Most people understand that exercise enhances the rate of weight loss, enhances body composition, and is vital in maintaining the lost weight. Not only will exercise maintain lean tissue, but advocates of the setpoint theory say that exercise resets the fat thermostat to a new, lower level.

Most people who struggle with weight management need 60 to 90 minutes of daily physical activity to effectively manage body weight. While accumulating 30 minutes of moderate-intensity activity per day provides substantial health benefits (the minimum daily recommended amount of activity), from a weight management point of view, however, the Institute of Medicine of the National Academy of Sciences recommends that people accumulate 60 minutes of moderate-intensity physical activity most days of the week.[23] The evidence shows that people who maintain recommended weight typically accumulate an hour or more of daily physical activity.

According to the American College of Sports Medicine position stand on strategies for weight loss and prevention of weight regain for adults (see Figure 5.9), greater weight loss is achieved by increasing the amount of weekly physical activity. Of even greater significance, physical activity is required for weight maintenance following weight loss. People who exercise regain less weight than those who do not. And those who exercise the most regain the least amount of weight. Individuals who remain physically active for 60 or more minutes per day are able to keep the weight off.

Further, data from the National Weight Control Registry (www.nwcr.ws) on more than 6,000 individuals who have lost at least 30 pounds and have kept them off for a minimum of 5 years indicate that they typically expend about 300 calories through daily moderate-intensity exercise.[24] Three hundred calories represents about three miles jogging in 30 minutes or walking briskly the same distance in 60 minutes. Individuals who completely stop physical activity regain almost 100 percent of the weight within 18 months of discontinuing the weight loss program. Most of the successful "weight maintainers" also show greater dietary restraint and follow a low-fat diet, consuming less than 30 percent of the total daily calories from fat.

Figure 5.9 Approximate decrease in body weight based on total weekly minutes of physical activity without caloric restrictions.

SOURCE: Adapted from American College of Sports Medicine, "Position Stand: Appropriate Physical Activity Intervention Strategies for Weight Loss and Prevention of Weight Regain for Adults," *Medicine and Science in Sports and Exercise* 41 (2009): 459–471.

Most experts and leading organizations now recognize that if weight management is not a consideration, 30 minutes of daily activity 5 days per week provides substantial health benefits. To prevent weight gain, nonetheless, 60 minutes of daily activity is recommended; to maintain substantial weight loss, 90 minutes may be required.

The most important reason why physical activity and exercise are so vital for weight loss maintenance is because sedentary living expends no additional energy (calories) over the resting metabolic rate. With limited physical activity throughout the day, sedentary people cannot afford to eat very many calories, perhaps only 1,000 to 1,200 calories per day. And such a low level of energy intake is not sufficient to keep the person from constantly feeling hungry. The only choice they now have is to go hungry every day, an impossible task to sustain. After terminating the diet, in just a few short days, energy intake climbs with an end result of weight regain. Thus, the only logical way to increase caloric intake and maintain weight loss is by burning more calories through exercise and incorporating physical activity throughout daily living.

If a person is trying to lose weight, a combination of aerobic and strength-training exercises works best. Aerobic exercise is the best exercise modality to offset the setpoint, and the continuity and duration of these types of activities cause many calories to be burned in the process. The role of aerobic exercise in successful lifetime weight management cannot be overestimated.

Behavior Modification Planning

Physical Activity Guidelines for Weight Management

The following physical activity guidelines are recommended to effectively manage body weight:

- 30 minutes of physical activity on most days of the week if you do not have difficulty maintaining body weight (more minutes and/or higher intensity if you choose to reach a high level of physical fitness).
- Between 30 and 60 minutes of light-to-moderate exercise on most days of the week if you are trying to lose weight. Incorporate as many light ambulatory activities as possible during the course of each day.
- 60 minutes of daily activity if you want to prevent weight gain.
- Between 60 and 90 minutes each day if you want to keep weight off following extensive weight loss (30 pounds of weight loss or more). Be sure to include some high-intensity/low impact activities at least twice a week in your program.

Try It

In your Behavior Change Planner Progress Tracker, Online Journal, or class notebook, record how many minutes of daily physical activity you accumulate on a regular basis and record your thoughts on how effectively your activity has helped you manage your body weight. Is there one thing you could do today to increase your physical activity?

Behavior Modification Planning

Weight Maintenance Benefits of a Lifetime Exercise Program

The authors of this book have been jogging together a minimum of 15 miles per week (3 miles/5 times per week) for the past 37 years. Without considering the additional energy expenditure from their regular strength-training program and their many other sport and recreational activities, the energy cost of this regular jogging program over 37 years has been approximately 2,886,000 calories (15 miles × 100 calories/mile × 52 weeks × 37 years) or the equivalent of 825 pounds of fat (2,886,000 ÷ 3,500). In essence, without this 30-minute jogging workout 5 times per week, the authors would weigh 967 and 941 pounds respectively. Such is the long-term gratification (reward) of a lifetime exercise program—not to mention the myriad health benefits, joy, and quality of life derived through this program.

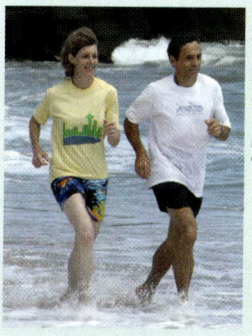

Try It

Ask yourself whether a regular aerobic exercise program is part of your long-term gratification and health enhancement program. If the answer is no, are you ready to change your behavior? Use the Behavior Change Planner to help you answer the question.

Strength training is critical in helping maintain and increase lean body mass. The number of calories burned during a typical hour-long strength-training session is much less than during an hour of aerobic exercise. Because of the high intensity of strength training, the person needs frequent rest intervals to recover from each set of exercises. In the long run, however, the person enjoys the benefits of gains in lean tissue. Guidelines for developing aerobic and strength-training programs are given in Chapters 6 and 7.

Although the increase in BMR through increased muscle mass is being debated in the literature and merits further research, data indicate that each additional pound of muscle tissue raises the BMR in the range of 6 to 35 calories per day.[25] The latter figure is based on calculations that an increase of 3 to 3.5 pounds of lean tissue through strength training increased BMR by about 105 to 120 calories per day.[26]

Most likely, the benefit of strength training goes beyond the new muscle tissue itself. Maybe a pound of muscle tissue requires only six calories per day to sustain itself, but as all muscles undergo strength training, they undergo increased protein synthesis to build and repair themselves, resulting in increased energy expenditure of 1 to 1.5 calories per pound in all trained muscle tissue. Such an increase would explain the 105- to 120-calorie BMR increase in this research study.

To examine the effects of a small increase in BMR on long-term body weight, let's use a very conservative estimate of an additional 50 calories per day as a result of a regular strength-training program. An increase of 50 calories represents an additional 18,250 calories per year (50 × 365), or the equivalent of 5.2 pounds of fat (18,250 ÷ 3,500). This increase in BMR would more than offset the typical adult weight gain of one to two pounds per year.

This figure of 18,250 calories per year does not include the actual energy cost of the strength-training workout. If we use an energy expenditure of only 150 calories per strength-training session, done twice per week, over a year's time it would represent 15,600 calories (150 × 2 × 52), or the equivalent of another 4.5 pounds of fat (15,600 ÷ 3,500).

In addition, although the amounts seem small, the previous calculations do not account for the increase in metabolic rate following the strength-training workout (the time it takes the body to return to its preworkout resting rate—about two hours). Depending on the training volume (see Chapter 7, page 245), this recovery energy expenditure ranges from 20 to 100 calories following each strength-training workout. All these "apparently small" changes make a big difference in the long run.

Although size (inches) and percent body fat both decrease when sedentary individuals begin an exercise program, body weight often remains the same or may even increase during the first couple of weeks of the program. Exercise helps to increase muscle tissue, connective tissue, blood volume (as much as 500 mL, or the equivalent of one pound, following the first week of aerobic exercise), enzymes and other structures within the cell, and glycogen (which binds water). All of these changes lead to a higher functional capacity of the human body. With exercise, most of the weight loss becomes apparent after a few weeks of training, when the lean component has stabilized.

We know that a negative caloric balance of 3,500 calories does not always result in a loss of one pound of fat, but the role of exercise in achieving a negative balance by burning additional calories is significant in weight reduction and maintenance programs. Sadly, some individuals claim that the number of calories burned during exercise is hardly worth the effort. They think that cutting their daily intake by 300 calories is easier than participating in some sort of exercise that would burn the same amount of calories. The problem is that the willpower to cut those 300 calories lasts only a few weeks, and then the person goes back to the old eating patterns.

If a person gets into the habit of exercising regularly, say 3 times a week, jogging 3 miles per exercise session (about 300 calories burned), this represents 900 calories in one week, about 3,600 calories in one month, or 46,800 calories per year. This minimal amount of exercise represents as many as 13.5 extra pounds of fat in 1 year, 27 in 2, and so on.

We tend to forget that our weight creeps up gradually over the years, not just overnight. Hardly worth the effort? And we have not even taken into consideration the increase in lean tissue, possible resetting of the setpoint, benefits to the cardiovascular system, and, most important, the improved quality of life. Fundamental reasons for excessive weight and obesity, few could argue, are sedentary living and lack of a regular exercise program.

In terms of preventing disease, many of the health benefits that people seek by losing weight are reaped through exercise alone, even without weight loss. Exercise offers protection against premature morbidity and mortality for everyone, including people who are overweight or already have risk factors for disease.

One additional benefit of exercise and physical activity is that it attenuates a person's predisposition to obesity. Genetic epidemiological studies have established that genetic factors play a role in obesity development in our 21st century obesogenic environment. Promoting physical activity, exercise, and an active lifestyle is especially critical for individuals genetically predisposed to obesity.

The Role of Exercise Intensity and Duration in Weight Management

A hotly debated and controversial current topic is the exercise volume required for adequate weight management. Depending on the degree of the initial weight problem and the person's fitness level, there appears to be a difference in the volume of exercise that is most conducive toward adequate weight loss, weight loss maintenance, and weight management.

We have known for years that compared with vigorous intensity, a greater proportion of calories burned during light-intensity exercise are derived from fat. The lower the intensity of exercise, the higher the percentage of fat utilization as an energy source. During light-intensity exercise, up to 50 percent of the calories burned may be derived from fat (the other 50 percent from glucose [carbohydrates]). With vigorous exercise, only 30 to 40 percent of the caloric expenditure comes from fat.

However, you can burn twice as many calories overall—and subsequently more fat—during vigorous exercise. Let's look at a practical illustration (also see Table 5.2). If you exercised for 30 to 40 minutes at light intensity and burned 200 calories, about 100 of those calories (50 percent) would come from fat. If you exercised at a vigorous intensity during those same 30 to 40 minutes, you could burn 400 calories, with 120 to 160 of the calories (30 to 40 percent) coming from fat. Thus, even though it is true that the percentage of fat used is greater during light-intensity exercise, the overall amount of fat used is still less during light-intensity exercise. Plus, if you were to exercise at a light intensity, you would have to do so twice as long to burn the same amount of calories.

Another benefit is that the metabolic rate remains at a slightly higher level longer after vigorous-intensity exercise, so you continue to burn a few extra calories following exercise. Studies indicate that very few calories are burned during recovery following a 45-minute moderate-intensity (50 percent of maximal capacity) exercise session, whereas exercising at or greater than 70 percent of the maximal capacity for the same 45 minutes, the individual will burn an additional 300 to 700 extra calories after the exercise session. Researchers believe that the extra caloric expenditure following vigorous exercise is because (a) the body uses more fat and less carbohydrates following a hard exercise session, and (b) additional energy is required to replenish glycogen stores used during intense exercise, and (c) hormones released during vigorous exercise remain high, maintaining an elevated metabolism for several hours thereafter.

This example does not mean that light-intensity exercise is ineffective. Light-intensity exercise provides substantial health benefits, including a decrease in premature morbidity among overweight individuals. Additionally, beginners are more willing to participate and stay with light-intensity programs. The risk of injury when starting out is quite low with this type of program. Light-intensity exercise does promote weight loss.

In terms of overall weight loss, there is controversy regarding the optimal exercise dose. Initial research indicated that vigorous-intensity exercise triggered more fat loss than light- to moderate-intensity exercise. Research conducted in the 1990s at Laval University in Quebec, Canada, using both men and women participants, showed that subjects who performed a high-intensity intermittent-training (HIIT) program lost more body fat than participants in a low- to moderate-intensity continuous aerobic endurance group.[27] Even more surprisingly, this finding occurred despite the fact that the vigorous-intensity group burned fewer total calories per exercise session. The researchers concluded that the "results reinforce the notion that for a given level of energy expenditure, vigorous exercise favors negative energy and lipid balance to a greater extent than exercise of low- to moderate-intensity. Moreover, the metabolic adaptations taking place in the skeletal muscle in response to the HIIT program appear to favor the process of "lipid oxidation." If time constrains do not allow much time for exercise, to increase energy expenditure, a vigorous 20- to 30-minute exercise programs is recommended.

Recently, it has been suggested that *when attempting to lose weight*, particularly for women, lengthy exercise sessions may not be helpful because they actually trigger greater food consumption following exercise, whereas shorter exercise sessions do not lead to a greater caloric intake. Thus, some people think that the potential weight reduction effect of lengthy exercise sessions may be attenuated because people end up eating more food when they exercise.

A 2009 study had postmenopausal women exercise at 50 percent of their maximal aerobic capacity for about 20 minutes, 40 minutes, or 60 minutes 3 to 4 times per week.[28] On average, the groups lost 3, 4.6, and, 3.3 pounds of weight, respectively. The data indicated that the 20- and 40-minute groups lost weight closely to what had been predicted, whereas the 60 minute group lost significantly less than predicted. The researchers concluded that 60 minutes of exercise led this group of women to compensate with greater food intake, possibly triggered by an increase in ghrelin levels. All three groups, nonetheless, exhibited a significant decrease in waist circumference, independent of total weight lost. Researchers theorize that the biological mechanism to maintain fat stores in women is stronger than in men.

Moderate-intensity exercise, nonetheless, is very effective for weight maintenance. A 2010 study of more than 34,000 women who were followed for 13 years, starting at an average age of 54, found that on average the women gained six pounds of weight; but a small group of them who reported 60 minutes of almost daily exercise at a moderate intensity closely maintained their body weight.[29] The exercise routine of the latter group was not something new to them, but rather exercise that they had been doing for years.

Table 5.2 Comparison of Approximate Energy Expenditure between 30–40 Minutes of Exercise at Three Intensity Levels

Exercise Intensity	Total Energy Expenditure (Calories)	Percent Calories from Fat	Total Fat Calories	Percent Calories from CHO*	Total CHO* Calories	Calories Burned per Minute	Calories per Pound per Minute
Light Intensity	200	50%	100	50%	100	6.67	0.045
Moderate Intensity	280	40%	112	60%	168	9.45	0.063
Vigorous Intensity	400	30%	120	70%	280	13.50	0.090

*CHO = Carbohydrates

© Cengage Learning

While the best exercise dose for optimal weight loss may not be a precise science, the research is quite clear that regular exercise is the best predictor of long-term weight maintenance. The data also indicate that even as little as 80 weekly minutes of aerobic or strength training exercise prevents regain of the harmful visceral fat (also see page 124 in Chapter 4).

The take-home message from these studies is that when trying to lose weight, initial lengthy exercise sessions (longer than 60 minutes) may not be the best approach to weight loss, *unless* you carefully monitor daily caloric intake and avoid caloric compensation. The data show that people who carefully monitor caloric intake, instead of "guesstimating" energy intake, are by far more successful with weight loss.

Caloric compensation in response to extensive exercise in overweight individuals may be related to a low initial fitness level and the already low caloric intake. Overall, inactive people tend to eat fewer calories, and a lengthy exercise session may very well trigger a greater appetite due to the large negative caloric balance. Research confirms that energy deficit, and not exercise, is the most significant regulator of the hormonal responses seen in previously inactive individuals who begin an exercise program.[30] In active/fit individuals, lengthy exercise sessions are not at all counterproductive. If such was the case, health clubs and jogging trails would be full of overweight and obese people.

New research is beginning to look into the role of increasing light-intensity ambulation (walking) and standing activities (doing some of the work on your feet instead of sitting the entire time) on weight loss. In essence, the individual will increase light-intensity physical activity throughout the day. Light-intensity activities do not seem to trigger the increase in ghrelin levels seen in previously inactive individuals who undertake long moderate- or vigorous-intensity exercise sessions. The difference in energy expenditure by increasing light-intensity activities throughout the day can represent several hundred calories. As you achieve a higher fitness level, you can combine light-intensity activities performed throughout the day with moderate- and/or vigorous-intensity exercise. A graphic illustration of such lifestyle patterns and the effects on the metabolic rate and overall energy expenditure is provided in Figure 5.10.

If you wish to engage in vigorous-intensity exercise to either maintain lost weight or for adequate weight management, a word of caution is in order: Be sure that it is medically safe for you to participate in such activities and that you build up gradually to that level. If you are cleared to participate in vigorous-intensity exercise, do not attempt to do too much too quickly, because you may incur injuries and become discouraged. You must allow your body a proper conditioning period of 8 to 12 weeks or even longer.

Also keep in mind that vigorous intensity does not mean high impact. High-impact activities are the most common cause of exercise-related injuries. Additional information on proper exercise prescription is presented in Chapter 6. And remember, when on a weight loss program, *always* carefully monitor your daily caloric intake to avoid food overconsumption.

Overweight and Fit Debate A hotly debated topic in the exercise and medical community is the topic most commonly referred to as "fit and fat." Can a person possibly be overweight/obese and still be fit?

Initially, the debate started with research indicating that the higher the aerobic fitness level, as measured by total treadmill-walking time, the lower the mortality rate, regardless of body weight. Most recently, fitness has been defined as "accumulating 30 minutes of moderate intensity activity on most days of the week." Many overweight people who reach this goal are not predisposed to premature death. In fact, data indicate that, on average, death rates for thin, but unfit, individuals are twice as high as that of obese and "fit" people. Furthermore, looking at every category of body composition, most "unfit" people have a higher rate of premature death than "fit" individuals. Thus, at least partially, lack of physical activity (fitness), and not the weight problem itself, may be the cause of premature death in most overweight people. It's not simply a matter of fitness or fatness, because both obesity and physical

FTO: The Obesity-Associated Gene

Researchers recently discovered a variant of the fat mass and obesity-associated (FTO) gene that appears to have a strong link to BMI and increases the risk that carriers will be overweight or obese. The strength of the genetic association depends on whether the individual has inherited one or two copies of the FTO gene variant. Having one copy of the variant has a corresponding modest effect on body weight. On average, such a person weighs an extra 2.5 pounds compared to those who do not have the variant. Someone with two copies of the variant typically weighs an extra 6.5 pounds. Nonetheless, obesity is only partially driven by genes, and the genetic code does not substantially change in just a few generations. In contrast, people's lifestyles and their environment have changed significantly over the last 100 years.

People with one or two variants of the gene are not destined to be obese. The gene variant does not cause a sluggish metabolism but rather causes them to eat more, in particular calorie-dense foods. And lifestyle plays a crucial role in enabling or minimizing susceptibility to weight gain. Physical activity is effective in controlling weight in people with this genetic predisposition toward obesity. Shortly after the discovery of FTO in 2007, researchers found that physical activity and exercise attenuate the effect of the gene on weight gain. As little as 60 minutes of moderate- to vigorous-intensity activity per week thwarts the genetic inheritance and reduces the effects of the FTO variant. Thus, the benefits of physical activity and exercise are strong enough to keep at recommended body weight people who could otherwise become seriously overweight.

inactivity are independent risk factors for heart disease, type 2 diabetes, and other chronic ailments.

The results of these studies, nonetheless, are encouraging because they show that many overweight/obese people who focus on healthy eating and become physically active can decrease the risk of premature mortality, regardless of whether they lose weight or not. Very few obese people, however, eat healthy and exercise regularly for 30 minutes on most days of the week. Most obese people either choose not to exercise or are unable to do so because of functional limitations as a result of the excessive body weight.

The answer to the question as to whether a person can be fit and fat depends on the definition of fitness. If cardiorespiratory fitness is determined by "accumulating 30 minutes of moderate-intensity activity on most days of the week," then the answer is a definite "yes." If one measures fitness based on maximal oxygen uptake (VO_{2max}—see Chapter 6, page 197), the answer is a clear "no." Many fitness experts do not agree with the concept of fit and fat. Exercise by itself will not remove all of the heart risks of being overweight, but it can blunt them. According to Dr. JoAnn Manson of the Harvard Medical School, "it's a rare bird" to find someone who is truly overweight and yet truly fit from a cardiorespiratory standpoint.

Most nutritionists and exercise scientists agree that healthy eating and healthy exercise contribute to healthy body weight. There are more than 50 medical conditions—from type 2 diabetes, acid reflux, arthritis, sleep apnea, and some types of cancers, that are directly related to excessive body weight. At this point, most fitness leaders do not support the notion that people can enjoy vibrant health and good quality of life while being overweight or obese.

Healthy Weight Gain

"Skinny" people, too, should realize that the only healthy way to gain weight is through exercise (mainly strength-training exercises) and a slight increase in caloric intake. Attempting to gain weight by overeating alone will raise the fat component and not the lean component—which is not the path to better health. Exercise is the best solution to weight (fat) reduction and weight (lean) gain alike.

A strength-training program such as explained in Chapter 7 is the best approach to add body weight. The training program should include at least two exercises of one to three sets for each major body part. Each set should consist of about 8 to 12 repetitions maximum.

Even though the metabolic cost of synthesizing a pound of muscle tissue is still unclear, consuming an estimated 500 additional calories per day is recommended to gain lean tissue. Your diet should include a daily total intake of about 1.5 grams of protein per kilogram of body weight. If your daily protein intake already exceeds 1.5 grams per day, the extra 500 calories should be primarily in the form of complex carbohydrates. The higher caloric intake must be accompanied by a strength-training program; otherwise, the increase in body weight will be in the form of fat, not muscle tissue. (Activity 5.4 can be used to monitor your caloric intake for healthy weight gain.) Additional information on nutrition to optimize muscle growth and strength development is provided in Chapter 7 in the section "Dietary Guidelines for Strength Development," page 251.

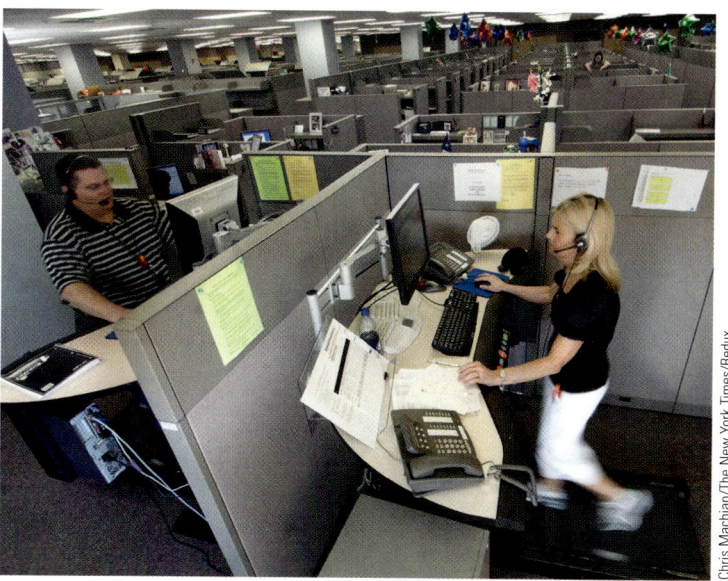

Increasing ambulatory activity throughout the day enhances fitness and is an excellent weight management strategy. These employees at Mutual of Omaha, working at Walkstations, typically walk five miles at a light-intensity level during the course of most days.

Weight Loss Myths

Cellulite and **spot reducing** are mythical concepts. Cellulite is caused by the herniation of subcutaneous fat within fibrous connective tissue, giving it a padded-like appearance.

Doing several sets of daily sit-ups will not get rid of fat in the midsection of the body. When fat comes off, it does so throughout the entire body, not just the exercised area. The greatest proportion of fat may come off the biggest fat deposits, but the caloric output of a few sets of sit-ups has practically no effect on reducing total body fat. A person has to exercise much longer to see results.

Other touted means toward quick weight loss, such as rubberized sweat suits, steam baths, and mechanical vibrators, are misleading. When a person wears a sweat suit or steps into a sauna, the weight lost is not fat but merely a significant amount of water. Sure, it looks nice when you step on the scale immediately afterward, but this represents a false loss of weight. As soon as you replace body fluids, you gain back the weight quickly.

Wearing rubberized sweat suits hastens the rate of

> **Cellulite** Term frequently used in reference to fat deposits that "bulge out"; caused by the herniation of subcutaneous fat within fibrous connective tissue, giving it a padded-like appearance.
>
> **Spot reducing** Fallacious theory proposing that exercising a specific body part will result in significant fat reduction in that area.

Figure 5.10 Effects of lifestyle patterns on overall daily expenditure.

body fluid that is lost—fluid that is vital during prolonged exercise—and raises core temperature at the same time. This combination puts a person in danger of dehydration, which impairs cellular function and, in extreme cases, can even cause death.

Similarly, mechanical vibrators are worthless in a weight-control program. Vibrating belts and turning rollers may feel good, but they require no effort whatsoever. Fat cannot be shaken off. It is lost primarily by burning it in muscle tissue.

5.11 Losing Weight the Sound and Sensible Way

Dieting never has been fun and never will be. People who are overweight and are serious about losing weight, however, have to include regular physical activity and exercise in their lives, along with proper food management and a sensible reduction in caloric intake.

Because excessive body fat is a risk factor for cardiovascular disease, some precautions are in order. Depending on the extent of the weight problem, a medical examination may be a good idea before undertaking the exercise program. Consult a physician in this regard.

Significantly overweight individuals need to choose activities in which they will not have to support their own body weight but that still will be effective in burning calories. Injuries to joints and muscles are common in excessively overweight individuals who participate in weight-bearing exercises such as walking, jogging, and aerobics.

Swimming may not be a good weight loss modality. Additional body fat makes a person more buoyant, and many people are not at the skill level required to swim fast enough to get a good training effect, thus limiting the number of calories burned as well as the benefits to the cardiorespiratory system. Additionally, swimmers often conduct "land training" to more effectively manage body weight. Research indicates that swimming has minimal effect on weight loss. The data further show that swimming in cold water stimulates appetite, so people tend to eat more following their exercise session. If your preferred mode of exercise is swimming, guard against eating more after you swim. During the initial stages of exercise, better alternatives include walking, riding a bicycle (either road or stationary), elliptical training, low-impact aerobics/Zumba, or walking in a warm shallow pool. These forms of exercise aid with weight loss without fear of injuries.

How long should each exercise session last? The amount of exercise needed to lose weight and maintain the weight loss is different from the amount of exercise needed to improve fitness. For health fitness, accumulating 30 minutes of physical activity a minimum of 5 days per week is recommended. To develop and maintain cardiorespiratory fitness, 20 to 60 minutes of vigorous-intensity exercise, 3 to 5 times per week, is suggested (see Chapter 6). For successful weight loss, however, 30 to 60 minutes of light to moderate exercise on most days of the week is recommended. Additional light-intensity ambulation and standing throughout the day are also strongly encouraged. To maintain substantial weight loss, 60 to 90 minutes of physical activity on a nearly daily basis is recommended.

A person should not try to do too much too fast. Unconditioned beginners should start with about 15 minutes of aerobic exercise 3 times a week, and during the next 3 to 4 weeks gradually increase the duration by approximately 5 minutes per week and the frequency by 1 day per week.

In addition to exercise and food management, a sensible reduction in caloric intake and careful monitoring of this intake are recommended. Research indicates that a negative caloric balance is required to lose weight because:

1. People tend to underestimate their caloric intake and are eating more than they should be eating.
2. Developing new behaviors takes time, and most people have trouble changing and adjusting to new eating habits.
3. Many individuals are in such poor physical condition that they take a long time to increase their activity level enough to offset the setpoint and burn enough calories to aid in losing body fat.
4. Most successful dieters carefully monitor their daily caloric intake.
5. A few people simply will not alter their food selection. For those who will not (which will increase their risk for chronic diseases), the only solution to lose weight successfully is a large increase in physical activity, a negative caloric balance, or a combination of the two.

Perhaps the only exception to a decrease in caloric intake for weight loss purposes is in people who already are eating too few calories. A nutrient analysis (see Chapter 3) often reveals that long-term dieters are not consuming enough calories. These people actually need to increase their daily caloric intake and combine it with an exercise program to get their metabolism to kick back up to a normal level.

You also must learn to make wise food choices. Think in terms of long-term benefits (weight management) instead of instant gratification (unhealthy eating and subsequent weight gain). Making healthful choices allows you to eat more food, eat more nutritious food, and ingest fewer calories. For example, instead of eating a high-fat, 700-calorie scone, you could eat as much as one orange, one cup of grapes, a hard-boiled egg, two slices of whole-wheat toast, two teaspoons of jam, one-half cup of honey-sweetened oatmeal, and one glass of skim milk (see Figure 5.11).

You can estimate your daily energy (caloric) requirement by consulting Tables 5.3 and 5.4 and completing Activity 5.1. Given that this is only an estimated value, individual adjustments related to many of the factors discussed in this chapter may be necessary to establish a more precise value. Nevertheless, the estimated value does offer beginning guidelines for weight control or reduction.

The EER without additional planned activity and exercise is based on age, total body weight, height, and gender. Individuals who hold jobs that require a lot of walking or heavy manual labor burn more calories during the day than those who have sedentary jobs (such as working behind a desk). To estimate your EER, refer to Table 5.3. For example, the EER computation for a 20-year-old man, 71 inches tall, who weighs 160 pounds, would be as follows:

1. Body weight (BW) in kilograms = 72.6 kg (160 lb ÷ 2.2046)
   Height (HT) in meters = 1.8 m (71 inches × .0254)
2. EER = $662 - (9.53 \times \text{Age}) + (15.91 \times \text{BW}) + (539 \times \text{HT})$
   EER = $662 - (9.53 \times 20) + (15.91 \times 72.6) + (539 \times 1.8)$
   EER = $662 - 190.6 + 1155 + 970$
   EER = 2,596 calories/day

Thus, the EER to maintain body weight for this individual would be 2,596 calories per day.

To determine the average number of calories you burn daily as a result of exercise, figure out the total number of minutes you exercise weekly, then figure the daily average exercise

Table 5.3 Estimated Energy Requirement (EER) Based on Age, Body Weight, and Height

Men	EER = $662 - (9.53 \times \text{Age}) + (15.91 \times \text{BW}) + (539 \times \text{HT})$
Women	EER = $354 - (6.91 \times \text{Age}) + (9.36 \times \text{BW}) + (726 \times \text{HT})$

Note: Includes activities of independent living only and no moderate physical activity or exercise.
BW = body weight in kilograms (divide BW in pounds by 2.2046).
HT = height in meters (multiply HT in inches by .0254).
© Cengage Learning

Figure 5.11 Making wise food choices.

Breakfast

1 banana nut muffin, 1 cafe mocha
Calories: 940
Percent fat calories: 48%

1 cup oatmeal, 1 English muffin with jelly,
1 slice whole wheat bread with honey,
½ cup peaches, 1 kiwi fruit, 1 orange,
1 apple, 1 cup skim milk
Calories: 900
Percent fat calories: 5%

Lunch

1 double-decker cheeseburger, 1 serving
medium French fries, 2 chocolate chip
cookies, 1 medium strawberry milkshake
Calories: 1,790
Percent fat calories: 37%

6-inch turkey breast/vegetable sandwich,
1 apple, 1 orange,
1 cup sweetened green tea
Calories: 500
Percent fat calories: 10%

Dinner

6 oz. popcorn chicken, 3 oz. barbecue
chicken wings, 1 cup potato salad,
1 12-oz. cola drink
Calories: 1,250
Percent fat calories: 42%

2 cups spaghetti with tomato sauce
and vegetables, a 2-cup salad bowl
with 2 tablespoons Italian dressing,
2 slices whole wheat bread, 1 cup
grapes, 3 large strawberries, 1 kiwi fruit,
1 peach, 1 12-oz. fruit juice drink
Calories: 1,240
Percent fat calories: 14%

These illustrations provide a comparsion of how much more food you can eat when you make healthy choices. You also get more vitamins, minerals, phythonutrients, antioxidants, and fiber by making healthy choices.

time. For instance, a person cycling at 10 miles per hour 5 times a week, 60 minutes each time, exercises 300 minutes per week (5 × 60). The average daily exercise time, therefore, is 42 minutes (300 ÷ 7, rounded off to the lowest unit).

Next, from Table 5.4, find the energy expenditure for the activity (or activities) chosen for the exercise program. In the case of cycling (10 miles per hour), the expenditure is .05 calories per pound of body weight per minute of activity (cal/lb/min). With a body weight of 160 pounds, this man would burn eight calories each minute (body weight × .05, or 160 × .05). In 42 minutes he would burn approximately 336 calories (42 × 8).

Now you can obtain the daily energy requirement, with exercise, needed to maintain body weight. To do this, add the EER obtained from Table 5.3 and the average calories burned through exercise. In our example, it is 2,932 calories (2,596 + 336).

Table 5.4 Caloric Expenditure of Selected Physical Activities

Activity*	Cal/lb/min	Activity*	Cal/lb/min
Aerobics		Jogging/running (on a level surface)	
Moderate	0.065	11.0 min/mile	0.070
Vigorous	0.095	8.5 min/mile	0.090
Step aerobics	0.070	7.0 min/mile	0.102
Archery	0.030	6.0 min/mile	0.114
Badminton		Deep water**	0.100
Recreation	0.038	Racquetball	0.065
Competition	0.065	Rope jumping	0.060
Baseball	0.031	Rowing (vigorous)	0.090
Basketball		Skating (moderate)	0.038
Moderate	0.046	Skiing	
Competition	0.063	Downhill	0.060
Bowling	0.030	Level (5 mph)	0.078
Calisthenics	0.033	Soccer	0.059
Cross-country skiing		Stationary cycling	
Moderate	0.090	Moderate	0.055
Vigorous	0.120	Vigorous	0.070
Circuit training		Strength training	0.050
Moderate	0.070	Swimming (crawl)	
Vigorous	0.100	20 yds/min	0.031
Cycling (on a level surface)		25 yds/min	0.040
5.5 mph	0.033	45 yds/min	0.057
10.0 mph	0.050	50 yds/min	0.070
13.0 mph	0.071	Table tennis	0.030
Dance		Tennis	
Moderate	0.030	Moderate	0.045
Vigorous	0.055	Competition	0.064
Elliptical training		Volleyball	0.030
Moderate	0.070	Walking	
Vigorous	0.090	4.5 mph	0.045
Golf	0.030	Shallow pool	0.090
Gymnastics		Water aerobics	
Light	0.030	Moderate	0.050
Heavy	0.056	Vigorous	0.070
Handball	0.064	Wrestling	0.085
High-intensity interval training	0.120	Zumba	
Hiking	0.040	Moderate	0.065
Judo/karate	0.086	Vigorous	0.095

*Values are for actual time engaged in the activity.
**Treading water

Adapted from: P. E. Allsen, J. M. Harrison, and B. Vance, *Fitness for Life: An Individualized Approach* (Dubuque, IA: Wm. C. Brown, 1989). C. A. Bucher and W. E. Prentice, Fitness for College and Life (St. Louis: Times Mirror/Mosby College Publishing, 1989). C. F. Consolazio, R. E. Johnson, and L. J. Pecora, *Physiological Measurements of Metabolic Functions in Man* (New York: McGraw-Hill, 1963). R. V. Hockey, *Physical Fitness: The Pathway to Healthy Living* (St. Louis: Times Mirror/Mosby College Publishing, 1989). W. W. K. Hoeger et al., Research conducted at Boise State University, 1986–2009.

If a negative caloric balance is recommended to lose weight, this person has to consume fewer than 2,932 calories daily to achieve the objective. Because of the many factors that play a role in weight control, this 2,932-calorie value is only an estimated daily requirement. Furthermore, we cannot predict that you will lose exactly 1 pound of fat in one week if you cut your daily intake by 500 calories (500 × 7 = 3,500 calories, or the equivalent of 1 pound of fat).

The daily energy requirement figure is only a target guideline for weight control. Periodic readjustments are necessary because individuals differ, and the daily requirement changes as you lose weight and modify your exercise habits.

To determine the target caloric intake to lose weight, multiply your current weight by 5 and subtract this amount from the total daily energy requirement (2,932 in our example) with exercise. For our example, this would mean 2,132 calories per day to lose weight (160 × 5 = 800 and 2,932 − 800 = 2,132 calories).

This final caloric intake to lose weight should not be less than 1,500 daily calories for most people. If distributed properly over the various food groups, 1,500 calories appears to be the lowest caloric intake that still provides the necessary nutrients the body needs. A multivitamin complex is recommended for diets that call for less than 1,500 calories. In terms of percentages of total calories, the daily distribution should be approximately 50–60 percent carbohydrates (mostly complex carbohydrates), about 20 percent fat, and 20 percent protein.

Many experts believe that a person can take off weight more efficiently by reducing the amount of daily fat intake to about 20 percent of the total daily caloric intake. Because 1 gram of fat supplies more than twice the amount of calories that carbohydrates and protein do, the tendency when someone eats less fat is to consume fewer calories. With fat intake at 20 percent of total calories, the individual will have sufficient fat in the diet to feel satisfied and avoid frequent hunger pangs.

Further, it takes only 3 to 5 percent of ingested calories to store fat as fat, whereas it takes approximately 25 percent of ingested calories to convert carbohydrates to fat. Some evidence indicates that if people eat the same number of calories as carbohydrate or as fat, those on the fat diet will store more fat. Long-term successful weight loss and weight management programs are low in fat content.

Many people have trouble adhering to a low–fat-calorie diet. During times of weight loss, however, you are strongly encouraged to do so. Refer to Table 5.5 to aid you in determining the grams of fat at 20 percent of the total calories for selected energy intakes. Also, use the form provided in Activity 3.2 (Chapter 3, page 94) to monitor your daily fat intake. For weight maintenance, individuals who have been successful in maintaining an average weight loss of 30 pounds for more than 6 years are consuming about 24 percent of calories from fat, 56 percent from carbohydrates, and 20 percent from protein.[31]

Breakfast is a critical meal while on a weight loss program. Many people skip breakfast because it's the easiest meal to skip. Evidence indicates that people who skip breakfast are hungrier later in the day and end up consuming more total daily calories than those who eat breakfast. Furthermore, regular breakfast

Table 5.5 Grams of Fat at 20 and 30 Percent of Total Calories for Selected Energy Intakes

Caloric Intake	Grams of Fat 20%	Grams of Fat 30%
1,200	27	40
1,300	29	43
1,400	31	47
1,500	33	50
1,600	36	53
1,700	38	57
1,800	40	60
1,900	42	63
2,000	44	67
2,100	47	70
2,200	49	73
2,300	51	77
2,400	53	80
2,500	56	83
2,600	58	87
2,700	60	90
2,800	62	93
2,900	64	97
3,000	67	100

© Cengage Learning

eaters have less of a weight problem, lose weight more effectively, and have less difficulty maintaining the weight loss.

If most of the daily calories are consumed during one meal (as in the typical evening meal), the body may perceive that something is wrong and will slow the metabolism so that it can store more calories in the form of fat. Also, eating most of the calories during one meal causes a person to go hungry the rest of the day, making it more difficult to adhere to the diet.

Consuming most of the calories earlier in the day seems helpful in losing weight and also in managing atherosclerosis. The time of day when most of the fats and cholesterol are consumed can influence blood lipids and coronary heart disease. Peak digestion time following a heavy meal is about seven hours after that meal. If most lipids are consumed during the evening meal, digestion peaks while the person is sound asleep, when the metabolism is at its lowest rate. Consequently, the body may not metabolize fats and cholesterol as well, leading to a higher blood lipid count and increasing the risk for atherosclerosis and coronary heart disease.

Before you proceed to develop a thorough weight-loss program, take a moment to identify, in Activity 5.2, your current stage of change as it pertains to your recommended body weight. If applicable—that is, if you are not at recommended weight—list also the processes and techniques for change that you will use to accomplish your goal. In Activity 5.2 you also outline your exercise program for weight management.

Monitoring Your Diet with Daily Food Logs To help you monitor and adhere to a weight loss program, use the daily food logs provided in Activity 5.3. If the goal is to maintain or increase body weight, use Activity 5.4.

Evidence indicates that people who monitor daily caloric intake are more successful at weight loss than those who don't self-monitor. "If you eat it, record it." Most people underestimate what they eat and wonder why they aren't losing weight. Before using the forms in Activity 5.3, make a master copy for

Behavior Modification Planning

Healthy Breakfast Choices

Breakfast is the most important meal of the day. Skipping breakfast makes you hungrier later in the day and leads to overconsumption and greater caloric intake throughout the rest of the day. Regular breakfast eaters have less of a weight problem, lose weight more effectively, have less difficulty maintaining lost weight, and live longer. Skipping breakfast also temporarily raises LDL (bad) cholesterol and lowers insulin sensitivity, changes that may increase the risk for heart disease and diabetes. Here are some healthy breakfast food choices:

- Fresh fruit
- Low-fat or skim milk
- Low-fat yogurt with berries
- Whole-grain cereal
- Whole-grain bread or bagel with fat-free cream cheese and slices of red or green pepper
- Hummus over a whole-grain bagel
- Peanut butter with whole-grain bread or bagel
- Low-fat cottage cheese with fruit
- Oatmeal
- Reduced-fat cheese
- Egg Beaters with salsa
- A scrambled egg with veggies (limit oil or butter use)

Try It

Select a healthy breakfast choice each day for the next 7 days. Evaluate how you feel the rest of the morning. What effect did eating breakfast have on your activities of daily living and daily caloric intake? Be sure to record your food choices, how you felt, and what activities you engaged in.

© Cengage Learning

your files so you can make future copies as needed. Guidelines are provided for 1,200-, 1,500-, 1,800-, and 2,000-calorie diet plans. These plans have been developed based on the MyPlate and the Dietary Guidelines for Americans to meet the Recommended Dietary Allowances.[32] The objective is to meet (not exceed) the number of servings allowed for each diet plan. Each time you eat a serving of a certain food, record it in the appropriate box.

To lose weight, you should use the diet plan that most closely approximates your target caloric intake. The plan is based on the following caloric allowances for these food groups:

- Grains: 80 calories per serving.
- Fruits: 60 calories per serving.
- Vegetables: 25 calories per serving.
- Dairy (use low-fat products): 120 calories per serving.
- Protein: Use low-fat (300 calories per serving) frozen entrees or an equivalent amount if you prepare your own main dish (see the following discussion).

As you start your diet plan, pay particular attention to food serving sizes. Take care with cup and glass sizes. A standard cup is 8 ounces, but most glasses nowadays contain between 12 and 16 ounces. If you drink 12 ounces of fruit juice, in essence you are getting two servings of fruit because a standard serving is three-fourths cup of juice.

Read food labels carefully to compare the caloric value of the serving listed on the label with the caloric guidelines provided above. Here are some examples:

- One slice of standard whole-wheat bread has about 80 calories. A plain bagel may have 200 to 350 calories. Although it is low in fat, a 350-calorie bagel is equivalent to almost four servings in the grains group.
- The standard serving size listed on the food label for most cereals is one cup. As you read the nutrition information, however, you will find that for the same cup of cereal, one type of cereal has 120 calories and another cereal has 200 calories. Because a standard serving in the grains group is 80 calories, the first cereal would be 1.5 servings and the second one 2.5 servings.
- A medium-size fruit is usually considered to be one serving. A large fruit provides more than one serving.
- In the dairy group, one serving represents 120 calories. A cup of whole milk has about 160 calories, compared with a cup of skim milk, which contains 88 calories. A cup of whole milk, therefore, would provide 1.33 servings in this food group.

Low-Fat Entrees To be more accurate with caloric intake and to simplify meal preparation, use commercially prepared low-fat frozen entrees as the main dish for lunch and dinner meals (only one entree per meal for the 1,200-calorie diet plan; see Activity 5.3). Look for entrees that provide about 300 calories and no more than 6 grams of fat per entree. These two entrees can be used as selections for the protein group and will provide most of your daily requirement.

Along with each entree, supplement the meal with some of your servings from the other food groups. This diet plan has been used successfully in weight loss research programs.[33] If you choose not to use these low-fat entrees, prepare a similar meal using three ounces (cooked) of lean meat, poultry, or fish with additional vegetables, rice, or pasta that will provide 300 calories with fewer than six grams of fat per dish.

In your daily logs, be sure to record the precise amount in each serving. You also can run a computerized nutrient analysis to verify your caloric intake and food distribution pattern (percent of total calories from carbohydrate, fat, and protein).

Protein Intake To minimize the loss of lean body mass and hunger pangs while dieting, it is extremely important that you consume sufficient protein with each meal. You need to ensure that you are consuming between 1.5 grams and 2.0 grams of protein per kilogram of body weight per day. As explained in Chapter 3, Table 3.4 (page 83), if you weigh 141 pounds (64 kg), your total daily protein intake would be between 96 and 128 grams per day (64 × 1.5 and 64 × 2.0) or the equivalent of 384 to 512 calories from protein every day (96 × 4 and 128 × 4), distributed in 32 to 43 grams of protein for each of your daily 3 meals. High-protein/low-calorie foods include fat-free or low-fat dairy products (milk, plain Greek yogurt, and cheese), eggs, lean meats and poultry, fish, soybeans and soy milk, tofu, quinoa, and beans. To help monitor your daily protein intake, you can calculate and record your daily intake in Activity 5.3 as well.

Effect of Food Choices on Long-Term Weight Gain Although still in its infancy, research published in 2011 on more than 120,000 people who were evaluated every 4 years over a 20-year period showed that food choices have a significant effect on weight gain.[34] On average, study participants gained 17 pounds over the course of 20 years. Regardless of other lifestyle habits, individuals who consumed unhealthy foods gained the most weight, whereas those who made healthy food choices gained the least amount of weight. Although more research is needed, in this study, four-year weight change was most strongly associated with the consumption of potato chips, potatoes, sugar-sweetened beverages, unprocessed and processed red meats and inversely associated with the consumption of vegetables, whole grains, fruits, nuts, and yogurt. The take-home message: Consume more fruits, vegetables, whole grains, low-fat dairy products, and nuts (the last in moderation because of their high caloric content).

Behavior Modification and Adherence to a Weight Management Program Achieving and maintaining recommended body composition is certainly possible, but it does require desire and commitment. If weight management is to become a priority, people must realize that they have to transform their behavior to some extent.

Activity 5.1: Computing Your Daily Caloric Requirement

Name _____ Date _____

Course _____ Section _____ Gender _____ Age _____

A. Current body weight (BW) in kilograms (body weight in pounds ÷ 2.2046).................................. [ ]

B. Current height (HT) in meters (HT in inches × .0254).. [ ]

C. Estimated energy requirement (EER) (Table 5.3, page 173)

    Men: EER = 663 − (9.53 × Age) + (15.91 × BW) + (539.6 × HT)

    Women: EER = 354 − (6.91 × Age) + (9.36 × BW) + (726 × HT)

EER = [ ] − ([ ] × [ ]) + ([ ] × [ ]) + ([ ] × [ ])

EER = [ ] − [ ] + [ ] + [ ] = [ ] calories

D. Selected physical activity (e.g., jogging)[a] .... [ ]

E. Number of exercise sessions per week... [ ]

F. Duration of exercise session (in minutes)... [ ]

G. Total weekly exercise time in minutes (E × F).. [ ]

H. Average daily exercise time in minutes (G ÷ 7)... [ ]

I. Caloric expenditure per pound per minute (cal/lb/min) of physical activity (use Table 5.4, page 175)............... [ ]

J. Body weight in pounds... [ ]

K. Total calories burned per minute of physical activity (I × J).................................. [ ]

L. Average daily calories burned as a result of the exercise program (H × K)..................... [ ]

M. Total daily energy requirement with exercise to maintain body weight (C + L).................. [ ]

Stop here if no weight loss is required, otherwise proceed to items N and O.

N. Number of calories to subtract from daily requirement to achieve a negative caloric balance (J × 5)............. [ ]

O. Target caloric intake to lose weight (M − N)[b].. [ ]

[a] If more than one physical activity is selected, you will need to estimate the average daily calories burned as a result of each additional activity (steps D through K) and add all of these figures to L above.
[b] This figure should never be below 1,200 calories for small women or 1,500 for everyone else. See Lab 5C for the 1,200-, 1,500-, and 2,000-calorie diet plans.

Activity 5.2: Weight-Loss Behavior Modification Plan

Name _____ Date _____

Course _____ Section _____ Gender _____ Age _____

1. Using Figure 2.5 (page 63) and Table 2.3 (page 62), identify your current stage of change regarding **recommended body weight:** [   ]
2. How much weight do you want to lose? [   ]   Is it a realistic goal? [   ]
3. Target caloric intake to lose weight (diet plan—see Activity 5.1, item O) [   ].
4. Based on the processes and techniques of change discussed in Chapter 2, indicate what you can do to help yourself implement a weight management program.

   _____
   _____

5. How much effort are you willing to put into reaching your weight loss goal? _____
   Indicate your feelings about participating in an exercise program.

   _____

6. Will you commit to participate in a combined aerobic and strength-training program?[a]   Yes [ ]   No [ ]
   If your answer is "Yes," proceed to the next question; if you answered "No," please read Chapters 3–9.
7. Select one or two aerobic activities in which you will participate regularly: [   ]
   List facilities available to you where you can carry out the aerobic and strength-training programs.

   _____

8. Indicate days and times you will set aside for your aerobic and strength-training program (5 or 6 days per week should be devoted to aerobic exercise and 1 to 3 nonconsecutive days per week to strength training).

   Monday: [   ]
   Tuesday: [   ]
   Wednesday: [   ]
   Thursday: [   ]
   Friday: [   ]
   Saturday: [   ]
   Sunday: A complete day of rest once a week is recommended to allow your body to fully recover from exercise.

Behavior Modification

Briefly describe whether you think you can meet the goals of your aerobic and strength-training program. What obstacles will you have to overcome, and how will you overcome them?

_____

[a] Flexibility programs are necessary for adequate fitness, possible injury prevention, and good health but do not help with weight loss. Stretching exercises can be conducted regularly during the cool-down phase of your aerobic and strength-training programs (see Chapter 8).

Behavior Modification Planning

Weight Loss Strategies

1. *Make a commitment to change.* The first necessary ingredient is the desire to modify your behavior. You have to stop precontemplating or contemplating change and get going! You must accept that you have a problem and decide by yourself whether you really want to change. Sincere commitment increases your chances for success.

2. *Set realistic goals.* The weight problem developed over several years. Similarly, new lifetime eating and exercise habits take time to develop. A realistic long-term goal also will include short-term objectives that allow for regular evaluation and help maintain motivation and renewed commitment to attain the long-term goal.

3. *Monitor caloric intake.* Keep an accurate daily record of food consumption. *"If you eat it, record it."* People who keep accurate food logs are more successful at weight loss.

4. *Plan on three small meals and possibly one to two snacks each day.* Eating less but more often helps keep your blood sugar levels steady and avoid hunger pangs. Include adequate protein intake with each meal and use primarily high-volume, low-calorie foods. Space your meals and snacks so that you eat every three to four hours. Snacks need to be nutrient-rich, including fruits, vegetables, low-fat/plain yogurt, or a small amount of nuts.

5. *Weigh yourself regularly,* preferably at the same time of day and under the same conditions. Do not adapt and accept a higher body weight as a new stable weight. Make dietary and physical activity adjustments accordingly.

6. *Incorporate exercise into the program.* Choosing enjoyable activities, places, times, equipment, and people to work out with will help you adhere to an exercise program (see Chapters 6–9). If time is a factor, you can easily create extra time in your day by recording your favorite TV programs and watching them later. You can then skip the commercials and end with extra time to fit in exercise.

7. *Differentiate hunger and appetite.* Hunger is the actual physical need for food. Appetite is a desire for food, usually triggered by factors such as stress, habit, boredom, depression, availability of food, or just the thought of food itself. Developing and sticking to a regular meal pattern will help control hunger.

8. *Eat less fat.* Each gram of fat provides nine calories, and protein and carbohydrates provide only four. In essence, you can eat more food on a low-fat diet because you consume fewer calories with each meal. Most of your fat intake should come from healthy unsaturated sources.

9. *Pay attention to calories.* Just because food is labeled "low-fat" does not mean you can eat as much as you want. When reading food labels—and when eating—don't just look at the fat content. Pay attention to calories as well. Many low-fat foods are high in calories.

10. *Cut unnecessary items from your diet.* Substituting water for a daily can of soda would cut 51,100 (140 × 365) calories yearly from the diet—the equivalent of 14.6 (51,000 ÷ 3,500) pounds of fat. If you always drink water instead of sugar-sweetened beverages when thirsty and with your meals, you can do even better and decrease caloric intake by an average of 300 daily calories. Studies also indicate that liquid calories do little to suppress hunger.

11. *Maintain a daily intake of calcium-rich foods,* especially low-fat or nonfat dairy products.

12. *Add foods to your diet that reduce cravings,* such as eggs; small amounts of red meat, fish, poultry, tofu, oils, fats; and nonstarchy vegetables such as lettuce, green beans, peppers, asparagus, broccoli, mushrooms, and Brussels sprouts. Also increasing the intake of low-glycemic carbohydrates with your meals helps you go longer before you feel hungry again.

13. *Avoid automatic eating.* Many people associate certain daily activities with eating, for example, cooking, watching television, or reading. Most foods consumed in these situations lack nutritional value or are high in sugar and fat.

14. *Stay busy.* People tend to eat more when they sit around and do nothing. Occupying the mind and body with activities not associated with eating helps take away the desire to eat. Some options are walking; cycling; playing sports; gardening; sewing; or visiting a library, a museum, or a park. You also might develop other skills and interests not associated with food.

15. *Plan meals and shop sensibly.* Always shop on a full stomach, because hungry shoppers tend to buy unhealthy foods impulsively—and then snack on the way home. Always use a shopping list, which should include 100 percent whole-grains (breads and cereals), fruits and vegetables, low-fat milk and dairy products, lean meats, fish, and poultry.

16. *Cook wisely:*
    - Use less fat and fewer refined foods in food preparation.
    - Trim all visible fat from meats and remove skin from poultry before cooking.

- Skim the fat off gravies and soups.
- Bake, broil, boil, or steam instead of frying.
- Sparingly use butter, cream, mayonnaise, and salad dressings.
- Avoid coconut oil, palm oil, and cocoa butter.
- Prepare plenty of foods that contain fiber.
- Include whole-grain breads and cereals, vegetables, and legumes in most meals.
- Eat fruits for dessert.
- Stay away from soda pop, fruit juices, and fruit-flavored drinks.
- Use less sugar, and cut down on other refined carbohydrates, such as corn syrup, malt sugar, dextrose, and fructose.
- Drink plenty of water—at least six glasses a day.

17. *Do not serve more food than you should eat.* Measure the food in portions and keep serving dishes away from the table. Do not force yourself or anyone else to "clean the plate" after they are satisfied (including children after they already have had a healthy, nutritious serving).

18. *Try "junior size" instead of "super size."* People who are served larger portions eat more, whether they are hungry or not. Use smaller plates, bowls, cups, and glasses. Try eating half as much food as you commonly eat. Watch for portion sizes at restaurants as well: Supersized foods create supersized people.

19. *Eat out infrequently.* The more often people eat out, the more body fat they have. People who eat out 6 or more times per week consume about 300 extra calories per day and 30 percent more fat than those who eat out less often.

20. *Eat slowly and at the table only.* Eating on the run promotes overeating because the body doesn't have enough time to "register" consumption and people overeat before the body perceives the fullness signal. Eating at the table encourages people to take time out to eat and deters snacking between meals. After eating, do not sit around the table but, rather, clean up and put away the food to avoid snacking.

21. *Avoid social binges.* Social gatherings tend to entice self-defeating behavior. Use visual imagery to plan ahead. Do not feel pressured to eat or drink and don't rationalize in these situations. Choose low-calorie foods and entertain yourself with other activities, such as dancing and talking.

22. *Do not place unhealthy foods within easy reach.* Ideally, avoid bringing high-calorie, high-sugar, or high-fat foods into the house. If they are there already, store them where they are hard to get to or see—perhaps the garage or basement.

23. *Avoid evening food raids.* Most people do really well during the day but then "lose it" at night. Take control. Stop and think. To avoid excessive nighttime snacking, stay busy after your evening meal. Go for a short walk, floss and brush your teeth, and get to bed earlier. Even better, close the kitchen after dinner and try not to eat anything three hours prior to going to sleep.

24. *Practice stress management techniques* (discussed in Chapter 12). Many people snack and increase their food consumption in stressful situations.

25. *Get support.* People who receive support from friends, relatives, and formal support groups are much more likely to lose and maintain weight loss than those without such support. The more support you receive, the better off you will be.

26. *Monitor changes and reward accomplishments.* Being able to exercise without interruption for 15, 20, 30, or 60 minutes; swimming a certain distance; running a mile—all these accomplishments deserve recognition. Create rewards that are not related to eating: new clothing, a tennis racquet, a bicycle, exercise shoes, or something else that is special and you would not have acquired otherwise.

27. *Prepare for slip-ups.* Most people will slip and occasionally splurge. Do not despair and give up. Reevaluate and continue with your efforts. An occasional slip won't make much difference in the long run.

28. *Think positive.* Avoid negative thoughts about how difficult changing past behaviors might be. Instead, think of the benefits you will reap, such as feeling, looking, and functioning better, plus enjoying better health and improving the quality of life. Avoid negative environments and unsupportive people.

Try It

In your Online Journal or class notebook, answer the following questions: How many of the previously listed strategies do you use to help you maintain recommended body weight? Do you feel that any of these strategies specifically help you manage body weight more effectively? If so, explain why.

Modifying old habits and developing new, positive behaviors take time. Individuals who apply the management techniques provided in the Behavior Modification Planning box (pages 180–181) are more successful at changing detrimental behavior and adhering to a positive lifetime weight-control program. In developing a retraining program, you are not expected to incorporate all of the strategies given but should note the ones that apply to you. The form provided in Activity 5.5 will allow you to evaluate and monitor your own weight-management behaviors.

Critical Thinking

What behavioral strategies have you used to properly manage your body weight? • How do you think those strategies would work for others?

Exercising with other people and in different places helps people maintain exercise regularity.

During the weight loss process, surround yourself with people who have the same goals as you do (weight loss). Data released in 2007 showed that obesity can spread through "social networks."[35] That is, if your friends, siblings, or spouse gain weight, you are more likely to gain weight as well. People tend to accept a higher weight standard if someone they are close to or care about gains weight.

In the study, the social ties of more than 12,000 individuals were examined over 32 years. The findings revealed that if a close friend becomes obese, your risk of becoming obese during the next 2 to 4 years increases 171 percent. The risk also increases 57 percent for casual friends, 40 percent for siblings, and 37 percent for the person's spouse. The reverse was also found to be true. When a person loses weight, the likelihood of friends, siblings, or spouse to lose weight is also enhanced.

Furthermore, the research found that gender plays a role in social networks. A male's weight has a greater effect on the weight of male friends and brothers than on female friends or sisters. Similarly, a woman's weight has a far greater influence on sisters and girlfriends than on brothers or male friends. Thus, if you are trying to lose weight, choose your friendships carefully: Do not surround yourself with people who either have a weight problem or are still gaining weight.

5.12 The Simple Truth

There is no quick and easy way to take off excess body fat and keep it off for good. Weight management is accomplished by making a lifetime commitment to physical activity and proper food selection. When taking part in a weight (fat) reduction program, people also have to decrease their caloric intake moderately, use portion control, be physically active, and implement strategies to modify unhealthy eating behaviors.

During the process, relapses into past negative behaviors are almost inevitable. The three most common reasons for relapse are:

1. Stress-related factors (such as major life changes, depression, job changes, illness)
2. Social reasons (entertaining, eating out, business travel)
3. Self-enticing behaviors (placing yourself in a situation to see how much you can get away with: "One small taste won't hurt" leads to "I'll eat just one slice" and finally to "I haven't done well, so I might as well eat some more").

Making mistakes is human and does not necessarily mean failure. Failure comes to those who give up and do not build on previous experiences and thereby develop skills that will prevent self-defeating behaviors in the future. Where there's a will, there's a way, and those who persist will reap the rewards.

Activity 5.3: Daily Food Intake Record

Name _____ Date _____

Course _____ Section _____ Gender _____ Age _____

1,200 CALORIE DIET PLAN
Instructions:
The objective of the diet plan is to meet (not exceed) the number of servings allowed for the food groups listed. Each time that you eat a particular food, record it in the space provided for each group along with the amount you ate. Refer to the number of calories below to find out what counts as one serving for each group listed. Instead of the meat, poultry, fish, dry beans, eggs, and nuts group, you are allowed to have a commercially available low-fat frozen entree for your main meal (this entree should provide no more than 300 calories and less than 6 grams of fat). You can make additional copies of this form as needed.

- Dairy: 2 servings
- Grains: 6 servings
- Fruits: 2 servings
- Veggies: 3 servings
- Protein: 1 low-fat frozen entree

Grains (80 calories/serving): 6 servings

1	
2	
3	
4	
5	
6	

Vegetables (25 calories/serving): 3 servings

1	
2	
3	

Fruits (60 calories/serving): 2 servings

1	
2	

Dairy (120 calories/serving, use low-fat milk and milk products): 2 servings

1	
2	

Low-fat Frozen Entree (300 calories and less than 6 grams of fat): 1 serving

1	

Today's physical activity: _____   Intensity: ___   Duration: ___ min   Number of steps: _____

1,500 CALORIE DIET PLAN

Instructions:
The objective of the diet plan is to meet (not exceed) the number of servings allowed for the food groups listed. Each time that you eat a particular food, record it in the space provided for each group along with the amount you ate. Refer to the number of calories below to find out what counts as one serving for each group listed. Instead of the meat, poultry, fish, dry beans, eggs, and nuts group, you are allowed to have two commercially available low-fat frozen entrees for your main meal (these entrees should provide no more than 300 calories and less than 6 grams of fat). You can make additional copies of this form as needed.

Dairy: 2 servings
Grains: 6 servings
Fruits: 2 servings
Veggies: 3 servings
Protein: 2 low-fat frozen entrees

Grains (80 calories/serving): 6 servings

1	
2	
3	
4	
5	
6	

Vegetables (25 calories/serving): 3 servings

1	
2	
3	

Fruits (60 calories/serving): 2 servings

1	
2	

Dairy (120 calories/serving, use low-fat milk and milk products): 2 servings

1	
2	

Two Low-fat Frozen Entrees (300 calories and less than 6 grams of fat): 2 servings

1	
2	

Today's physical activity: ☐   Intensity: ☐   Duration: ☐ min   Number of steps: ☐

1,800 CALORIE DIET PLAN

Instructions:
The objective of the diet plan is to meet (not exceed) the number of servings allowed for the food groups listed. Each time that you eat a particular food, record it in the space provided for each group along with the amount you ate. Refer to the number of calories below to find out what counts as one serving for each group listed. Instead of the meat, poultry, fish, dry beans, eggs, and nuts group, you are allowed to have two commercially available low-fat frozen entrees for your main meal (these entrees should provide no more than 300 calories and less than 6 grams of fat). You can make additional copies of this form as needed.

Dairy: 2 servings
Grains: 8 servings
Fruits: 3 servings
Veggies: 5 servings
Protein: 2 low-fat frozen entrees

Grains (80 calories/serving): 8 servings

1.
2.
3.
4.
5.
6.
7.
8.

Vegetables (25 calories/serving): 5 servings

1.
2.
3.
4.
5.

Fruits (60 calories/serving): 3 servings

1.
2.
3.

Dairy (120 calories/serving, use low-fat milk and milk products): 2 servings

1.
2.

Two Low-fat Frozen Entrees (300 calories and less than 6 grams of fat): 2 servings

1.
2.

Today's physical activity: ☐ Intensity: ☐ Duration: ☐ min Number of steps: ☐

2,000 CALORIE DIET PLAN

Instructions:
The objective of the diet plan is to meet (not exceed) the number of servings allowed for the food groups listed. Each time that you eat a particular food, record it in the space provided for each group along with the amount you ate. Refer to the number of calories below to find out what counts as one serving for each group listed. Instead of the meat, poultry, fish, dry beans, eggs, and nuts group, you are allowed to have two commercially available low-fat frozen entrees for your main meal (these entrees should provide no more than 300 calories and less than 6 grams of fat). You can make additional copies of this form as needed.

Dairy: 2 servings
Grains: 10 servings
Fruits: 4 servings
Veggies: 5 servings
Protein: 2 low-fat frozen entrees

Grains (80 calories/serving): 10 servings

1.
2.
3.
4.
5.
6.
7.
8.
9.
10.

Vegetables (25 calories/serving): 5 servings

1.
2.
3.
4.
5.

Fruits (60 calories/serving): 4 servings

1.
2.
3.
4.

Dairy (120 calories/serving, use low-fat milk and milk products): 2 servings

1.
2.

Two Low-fat Frozen Entrees (300 calories and less than 6 grams of fat): 2 servings

1.
2.

Today's physical activity: ____   Intensity: ____   Duration: ____ min   Number of steps: ____

Activity 5.4: Healthy Plan for Weight Maintenance or Weight Gain

Name _____ Date _____

Course _____ Section _____ Gender _____ Age _____

I. Daily Caloric Requirement

A. Current body weight in pounds .... ☐

B. Current percent body fat .... ☐

C. Current body composition classification (Table 4.10, page 138) .... ☐

D. Total daily energy requirement with exercise to maintain body weight (use item M from Activity 5.1). Use this figure and stop further computations if the goal is to maintain body weight .... ☐

E. Target body weight (if your goal is to increase body weight) .... ☐

F. Number of additional daily calories to increase body weight (combine this increased caloric intake with a strength-training program, see Chapter 7) 500

G. Total daily energy (caloric) requirement with exercise to increase body weight (D + 500) ☐

II. Strength-Training Program

For weight gain purposes, indicate three days during the week and the time when you will engage in a strength-training program.

_____

_____

III. Healthy Diet Plan

Design a sample healthy daily diet plan according to the total daily energy requirement computed in D (maintenance) or G (weight gain) in Part I. Using Appendix A, list all individual food items that you can consume on that day, along with their caloric, carbohydrate, fat, and protein content. Be sure that the diet meets the recommended number of servings from the five food groups.

Breakfast

	Food item	Amount	Calories	Carbohydrates (gr)	Fat (gr)	Protein (gr)
1.						
2.						
3.						
4.						
5.						
6.						
7.						
8.						

Lunch	Food item	Amount	Calories	Carbohydrates (gr)	Fat (gr)	Protein (gr)
1.						
2.						
3.						
4.						
5.						
6.						
7.						
8.						
Snack						
1.						
Dinner						
1.						
2.						
3.						
4.						
5.						
6.						
7.						
8.						
		Totals:				

IV. Percent of Macronutrients

Determine the percent of total calories that are derived from carbohydrates, fat, and protein.

A. Total calories = ☐

B. Grams of carbohydrates ☐ × 4 ÷ ☐ (total calories) = ☐ %

C. Grams of fat ☐ × 9 ÷ ☐ (total calories) = ☐ %

D. Grams of protein ☐ × 4 ÷ ☐ (total calories) = ☐ %

E. Body weight (BW) in kilograms (BW in pounds divided by 2.2046) = ☐ kg

F. Grams of protein per kilogram of body weight ☐ (grams of protein) ÷ ☐ (BW in kg) = ☐ gr/kg

G. Please summarize your diet and protein intake to either maintain or gain weight.

_____

_____

Activity 5.5: Weight Management: Measuring Progress

Name _____ Date _____

Course _____ Section _____ Gender _____ Age _____

I. Please answer all of the following:

1. State your own feelings regarding your current body weight, your target body composition, and a completion date for this goal.

   _____
   _____
   _____
   _____

2. Do you have an eating disorder? If so, express your feelings about it. Can your instructor help you find professional advice so that you can work toward resolving this problem?

   _____
   _____
   _____
   _____

3. Is your present diet adequate according to the nutrient analysis? Yes _____ No _____

4. State dietary changes necessary to achieve a balanced diet and/or to lose weight (increase or decrease caloric intake, decrease fat intake, increase intake of complex carbohydrates, etc.). List specific foods that will help you improve in areas where you may have deficiencies and food items to avoid or consume in moderation to help you achieve better nutrition.

   Changes to make: _____
   _____

   Foods that will help: _____
   _____

   Foods to avoid: _____
   _____

II. Behavior Modification Progress Form

Instructions: Read the section on tips for behavior modification and adherence to a weight management program (pages 180–181). On a weekly or biweekly basis, go through the list of strategies and provide a "Yes" or "No" answer to each statement. If you are able to answer "Yes" to most questions, you have been successful in implementing positive weight management behaviors. (Make additional copies of this page as needed.)

Strategy	Date						
1. I have made a commitment to change.							
2. I set realistic goals.							
3. I monitor body weight on a regular basis.							
4. I exercise regularly.							
5. I exercise control over my appetite.							
6. I am consuming less fat in my diet.							
7. I pay attention to the number of calories in food.							
8. I have eliminated unnecessary food items from my diet.							
9. I include calcium-rich foods in my diet.							
10. I use craving-reducing foods in my diet.							
11. I avoid automatic eating.							
12. I stay busy.							
13. I plan meals ahead of time and shop sensibly.							
14. I cook wisely.							
15. I do not serve more food than I should eat.							
16. I use portion control in my diet and when dining out.							
17. I do not eat out more than once per week. When I do, I eat low-fat meals.							
18. I eat slowly and at the table only.							
19. I avoid social binges.							
20. I avoid temptation by relocating or removing unhealthy foods.							
21. I avoid evening food raids.							
22. I practice stress management.							
23. I have a strong support group.							
24. I monitor changes and reward my accomplishments.							
25. I prepare for lapses/relapses.							
26. I think positive.							
27. I make sensible adjustments in caloric intake and physical activity if my weight increases and stabilizes there for several days.							

ASSESS YOUR BEHAVIOR

CENGAGEbrain To access course materials, including companion resources, please visit www.cengagebrain.com.

1. Are you satisfied with your current body composition (including body weight) and quality of life? If not, are you willing to do something about it to properly resolve the problem?
2. Are physical activity, aerobic exercise, and strength training a regular part of your lifetime weight management program?
3. Do you weigh yourself regularly and make adjustments in energy intake and physical activity habits if your weight starts to slip upward?
4. Do you exercise portion control, watch your overall fat intake, and plan ahead before you eat out or attend social functions that entice overeating?

ASSESS YOUR KNOWLEDGE

Evaluate how well you understand the concepts presented in this chapter using the chapter-specific quizzing available in the online materials at www.cengagebrain.com.

1. During the last decade, the rate of obesity in the United States has
   a. been on the decline.
   b. increased at an alarming rate.
   c. increased slightly.
   d. remained steady.
   e. increased in men and decreased in women.

2. Obesity is defined as a body mass index (BMI) equal to or greater than
   a. 10.
   b. 25.
   c. 30.
   d. 45.
   e. 50.

3. Obesity increases the risk for
   a. hypertension.
   b. congestive heart failure.
   c. atherosclerosis.
   d. type 2 diabetes.
   e. all of the above.

4. Tolerable weight is a body weight
   a. that is not ideal but one that you can live with.
   b. that will tolerate the increased risk for chronic diseases.
   c. with a BMI range between 25 and 30.
   d. that meets both ideal values for percent body weight and BMI.
   e. All are correct choices.

5. When the body uses protein instead of a combination of fats and carbohydrates as a source of energy,
   a. weight loss is very slow.
   b. a large amount of weight loss is in the form of water.
   c. muscle turns into fat.
   d. fat is lost very rapidly.
   e. fat cannot be lost.

6. Eating disorders
   a. are characterized by an intense fear of becoming fat.
   b. are physical and emotional conditions.
   c. almost always require professional help for successful treatment of the disease.
   d. are common in societies that encourage thinness.
   e. All are correct choices.

7. The mechanism that seems to regulate how much a person weighs is known as
   a. setpoint.
   b. weight factor.
   c. basal metabolic rate.
   d. metabolism.
   e. energy-balancing equation.

8. The key to maintaining weight loss successfully is
   a. frequent dieting.
   b. very low calorie diets when "normal" dieting doesn't work.
   c. a lifetime physical activity program.
   d. regular high-protein/low-carbohydrate meals.
   e. All are correct choices.

9. The daily amount of physical activity recommended for weight loss purposes is
   a. 15 to 20 minutes.
   b. 20 to 30 minutes.
   c. 30 to 60 minutes.
   d. 60 to 90 minutes.
   e. Any amount is sufficient as long as it is done daily.

10. A daily energy expenditure of 300 calories through physical activity is the equivalent of approximately ___ pounds of fat per year.
    a. 12
    b. 15
    c. 22
    d. 27
    e. 31

Correct answers can be found at the back of the book.

Cardiorespiratory Endurance

Daily physical activity is the miracle medication that people are looking for. It makes you look and feel younger, boosts energy, provides lifetime weight management, improves self-confidence and self-esteem, and enhances independent living, health, and quality of life. It further allows you to enjoy a longer life by decreasing the risk of many chronic conditions, including heart disease, high blood pressure, stroke, diabetes, some cancers, and osteoporosis.

Objectives

- **Define** cardiorespiratory endurance and describe the benefits of cardiorespiratory endurance training in maintaining health and well-being.
- **Define** aerobic and anaerobic exercise, and give examples.
- **Be able** to assess cardiorespiratory fitness through five different test protocols: 1.5-Mile Run Test, 1.0-Mile Walk Test, Step Test, Astrand-Ryhming Test, and 12-Minute Swim Test.
- **Be able** to interpret the results of cardiorespiratory endurance assessments according to health fitness and physical fitness standards.
- **Determine** your readiness to start an exercise program.
- **Explain** the principles that govern cardiorespiratory exercise prescription: intensity, mode, duration, frequency, volume, and rate of progression.
- **Learn** how to write a comprehensive cardiorespiratory exercise prescription.
- **Learn** some ways to foster adherence to exercise.
- **Assess** your cardiorespiratory endurance.
- **Maintain** a log of all your fitness activities.

CENGAGEbrain.com
Visit www.cengagebrain.com to access course materials and companion resources for this text, including quiz questions designed to check your understanding of the chapter contents. See the preface on page ix for more information.

Does aerobic exercise make a person immune to heart and blood vessel disease?

Although aerobically fit individuals as a whole have a lower incidence of cardiovascular disease, a regular aerobic exercise program by itself does not offer an absolute guarantee against cardiovascular disease. The best way to minimize the risk for cardiovascular disease is to manage the risk factors. Many factors, including a genetic predisposition, can increase the risk. Research data, however, indicate that a regular aerobic exercise program will delay the onset of cardiovascular problems and will improve the chances of surviving a heart attack. Even moderate increases in aerobic fitness significantly lower the incidence of premature cardiovascular deaths. Data from the research study on death rates by physical fitness groups (illustrated in Figure 1.11, page 20) indicate that the decrease in cardiovascular mortality is greatest between the unfit and the moderately fit groups. A further decrease in cardiovascular mortality is observed between the moderately fit and the highly fit groups.

Is light-intensity aerobic exercise more effective in burning fat?

During light-intensity and moderate-intensity exercise a greater percentage of the energy is derived from fat. It is also true, however, that an even greater percentage of the energy comes from fat when doing absolutely nothing (resting/sleeping). And when one does nothing, as in a sedentary lifestyle, one doesn't burn many calories.

Let's examine this issue. During resting conditions, the human body is a very efficient "fat-burning machine." That is, most of the energy, approximately 70 percent, is derived from fat and only 30 percent from carbohydrates. But we burn few calories at rest, about 1.5 calories per minute compared with 3 to 4 calories during light-intensity exercise, 5 to 7 calories during moderate-intensity exercise, and 8 to 10 (or more) calories per minute during vigorous-intensity exercise. As we begin to exercise and subsequently increase its intensity, we progressively rely more on carbohydrates and less on fat for energy, until we reach maximal intensity, when 100 percent of the energy is derived from carbohydrates. Even though a lower percentage of the energy is derived from fat during vigorous-intensity exercise, the total caloric expenditure is so much greater (twice as high or more) that overall the total fat burned is still higher than during moderate intensity.

A word of caution, nonetheless: Do not start vigorous-intensity exercise without several weeks of proper and gradual conditioning. Even worse is if such exercise is a weight-bearing activity. If you do such exercise from the outset, you increase the risk of injury and may have to stop exercising altogether. Also, people with an initial low level of fitness often compensate with greater caloric intake following vigorous-intensity exercise, thus defeating the added energy expenditure obtained through exercise (additional information on this subject is provided on pages 170-171).

Do energy drinks enhance performance?

People associate energy with work. If an energy drink can enhance work capacity, the benefits of such drinks would surpass plain thirst-quenching drinks. Energy drinks typically contain sugar, herbal extracts, large amounts of caffeine, and water-soluble vitamins. Consumers are led to believe that these ingredients increase energy metabolism, provide an energy boost, improve endurance, and aid in weight loss. These purported benefits are yet to be proven through scientific research.

The energy content of many of these drinks is around 60 grams of sugar and 240 calories in a 16-ounce drink, with little additional nutritive value. If you are going to participate in an intense and lengthy workout, the carbohydrate content can boost performance and help you get through the workout. If, however, you are concerned with weight management, 240 calories is an extraordinarily large amount of calories in a two-cup drink. Weight gain may be the end result if you drink a few of these throughout the day to give you a boost while studying or while at work. Sugar-free energy drinks provide little or no energy (calories), although they are packed with nervous system stimulants.

The high caffeine content in energy drinks can cause adverse health effects. Caffeine intake greater than 400 mg can precipitate adverse health effects. Many of the popular energy drinks (Red Bull, Sobe Adrenaline Rush, Full Throttle, Rip It Energy Fuel) contain about 80 mg of caffeine per 8-ounce cup. If you drink two 16-ounce cans, you'll end up with upward of 300 mg of caffeine through these drinks alone. You may also have to consider additional caffeine intake from other beverages that you routinely consume during the day (coffee, tea, sodas).

Consumption of energy drinks has been linked with many a rapid heart rate (palpitations and tachycardia), ischemia (lack of blood flow to the heart muscle), chest pain, increased blood pressure, tremors, jitters, convulsions, agitation, restlessness, gastrointestinal disturbance, increase urination, nausea, dizziness, irritability, nervousness, syncope (loss of consciousness), paraesthesia (tingling or numbing of the skin), insomnia, respiratory distress, headaches; and most seriously, based on circumstantial evidence, myocardial infarctions and sudden cardiac deaths. At least one sudden cardiac death has been reported in a 28-year-old man who consumed 8 cans of an energy drink containing

(continued)

80 mg of caffeine each over a 7-hour span of time. Between 2008 and 2012, the Food and Drug Administration (FDA) received reports of 13 deaths possibly linked to the highly caffeinated drink 5-Hour Energy (215 milligrams of caffeine per drink—about two cups of coffee) and more than 90 filings of adverse effects, including more than 30 citing life-threatening complications.

Energy drinks manufacturers state that the products are safe when used as directed. The potential for excessive use or abuse, however, is real because the FDA does not regulate the products. As with most addictive substances, invariably a sugar and caffeine rush is likely to end up in a physiological crash, requiring a subsequent larger intake to obtain a similar "physical high," thus augmenting the risk for adverse and life-threatening effects.

Real Life Story | Yumiko's Experience

I never really noticed how much walking I did (or did not do) each day until our whole class got pedometers and started tracking our steps as part of an assignment for health class. At first I was shocked that my number of steps was so low. I would have guessed that I was a lot more active than that. But after a while, wearing the pedometer made me want to walk more so that I could break my previous record. I set a goal each day for the number of steps I was aiming for. I started taking the stairs instead of elevators, parking farther away from wherever I was going, and walking to friends' dorm rooms to talk to them rather than calling or texting them, just to try to get more steps in. If at the end of the day my total number of steps was under the goal, I would go outside and walk around the block until I got to the goal number. I was surprised to find how much seeing that number on the pedometer would motivate me. Eventually, after continuing to increase my number of steps over the semester, I started hitting the recommended amount of 10,000 steps per day, and even increased to 12,000. Though the semester has ended and I am no longer in the fitness class, I have still kept up my walking habit, hitting my goal number most days, and sometimes jogging a portion of my steps. I have really noticed a difference in my cardiorespiratory fitness, and am hoping to keep my new habit up for life. I would recommend that anyone else who has trouble getting motivated purchase a pedometer and start walking!

© Photodisc/Jupiter Images

PERSONAL PROFILE: Personal Cardiorespiratory Fitness Profile

I. Have you ever experienced the feeling of being aerobically fit? If so, can you describe that feeling?

II. Do you understand the concept of oxygen uptake and the difference between absolute and relative oxygen uptake? What are the applications of the latter two?

III. At 70 percent training intensity, your exercise prescription requires a heart rate of 156 beats per minute. Is there a difference between jogging and doing Zumba when exercising at this same heart rate? Please expound on your response.

IV. Can you identify and relate to the factors that motivated Yukimo to become aerobically fit and what helped him stay with the exercise program? What factors do you think can help you start or stay with aerobic exercise?

V. Your cardiorespiratory fitness test indicates that your VO_{2max} is 48 mL/kg/min. If you chose to exercise at 50 percent of your VO_{2max} (moderate intensity, as most people like to do during aerobic exercise), can you compute how many calories you burn per minute at this intensity level and the total minutes that you'd have to exercise to burn the equivalent of one pound of fat?

Cardiorespiratory endurance is the single most important component of health-related physical fitness. The exception occurs among older adults, for whom muscular strength is particularly important. In any case, people can get by without high levels of strength and flexibility, but we cannot do without a good cardiorespiratory (CR) system, facilitated by aerobic exercise.

Aerobic exercise is especially important in preventing cardiovascular disease. A poorly conditioned heart, which has to pump more often just to keep a person alive, is subject to more wear and tear than a well-conditioned heart. In situations that place strenuous demands on

> **Cardiorespiratory endurance** The ability of the lungs, heart, and blood vessels to deliver adequate amounts of oxygen to the cells to meet the demands of prolonged physical activity.

The epitome of physical inactivity: driving around a parking lot for several minutes in search of a parking spot 20 yards closer to the store's entrance.

Advances in modern technology have almost completely eliminated the need for physical activity, but you can choose to be physically active and greatly decrease the risk for premature mortality.

the heart, such as doing yard work, lifting heavy objects or weights, or running to catch a bus, the unconditioned heart may not be able to sustain the strain. Regular participation in CR endurance activities also helps a person achieve and maintain recommended body weight—the fourth component of health-related physical fitness.

Physical activity, unfortunately, is no longer a natural part of our existence. Technological developments have driven most people in developed countries into sedentary lifestyles. For instance, when many people go to a store only a couple of blocks away, they drive their automobiles and then spend a couple of minutes driving around the parking lot to find a spot 20 yards closer to the store's entrance. At times, they don't even have to carry the groceries to the car, as an employee working at the store offers to do this for them.

Similarly, during a visit to a multilevel shopping mall, almost everyone chooses to take the escalator instead of the stairs (which tend to be inaccessible). Automobiles, elevators, escalators, telephones, intercoms, remote controls, electric garage door openers—all are modern-day conveniences that minimize the amount of movement and effort required of the human body.

One of the most harmful effects of modern-day technology is an increase in chronic conditions related to a lack of physical activity. These **hypokinetic diseases** include hypertension, heart disease, chronic low back pain, and obesity. (The term "hypo" means low or little, and "kinetic" implies motion.) Lack of adequate physical activity is a fact of modern life that most people can avoid no longer. To enjoy modern-day conveniences and still expect to live life to its fullest, however, one has to make a personalized lifetime exercise program a part of daily living.

6.1 Basic Cardiorespiratory Physiology: A Quick Survey

Before we begin to overhaul our bodies with an exercise program, we should understand the mechanisms that we propose to alter and survey the ways by which to measure how well we perform them. CR endurance is a measure of how the pulmonary (lungs), cardiovascular (heart and blood vessels), and muscular systems work together during aerobic activities. As a person breathes, part of the oxygen in the air is taken up by the **alveoli** in the lungs. As blood passes through the alveoli, oxygen is picked up by **hemoglobin** and transported in the blood to the heart. The heart then is responsible for pumping the oxygenated blood through the circulatory system to all organs and tissues of the body.

At the cellular level, oxygen is used to convert food substrates (primarily carbohydrates and fats) through aerobic metabolism into **adenosine triphosphate (ATP)**. This compound provides the energy for physical activity, body functions, and maintenance of a constant internal equilibrium. During physical exertion, more ATP is needed to perform the activity. As a

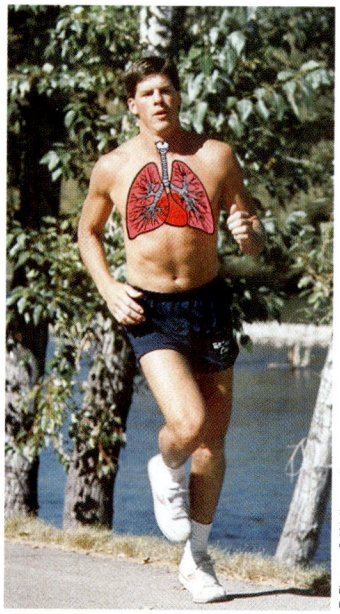

Cardiorespiratory endurance refers to the ability of the lungs, heart, and blood vessels to deliver adequate amounts of oxygen to the cells to meet the demands of prolonged physical activity.

Critical Thinking

Your friend Joe is not physically active and doesn't exercise. He manages to keep his weight down by dieting and tells you that because he feels and looks good, he doesn't need to exercise.
- How do you respond to your friend?

result, the lungs, heart, and blood vessels have to deliver more oxygen to the muscle cells to supply the required energy.

During prolonged exercise, an individual with a high level of CR endurance is able to deliver the required amount of oxygen to the tissues with relative ease. In contrast, the CR system of a person with a low level of endurance has to work much harder; the heart has to work at a higher rate; less oxygen is delivered to the tissues; and consequently, the individual fatigues faster. Hence, a higher capacity to deliver and utilize oxygen—called **oxygen uptake**, or VO_2—indicates a more efficient CR system. Measuring VO_2, therefore, is an important way by which to evaluate our CR health.

6.2 Aerobic and Anaerobic Exercise

Cardiorespiratory endurance activities often are called **aerobic** exercises. Examples are walking, jogging, swimming, cycling, cross-country skiing, aerobics (including water aerobics), and rope skipping. By contrast, the intensity of **anaerobic** exercise is so high that oxygen cannot be delivered and utilized to produce energy. Because energy production is limited in the absence of oxygen, anaerobic activities can be carried out for only short periods—two to three minutes. The higher the intensity of the activity, the shorter the duration.

Good examples of anaerobic activities are the 100, 200, and 400 meters in track and field, the 100 meters in swimming, gymnastics routines, and strength training. Anaerobic activities do not contribute much to developing the CR system. Only aerobic activities will increase CR endurance. The basic guidelines for CR exercise prescription are set forth later in this chapter.

Benefits of Aerobic Training Everyone who participates in a CR or aerobic exercise program can expect a number of beneficial physiological adaptations from training (Figure 6.1). Among them are the following:

1. A higher **maximal oxygen uptake (VO_{2max})**. The amount of oxygen that the body is able to use during exercise increases significantly. This allows the individual to exercise longer and more intensely before becoming fatigued. Depending on the initial fitness level, the increases in VO_{2max} average 15 to 20 percent, although increases greater than 50 percent have been reported in people who have very low initial levels of fitness or who were significantly overweight prior to starting the aerobic exercise program.

2. An increase in the oxygen-carrying capacity of the blood. As a result of training, the red blood cell count goes up. Red blood cells contain hemoglobin, which transports oxygen in the blood.

3. A decrease in **resting heart rate (RHR)** and an increase in cardiac muscle strength.

Hypokinetic diseases "Hypo" denotes "lack of"; therefore, illnesses related to a lack of physical activity.

Alveoli Air sacs in the lungs where oxygen is taken up and carbon dioxide (produced by the body) is released from the blood.

Hemoglobin Iron-containing compound, found in red blood cells, that transports oxygen.

Adenosine triphosphate (ATP) A high-energy chemical compound that the body uses for immediate energy.

Oxygen uptake (VO_2) The amount of oxygen the human body uses.

Aerobic Describes exercise that requires oxygen to produce the necessary energy (ATP) to carry out the activity.

Anaerobic Describes exercise that does not require oxygen to produce the necessary energy (ATP) to carry out the activity.

Maximal oxygen uptake (VO_{2max}) Maximum amount of oxygen the body is able to utilize per minute of physical activity, commonly expressed in milliliters per kilogram per minute (mL/kg/min); the best indicator of cardiorespiratory or aerobic fitness.

Resting heart rate (RHR) Heart rate after a person has been sitting quietly for 15 to 20 minutes.

During resting conditions, the heart ejects between five and six liters of blood per minute (a liter is slightly larger than a quart). This amount of blood, also referred to as **cardiac output**, meets the body's energy demands in the resting state. Like any other muscle, the heart responds to training by increasing in strength and size. As the heart gets stronger, the muscle can produce a more forceful contraction, which helps the heart to eject more blood with each beat. This **stroke volume** yields a lower heart rate. The lower heart rate also allows the heart to rest longer between beats. Average resting and maximal cardiac outputs, stroke volumes, and heart rates for sedentary, trained, and highly trained (elite) males are shown in Table 6.1. Resting heart rates frequently decrease by 10 to 20 beats per minute (bpm) after only 6 to 8 weeks of training. A reduction of 20 bpm saves the heart about 10,483,200 beats per year. The average heart beats between 70 and 80 bpm. As seen in Table 6.1, RHRs in highly trained athletes are often around 45 bpm.

4. A lower heart rate at given workloads. When compared with untrained individuals, a trained person has a lower heart rate response to a given task because of greater efficiency of the CR system. Individuals are surprised to find that following several weeks of training, a given **workload** (let's say a 10-minute mile) elicits a much lower heart rate response than their response when they first started training.

5. An increase in the number, size, and capacity of mitochondria. All energy necessary for cell function is produced in the **mitochondria**. As their size and numbers increase, so does their potential to produce energy for muscular work.

6. An increase in the number of functional capillaries. **Capillaries** allow for the exchange of oxygen and carbon dioxide between the blood and the cells. As more vessels open up, more gas exchange can take place, delaying the onset of fatigue during prolonged exercise. This increase in capillaries also speeds the rate at which waste products of cell metabolism can be removed. This increased capillarization also occurs in the heart, which enhances the oxygen delivery capacity to the heart muscle itself.

7. Ability to recover rapidly. Trained individuals have a faster **recovery time** after exercising. A fit system is able to more quickly restore any internal equilibrium disrupted during exercise.

8. Lower blood pressure and blood lipids. A regular aerobic exercise program leads to lower blood pressure (thereby reducing a major risk factor for stroke) and lower levels of fats (such as cholesterol and triglycerides) that have been linked to the formation of atherosclerotic plaque, which obstructs the arteries. This decreases the risk for coronary heart disease (see Chapter 10).

9. An increase in fat-burning enzymes. These enzymes are significant because fat is lost primarily by burning it in

Aerobic activities.

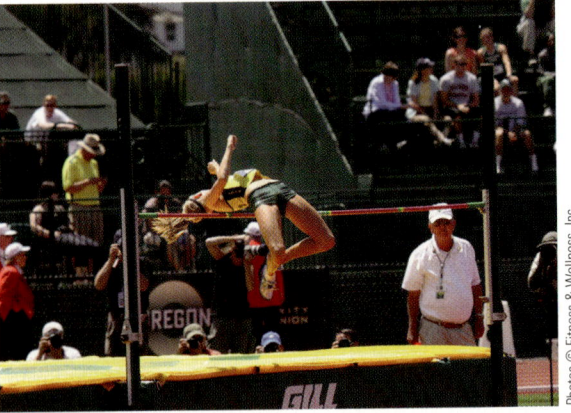

Anaerobic activities.

Table 6.1 Average Resting and Maximal Cardiac Output, Stroke Volume, and Heart Rate for Sedentary, Trained, and Highly Trained Young Males

	Resting			Maximal		
	Cardiac Output (L/min)	Stroke Volume (mL)	Heart Rate (bpm)	Cardiac Output (L/min)	Stroke Volume (mL)	Heart Rate (bpm)
Sedentary	5–6	68	74	20	100	200
Trained	5–6	90	56	30	150	200
Highly trained	5–6	110	45	35	175	200

NOTE: Cardiac output and stroke volume in women are about 25 percent lower than in men.
© Cengage Learning

Figure 6.1 Selected benefits of cardiorespiratory (aerobic) fitness.

- Improved brain function. Lower risk for stroke and depression.
- A higher maximal oxygen uptake (VO_{2max}).
- Decreased risk for several types of cancer.
- Improved functional capacity.
- Lower risk for type 2 diabetes.
- Decreased risk for osteoporosis and fractures.
- Increase in the number, size, and activity of the mitochondria.
- Increase in the number of functional capillaries.
- Higher academic performance.
- Lower risk for heart disease.
- Lower blood pressure.
- Better health and a higher quality of life.
- Improved balance and decreased risk for falls.
- Decreased pain and disability from arthritis.

muscle. As the concentration of the enzymes increases (along with the number and size of mitochondria), so does the ability to burn fat (triglycerides) as opposed to carbohydrates (glucose/glycogen) during submaximal workloads (below a pace that you can comfortably sustain for at least 20 minutes).

6.3 Physical Fitness Assessment

The assessment of physical fitness serves several purposes:

- To educate participants regarding their present fitness levels and compare them with health fitness and physical fitness standards
- To motivate individuals to participate in exercise programs
- To provide a starting point for an individualized exercise prescription and to establish realistic goals
- To evaluate improvements in fitness achieved through exercise programs and adjust exercise prescription and fitness goals accordingly
- To monitor changes in fitness throughout the years

Responders versus Nonresponders Individuals who follow similar training programs show a

> **Cardiac output** Amount of blood pumped by the heart in one minute.
> **Stroke volume** Amount of blood pumped by the heart in one beat.
> **Workload** Load (or intensity) placed on the body during physical activity.
> **Mitochondria** Structures within the cells where energy transformations take place.
> **Capillaries** Smallest blood vessels carrying oxygenated blood to the tissues in the body.
> **Recovery time** Amount of time that the body takes to return to resting levels after exercise.

Behavior Modification Planning

Tips to Increase Daily Physical Activity

Adults need recess, too! There are 1,440 minutes in every day. Schedule a minimum of 30 of these minutes for physical activity. With a little creativity and planning, even the person with the busiest schedule can make room for physical activity. For many folks, before or after work or meals is often an available time to cycle, walk, or play. Think about your weekly or daily schedule and look for or make opportunities to be more active. Every little bit helps. Consider the following suggestions:

I PLAN TO / I DID IT

- ☐ ☐ Walk, cycle, jog, or skate to school, work, the store, or place of worship.
- ☐ ☐ Use a pedometer to count your daily steps.
- ☐ ☐ Walk while doing errands.
- ☐ ☐ Get on or off the bus several blocks away.
- ☐ ☐ Park the car farther away from your destination.
- ☐ ☐ At work, walk to nearby offices instead of sending e-mails or using the phone.
- ☐ ☐ Walk or stretch a few minutes every hour that you are at your desk.
- ☐ ☐ Take fitness breaks—walking or doing desk exercises—instead of taking cigarette breaks or coffee breaks.
- ☐ ☐ Incorporate activity into your lunch break (walk to the restaurant).
- ☐ ☐ Take the stairs instead of the elevator or escalator.
- ☐ ☐ Play with children, grandchildren, or pets. Everybody wins. If you find it too difficult to be active after work, try it before work.
- ☐ ☐ Do household tasks.
- ☐ ☐ Work in the yard or garden.
- ☐ ☐ Avoid labor-saving devices. Turn off the self-propelled option on your lawnmower or vacuum cleaner.
- ☐ ☐ Use leg power. Take small trips on foot to get your body moving.
- ☐ ☐ Exercise while watching TV (for example, use hand weights, stationary bicycle/treadmill, elliptical training, or stretch).
- ☐ ☐ Spend more time playing sports than sitting in front of the TV or the computer.
- ☐ ☐ Dance to music.
- ☐ ☐ Keep a pair of comfortable walking or running shoes in your car and office. You'll be ready for activity wherever you go!
- ☐ ☐ Make a Saturday morning walk a group habit.
- ☐ ☐ Learn a new sport or join a sports team.
- ☐ ☐ Avoid carts when golfing.
- ☐ ☐ When out of town, stay in hotels with fitness centers.

Try It

Keep a three-day log of all your activities. List the activities performed, time of day, and how long you were engaged in these activities. You may be surprised by your findings.

SOURCE: Adapted from Centers for Disease Control and Prevention, Atlanta.

---

wide variation in physiological responses. Heredity plays a crucial role in how each person responds to and improves after beginning an exercise program. Several studies have documented that following exercise training, most individuals, called **responders**, readily show improvements, but a few, **nonresponders**, exhibit small or no improvements at all. This concept is referred to as the **principle of individuality**.

After several months of aerobic training, increases in VO_{2max} are between 15 and 20 percent on the average, although individual responses can range from 0 percent (in a few selected cases) to more than 50 percent improvement, even when all participants follow exactly the same training program. Nonfitness and low-fitness participants, however, should not label themselves as nonresponders based on the previous discussion. Nonresponders constitute less than 5 percent of exercise participants. Although additional research is necessary, lack of improvement in CR endurance among nonresponders might be related to low levels of leg strength. A lower-body strength-training program has been shown to help these individuals improve VO_{2max} through aerobic exercise.[1]

Following your self-assessment of CR fitness, if your fitness level is less than adequate, do not let that discourage you, but do set a priority to be physically active every day. In addition to regular exercise, lifestyle behaviors—walking, taking stairs, cycling to work, parking farther from the office, doing household tasks, gardening, and doing yard work, for example—provide substantial benefits. In this regard, daily **physical activity** and **exercise** habits should be monitored in conjunction with fitness testing to evaluate adherence among nonresponders. After all, it is through increased daily activity that we reap the health benefits that improve our quality of life.

6.4 Assessment of Cardiorespiratory Endurance

Cardiorespiratory endurance, CR fitness, or aerobic capacity is determined by the maximal amount of oxygen the human body is able to utilize (the oxygen uptake) per minute of physical activity (VO_{2max}). This value can be expressed in liters per minute (L/min) or milliliters per kilogram per minute (mL/kg/min). The relative value in mL/kg/min is used most often because it considers total body mass (weight) in kilograms. When comparing two individuals with the same absolute value, the one with the lesser body mass will have a higher relative value, indicating that more oxygen is available to each kilogram (2.2 pounds) of body weight. Because all tissues and organs of the body need oxygen to function, higher oxygen consumption indicates a more efficient CR system.

VO_2 expressed in L/min is valuable in determining the caloric expenditure of physical activity. The human body burns about five calories for each liter of oxygen consumed. During aerobic exercise the average person trains around 50 percent of VO_{2max}.

A person with a VO_{2max} of 3.5 L/min who trains at 60 percent of maximum uses 2.1 (3.5 × .60) liters of oxygen per minute of physical activity. This indicates that 10.5 calories are burned during each minute of exercise (2.1 × 5). If the activity is carried out for 30 minutes, 315 calories (10.5 × 30) have been burned. Because a pound of body fat represents about 3,500 calories, the previous example indicates that this individual would have to exercise for a total of 333 minutes (3,500 ÷ 10.5) to burn the equivalent of a pound of body fat. At 30 minutes per exercise session, approximately 11 sessions would be required to expend the 3,500 calories.

Components of Oxygen Uptake (VO_2)
The amount of oxygen the body actually uses at rest or during submaximal (VO_2) or maximal (VO_{2max}) exercise is determined by the heart rate, the stroke volume, and the amount of oxygen removed from the vascular system (for use by all organs and tissues of the body, including the muscular system).

Heart Rate
Normal heart rate ranges from about 40 bpm during resting conditions in trained athletes to 200 bpm or higher during maximal exercise. The **maximal heart rate (MHR)** that a person can achieve starts to drop by about one beat per year beginning at about 12 years of age. Maximal heart rate in trained endurance athletes is sometimes slightly lower than in untrained individuals. This adaptation to training is thought to allow the heart more time to effectively fill with blood so as to produce a greater stroke volume.

Aerobic fitness leads to better health and a higher quality of life.

Stroke Volume
Stroke volume ranges from 50 mL per beat (stroke) during resting conditions in untrained individuals to 200 mL at maximum in endurance-trained athletes (see Table 6.1). Following endurance training, stroke volume increases significantly. Some of the increase is the result of a stronger heart muscle, but it also is related to an increase in total blood volume and a greater filling capacity of the ventricles during the resting phase (diastole) of the cardiac cycle. As more blood enters the heart, more blood can be ejected with each heartbeat (systole). The in-

> **Responders** Individuals who exhibit improvements in fitness as a result of exercise training.
>
> **Nonresponders** Individuals who exhibit small or no improvements in fitness as compared to others who undergo the same training program.
>
> **Principle of individuality** Training concept holding that genetics plays a major role in individual responses to exercise training and these differences must be considered when designing exercise programs for different people.
>
> **Physical activity** Bodily movement produced by skeletal muscles; requires expenditure of energy and produces progressive health benefits. Examples include walking, taking the stairs, dancing, gardening, yard work, house cleaning, snow shoveling, washing the car, and all forms of structured exercise.
>
> **Exercise** A type of physical activity that requires planned, structured, and repetitive bodily movement with the intent of improving or maintaining one or more components of physical fitness.
>
> **Maximal heart rate (MHR)** Highest heart rate for a person, related primarily to age.

crease in stroke volume is primarily responsible for the increase in VO_{2max} with endurance training.

Amount of Oxygen Removed from Blood

The amount of oxygen removed from the vascular system is known as the **arterial-venous oxygen difference** ($a\text{-}\bar{v}O_{2diff}$). The oxygen content in the arteries at sea level is typically 20 mL of oxygen per 100 cubic centimeters (cc) of blood. (This value decreases at higher altitudes because of the drop in barometric pressure, which affects the amount of oxygen picked up by hemoglobin.) The oxygen content in the veins during a resting state is about 15 mL per 100 cc. Thus, the ($a\text{-}\bar{v}O_{2diff}$)—the amount of oxygen in the arteries minus the amount in the veins—at rest is 5 mL per 100 cc. The arterial value remains constant during both resting and exercise conditions. Because of the additional oxygen removed during maximal exercise, the venous oxygen content drops to about 5 mL per 100 cc, yielding an ($a\text{-}\bar{v}O_{2diff}$) of 15 mL per 100 cc. The latter value may be slightly higher in endurance athletes.

These three factors are used to compute VO_2 using the following equation:

$$VO_2 \text{ in L/min} = (HR \times SV \times a\text{-}\bar{v}O_{2diff}) \div 100{,}000$$

where

$$HR = \text{heart rate}$$

$$SV = \text{stroke volume}$$

For example, the resting VO_2 (also known as the resting metabolic rate) of an individual with a RHR of 76 bpm and a stroke volume of 79 mL would be

$$VO_2 \text{ in L/min} = (76 \times 79 \times 5) \div 100{,}000 = .3 \text{ L/min}.$$

Likewise, the VO_{2max} of a person exercising maximally who achieves a heart rate of 190 bpm and a maximal stroke volume of 120 mL would be

$$VO_{2max} \text{ in L/min} = (190 \times 120 \times 15) \div 100{,}000$$
$$= 3.42 \text{ L/min}.$$

To convert L/min to mL/kg/min, multiply the L/min value by 1,000 and divide by body weight in kilograms. In the previous example, if the person weighs 70 kilograms, the VO_{2max} would be 48.9 mL/kg/min ($3.42 \times 1000 \div 70$).

> **Critical Thinking**
>
> You can improve your relative VO_{2max} without engaging in an aerobic exercise program. • How do you accomplish this? • Would you benefit from doing so?

Because the actual measurement of the stroke volume and the $a\text{-}\bar{v}O_{2diff}$ is impractical in the fitness setting, VO_2 also is determined through gas (air) analysis. The person being tested breathes into a metabolic cart that measures the difference in oxygen content between the person's exhaled air and the atmosphere. The air we breathe contains 21 percent oxygen; thus, VO_2 can be assessed by establishing the difference between 21 percent and the percent of oxygen left in the air the person exhales, according to the total volume of air taken into the lungs. This type of equipment, however, is expensive. Consequently, several alternative methods of estimating VO_{2max} using limited equipment have been developed. These methods are discussed next.

VO_{2max} is affected by genetics, training, gender, age, and body composition. Although aerobic training can help people attain good or excellent CR fitness, only those with a strong genetic component are able to reach an "elite" level of aerobic capacity (60 to 80 mL/kg/min). Further, VO_{2max} is 15 to 30 percent higher in men. This is related to a greater hemoglobin content, lower body fat (see "Essential and Storage Fat" in Chapter 4, page 126), and larger heart size in men (a larger heart pumps more blood, and thus produces a greater stroke volume). VO_{2max} also decreases by about 1 percent per year starting at age 25. This decrease, however, is only .5 percent per year in physically active individuals.

Tests to Estimate VO_{2max} Even though most CR endurance tests probably are safe to administer to apparently healthy individuals (those with no major coronary risk factors or symptoms), a health history questionnaire (including the PAR-Q), such as found in Activity 1.3 in Chapter 1, should be used as a minimum screening tool prior to exercise testing or participation. The American College of Sports Medicine (ACSM) also recommends that individuals at risk, or diagnosed with cardiovascular disease, undergo a medical examination prior to exercise testing or exercise participation.[2]

Five exercise tests used to assess CR fitness are introduced in this chapter: the 1.5-Mile Run Test, the 1.0-Mile Walk Test, the Step Test, the Astrand-Ryhming Test, and the 12-Minute Swim Test. The procedures for each test are explained in detail in Figures 6.2, 6.3, 6.4, 6.5, and 6.6, respectively. The 1.5-Mile Run Test and the Swim Test are considered maximal tests, as they require an all-out or nearly all-out effort on the part of the participant. Submaximal exercise tests do not require all-out efforts.

Several tests are provided in this chapter, so you may choose one depending on time, equipment, and individual physical limitations. For example, people who can't jog or walk can take the Astrand-Ryhming (bicycle) or swim test. You may perform more than one test, but because they are different and they estimate VO_{2max}, they will not necessarily yield the same results. Therefore, to make valid comparisons, you should take the same test when doing pre- and post-assessments. You may record the results of your test(s) in Activity 6.1.

1.5-Mile Run Test

The 1.5-Mile Run Test is used most frequently to predict VO_{2max} according to the time the person takes to run or walk a 1.5-mile course (see Figure 6.2). VO_{2max} is estimated based on the time the person takes to cover the distance (see Table 6.2).

The only equipment necessary to conduct this test is a stopwatch and a track or premeasured 1.5-mile course. This

Figure 6.2 Procedure for the 1.5-Mile Run Test.

1. Make sure you qualify for this test. This test is contraindicated for unconditioned beginners, individuals with symptoms of heart disease, and those with known heart disease or risk factors.
2. Select the testing site. Find a school track (each lap is one-fourth of a mile) or a premeasured 1.5-mile course.
3. Have a stopwatch available to determine your time.
4. Conduct a few warm-up exercises prior to the test. Do some stretching exercises, some walking, and slow jogging.
5. Initiate the test and try to cover the distance in the fastest time possible (walking or jogging). Time yourself during the run to see how fast you have covered the distance. If any unusual symptoms arise during the test, do not continue. Stop immediately and retake the test after another 6 weeks of aerobic training.
6. At the end of the test, cool down by walking or jogging slowly for another 3 to 5 minutes. Do not sit or lie down after the test.
7. According to your performance time, look up your estimated maximal oxygen uptake (VO_{2max}) in Table 6.2.

Example: A 20-year-old male runs the 1.5-mile course in 10 minutes and 20 seconds. Table 6.2 shows a VO_{2max} of 49.5 mL/kg/min for a time of 10:20. According to Table 6.8, this VO_{2max} would place him in the "good" cardiorespiratory fitness category.

Table 6.2 Estimated Maximal Oxygen Uptake (VO_{2max}) for the 1.5-Mile Run Test

Time	VO_{2max} (mL/kg/min)	Time	VO_{2max} (mL/kg/min)
6:10	80.0	12:40	39.8
6:20	79.0	12:50	39.2
6:30	77.9	13:00	38.6
6:40	76.7	13:10	38.1
6:50	75.5	13:20	37.8
7:00	74.0	13:30	37.2
7:10	72.6	13:40	36.8
7:20	71.3	13:50	36.3
7:30	69.9	14:00	35.9
7:40	68.3	14:10	35.5
7:50	66.8	14:20	35.1
8:00	65.2	14:30	34.7
8:10	63.9	14:40	34.3
8:20	62.5	14:50	34.0
8:30	61.2	15:00	33.6
8:40	60.2	15:10	33.1
8:50	59.1	15:20	32.7
9:00	58.1	15:30	32.2
9:10	56.9	15:40	31.8
9:20	55.9	15:50	31.4
9:30	54.7	16:00	30.9
9:40	53.5	16:10	30.5
9:50	52.3	16:20	30.2
10:00	51.1	16:30	29.8
10:10	50.4	16:40	29.5
10:20	49.5	16:50	29.1
10:30	48.6	17:00	28.9
10:40	48.0	17:10	28.5
10:50	47.4	17:20	28.3
11:00	46.6	17:30	28.0
11:10	45.8	17:40	27.7
11:20	45.1	17:50	27.4
11:30	44.4	18:00	27.1
11:40	43.7	18:10	26.8
11:50	43.2	18:20	26.6
12:00	42.3	18:30	26.3
12:10	41.7	18:40	26.0
12:20	41.0	18:50	25.7
12:30	40.4	19:00	25.4

Source: Adapted from K. H. Cooper, "A Means of Assessing Maximal Oxygen Intake," *Journal of the American Medical Association,* 203 (1968): 201–204; M. L. Pollock, J. H. Wilmore, and S. M. Fox III, *Health and Fitness Through Physical Activity* (New York: John Wiley & Sons, 1978); and J. H. Wilmore and D. L. Costill, *Training for Sport and Activity* (Dubuque, IA: Wm. C. Brown Publishers, 1988).

---

perhaps is the easiest test to administer, but a note of caution is in order when conducting the test: Given that the objective is to cover the distance in the shortest time, it is considered a maximal exercise test. The 1.5-Mile Run Test should be limited to conditioned individuals who have been cleared for exercise. The test is not recommended for unconditioned beginners, men older than age 45 and women older than age 55 without proper medical clearance, symptomatic individuals, and those with known disease or risk factors for coronary heart disease. A program of at least 6 weeks of aerobic training is recommended before unconditioned individuals take this test.

1.0-Mile Walk Test

The 1.0-Mile Walk Test can be used by individuals who are unable to run because of low fitness levels or injuries. All that is required is a brisk 1.0-mile walk that will elicit an exercise heart rate of at least 120 bpm at the end of the test.

You will need to know how to take your heart rate by counting your pulse. You can do this by gently placing the middle and index fingers over the radial artery on the inside of the wrist on the side of the thumb or over the carotid artery in the neck just below the jaw next to the voice box. You should not use the thumb to check the pulse because it has a strong pulse of its own, which can make you miscount. When checking the carotid pulse, do not press too hard, because it may cause a reflex action that slows the heart. For checking the pulse over the carotid artery, some exercise experts recommend that the hand on the same side of the neck (right hand over right carotid artery) be used to avoid excessive pressure on the artery. With minimum experience, however, you can be accurate using either hand as long as you apply only gentle pressure. If available, heart rate monitors can be used to increase the accuracy of heart rate assessment.

VO_{2max} is estimated according to a prediction equation that requires the following data: 1.0-mile

Arterial-venous oxygen difference ($a-\bar{v}O_{2diff}$) The amount of oxygen removed from the blood as determined by the difference in oxygen content between arterial and venous blood.

Oxygen uptake (VO_2), as determined through direct gas analysis.

Pulse taken at the radial artery.   Pulse taken at the carotid artery.

walk time, exercise heart rate at the end of the walk, gender, and body weight in pounds. The procedure for this test and the equation are given in Figure 6.3.

Step Test

The Step Test requires little time and equipment and can be administered to almost anyone because a submaximal workload is used to estimate VO_{2max}. Symptomatic and diseased individuals should not take this test. Significantly overweight individuals and those with joint problems in the lower extremities may have difficulty performing the test.

The actual test takes only three minutes. A 15-second recovery heart rate is taken between 5 and 20 seconds following the test (see Figure 6.4 and Table 6.3). The required equipment consists of a bench or gymnasium bleacher 16¼ inches high, a stopwatch, and a metronome.

You also will need to know how to take your heart rate by counting your pulse, as we have just discussed. Once people learn to take their own heart rate, a large group of people can be tested at once, using gymnasium bleachers for the steps.

Astrand-Ryhming Test

Because of its simplicity and practicality, the Astrand-Ryhming Test is one of the most popular tests used to estimate VO_{2max} in the laboratory setting. The test is conducted on a bicycle ergometer and, similar to the Step Test, requires only submaximal workloads and little time to administer.

The cautions given for the Step Test also apply to the Astrand-Ryhming Test. Nevertheless, because the participant does not have to support his or her own body weight while riding the bicycle, overweight individuals and those with limited joint problems in the lower extremities can take this test.

Figure 6.3 Procedure for the 1.0-Mile Walk Test.

1. Select the testing site. Use a 440-yard track (4 laps to a mile) or a premeasured 1.0-mile course.
2. Determine your body weight in pounds prior to the test.
3. Have a stopwatch available to determine total walking time and exercise heart rate.
4. Walk the 1.0-mile course at a brisk pace (the exercise heart rate at the end of the test should be above 120 beats per minute).
5. At the end of the 1.0-mile walk, check your walking time and immediately count your pulse for 10 seconds. Multiply the 10-second pulse count by 6 to obtain the exercise heart rate in beats per minute.
6. Convert the walking time from minutes and seconds to minute units. Because each minute has 60 seconds, divide the seconds by 60 to obtain the fraction of a minute. For instance, a walking time of 12 minutes and 15 seconds would equal 12 + (15 ÷ 60), or 12.25 minutes.
7. To obtain the estimated maximal oxygen uptake (VO_{2max}) in mL/kg/min, plug your values in the following equation:
   $VO_{2max} = 88.768 − (0.0957 × W) + (8.892 × G) − (1.4537 × T) − (0.1194 × HR)$

Where:
- W = Weight in pounds
- G = Gender (use 0 for women and 1 for men)
- T = Total time for the one-mile walk in minutes (see item 6)
- HR = Exercise heart rate in beats per minute at the end of the 1.0-mile walk

Example: A 19-year-old female who weighs 140 pounds completed the 1.0-mile walk in 14 minutes 39 seconds with an exercise heart rate of 148 beats per minute. Her estimated VO_{2max} would be:

W = 140 lbs
G = 0 (female gender = 0)
T = 14:39 = 14 + (39 ÷ 60) = 14.65 min
HR = 148 bpm
$VO_{2max} = 88.768 − (0.0957 × 140) + (8.892 × 0) − (1.4537 × 14.65) − (0.1194 × 148)$
$VO_{2max} = 36.4$ mL/kg/min

SOURCE: Dolgener, F.A., et al. "Validation of the Rockport Fitness Walking Test in College Males and Females," *Research Quarterly for Exercise and Sport* 65 (1994): 152–158.

Figure 6.4 Procedure for the Step Test.

1. Conduct the test with a bench or gymnasium bleacher 16¼ inches high.
2. Perform the stepping cycle to a four-step cadence (up-up-down-down). Men should perform 24 complete step-ups per minute, regulated with a metronome set at 96 beats per minute. Women perform 22 step-ups per minute, or 88 beats per minute on the metronome.
3. Allow a brief practice period of 5 to 10 seconds to familiarize yourself with the stepping cadence.
4. Begin the test and perform the step-ups for exactly 3 minutes.
5. Upon completing the 3 minutes, remain standing and take your heart rate for a 15-second interval from 5 to 20 seconds into recovery. Convert recovery heart rate to beats per minute (multiply 15-second heart rate by 4).
6. Maximal oxygen uptake (VO_{2max}) in mL/kg/min is estimated according to the following equations:

Men:
$VO_{2max} = 111.33 - (0.42 \times$ recovery heart rate in bpm$)$
Women:
$VO_{2max} = 65.81 - (0.1847 \times$ recovery heart rate in bpm$)$

Example: The recovery 15-second heart rate for a male following the 3-minute step test is found to be 39 beats. His VO_{2max} is estimated as follows:

15-second heart rate = 39 beats
Minute heart rate = 39 × 4 = 156 bpm
$VO_{2max} = 111.33 - (0.42 \times 156) = 45.81$ mL/kg/min
VO_{2max} also can be obtained according to recovery heart rates in Table 6.3.

SOURCE: McArdle, W.D., et al. *Exercise Physiology: Energy, Nutrition, and Human Performance* (Philadelphia: Lea & Febiger, 1986).

Table 6.3 Predicted Maximal Oxygen Uptake for the Step Test

15-Sec HR	HR (bpm)	Men (mL/kg/min)	Women (mL/kg/min)
30	120	60.9	43.6
31	124	59.3	42.9
32	128	57.6	42.2
33	132	55.9	41.4
34	136	54.2	40.7
35	140	52.5	40.0
36	144	50.9	39.2
37	148	49.2	38.5
38	152	47.5	37.7
39	156	45.8	37.0
40	160	44.1	36.3
41	164	42.5	35.5
42	168	40.8	34.8
43	172	39.1	34.0
44	176	37.4	33.3
45	180	35.7	32.6
46	184	34.1	31.8
47	188	32.4	31.1
48	192	30.7	30.3
49	196	29.0	29.6
50	200	27.3	28.9

© Cengage Learning

The bicycle ergometer to be used for this test should allow for the regulation of workloads (see the test procedure in Figure 6.5). Besides the bicycle ergometer, a stopwatch and an additional technician to monitor the heart rate are needed to conduct the test.

The heart rate is taken every minute for six minutes. At the end of the test, the heart rate should be in the range given for each workload in Table 6.5 (generally between 120 and 170 bpm).

When administering the test to older people, good judgment is essential. Low workloads should be used, because if the higher heart rates (around 150 to 170 bpm) are reached, these individuals could be working near or at their maximal capacity, making this an unsafe test without adequate medical supervision. When testing older people, choose workloads so that the final exercise heart rates do not exceed 130 to 140 bpm.

12-Minute Swim Test

Similar to the 1.5-Mile Run Test, the 12-Minute Swim Test is considered a maximal exercise test, and the same precautions apply. The objective is to swim as far as possible during the 12-Minute Swim Test (see Figure 6.6).

Unlike land-based tests, predicting VO_{2max} through a swimming test is difficult. A swimming test is practical only for those who are planning to take part in a swimming program or who cannot perform any of the other tests. Differences in skill level, swimming conditioning, and body composition greatly affect the energy requirements (oxygen uptake) of swimming.

Unskilled and unconditioned swimmers can expect lower CR fitness ratings than can be obtained with a land-based test. A skilled swimmer is able to swim more efficiently and expend much less energy than an unskilled swimmer. Improper breathing patterns cause premature fatigue. Overweight individuals are more buoyant in the water, and the larger surface area (body size) produces more friction against movement in the water medium.

Lack of conditioning affects swimming test results as well. An unconditioned skilled swimmer who is in good CR shape because of a regular jogging program will not perform as effectively in a swimming test. Swimming conditioning is important for adequate performance on this test.

Because of these limitations, VO_{2max} cannot be estimated for a swimming test, and the fitness categories given in Table 6.7 are only estimated ratings.

Figure 6.5 Procedure for the Astrand-Ryhming Test.

1. Adjust the bike seat so the knees are almost completely extended as the foot goes through the bottom of the pedaling cycle.
2. During the test, keep the speed constant at 50 revolutions per minute. Test duration is 6 minutes.
3. Select the appropriate workload for the bike based on gender, age, weight, health, and estimated fitness level. For unconditioned individuals: women, use 300 kpm (kilopounds per meter) or 450 kpm; men, 300 kpm or 600 kpm. Conditioned adults: women, 450 kpm or 600 kpm; men, 600 kpm or 900 kpm.*
4. Ride the bike for 6 minutes and check the heart rate every minute, during the last 15 seconds of each minute. Determine heart rate by recording the time it takes to count 30 pulse beats and then converting to beats per minute using Table 6.4.
5. Average the final two heart rates (5th and 6th minutes). If these two heart rates are not within 5 beats per minute of each other, continue the test for another few minutes until this is accomplished. If the heart rate continues to climb significantly after the 6th minute, stop the test and rest for 15 to 20 minutes. You may then retest, preferably at a lower workload. The final average heart rate should also fall between the ranges given for each workload in Table 6.5 (men: 300 kpm = 120 to 140 beats per minute; 600 kpm = 120 to 170 beats per minute).
6. Based on the average heart rate of the final 2 minutes and your workload, look up the maximal oxygen uptake (VO_{2max}) in Table 6.5 (for example: men: 600 kpm and average heart rate = 145, VO_{2max} = 2.4 L/min).
7. Correct VO_{2max} using the correction factors found in Table 6.6 (if VO_{2max} = 2.4 and age 35, correction factor = .870. Multiply 2.4 × .870 and final corrected VO_{2max} = 2.09 L/min).
8. To obtain VO_{2max} in mL/kg/min, multiply the VO_{2max} by 1,000 (to convert liters to milliliters) and divide by body weight in kilograms (to obtain kilograms, divide your body weight in pounds by 2.2046).

Example: Corrected VO_{2max} = 2.09 L/min
Body weight = 132 pounds ÷ 2.2046 = 60 kilograms

$$VO_{2max} \text{ in mL/kg/min} = \frac{2.09 \times 1,000}{60} = 34.8 \text{ mL/kg/min}$$

*On the Monark bicycle ergometer, at a speed of 50 revolutions per minute, a load of 1 kp = 300 kpm, 1.5 kp = 450 kpm, 2 kp = 600 kpm, and so forth, with increases of 150 kpm to each half kp.

Critical Thinking

Should fitness testing be a part of a fitness program? • Why or why not? • Does preparticipation fitness testing have benefits, or should fitness testing be done at a later date?

Interpreting the Results of Your Maximal Oxygen Uptake After obtaining your VO_{2max}, you can determine your current level of CR fitness by consulting Table 6.8. Locate the VO_{2max} in your age category, and on the top row you will find your present level of CR fitness. For example, a 19-year-old male with a VO_{2max} of 35 mL/kg/min would be classified in the "average" CR fitness category. After you initiate your personal CR exercise program (see Activity 6.4), you may wish to retest yourself periodically to evaluate your progress.

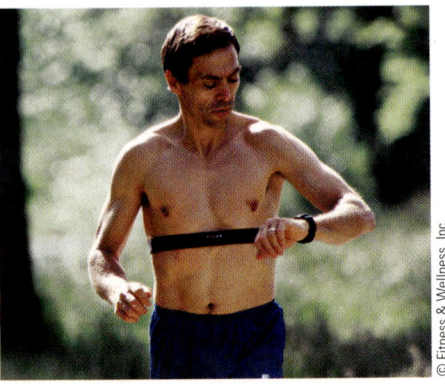

Heart rate monitors increase the accuracy of heart rate assessment.

6.5 Principles of CR Exercise Prescription

Before proceeding with the principles of exercise prescription, you should ask yourself if you are willing to give exercise a try. A low percentage of the U.S. population is truly committed to exercise. The first six weeks of the program are most critical. Adherence to exercise is greatly enhanced if you are able to make it through four to six weeks of training. Keep in mind, that all of the benefits of exercise cannot help unless you commit and participate in a lifetime program of physical activity.

Readiness for Exercise The first step is to ask yourself: Am I ready to start an exercise program? The information provided in Activity 6.2 can help you answer this question. You are evaluated in four categories: mastery (self-control), attitude, health, and commitment. The higher you score in any category—mastery, for example—the more important that reason is for you to exercise.

Scores can vary from 4 to 16. A score of 12 or greater is a strong indicator that the factor is important to you, whereas less than 8 is low. If you score 12 or more points in each category, your chances of initiating and sticking to an exercise program are good. If you do not score at least 12 points in each of any three categories, your chances of succeeding at exercise may be slim. You need to be better informed about the benefits of exercise, and a retraining process might be helpful to change core values regarding exercise. More tips on how you can become committed to exercise are provided in "Getting Started and Adhering to a Lifetime Exercise Program" (page 224).

Table 6.4 Conversion of the Time for 30 Pulse Beats to Pulse Rate per Minute

Sec	bpm	Sec	bpm	Sec	bpm
22.0	82	17.3	104	12.6	143
21.9	82	17.2	105	12.5	144
21.8	83	17.1	105	12.4	145
21.7	83	17.0	106	12.3	146
21.6	83	16.9	107	12.2	148
21.5	84	16.8	107	12.1	149
21.4	84	16.7	108	12.0	150
21.3	85	16.6	108	11.9	151
21.2	85	16.5	109	11.8	153
21.1	85	16.4	110	11.7	154
21.0	86	16.3	110	11.6	155
20.9	86	16.2	111	11.5	157
20.8	87	16.1	112	11.4	158
20.7	87	16.0	113	11.3	159
20.6	87	15.9	113	11.2	161
20.5	88	15.8	114	11.1	162
20.4	88	15.7	115	11.0	164
20.3	89	15.6	115	10.9	165
20.2	89	15.5	116	10.8	167
20.1	90	15.4	117	10.7	168
20.0	90	15.3	118	10.6	170
19.9	90	15.2	118	10.5	171
19.8	91	15.1	119	10.4	173
19.7	91	15.0	120	10.3	175
19.6	92	14.9	121	10.2	176
19.5	92	14.8	122	10.1	178
19.4	93	14.7	122	10.0	180
19.3	93	14.6	123	9.9	182
19.2	94	14.5	124	9.8	184
19.1	94	14.4	125	9.7	186
19.0	95	14.3	126	9.6	188
18.9	95	14.2	127	9.5	189
18.8	96	14.1	128	9.4	191
18.7	96	14.0	129	9.3	194
18.6	97	13.9	129	9.2	196
18.5	97	13.8	130	9.1	198
18.4	98	13.7	131	9.0	200
18.3	98	13.6	132	8.9	202
18.2	99	13.5	133	8.8	205
18.1	99	13.4	134	8.7	207
18.0	100	13.3	135	8.6	209
17.9	101	13.2	136	8.5	212
17.8	101	13.1	137	8.4	214
17.7	102	13.0	138	8.3	217
17.6	102	12.9	140	8.2	220
17.5	103	12.8	141	8.1	222
17.4	103	12.7	142	8.0	225

© Cengage Learning

Table 6.5 Maximal Oxygen Uptake (VO_{2max}) Estimates for the Astrand-Ryhming Test

Heart Rate	Men Workload					Women Workload				
	300	600	900	1200	1,500	300	450	600	750	900
120	2.2	3.4	4.8			2.6	3.4	4.1	4.8	
121	2.2	3.4	4.7			2.5	3.3	4.0	4.8	
122	2.2	3.4	4.6			2.5	3.2	3.9	4.7	
123	2.1	3.4	4.6			2.4	3.1	3.9	4.6	
124	2.1	3.3	4.5	6.0		2.4	3.1	3.8	4.5	
125	2.0	3.2	4.4	5.9		2.3	3.0	3.7	4.4	
126	2.0	3.2	4.4	5.8		2.3	3.0	3.6	4.3	
127	2.0	3.1	4.3	5.7		2.2	2.9	3.5	4.2	
128	2.0	3.1	4.2	5.6		2.2	2.8	3.5	4.2	4.8
129	1.9	3.0	4.2	5.6		2.2	2.8	3.4	4.1	4.8
130	1.9	3.0	4.1	5.5		2.1	2.7	3.4	4.0	4.7
131	1.9	2.9	4.0	5.4		2.1	2.7	3.4	4.0	4.6
132	1.8	2.9	4.0	5.3		2.0	2.7	3.3	3.9	4.5
133	1.8	2.8	3.9	5.3		2.0	2.6	3.2	3.8	4.4
134	1.8	2.8	3.9	5.2		2.0	2.6	3.2	3.8	4.4
135	1.7	2.8	3.8	5.1		2.0	2.6	3.1	3.7	4.3
136	1.7	2.7	3.8	5.0		1.9	2.5	3.1	3.6	4.2
137	1.7	2.7	3.7	5.0		1.9	2.5	3.0	3.6	4.2
138	1.6	2.7	3.7	4.9		1.8	2.4	3.0	3.5	4.1
139	1.6	2.6	3.6	4.8		1.8	2.4	2.9	3.5	4.0
140	1.6	2.6	3.6	4.8	6.0	1.8	2.4	2.8	3.4	4.0
141		2.6	3.5	4.7	5.9	1.8	2.3	2.8	3.4	3.9
142		2.5	3.5	4.6	5.8	1.7	2.3	2.8	3.3	3.9
143		2.5	3.4	4.6	5.7	1.7	2.2	2.7	3.3	3.8
144		2.5	3.4	4.5	5.7	1.7	2.2	2.7	3.2	3.8
145		2.4	3.4	4.5	5.6	1.6	2.2	2.7	3.2	3.7
146		2.4	3.3	4.4	5.6	1.6	2.2	2.6	3.2	3.7
147		2.4	3.3	4.4	5.5	1.6	2.1	2.6	3.1	3.6
148		2.4	3.2	4.3	5.4	1.6	2.1	2.6	3.1	3.6
149		2.3	3.2	4.3	5.4		2.1	2.6	3.0	3.5
150		2.3	3.2	4.2	5.3		2.0	2.5	3.0	3.5
151		2.3	3.1	4.2	5.2		2.0	2.5	3.0	3.4
152		2.3	3.1	4.1	5.2		2.0	2.5	2.9	3.4
153		2.2	3.0	4.1	5.1		2.0	2.4	2.9	3.3
154		2.2	3.0	4.0	5.1		2.0	2.4	2.8	3.3
155		2.2	3.0	4.0	5.0		1.9	2.4	2.8	3.2
156		2.2	2.9	4.0	5.0		1.9	2.3	2.8	3.2
157		2.1	2.9	3.9	4.9		1.9	2.3	2.7	3.2
158		2.1	2.9	3.9	4.9		1.8	2.3	2.7	3.1
159		2.1	2.8	3.8	4.8		1.8	2.2	2.7	3.1
160		2.1	2.8	3.8	4.8		1.8	2.2	2.6	3.0
161		2.0	2.8	3.7	4.7		1.8	2.2	2.6	3.0
162		2.0	2.8	3.7	4.6		1.8	2.2	2.6	3.0
163		2.0	2.8	3.7	4.6		1.7	2.2	2.6	2.9
164		2.0	2.7	3.6	4.5		1.7	2.1	2.5	2.9
165		2.0	2.7	3.6	4.5		1.7	2.1	2.5	2.9
166		1.9	2.7	3.6	4.5		1.7	2.1	2.5	2.8
167		1.9	2.6	3.5	4.4		1.6	2.1	2.4	2.8
168		1.9	2.6	3.5	4.4		1.6	2.0	2.4	2.8
169		1.9	2.6	3.5	4.3		1.6	2.0	2.4	2.8
170		1.8	2.6	3.4	4.3		1.6	2.0	2.4	2.7

SOURCE: I. Astrand, *Acta Physiologica Scandinavica* 49 (1960). Supplementum 169: 45–60.

Table 6.6 Age-Based Correction Factors for Maximal Oxygen Uptake

Age	Correction Factor	Age	Correction Factor	Age	Correction Factor	Age	Correction Factor	Age	Correction Factor	Age	Correction Factor
14	1.11	23	1.02	32	.909	41	.820	50	.750	59	.686
15	1.10	24	1.01	33	.896	42	.810	51	.742	60	.680
16	1.09	25	1.00	34	.883	43	.800	52	.734	61	.674
17	1.08	26	.987	35	.870	44	.790	53	.726	62	.668
18	1.07	27	.974	36	.862	45	.780	54	.718	63	.662
19	1.06	28	.961	37	.854	46	.774	55	.710	64	.656
20	1.05	29	.948	38	.846	47	.768	56	.704	65	.650
21	1.04	30	.935	39	.838	48	.762	57	.698		
22	1.03	31	.922	40	.830	49	.756	58	.692		

Adapted from I. Astrand, *Acta Physiologica Supplementum* 169: 45–60.

Table 6.7 12-Minute Swim Test Fitness Categories

Distance (yards)	Fitness Category
≥700	Excellent
500–700	Good
400–500	Average
200–400	Fair
≤200	Poor

Adapted from K. H. Cooper, *The Aerobics Program for Total Well-Being* (New York: Bantam Books, 1982).

Figure 6.6 Procedure for the 12-Minute Swim Test.

1. Enlist a friend to time the test. The only other requisites are a stopwatch and a swimming pool. Do not attempt to do this test in an unsupervised pool.
2. Warm up by swimming slowly and doing a few stretching exercises before taking the test.
3. Start the test and swim as many laps as possible in 12 minutes. Pace yourself throughout the test and do not swim to the point of complete exhaustion.
4. After completing the test, cool down by swimming another 2 or 3 minutes at a slower pace.
5. Determine the total distance you swam during the test and look up your fitness category in Table 6.7.

© Cengage Learning

Table 6.8 Cardiorespiratory Fitness Classification According to Maximal Oxygen Uptake (VO$_{2max}$)

Gender	Age	Fitness Category (based on VO$_{2max}$ in mL/kg/min)				
		Poor	Fair	Average	Good	Excellent
Men	<29	<24.9	25–33.9	34–43.9	44–52.9	>53
	30–39	<22.9	23–30.9	31–41.9	42–49.9	>50
	40–49	<19.9	20–26.9	27–38.9	39–44.9	>45
	50–59	<17.9	18–24.9	25–37.9	38–42.9	>43
	60–69	<15.9	16–22.9	23–35.9	36–40.9	>41
	≥70	≤12.9	13–20.9	21–32.9	33–37.9	≥38
Women	<29	<23.9	24–30.9	31–38.9	39–48.9	>49
	30–39	<19.9	20–27.9	28–36.9	37–44.9	>45
	40–49	<16.9	17–24.9	25–34.9	35–41.9	>42
	50–59	<14.9	15–21.9	22–33.9	34–39.9	>40
	60–69	<12.9	13–20.9	21–32.9	33–36.9	>37
	≥70	≤11.9	12–19.9	20–30.9	31–34.9	≥35

High physical fitness standard   Health fitness standard

NOTE: See the Chapter 1 discussion on health fitness versus physical fitness.

© Cengage Learning

Monitoring heart rate on the carotid artery during the Astrand-Ryhming Test.

Activity 6.1: Cardiorespiratory Endurance Test Results

Name _____ Date _____

Course _____ Section _____ Gender _____ Age _____

NECESSARY EQUIPMENT
1.5-Mile Run: School track or premeasured course and a stopwatch.
1.0-Mile Walk Test: School track or premeasured course and a stopwatch.
STEP TEST: A bench or gymnasium bleachers 16¼ inches high, a metronome, and a stopwatch.
ASTRAND-RYHMING TEST: A bicycle ergometer that allows for regulation of workloads in kilopounds per meter (or watts) and a stopwatch.
12-MINUTE SWIM TEST: Swimming pool and a stopwatch.

OBJECTIVE
To estimate maximal oxygen uptake (VO_{2max}) and cardiorespiratory endurance classification.

PREPARATION
Wear appropriate exercise clothing including jogging shoes and a swimsuit if required. Be prepared to take the 1.0-Mile Walk Test, the Step Test, the Astrand–Ryhming Test, the 1.5-Mile Run Test, and/or the 12-Minute Swim Test. If more than one test will be conducted, perform them in the order just listed and allow at least 15 minutes between tests. Avoid vigorous physical activity 24 hours prior to this activity.

I. 1.5-Mile Run Test

1.5-Mile Run Time: _____ min and _____ sec VO_{2max} (see Table 6.2, page 203): _____ mL/kg/min

Cardiorespiratory Fitness Category (Table 6.8, page 208): _____

II. 1.0-Mile Walk Test

Weight (W) = _____ lbs   Gender (G) = _____ (female = 0, male = 1)   Time = _____ min and _____ sec

Heart Rate (HR) = _____ bpm

Time in minutes (T) = min + (sec ÷ 60) or T = _____ + (_____ ÷ 60) = _____ min

$VO_{2max} = 88.768 - (0.0957 \times W) + (8.892 \times G) - (1.4537 \times T) - (0.1194 \times HR)$

$VO_{2max} = 88.768 - (0.0957 \times \_\_\_\_) + (8.892 \times \_\_\_\_) - (1.4537 \times \_\_\_\_) - (0.1194 \times \_\_\_\_)$

$VO_{2max} = 88.768 - (\_\_\_\_) + (\_\_\_\_) - (\_\_\_\_) - (\_\_\_\_) = \_\_\_\_$ mL/kg/min

Cardiorespiratory Fitness Category (Table 6.8, page 208): _____

III. Step Test

15-second recovery heart rate: _____ beats VO_{2max} (Table 6.3, page 205): _____ mL/kg/min

Cardiorespiratory Fitness Category (Table 6.8, page 208): _____

IV. Astrand–Ryhming Test

Weight (W) = _____ lbs   Weight (BW) in kilograms = (W ÷ 2.2046) = _____ kg   Workload = _____ kpm

Exercise Heart Rates	Time to count 30 beats	Heart Rate (bpm) (from Table 6.4, page 207)		Time to count 30 beats	Heart Rate (bpm) (from Table 6.4, page 207)
First minute:			Fourth minute:		
Second minute:			Fifth minute:		
Third minute:			Sixth minute:		

Average heart rate for the fifth and sixth minutes = _____ bpm

VO_{2max} in L/min (Table 6.5, page 207) = _____ L min   Correction factor (from Table 6.6, page 208) = _____

Corrected VO_{2max} = VO_{2max} in L/min × correction factor = _____ × _____ = _____ L/min

VO_{2max} in mL/kg/min = corrected VO_{2max} in L/min × 1000 ÷ BW in kg = _____ × 1000 ÷ _____ = _____ mL/kg/min

Cardiorespiratory Fitness Category (Table 6.8, page 208): _____

V. 12-Minute Swim Test

Distance swum in 12 minutes: _____ yards

Cardiorespiratory Fitness Category (Table 6.7, page 208): _____

VI. What I Learned and Where I Go from Here:

1. Interpret the results of your cardiorespiratory endurance test(s). Indicate the cardiorespiratory fitness classification you would like to achieve by the end of the term and explain how you are planning to achieve this goal.

2. Briefly discuss the advantages and disadvantages of the cardiorespiratory endurance tests used in this activity.

Activity 6.2: Exercise Readiness Questionnaire

Name _____ Date _____

Course _____ Section _____ Gender _____ Age _____

> Carefully read each statement and circle the number that best describes your feelings in each statement. Please be completely honest with your answers.

I.	Strongly Agree	Mildly Agree	Mildly Disagree	Strongly Disagree
1. I can walk, ride a bike (or use a wheelchair), swim, or walk in a shallow pool.	4	3	2	1
2. I enjoy exercise.	4	3	2	1
3. I believe exercise can help decrease the risk for disease and premature mortality.	4	3	2	1
4. I believe exercise contributes to better health.	4	3	2	1
5. I have previously participated in an exercise program.	4	3	2	1
6. I have experienced the feeling of being physically fit.	4	3	2	1
7. I can envision myself exercising.	4	3	2	1
8. I am contemplating an exercise program.	4	3	2	1
9. I am willing to stop contemplating and give exercise a try for a few weeks.	4	3	2	1
10. I am willing to set aside time at least three times a week for exercise.	4	3	2	1
11. I can find a place to exercise (the streets, a park, a YMCA, a health club).	4	3	2	1
12. I can find other people who would like to exercise with me.	4	3	2	1
13. I will exercise when I am moody, fatigued, and even when the weather is bad.	4	3	2	1
14. I am willing to spend a small amount of money for adequate exercise clothing (shoes, shorts, leotards, swimsuit).	4	3	2	1
15. If I have any doubts about my present state of health, I will see a physician before beginning an exercise program.	4	3	2	1
16. Exercise will make me feel better and improve my quality of life.	4	3	2	1

Scoring Your Test:

This questionnaire allows you to examine your readiness for exercise. You have been evaluated in four categories: mastery (self-control), attitude, health, and commitment. Mastery indicates that you can be in control of your exercise program. Attitude examines your mental disposition toward exercise. Health measures the strength of your convictions about the wellness benefits of exercise. Commitment shows dedication and resolution to carry out the exercise program. Write the number you circled after each statement in the corresponding spaces below. Add the scores on each line to get your totals. Scores can vary from 4 to 16. A score of 12 and above is a strong indicator that that factor is important to you, and 8 and below is low. If you score 12 or more points in each category, your chances of initiating and adhering to an exercise program are good. If you fail to score at least 12 points in three categories, your chances of succeeding at exercise may be slim. You need to be better informed about the benefits of exercise, and a retraining process may be required.

Mastery: 1. _____ + 5. _____ + 6. _____ + 9. _____ = _____

Attitude: 2. _____ + 7. _____ + 8. _____ + 13. _____ = _____

Health: 3. _____ + 4. _____ + 15. _____ + 16. _____ = _____

Commitment: 10. _____ + 11. _____ + 12. _____ + 14. _____ = _____

Activity 6.3: Behavior Modification Plan for Cardiorespiratory Endurance

Name _____ Date _____

Course _____ Section _____ Gender _____ Age _____

I. Advantages and Disadvantages of Starting an Exercise Program

Advantages: _____
_____
_____
_____
_____

Disadvantages: _____
_____
_____
_____
_____
_____

II. Stage of Change for Cardiorespiratory Endurance Exercise

Using Figure 2.5 (page 63) and Table 2.3 (page 62), identify your current stage of change in regard to participation in a cardiorespiratory endurance exercise program: [   ]

III. Processes and Techniques for Change

Identify the processes of change (Table 2.1, page 56) that may help you implement a cardiorespiratory endurance exercise program and list a minimum of three techniques (Table 2.2, page 62) that you will use with each process of change.

Advantages: _____
_____
_____
_____
_____

Disadvantages: _____
_____
_____
_____
_____
_____

Next you will have to decide positively that you will try. Using Activity 6.3, you can list the advantages and disadvantages of incorporating exercise into your lifestyle. Your list might include advantages such as:

- It will make me feel better.
- I will lose weight.
- I will have more energy.
- It will lower my risk for chronic diseases.

Your list of disadvantages might include the following:

- I don't want to take the time.
- I'm too out of shape.
- There's no good place to exercise.
- I don't have the willpower to do it.

When your reasons for exercising outweigh your reasons for not exercising, you will find it easier to try. In Activity 6.3 you will also determine your stage of change for aerobic exercise. Using the information learned in Chapter 2, you can outline specific processes and techniques for change (also see the example in Chapter 9, pages 330-332).

6.6 Guidelines for CR Exercise Prescription

In spite of the release of the U.S. Surgeon General's statement on physical activity and health in 1996 indicating that regular moderate physical activity provides substantial health benefits[3] and the overwhelming evidence validating the benefits of exercise on health, longevity, and quality of life, the majority of adults in the United States still do not meet the minimum recommendations for the improvement and maintenance of CR fitness. According to the most recent survey released in 2013 by the Centers for Disease Control and Prevention (CDC), overall, only 46.1 percent of adults (50.4 percent of men and 42.1 percent of women) in the U. S. meet the 2008 federal guidelines for aerobic physical activity. Furthermore, almost 34 percent did not engage in any leisure-time physical activities.

Most people are not familiar with the basic principles of CR exercise prescription. Thus, although they exercise regularly, they do not reap significant improvements in CR endurance.

To develop the CR system, the heart muscle has to be overloaded like any other muscle in the human body. Just as the biceps muscle in the upper arm is developed through strength-training exercises, the heart muscle has to be exercised to increase in size, strength, and efficiency. To better understand how the CR system can be developed, you have to be familiar with the different variables that govern exercise prescription.[4]

First, however, you should be aware that the ACSM recommends that individuals with two or more risk factors for cardiovascular disease (men 45 or older and women 55 or older, family history, cigarette smoking, sedentary lifestyle, obesity, high blood pressure, high LDL cholesterol, low HDL cholesterol [see Chapter 10], or prediabetes) get a medical exam prior to **vigorous exercise**.[5] They may, however, initiate a light-to-moderate intensity exercise program without medical clearance. The ACSM has defined vigorous exercise as exercise intensity greater than 60 percent of maximal capacity. For individuals initiating an exercise program, this intensity is the equivalent of exercise that "substantially increases heart rate and breathing." Anyone at high risk, symptomatic, or diagnosed with disease should undergo a medical examination prior to initiating even a moderate exercise program (one that noticeably increases heart rate and breathing or between 40 percent and 60 percent of maximal capacity).

For exercise prescription purposes, the ACSM uses the **FITT-VP** principle. This acronym stands for Frequency, Intensity, Time (duration), Type (mode), Volume, and Progression. A discussion of each of these variables follows. For practicability and ease of understanding, the variables are discussed in a different order.

Intensity of Exercise

When trying to develop the CR system, many people ignore **intensity** of exercise. For muscles to develop, they have to be overloaded to a given point. The training stimulus to develop the biceps muscle, for example, can be accomplished with arm curl exercises with increasing weights. Likewise, the CR system is stimulated by making the heart pump faster for a specified period.

Health and CR fitness benefits result when the person is working between 30 and 90 percent of **heart rate reserve (HRR)** combined with an appropriate duration and frequency of training (see how to calculate intensity, on page 214).[6] Health benefits are achieved when training at a lower exercise intensity, that is, between 30 and 60 percent of the person's HRR. Even greater health and cardioprotective benefits, and higher and faster improvements in CR fitness (VO_{2max}), however, are achieved primarily through vigorous-intensity programs.[7]

Most people who initiate exercise programs have a difficult time adhering to vigorous-intensity exercise. Thus, unconditioned individuals (those in the "poor" CR fitness category) and older adults should start at a 30 to 40 percent training intensity (TI). For persons in "fair" fitness, training is recommended between 40 and 50 percent TI. For those in the "average" category, a 50 to 60 percent TI is recommended. Active and fit people in the "good" category should exercise between 60 and 70 percent TI, while active persons in the "excel-

> **Vigorous exercise** CR exercise that requires an intensity level of approximately 70 percent of capacity.
>
> **FITT-VP** An acronym used to describe the cardiorespiratory exercise prescription variables: frequency, intensity, time (duration), type (mode), volume, and progression.
>
> **Intensity** In cardiorespiratory exercise, how hard a person has to exercise to improve or maintain fitness.
>
> **Heart rate reserve (HRR)** The difference between maximal heart rate and resting heart rate.

lent" fitness category can exercise at the higher TIs between 70 and 90 percent.

Following 4 to 8 weeks of progressive training (depending on your starting TI) at light to moderate (30 to 60 percent) intensities, exercise can be performed between 60 and 90 percent TI. Increases in VO_{2max} are accelerated when the heart is working closer to 90 percent of HRR. Exercise training greater than 90 percent is recommended only for healthy, performance-oriented individuals and competitive athletes. For most people, training greater than 90 percent is discouraged to avoid potential cardiovascular problems associated with very-hard-intensity exercise. As intensity increases, exercise adherence decreases and the risk of orthopedic injuries increases.

Intensity of exercise can be calculated easily, and training can be monitored by checking your pulse. To determine the intensity of exercise or **cardiorespiratory training zone** according to heart rate reserve, follow these steps (also refer to Activity 6.4):

1. Estimate your maximal heart rate (MHR)* according to the following formula[8]:

   $$MHR = 207 - (.7 \times age)$$

2. Check your resting heart rate (RHR) for a full minute in the evening, after you have been sitting quietly for about 30 minutes reading or watching a relaxing TV show. As explained on page 203, you can check your pulse on the wrist by placing two or three fingers over the radial artery or in the neck, using the carotid artery.

3. Determine the heart rate reserve (HRR) by subtracting the resting heart rate from the maximal heart rate:

   $$HRR = MHR - RHR$$

4. Calculate the TIs at 30, 40, 50, 60, 70, and 90 percent. Multiply the heart rate reserve by the respective .30, .40, .50, .60, and .90, and then add the resting heart rate to all four of these figures (e.g., 60% TI = HRR × .60 + RHR).

Example. The 30, 40, 50, 60, 70, and 90 percent TIs for a 20-year-old with a resting heart rate of 68 bpm would be as follows:

MHR: 207 − (.70 × 20) = 193 bpm
RHR = 68 bpm
HRR = 193 − 68 = 125 beats
30% TI = (125 × .30) + 68 = 106 bpm
40% TI = (125 × .40) + 68 = 118 bpm
50% TI = (125 × .50) + 68 = 131 bpm
60% TI = (125 × .60) + 68 = 143 bpm
70% TI = (125 × .70) + 68 = 155 bpm
90% TI = (125 × .90) + 68 = 181 bpm

*Research indicates that the traditional equation of 220 − age overpredicts MHR in people 40 years and younger and underpredicts MHR in older individuals.

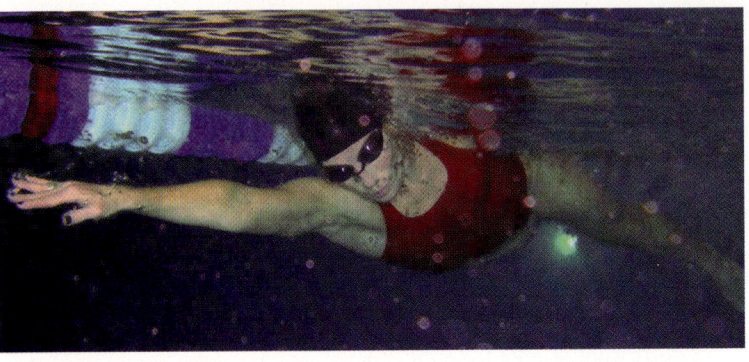

Only those with swimming skill and proper conditioning should take the 12-Minute Swimming Test.

Light-intensity CR training zone: 106 to 118 bpm
Moderate-intensity CR training zone: 118 to 143 bpm
Vigorous-intensity CR training zone: 143 to 181 bpm

Once you reach the vigorous-intensity CR training zone, continue to exercise between the 60 and 90 TIs to further improve or maintain your CR fitness (see Figure 6.7).

Following a few weeks of training, you may have a considerably lower resting heart rate (10 to 20 beats fewer in 8 to 12 weeks). Therefore, you should recompute your target zone periodically. You can compute your own CR training zone using Activity 6.4. Once you have reached an ideal level of CR endurance, frequent training in the 60 to 90 percent range will allow you to maintain your fitness level.

Moderate- versus Vigorous-Intensity Exercise

As fitness programs became popular in the 1970s, vigorous-intensity exercise (about 70 percent TI) was routinely prescribed for all fitness participants. Following extensive research in the late 1980s and 1990s, we learned that moderate-intensity physical activity (about 50 percent TI) provided many health benefits, including decreased risk for cardiovascular mortality; a statement endorsed by the U.S. Surgeon General in 1996.[9] Thus, the emphasis switched from vigorous- to moderate-intensity training in the late 1990s. In the 1996 report, the surgeon general also stated that vigorous-intensity exercise would provide even greater benefits. Limited attention, however, was paid to this recommendation.

Vigorous-intensity programs yield higher improvements in VO_{2max} than do moderate-intensity programs, especially in people with higher fitness levels.[10] Furthermore, a comprehensive review of research articles looking at the protective benefits of physical fitness versus weekly amount of physical activity found that higher levels of aerobic fitness are associated with a lower incidence of cardiovascular disease (see Figure 6.8), even when the duration of moderate-intensity activity is prolonged to match the energy expenditure performed during a shorter vigorous-

> **Cardiorespiratory training zone** Recommended training intensity range, in terms of exercise heart rate, to obtain adequate cardiorespiratory endurance development.

Figure 6.7 Recommended cardiorespiratory or aerobic training pattern.

Health and Fitness Apps

An app is an application, or computer software, designed to help the user perform a specific task related to accounting, graphics, office suites, education, media, or music and entertainment, among others. In the fitness industry, apps are available for a variety of exercise programs, weight loss, and nutrition, as well as to track workouts (exercise logs). Be careful, however, when selecting apps. Many people are designing apps with limited or no knowledge in the related field. When it comes to fitness, one size doesn't fit all, because fitness levels and needs vary widely among participants. An instructor or personal trainer may be a better option when getting started. If you are looking for apps, search for those designed by health experts who hold degrees and certifications in the related field. A good place to start is the government's app store (apps.usa.gov) that lists apps designed by experts. Furthermore, the U.S. Surgeon General ran an app health challenge contest in 2012. The winners were selected from among apps that provide tailored health information and empower users to engage in and enjoy healthy behavior. The winners were

- Lose it! in the category of fitness/physical activity
- GoodGuide and Fooducate in the category of nutrition/healthy eating
- Healthy Habits in the category of integrative health
- Additionally, Fit Friendzy and MapMyFitness were also recommended for fitness/physical activity.

As a consumer, you are strongly encouraged to research available apps and search for the best that fit your interests but still follow recommended exercise guidelines by leading national health, fitness, and sports medicine organizations.

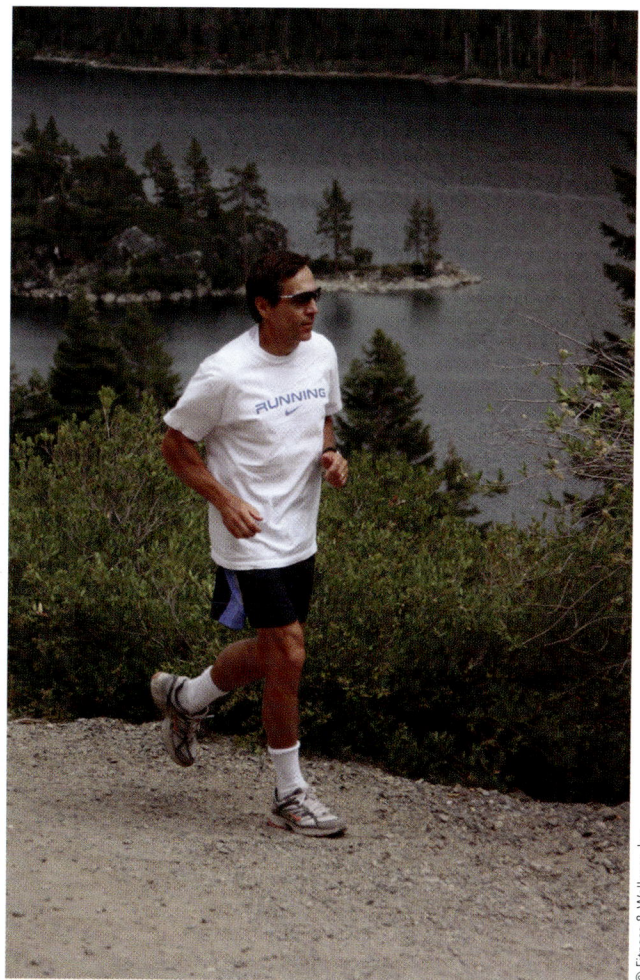

Vigorous-intensity aerobic exercise is required to achieve the high physical fitness standard (excellent category) for cardiorespiratory endurance.

intensity effort.[11] The results showed that persons who accumulate the greatest amount of weekly physical activity (100th percentile rank in Figure 6.8) have a 28 percent reduction in the risk of cardiovascular disease, whereas the individuals with the highest level of aerobic fitness (also see 100th percentile rank in Figure 6.8) reduce their risk by 64 percent, more than twice the level of risk reduction in the most active group.

Another review of several clinical studies substantiated that vigorous-intensity-exercise, compared with moderate-intensity exercise, leads to better improvements in coronary heart disease risk factors, including aerobic endurance, blood pressure, and blood glucose control.[12] As a result, the pendulum is again swinging toward vigorous intensity because of the added aerobic benefits, greater protection against disease, and larger energy expenditure that helps with weight management.

Monitoring Exercise Heart Rate

During the first few weeks of an exercise program, you should monitor your exercise heart rate regularly to make sure you are training in the proper zone. Wait until you are about five minutes into the aerobic phase of your exercise session before taking your first reading. When you check your heart rate, count your pulse for 10 seconds, then multiply by six to get the per minute pulse rate. The exercise heart rate will remain at the same level for about 15 seconds following aerobic exercise, then drops rapidly. Do not hesitate to stop during your exercise bout to check your pulse. If the rate is too low, increase the intensity of exercise. If the rate is too high, slow down.

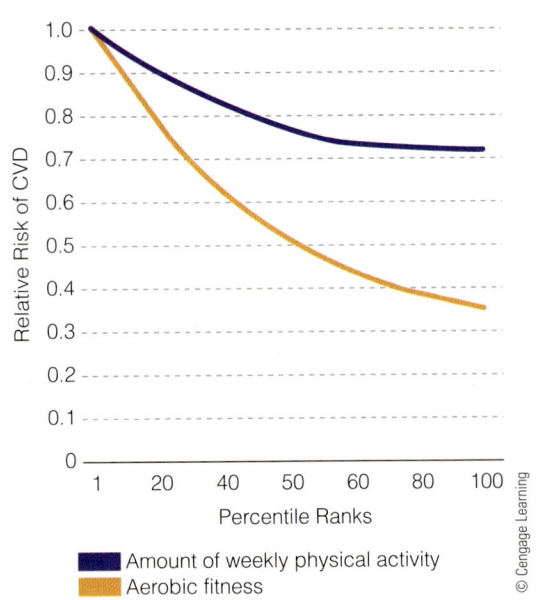

Figure 6.8 Relative risk of cardiovascular disease (CVD) based on weekly volume of physical activity and aerobic fitness.

When determining the TI for your own program, you need to consider your personal fitness goals and possible cardiovascular risk factors. Individuals who exercise at around the 50 percent TI still reap significant health benefits—in particular, improvements in the metabolic profile (see "Health Fitness Standards" in Chapter 1, page 21). Training at this lower percentage, however, may place you in only the "average" (moderate fitness) category (see Table 6.8). Exercising at this lower intensity will not allow you to achieve a "good" or "excellent" CR endurance fitness rating (the physical fitness standard). The latter ratings, and even greater health benefits, are obtained by exercising closer to the 90 percent threshold.

Rate of Perceived Exertion

Because many people do not check their heart rate during exercise, an alternative method of prescribing intensity of exercise has been devised using the **physical activity perceived exertion (H-PAPE) scale** (Figure 6.9). This scale uses phrases based on common terminology used in physical activity and exercise prescription guidelines. Using the scale, a person subjectively rates the perceived exertion or difficulty of exercise when training at different intensity levels. The exercise heart rate then is associated with the corresponding perceived exertion phrase provided.

For example, if training between 143 (60% TI) and 155 (70% TI) bpm, the person may associate this with training between "somewhat hard" and "vigorous." Some individuals perceive less exertion than others when training at a certain intensity level. Therefore, you have to associate your own inner perception of the task with the phrases given on the scale. You then may proceed to exercise at that rate of perceived exertion.

Be sure to crosscheck your target zone with your perceived exertion during the first weeks of your exercise program. To help you develop this association, you should regularly keep a record of your activities, using the form provided in Activity 6.5. After several weeks of training, you should be able to predict your exercise heart rate just by your own perceived exertion of the intensity of exercise.

Whether you monitor the intensity of exercise by checking your pulse or through the H-PAPE rate, you should be aware that changes in normal exercise conditions will affect the TI. For example, exercising on a hot, humid day or at high altitude increases the heart rate response to a given task, requiring adjustments in the intensity of your exercise.

Mode (Type) of Exercise

The **mode**, or type, of exercise that develops the CR system has to be aerobic in nature. Once you have established your CR training zone, any activity or combination of activities that will get

> **Physical activity perceived exertion (H-PAPE)** A perception scale to monitor or interpret the intensity of aerobic exercise.
>
> **Mode** Form or type of exercise.

Chapter 6 Cardiorespiratory Endurance   217

Activity 6.4: Personalized Cardiorespiratory Exercise Prescription

Name _____ Date _____

Course _____ Section _____ Gender _____ Age _____

I. Intensity of Exercise

1. Estimate your own maximal heart rate (MHR)

   MHR = 207 − (.70 × age)

   MHR = 207 − (.70 × [____]) = [____] bpm

2. Resting Heart Rate (RHR). Determine your RHR by counting your pulse for a full minute in the evening after you have been sitting quietly, reading, or watching a relaxing TV show.

   RHR = [____] bpm

3. Heart Rate Reserve (HRR) = MHR − RHR

   HRR = [____] − [____] = [____] beats

4. Training Intensities (TI) = HRR × TI + RHR

   30 Percent TI = [____] × .30 + [____] = [____] bpm
   40 Percent TI = [____] × .40 + [____] = [____] bpm
   50 Percent TI = [____] × .50 + [____] = [____] bpm
   60 percent TI = [____] × .60 + [____] = [____] bpm
   70 percent TI = [____] × .70 + [____] = [____] bpm
   85 Percent TI = [____] × .90 + [____] = [____] bpm

5. Current cardiorespiratory fitness category (see Activity 6.1, pp. 209–210): [____]

   Cardiorespiratory Training Zone: unconditioned individuals, persons in the poor cardiorespiratory fitness category, and older adults starting an exercise program should use a 30 to 40 percent TI. Individuals in fair and average fitness are encouraged to exercise between 40 and 60 percent TI. Active individuals in the good or excellent categories should exercise between 60 and 90 percent TI.

   Light-intensity cardiorespiratory training zone (30% to 40% TI): [____] to [____] bpm

   Moderate-intensity cardiorespiratory training zone (40% to 60% TI): [____] to [____] bpm

   Vigorous-intensity cardiorespiratory training zone (60% to 90% TI): [____] to [____] bpm

II. Mode of Exercise

Select any activity or combination of activities that you enjoy doing. The activity has to be continuous in nature and must get your heart rate up to the cardiorespiratory training zone and keep it there for as long as you exercise. Indicate your preferred mode(s) of exercise:

1. [____]   2. [____]   3. [____]
4. [____]   5. [____]   6. [____]

III. Cardiorespiratory Exercise Program

The following is your weekly program for development of cardiorespiratory endurance. If you are in the poor or fair cardiorespiratory fitness category, start with week 1. If you are in the average category, you may start at week 5. If you are already active and in the good or excellent category, you may start at week 9 (otherwise start at week 5). After completing the goal for week 12, you can maintain fitness by training between a 70 and 85 percent TI for about 20 to 30 minutes, a minimum of three times per week, on nonconsecutive days. You should also recompute your TIs periodically because you will experience a significant reduction in resting heart rate with aerobic training (approximately 10 to 20 beats in 8 to 12 weeks).

Week	Duration (min)	Frequency	Training Intensity	Heart Rate (bpm)	Physical Activity Perceived Exertion*
1	15	3	Between 30% and 40%	☐ to ☐	☐ to ☐ beats
2	15	4	Between 30% and 40%		
3	20	4	Between 30% and 40%		
4	20	5	Between 30% and 40%		
5	20	4	Between 40% and 60%	☐ to ☐	☐ to ☐ beats
6	20	5	Between 40% and 60%		
7	30	4	Between 40% and 60%		
8	30	5	Between 40% and 60%		
9	30	4	Between 60% and 90%	☐ to ☐	☐ to ☐ beats
10	30	5	Between 60% and 90%		
11	30–40	5	Between 60% and 90%		
12	30–40	5	Between 60% and 90%		

*See Figure 6.9, page 219.

Maintenance cardiorespiratory training zone (60% to 90% TI): ☐ to ☐ bpm

IV. Briefly State Your Experiences and Feelings Regarding Aerobic Exercise:

V. Monitoring Daily Physical Activity

What is your average total number of daily steps (use a 7-day average): ☐

Do you accumulate 10,000 steps on most days of the week (at least five days)? ☐ Yes ☐ No

Figure 6.9 Physical activity perceived exertion scale.

The H-PAPE (Hoeger-Physical Activity Perceived Exertion) Scale provides a subjective rating of the perceived exertion or difficulty of physical activity and exercise when training at a given intensity level. The intensity level is associated with the corresponding perceived exertion phrase provided. These phrases are based on common terminology used in physical activity and exercise prescription guidelines.

Perceived exertion	Training intensity
Light	40%
Moderate	50%
Somewhat hard	60%
Vigorous	70%
Hard	80%
Very hard	90%
All-out effort	100%

SOURCE: Adapted from Hoeger, Werner W. K. "Training for a Walkathon," *Diabetes Self-Management* 24 no. 4 (2007): 56-68.

your heart rate up to that zone and keep it there for as long as you exercise will give you adequate development. Examples of these activities are walking, jogging, elliptical training, aerobics, water aerobics, road cycling, spinning, stair climbing, and stationary jogging or cycling. The latter activities require little skill to perform and can be enjoyed by most adults to improve health and fitness. Other aerobic activities such as swimming, cross-country skiing, mountain cycling, rope skipping, racquetball, basketball, and soccer can also be used and are recommended for individuals who already possess the skills to perform these activities or have adequate fitness to learn the necessary skills to safely perform the activity.

Aerobic exercise has to involve the major muscle groups of the body, and it has to be rhythmic and continuous. As the amount of muscle mass involved during exercise increases, so do the demands on the CR system. The activity you choose should be based on your personal preferences, what you most enjoy doing, and your physical limitations. Low-impact activities greatly reduce the risk for injuries. Most injuries to beginners result from high-impact activities. Also, general strength conditioning (see Chapter 7) is recommended prior to initiating an aerobic exercise program for individuals who have been inactive. Strength conditioning can significantly reduce the incidence of injuries.

The amount of strength or flexibility you develop through various activities differs. In terms of CR development, though, the heart doesn't know whether you are walking, swimming, or cycling. All the heart knows is that it has to pump at a certain rate, and as long as that rate is in the desired range, your CR fitness will improve. From a health fitness point of view, training in the lower end of the CR zone will yield substantial health benefits. The closer the heart rate is to the higher end of the CR training zone, however, the greater will be the health benefits and improvements in VO_{2max} (high physical fitness).

Because of the specificity of training, to ascertain changes in fitness, it is recommended that you use the same mode of exercise for training and testing. If your primary mode of training is cycling, it is recommended that you assess VO_{2max} using a bicycle test. For joggers, a field or treadmill running test is best. Swimmers should use a swim test.

Duration (Time) of Exercise The general recommendation is that a person exercise between 20 and 60 minutes per session. For vigorous-intensity exercise, a minimum of 75 total minutes per week is recommended, while those in a moderate-intensity program should accumulate at least 150 minutes per week.

The duration of exercise is based on how intensely a person trains. The variables are inversely related. If the training is done at around 90 percent, a session of 20 to 30 minutes is sufficient. At about 50 percent intensity, the person should train close to 60 minutes. As mentioned under "Intensity of Exercise," unconditioned people and older adults should train at lower percentages and, therefore, the activity should be carried out over a longer time.

Although the recommended guideline is 20 to 60 minutes of aerobic exercise per session, in the early stages of conditioning and for individuals who are pressed for time, accumulating 30 minutes or more of moderate-intensity physical activity throughout the day does provide health benefits. Three 10-minute exercise sessions per day (separated by at least 4 hours), at approximately 70 percent of maximal heart rate, have been shown to produce training benefits.[13] Although the increases in VO_{2max} with the latter program were not as large (57 percent) as those found in a group performing a continuous 30-minute bout of exercise per day, the researchers concluded that the accumulation of 30 minutes of moderate-intensity physical activity, conducted for *at least 10 minutes* 3 times per day, benefits the CR system significantly. Activity bouts of less than 10 minutes in duration do not count toward the 30-minute daily guideline.

Results of this and other similar studies are meaningful because people often mention lack of time as the reason they do not take part in an exercise program. Many think they have to exercise at least 20 continuous minutes to get any benefits at all. Even though 20 to 30 minutes of continuous vigorous-intensity activity is ideal, short, intermittent physical activity bouts, of at least 10 minutes long each, are beneficial to the CR system.

The 2008 Federal Guidelines for Physical Activity measure duration of exercise in terms of the total quantity of physical activity performed on a weekly basis. Two hours and 30 minutes (150 minutes) of moderate-intensity aerobic activity or 1 hour and 15 minutes (75 minutes) of vigorous-intensity aerobic activity per week, or an equivalent combination of the two are recommended (30 minutes of moderate-intensity twice per week combined with 20 minutes of vigorous-intensity another 2 times per week).

Two hours and 30 minutes per week represents the accumulation of 30 minutes of moderate-intensity aerobic activity (done in bouts of at least 10 minutes each) per session/day performed 5 days per week, whereas 1 hour and 15 minutes is approximately 25 minutes of vigorous-intensity aerobic activity done 3 times per week. The federal guidelines also indicate that 5 hours of moderate-intensity activity, or 2 hours and 30 minutes of vigorous-intensity activity per week provide additional benefits. Thus, when possible, people are encouraged to go beyond the minimum recommendation.

From a weight management point of view, the recommendation to prevent weight gain is for people to accumulate 60 minutes of moderate-intensity physical activity most days of the week,[14] whereas 60 to 90 minutes of daily moderate-intensity activity is necessary to prevent weight regain.[15] These recommendations are based on evidence that people who maintain healthy weight typically accumulate between 1 and 1½ hours of physical activity at least 5 times per week. The duration of exercise should be increased gradually to avoid undue fatigue and exercise-related injuries.

If lack of time is a concern, you should exercise at a vigorous intensity for about 30 minutes, which can burn as many calories as 60 minutes of moderate-intensity exercise (also see "The Role of Exercise Intensity and Duration in Weight Management," Chapter 5, page 168), but only 19 percent of adults in the United States typically exercise at a vigorous-intensity level. Novice and overweight exercisers also need proper conditioning prior to vigorous-intensity exercise to avoid injuries or cardiovascular-related problems.

Exercise sessions always should be preceded by a 5- to 10-minute **warm-up** and be followed by a 10-minute **cool-down** period (see Figure 6.7). The purpose of the warm-up is to aid in the transition from rest to exercise. A good warm-up increases extensibility of the muscles and connective tissue, extends joint range of motion, and enhances muscular activity. A warm-up consists of general calisthenics, mild stretching exercises, and walking/jogging/cycling for a few minutes at a lower intensity than the actual target zone. The concluding phase of the warm-up is a gradual increase in exercise intensity to the lower end of the target training zone.

In the cool-down, the intensity of exercise is decreased gradually to help the body return to near resting levels, followed by stretching and relaxation activities. Stopping abruptly causes blood to pool in the exercised body parts, diminishing the return of blood to the heart. Less blood return can cause a sudden drop in blood pressure, dizziness, and faintness, or it can bring on cardiac abnormalities. The cool-down phase also helps dissipate body heat and aid in removing the lactic acid produced during high-intensity exercise.

In its latest guidelines, the ACSM recommends at least 10 minutes of stretching exercises performed immediately following the warm-up phase (prior to exercising in the appropriate target zone) or after the cool-down phase. The purpose of stretching following either the warm-up or the cool-down phase is because warm muscles achieve a greater range of motion, thus helping enhance the flexibility program (discussed in Chapter 8). While two to three stretching sessions per week are recommended, near daily stretching is most effective.

Behavior Modification Planning

Tips for People Who Have Been Physically Inactive

I PLAN TO / **I DID IT**

- ❑ ❑ Take the sensible approach by starting slowly.
- ❑ ❑ Begin by choosing moderate-intensity activities you enjoy the most. By choosing activities you enjoy, you'll be more likely to stick with them.
- ❑ ❑ Gradually build up the time spent exercising by adding a few minutes every few days or so until you can comfortably perform a minimum recommended amount of exercise (20 minutes per day).
- ❑ ❑ As the minimum amount becomes easier, gradually increase either the length of time exercising or increase the intensity of the activity, or both.
- ❑ ❑ Vary your activities, both for interest and to broaden the range of benefits.
- ❑ ❑ Explore new physical activities.
- ❑ ❑ Reward and acknowledge your efforts.

Try It

Fill out the cardiorespiratory exercise prescription either in Activity 6.4 or online. In your Online Journal or class notebook, describe how well you implement these suggestions.

SOURCE: Adapted from: Centers for Disease Control and Prevention, Atlanta, 2013.

Frequency of Exercise

The recommended exercise **frequency** for aerobic exercise is three to five days per week. When performing vigorous-intensity exercise, three 20- to 30-minute exercise sessions per week, on nonconsecutive days, are sufficient to improve or maintain VO_{2max}. When exercising at a moderate intensity, 30 to 60 minutes five days per week are required. A combination of moderate- and vigorous-intensity exercises may also be used three to five days per week. Research indicates that when vigorous training is conducted more than five days a week, further improvements in VO_{2max} are minimal. Although endurance athletes often train six or seven days per week (often twice per day), their training programs are designed to increase training mileage to endure long-distance races (6 to 100 miles) at a high percentage of VO_{2max}, frequently at or greater than the **anaerobic threshold**.

Although three exercise sessions per week will maintain CR fitness, the importance of almost daily physical activity in preventing disease and enhancing quality of life has been pointed out clearly by the ACSM, the U.S. Centers for Disease Control and Prevention, and by the President's Council on Physical Fitness and Sports. These organizations along with the U.S. Surgeon General advocate at least 30 minutes of moderate-intensity physical activity on most (defined as five days per week) or preferably all days of the week. This routine has been promoted as an effective way to improve health and quality of life. Further, the Surgeon General states that no one, including older adults, is too old to enjoy the benefits of regular physical activity. Also, be aware that most of the benefits of exercise and activity diminish within two weeks of substantially decreased physical activity, and the benefits are completely lost within a few months of inactivity.

Excessive Sitting: A Deadly Proposition

As introduced in Chapter 1 under "Sitting Disease" (page 13), if you meet the guidelines and exercise five times per week, but spend most of your day sitting, your lifestyle may be voiding the health benefits of exercise. Our society, however, is primarily a sedentary society that lulls people into physical inactivity. Most Americans spend more than half their waking hours sitting. The research indicates that people who spend most of their day sitting have a greater risk of dying prematurely from all causes and an even greater risk of dying from cardiovascular disease.[16] The data further indicate that death rates are still high for people who spend most of their day sitting, even though they meet the current minimum moderate-physical activity recommendations (30 minutes, at least 5 times per week).[17] Thus, people are strongly encouraged to incorporate as many physical activities throughout the day, at least 10 minutes every waking hour of the day.

Exercise Volume

A relatively new concept, volume of exercise is the product of frequency, intensity, and duration. The recommended absolute minimum volume is an energy expenditure of 1,000 calories per week or the equivalent of 150 minutes of moderate-intensity exercise each week. Volume can also be measured using a pedometer and achieving 10,000 or more steps each day. This minimal amount of volume is essential to achieve health benefits. A minimum of 75 minutes of vigorous-intensity aerobic activity per week (conducted over three nonconsecutive days), along with at least 2 additional days of 30 minutes each of moderate-intensity physical activity are necessary for substantial fitness benefits.

Training volume is also used as an indicator of excessive exercise. Too much exercise and physical activity lead to overtraining, muscle soreness, undue fatigue, shortness of breath, and increase the risk for injury. Should you experience any adverse effects as a result of your physical activity/exercise program, downward adjustments are recommended to the exercise prescription, including the rate of exercise progression (discussed next).

Rate of Progression

How quickly an individual progresses through an exercise program depends on the person's health status, fitness status, exercise tolerance, training responses, and exercise program goals. Initially, only 3 weekly training sessions of 15 to 20 minutes are recommended to avoid excessive muscle soreness and musculoskeletal injuries. You may then increase the duration by 5 to 10 minutes per week and the frequency so that by the fourth or fifth week you are exercising five times per week (see Activity 6.4). Thereafter, you can adjust frequency, duration, and intensity of exercise until you reach your fitness and maintenance goals. All increases in FITT-VP variables should be gradual to minimize the risk of overtraining and injuries.

To sum up: Ideally, a person should engage in physical activity six or seven times per week. Based on the previous discussion, to reap both the high-fitness and health-fitness benefits of exercise, a person should do vigorous exercise three times per week for high fitness maintenance, and two to four additional times per week in moderate-intensity activities (see Figure 6.10) to maintain good health. Depending on the intensity of the activity and the health/fitness goals, all exercise sessions should last between 20 and 60 minutes. For adequate weight-management purposes, additional daily physical activity, up to 90 minutes, may be necessary. A summary of the CR exercise prescription guidelines according to the ACSM is provided in Figure 6.11.

> **Warm-up** Starting a workout slowly.
>
> **Cool-down** Tapering off an exercise session slowly.
>
> **Frequency** Number of times per week a person engages in exercise.
>
> **Anaerobic threshold** The highest percentage of the VO_{2max} at which an individual can exercise (maximal steady state) for an extended time without accumulating significant amounts of lactic acid (accumulation of lactic acid forces an individual to slow down the exercise intensity or stop altogether).

Figure 6.10 The physical activity pyramid.

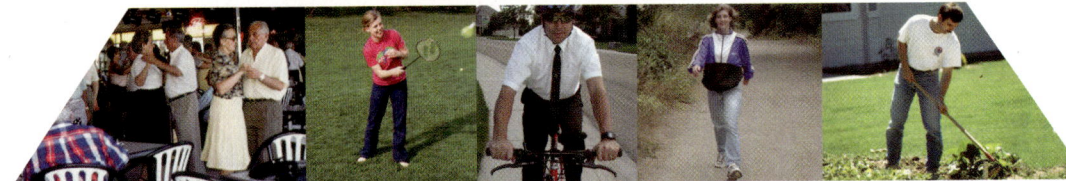

Minimize inactivity

Strength and flexibility: 2–3 days/week

Cardiorespiratory endurance: Exercise 20–60 minutes 3–5 days/week

Physical activity: Accumulate 60 to 90 minutes of moderate-intensity activity nearly every day.

© Cengage Learning
Photos © Fitness & Wellness, Inc.

6.7 Fitness Benefits of Aerobic Activities

The contributions of different aerobic activities to the health-related components of fitness vary. Although an accurate assessment of the contributions to each fitness component is difficult to establish, a summary of likely benefits of several activities is provided in Table 6.9. Instead of a single rating or number, ranges are given for some of the categories. The benefits derived are based on the person's effort while participating in the activity.

The nature of the activity often dictates the potential aerobic development. For example, jogging is much more strenuous than walking. The effort during exercise also affects the amount of physiological development. For example, during a low-impact aerobics routine, accentuating all movements (instead of just going through the motions) increases training benefits by orders of magnitude.

Table 6.9 indicates a starting fitness level for each aerobic activity. Attempting to participate in vigorous-intensity activities without proper conditioning often leads to injuries, not to mention discouragement. Beginners should start with light-intensity activities that carry a minimum risk for injuries.

In some cases, such as high-impact aerobics, the risk for orthopedic injuries remains high even if the participants are

Figure 6.11 Cardiorespiratory exercise prescription guidelines.

- Mode: Moderate- or vigorous-intensity aerobic activity (examples: walking, jogging, stair climbing, elliptical activity, aerobics, water aerobics, cycling, stair climbing, swimming, cross-country skiing, racquetball, basketball, and soccer)
- Intensity: 30% to 90% of heart rate reserve (the training intensity is based on age, health status, initial fitness level, exercise tolerance, and exercise program goals)
- Duration: Be active 20 to 90 minutes. At least 20 minutes of continuous vigorous-intensity or 30 minutes of moderate-intensity aerobic activity (the latter may be accumulated in segments of at least 10 minutes in duration each over the course of the day)
- Frequency: 3 to 5 days per week for vigorous-intensity aerobic activity to accumulate at least 75 minutes per week, or 5 days per week of moderate-intensity aerobic activity for a minimum total of 150 minutes weekly
- Rate of progression:
  - Start with three training sessions per week of 15 to 20 minutes
  - Increase the duration by 5 to 10 minutes per week and the frequency so that by the fourth or fifth week you are exercising five times per week
  - Progressively increase frequency, duration, and intensity of exercise until you reach your fitness goal prior to exercise maintenance

SOURCE: Adapted from American College of Sports Medicine, *ACSM's Guidelines for Exercise Testing and Prescription* (Philadelphia: Wolters Kluwer/Lippincott Williams & Wilkins, 2014).

Table 6.9 Ratings of Selected Aerobic Activities

Activity	Recommended Starting Fitness Level[1]	Injury Risk[2]	Potential Cardiorespiratory Endurance Development (VO_{2MAX})[3,4]	Upper Body Strength Development[3]	Lower Body Strength Development[3]	Upper Body Flexibility Development[3]	Lower Body Flexibility Development[3]	Weight Management[3]	MET Level[4,5,6]	Caloric Expenditure (cal/hour)[4,6]
Aerobics										
High-Impact Aerobics	A	H	3–4	2	4	3	2	4	6–12	450–900
Moderate-Impact Aerobics	I	M	2–4	2	3	3	2	3	6–12	450–900
Low-Impact Aerobics	B	L	2–4	2	3	3	2	3	5–10	375–750
Step Aerobics	I	M	2–4	2	3–4	3	2	3–4	5–12	375–900
Circuit Training	B	M	2–3	3–4	3–4	2	2–3	3–4	5–12	375–900
Cross-Country Skiing	B	M	4–5	4	4	2	2	4–5	8–16	600–1,200
Cross-Training	I	M	3–5	2–3	3–4	2–3	1–2	3–5	6–15	450–1,125
Cycling										
Road	I	M	2–5	1	4	1	1	3	6–12	450–900
Stationary	B	L	2–4	1	4	1	1	3	6–10	450–750
Functional Fitness	B	L	2–3	2–3	2–3	2–3	2–3	2–3	5–10	375–750
High-Intensity Interval Training	I	M	4–5	2	3–4	1	1	4–5	8–16	600–1,200
Jogging	I	M	3–5	1	3	1	1	5	6–15	450–1,125
Jogging, Deep Water	I	L	3–5	2	2	1	1	5	5–12	375–900
Racquet Sports	I	M	2–4	3	3	3	2	3	6–10	450–750
Rowing	B	L	3–5	4	2	3	1	4	8–14	600–1,050
Elliptical training/Stair Climbing	B	L	3–5	1	4	1	1	4–5	8–15	600–1,125
Strength Training	B	L	1	4–5	4–5	2–3	2–3	3–4	4–8	300–600
Swimming (front crawl)	B	L	3–5	4	2	3	1	3	6–12	450–900
Walking	B	L	1–2	1	2	1	1	3	4–6	300–450
Walking, Water, Chest-Deep	I	L	2–4	2	3	1	1	3	5–10	375–750
Water Aerobics	B	L	2–4	3	3	3	2	3	6–10	450–750
Yoga	B	L	1	1–2	1–2	3–5	3–5	1–3	4–8	300–600
Zumba	B	M	3–4	2	3	3	2	3–4	6–12	450–900

[1] B = Beginner, I = Intermediate, A = Advanced
[2] L = Low, M = Moderate, H = High
[3] 1 = Low, 2 = Fair, 3 = Average, 4 = Good, 5 = Excellent
[4] Varies according to the person's effort (intensity) during exercise.
[5] 1 MET represents the rate of energy expenditure at rest (3.5 mL/kg/min). Each additional MET is a multiple of the resting value. For example, 5 METs represents an energy expenditure equivalent to five times the resting value, or about 17.5 mL/kg/min.
[6] Varies according to body weight.
© Cengage Learning

adequately conditioned. These activities should be supplemental only and are not recommended as the sole mode of exercise. Most exercise-related injuries occur as a result of high-impact activities, not high intensity of exercise.

An alternative method of prescribing exercise intensity is through metabolic equivalents (**METs**). One MET represents the rate of energy expenditure at rest, that is, 3.5 mL/kg/min. METs are used to measure the intensity of physical activity and exercise in multiples of the resting metabolic rate. At an intensity level of 10 METs, the activity requires a 10-fold increase in the resting energy requirement (or approximately 35 mL/kg/min). MET levels for a given activity vary according to the effort expended. The MET range for various activities is included in Table 6.9. The harder a person exercises, the higher the MET level.

The effectiveness of various aerobic activities in weight management is charted in Table 6.9. As a general rule, the

> **MET** Short for metabolic equivalent, the rate of energy expenditure at rest; 1 MET is the equivalent of a VO_2 of 3.5 mL/kg/min.

Cross-country skiing requires more oxygen and energy than most other aerobic activities.

greater the muscle mass involved in exercise, the better the results. Rhythmic and continuous activities that involve large amounts of muscle mass are most effective in burning calories.

Vigorous-intensity activities increase caloric expenditure as well. Exercising longer, however, compensates for lower intensities. If carried out long enough (45 to 60 minutes 5 or 6 times per week), even walking can be a good exercise mode for weight management. Additional information on a comprehensive weight management program can be given in Chapter 5.

Critical Thinking

Mary started an exercise program last year as a means to lose weight and enhance her body image. She now runs about six miles every day, strength-trains daily, participates in step aerobics twice per week, and plays tennis or racquetball twice a week. Evaluate her program and make suggestions for improvements.

Getting Started and Adhering to a Lifetime Exercise Program Following the guidelines provided in Activity 6.4, you may proceed to initiate your own CR endurance program. If you have not been exercising regularly, you might begin by attempting to train 5 or 6 times a week for 30 minutes at a time. You might find this discouraging, however, and drop out before getting too far, because you will probably develop some muscle soreness and stiffness and possibly incur minor injuries. Muscle soreness and stiffness and the risk for injuries can be lessened or eliminated by increasing the intensity, duration, and frequency of exercise progressively, as outlined in Activity 6.4.

Once you have determined your exercise prescription, the difficult part begins: starting and sticking to a lifetime exercise program. Although you may be motivated after reading about the benefits to be gained from physical activity, lifelong dedication and perseverance are necessary to reap and maintain good fitness.

The first few weeks probably will be the most difficult for you, but where there's a will, there's a way. Once you begin to see positive changes, it won't be as hard. Soon you will develop a habit of exercising that will be deeply satisfying and will bring about a sense of self-accomplishment. The suggestions provided in the accompanying Behavior Modification Planning box (see page 224) have been used successfully to help change behavior and adhere to a lifetime exercise program.

6.8 A Lifetime Commitment to Fitness

The benefits of fitness can be maintained only through a regular lifetime program. Exercise is not like putting money in the bank. It doesn't help much to exercise four or five hours on Saturday and not do anything else the rest of the week. If anything, exercising only once a week is not safe for unconditioned adults.

Physically challenged people can participate and derive health and fitness benefits through a vigorous-intensity exercise program.

Behavior Modification Planning

Tips to Enhance Exercise Compliance

I PLAN TO / **I DID IT**

☐ ☐ 1. Set aside a regular time for exercise. If you don't plan ahead, it is a lot easier to skip. On a weekly basis, using red ink, schedule your exercise time into your day planner. Next, hold your exercise hour "sacred." Give exercise priority equal to the most important school or business activity of the day. If you are too busy, attempt to accumulate 30 to 60 minutes of daily activity by doing separate 10-minute sessions throughout the day. Try reading the mail while you walk, taking stairs instead of elevators, walking the dog, or riding the stationary bike as you watch the evening news.

☐ ☐ 2. Exercise early in the day, when you will be less tired and the chances of something interfering with your workout are minimal; thus, you will be less likely to skip your exercise session.

☐ ☐ 3. Select aerobic activities you enjoy. Exercise should be as much fun as your favorite hobby. If you pick an activity you don't enjoy, you will be unmotivated and less likely to keep exercising. Don't be afraid to try out a new activity, even if that means learning new skills.

☐ ☐ 4. Combine different activities. You can train by doing two or three different activities the same week. This cross-training may reduce the monotony of repeating the same activity every day. Try lifetime sports. Many endurance sports, such as racquetball, basketball, soccer, badminton, roller-skating, cross-country skiing, and body surfing (paddling the board), provide a nice break from regular workouts.

☐ ☐ 5. Use the proper clothing and equipment for exercise. A poor pair of shoes, for example, can make you more prone to injury, discouraging you from the beginning.

☐ ☐ 6. Find a friend or group of friends to exercise with. Social interaction will make exercise more fulfilling. Besides, exercise is harder to skip if someone is waiting to go with you.

☐ ☐ 7. Set goals and share them with others. Quitting is tougher when someone else knows what you are trying to accomplish. When you reach a targeted goal, reward yourself with a new pair of shoes or a jogging suit.

☐ ☐ 8. Purchase a pedometer (step counter) and build up to 10,000 steps per day. These 10,000 steps may include all forms of daily physical activity combined. Pedometers motivate people toward activity because they track daily activity, provide feedback on activity level, and remind the participant to enhance daily activity.

☐ ☐ 9. Don't become a chronic exerciser. Overexercising can lead to chronic fatigue and injuries. Exercise should be enjoyable, and in the process you should stop and smell the roses.

☐ ☐ 10. Exercise in different places and facilities. This will add variety to your workouts.

☐ ☐ 11. Exercise to music. People who listen to fast-tempo music tend to exercise more vigorously and longer. Using headphones when exercising outdoors, however, can be dangerous. Even indoors, it is preferable not to use headphones so that you are still aware of your surroundings.

☐ ☐ 12. Keep a regular record of your activities. Keeping a record allows you to monitor your progress and compare it against previous months and years (see Figure 6.11, page 222)

☐ ☐ 13. Conduct periodic assessments. Improving to a higher fitness category is often a reward in itself, and creating your own rewards is even more motivating.

☐ ☐ 14. Listen to your body. If you experience pain or unusual discomfort, stop exercising. Pain and aches are an indication of potential injury. If you do suffer an injury, don't return to your regular workouts until you are fully recovered. You may cross-train using activities that don't aggravate your injury (e.g., swimming instead of jogging).

☐ ☐ 15. If a health problem arises, see a physician. When in doubt, it's better to be safe than sorry.

Try It

The most difficult challenge about exercise is to keep going once you start. These behavioral change tips will enhance your chances for exercise adherence. In your Online Journal or class notebook, describe which suggestions were most useful.

Activity 6.5: Cardiorespiratory Exercise Record Form

Name: _____ Date: _____ Course: _____ Section: _____ Gender: _____ Age: _____

Month: _____

Date	Body Weight	Exercise HR	Type of Activity	Dist. in Miles	Time in Min.	H-PAPE*	Daily Steps
1							
2							
3							
4							
5							
6							
7							
8							
9							
10							
11							
12							
13							
14							
15							
16							
17							
18							
19							
20							
21							
22							
23							
24							
25							
26							
27							
28							
29							
30							
31							
						Total	

*Physical activity perceived exertion.

Month: _____

Date	Body Weight	Exercise HR	Type of Activity	Dist. in Miles	Time in Min.	H-PAPE*	Daily Steps
1							
2							
3							
4							
5							
6							
7							
8							
9							
10							
11							
12							
13							
14							
15							
16							
17							
18							
19							
20							
21							
22							
23							
24							
25							
26							
27							
28							
29							
30							
31							
						Total	

*Physical activity perceived exertion.

© Cengage Learning

Chapter 6 Cardiorespiratory Endurance 227

Name: _____ Date: _____ Course: _____ Section: _____ Gender: _____ Age: _____

Month: ☐

Date	Body Weight	Exercise HR	Type of Activity	Dist. in Miles	Time in Min.	H-PAPE*	Daily Steps
1							
2							
3							
4							
5							
6							
7							
8							
9							
10							
11							
12							
13							
14							
15							
16							
17							
18							
19							
20							
21							
22							
23							
24							
25							
26							
27							
28							
29							
30							
31							

Total

*Physical activity perceived exertion.
© Cengage Learning

Month: ☐

Date	Body Weight	Exercise HR	Type of Activity	Dist. in Miles	Time in Min.	H-PAPE*	Daily Steps
1							
2							
3							
4							
5							
6							
7							
8							
9							
10							
11							
12							
13							
14							
15							
16							
17							
18							
19							
20							
21							
22							
23							
24							
25							
26							
27							
28							
29							
30							
31							

Total

*Physical activity perceived exertion.

The time involved in losing the benefits of exercise varies among the different components of physical fitness and also depends on the person's condition before the interruption. In regard to CR endurance, it has been estimated that four weeks of aerobic training are completely reversed in two consecutive weeks of physical inactivity. But if you have been exercising regularly for months or years, two weeks of inactivity won't hurt you as much as it will someone who has exercised only a few weeks. As a rule, after 48 to 72 hours of aerobic inactivity, the CR system starts to lose some of its capacity.

To maintain fitness, you should keep up a regular exercise program, even during vacations. If you have to interrupt your program for reasons beyond your control, you should not attempt to resume training at the same level you left off but, rather, build up gradually again.

Even the greatest athletes on earth, if they were to stop exercising, would be, after just a few years, at about the same risk for disease as someone who has never done any physical activity. Staying with a physical fitness program long enough brings about positive physiological and psychological changes. Once you are there, you will not want to have it any other way.

ASSESS YOUR BEHAVIOR

CENGAGEbrain.com To access course materials, including companion resources, please visit www.cengagebrain.com.

1. Do you consciously attempt to incorporate as much physical activity as possible in your daily living (walk, take stairs, cycle, participate in sports and recreational activities)?
2. Are you accumulating at least 30 minutes of moderate-intensity physical activity over a minimum of five days per week?
3. Is aerobic exercise in the appropriate target zone a priority in your life a minimum of three times per week for at least 20 minutes per exercise session?
4. Do you own a pedometer and do you accumulate 10,000 or more steps on most days of the week?
5. Have you evaluated your aerobic fitness, and do you meet at least the health fitness category?

ASSESS YOUR KNOWLEDGE

Evaluate how well you understand the concepts presented in this chapter using the chapter-specific quizzing available in the online materials at www.cengagebrain.com.

1. CR endurance is determined by
   a. the amount of oxygen the body is able to utilize per minute of physical activity.
   b. the length of time it takes the heart rate to return to 120 bpm following the 1.5-Mile Run Test.
   c. the difference between the maximal heart rate and the resting heart rate.
   d. the product of the heart rate and blood pressure at rest versus exercise.
   e. the time it takes a person to reach a heart rate between 120 and 170 bpm during the Astrand-Ryhming test.

2. Which of the following is not a benefit of aerobic training?
   a. higher VO_{2max}
   b. increase in red blood cell count
   c. decrease in resting heart rate
   d. increase in heart rate at a given workload
   e. increase in functional capillaries

3. The VO_2 for a person with an exercise heart rate of 130, a stroke volume of 100, and an a-$\bar{v}O_{2diff}$ of 10 is
   a. 130,000 mL/kg/min.
   b. 1,300 L/min.
   c. 1.3 L/min.
   d. 130 mL/kg/min.
   e. 13 mL/kg/min.

4. The VO_2, in mL/kg/min, for a person with a VO_2 of 2.0 L/min who weighs 60 kilograms is
   a. 120.
   b. 26.5.
   c. 33.3.
   d. 30.
   e. 120,000.

5. The Step Test estimates VO_{2max} according to
   a. how long a person is able to sustain the proper Step Test cadence.
   b. the lowest heart rate achieved during the test.
   c. the recovery heart rate following the test.
   d. the difference between the maximal heart rate achieved and the resting heart rate.
   e. the exercise heart rate and the total stepping time.

6. An "excellent" CR fitness rating, in mL/kg/min, for young male adults is about
   a. 10.
   b. 20.
   c. 30.
   d. 40.
   e. 50.

7. How many minutes would a person training at 2.0 L/min have to exercise to burn the equivalent of one pound of fat?
   a. 700
   b. 350
   c. 120
   d. 60
   e. 20

8. The vigorous-intensity CR training zone for a 22-year-old individual with a resting heart rate of 68 bpm is
   a. 120 to 148.
   b. 132 to 156.
   c. 138 to 164.
   d. 146 to 179.
   e. 154 to 188.

9. Which of the following activities does not contribute to the development of CR endurance?
   a. light-impact aerobics
   b. jogging
   c. 400-yard dash
   d. racquetball
   e. All of these activities contribute to its development.

10. The recommended duration for each cardiorespiratory training session is
    a. 10 to 20 minutes.
    b. 15 to 30 minutes.
    c. 20 to 60 minutes.
    d. 45 to 70 minutes.
    e. 60 to 120 minutes.

Correct answers can be found at the back of the book.

Muscular Fitness: Strength and Endurance

7

Progressive resistance strength training provides significant improvements in functional capacity, fitness, health, self-esteem and self-confidence, and overall well-being.

Objectives

- **Explain** the importance of adequate muscular fitness in maintaining good health and well-being.
- **Clarify** misconceptions about strength fitness.
- **Define** muscular fitness, muscular strength, and muscular endurance.
- **Be able to assess** muscular strength and endurance and learn to interpret test results according to health fitness and physical fitness standards.
- **Identify** the factors that affect strength.
- **Understand** the principles of overload and specificity of training for strength development.
- **Learn** dietary guidelines for optimum strength development.
- **Become** familiar with core strength training and realize its importance for overall quality of life.
- **Become acquainted** with two distinct strength-training programs—with weights and without weights.
- **Chart** your achievements for strength tests.

CENGAGEbrain.com

Visit www.cengagebrain.com to access course materials and companion resources for this text, including quiz questions designed to check your understanding of the chapter contents. See the preface on page ix for more information.

FAQ

Which is more important for good health: aerobic fitness or muscular fitness?

They are both important. During the initial fitness boom in the 1970s and 1980s, the emphasis was almost exclusively on aerobic fitness. We now know that both aerobic fitness and muscular fitness (muscular strength and muscular endurance) contribute to health, overall fitness, work capacity, and overall quality of life. Among many health benefits, aerobic fitness is important in the prevention of cardiovascular diseases and some types of cancer, whereas muscular fitness will build strong muscles and bones, increase functional capacity, prevent osteoporosis and type 2 diabetes, and decrease the risk for low back pain and other musculoskeletal injuries.

Should I do aerobic exercise or strength training first?

Ideally, allow some recovery hours between the two types of training. If you can't afford the time, the training order should be based on your fitness goals and preferences. Unless extremely exhausting, aerobics provides a good lead into strength training. Excessive fatigue can lead to bad form while lifting and may result in injury. If your primary goal is strength development, lift first, as you'll be less fatigued and will end up with a more productive workout. On the other hand, if you are trying to develop the cardiorespiratory system or enhance caloric expenditure for weight-loss purposes, heavy lower body lifting will make it very difficult to sustain a good cardio workout thereafter. Thus, evaluate your goals, and select the training order accordingly.

Do big muscles turn into fat when the person stops training?

Muscle and fat tissue are two completely different types of tissue. Just as an apple will not turn into an orange, muscle tissue cannot turn into fat or vice versa. Muscle cells increase and decrease in size according to your training program. If you train quite hard, muscle cells increase in size. This increase is limited in women due to hormonal differences compared with men. When one stops training, muscle cells again decrease in size. If the person maintains a high caloric intake without physical training, however, fat cells will increase in size as weight (fat) is gained.

What strength-training exercises are best to get an abdominal "six-pack"?

Most men tend to store body fat around the waist, while women do so around the hips. There are, however, no "miracle" exercises to spot-reduce. Multiple sets of abdominal curl-ups, crunches, reverse crunches, or sit-ups performed three to five times per week will strengthen the abdominal musculature but will not be sufficient to allow the muscles to appear through the layer of fat between the skin and the muscles. The total energy (caloric) expenditure of a few sets of abdominal exercises will not be sufficient to lose a significant amount of weight (fat). If you want to get a "washboard stomach" (or, for women, achieve shapely hips), you need to engage in a moderate to vigorous aerobic and strength-training program combined with a moderate reduction in daily caloric intake (diet).

Real Life Story | Nathan's Experience

I started strength training two years ago because I wanted to get stronger and have a more muscular build. I got a membership to a gym near my house, and started using the free weights and machines there. The problem was, after a year of going off and on, I still didn't see the improvements I was hoping for. I then decided to take a strength training course at my college, and there I learned all the things that I had been doing wrong that had prevented me from getting results. My biggest mistake was that when I would go to the gym, I would try to do too much, working out for almost two hours, pushing myself to use heavy weights, and doing 20 different exercises. Afterwards, I would get very sore, and sometimes I wouldn't feel like going back to the gym for the rest of the week or even a couple weeks. So my workouts were off and on, and I was never consistent enough to really progress in the amount of weight I could lift. Another big mistake I made was that I didn't watch what I ate. In fact, since I had started to lift weights, I figured I could eat whatever I wanted, so I would go ahead and take an extra slice of pizza or two. The only thing I did, nutrition-wise, to try to help my efforts to get a stronger body was to buy a box of chocolate and peanut butter supplement bars that my gym sells and eat a couple a day. But my weight lifting teacher says that the ones I was buying were not much better than candy bars, and eating them in that amount was just causing me to take in way more sugar and calories than I needed. Once I changed my habits to work out moderately and consistently, to slowly increase the amount of weight I lift, and to support my routine with healthy meals and snacks, I really started to get the toned and muscular body I want!

Chapter 7 Muscular Fitness: Strength and Endurance

PERSONAL PROFILE: Personal Understanding of Muscular Fitness Concepts

I. Good muscular fitness (muscular strength and muscular endurance) is not a critical component for adequate health fitness. ___ Yes ___ No

II. Body weight may not drop or even increase as a result of a progressive resistance strength-training program, nonetheless, circumference measurements (inches) and percent body fat may decrease. ___ True ___ False
Can you explain why?

III. Performing at least one set within the repetition maximum (RM) zone for each exercise produces substantial strength development. ___ Yes ___ No

IV. A periodized strength-training program is frequently used to maximize muscular strength and endurance gains. ___ Yes ___ No

V. Single-joint exercises are more effective than multiple-joint exercises for strength development. ___ Yes ___ No

---

The benefits of **muscular fitness**, achieved through **strength training** or **resistance training**, on health and well-being are well documented. Muscular fitness, achieved through **progressive resistance training**, involves both muscular strength and muscular endurance, with the corresponding improvements in muscle tone and power.

The need for muscular fitness is not confined to highly trained athletes, fitness enthusiasts, and individuals who have jobs that require heavy muscular work. All people need adequate muscular fitness for good health, improved functional capacity, and a better quality of life. Unfortunately, according to the 2013 survey released by the Centers for Disease Control and Prevention (CDC), only 27 percent of men and 19 percent of women met the 2008 Federal Physical Activity Guidelines for muscular fitness. Worse yet, almost 74 percent or nearly 3 out of every 4 American adults, did not participate in any type of muscular fitness activity; that is, they did not strength train or take a class that required some sort of muscular strength activity such as cardio/strength training, Pilates, boot camp, PX90, CrossFit, or even a single push-up during their available leisure time.

7.1 Strength-Training Benefits

A well-planned strength-training program leads to increased muscle strength and endurance, power, muscle tone, and tendon and ligament strength—all of which help to improve and maintain everyday functional physical capacity. Muscular fitness is a basic health-related fitness component and is an important wellness component for optimal performance in daily activities such as sitting, walking, running, lifting and carrying objects, doing housework, and enjoying recreational activities. Strength also is of great value in improving posture, personal appearance, and self-image; in developing sports skills; in promoting stability of joints; and in meeting certain emergencies in life.

From a health standpoint, increasing strength helps to increase or maintain muscle and a higher resting metabolic rate; encourages weight loss and maintenance, which prevents obesity; lessens the risk for injury; reduces chronic low back pain; reduces pressure on the joints alleviating arthritic pain; aids in childbearing; improves bone density, which prevents osteoporosis; improves cholesterol levels, decreases triglyceride levels, and reduces high blood pressure, thus reducing the risk for cardiovascular disease and premature mortality; and promotes psychological well-being. Furthermore, it decreases the risk of developing physical function limitations and the overall risk of nonfatal disease.[1]

Regular strength training also helps control blood sugar. Much of the blood glucose from food consumption goes to the muscles, where it is stored as glycogen. When muscles are not used, muscle cells may become insulin resistant, and glucose cannot enter the cells, thereby increasing the risk for type 2 diabetes. Research indicates that even a single strength-training exercise session enhances insulin sensitivity for the next 24 hours. Additionally, following 16 weeks of strength training, a group of diabetic men and women improved their blood sugar control, gained strength, increased lean body mass, lost body fat, and lowered blood pressure.[2]

Furthermore, with time, the heart rate and blood pressure response to lifting a heavy resistance (a weight) decreases. This adaptation reduces the demands on the cardiovascular system when you perform activities such as carrying a child, the groceries, or a suitcase.

Because of the many health benefits provided by a regular muscular fitness training program, both the American Medical Association (AMA) and the CDC have offered strong support of strength training as an exercise modality to improve people's overall health.

Muscular Fitness and Aging In the older adult population (65 and older), muscular fitness may be the most important health-related component of physical fitness. Although proper cardiorespiratory endurance is necessary to help maintain a healthy heart, good strength contributes more to independent living than any other fit-

> **Muscular fitness** A term used in reference to the general health, strength, and endurance of a person's muscular system.
>
> **Strength training** A program designed to improve muscular strength and/or endurance through a series of progressive resistance (weight) training exercises that overload the muscle system and cause physiological development.
>
> **Resistance training** See Strength training.
>
> **Progressive resistance training** A gradual increase of resistance used during strength training over a period of time.

ness component. Studies indicate that an average 30-year-old loses 25 percent of muscle strength by age 70 and about half by age 90. Once in the 50s, older adults with good strength levels can successfully perform most **activities of daily living**.

A common occurrence as people age is **sarcopenia**, the loss of lean body mass, strength, and function. How much of this loss is related to the aging process itself or to actual physical inactivity and faulty nutrition is unknown. Studies[3] indicate, nonetheless, that adults who do not strength train lose between 4 and 6 pounds of muscle tissue per decade of life. As a result, a person who has maintained body weight but did not strength train between the ages of 40 and 60, can remain at the same body mass index (BMI), but percent body fat can easily go up 7 to 10 percentage points (i.e., from 20 percent to 27 to 30 percent). A summary of 49 research studies also indicates that older adults gain an average of 2.42 pounds of lean body mass following 20 weeks of strength training.[4] The findings are significant because so many older adults are affected by sarcopenia, and strength training can prevent much of this loss and allow these older adults to preserve independent living throughout the aging process.

Currently, according to the CDC report of 2013, less than 20 percent of older adults engage in strength-training exercises. Whereas thinning of the bones from osteoporosis renders them prone to fractures, the gradual loss of muscle mass and ensuing frailty are what lead to falls and subsequent loss of function in older adults. Strength training helps to slow the age-related loss of muscle function. Protein deficiency, seen in some older adults, also contributes to loss of lean tissue.

More than anything else, older adults want to enjoy good health and to function independently. Many of them, however, are confined to nursing homes because they lack sufficient strength to move about. They cannot walk very far, and many have to be helped in and out of beds, chairs, and tubs.

A strength-training program can enhance quality of life tremendously, and nearly everyone can benefit from it. Only people with advanced heart disease are advised to refrain from strength training. Inactive adults between the ages of 56 and 86 who participated in a 12-week strength-training program increased their lean body mass by about 3 pounds, lost about 4 pounds of fat, and increased their resting metabolic rate by almost 7 percent.[5] In other research, leg strength improved by as much as 200 percent in previously inactive adults older than age 90.[6] As strength improves, so does the ability to move about, the capacity for independent living, and enjoyment of life during the "golden years." More specifically, good strength enhances quality of life by

- improving balance and restoring mobility,
- making lifting and reaching easier,
- decreasing the risk for injuries and falls, and
- stressing the bones and preserving bone mineral density, thereby decreasing the risk for osteoporosis.

Another benefit of maintaining a good strength level is its relationship to human **metabolism**. A primary outcome of a strength-training program is an increase in muscle mass or size (lean body mass), known as muscle **hypertrophy**.

Muscle tissue uses more energy than does fatty tissue. That is, your body expends more calories to maintain muscle than to maintain fat. All other factors being equal, if two individuals both weigh 150 pounds but have different amounts of muscle mass, the one with more muscle mass will have a higher **resting metabolism**. Even small increases in muscle mass have a long-term positive effect on metabolism.

Loss of lean tissue also is thought to be a primary reason for the decrease in metabolism as people grow older. Contrary to some beliefs, metabolism does not have to slow down significantly with aging. It is not so much that metabolism slows down; it's that we slow down. Lean body mass decreases with sedentary living, which in turn slows down the resting metabolic rate. Thus, if people continue eating at the same rate as they age, body fat increases.

Daily energy requirements decrease an average of 360 calories between age 26 and age 60.[7] Participating in a strength-training program can offset much of the decline and prevent and reduce excess body fat. One research study found an increase in resting metabolic rate of 35 calories per pound of muscle mass in older adults who participated in a strength-training program.[8]

Gender Differences
A common misconception about physical fitness concerns women and strength training. Because of the increase in muscle mass typically seen in men, some women think that a strength-training program will result in their developing large musculature.

Even though the quality of muscle in men and women is the same, endocrinological differences do not allow women to achieve the same amount of muscle hypertrophy (size) as men. Men also have more muscle fibers, and because of the sex-specific male hormones, each individual fiber has more potential for hypertrophy. On the average, following 6 months of training, women can achieve up to a 50-percent increase in strength but only a 10-percent increase in muscle size.

The idea that strength training allows women to develop muscle hypertrophy to the same extent as men is as false as the notion that playing basketball will turn women into giants. Masculinity and femininity are established by genetic inheritance, not by the amount of physical activity. Variations in the extent of masculinity and femininity are determined by individual differences in hormonal secretions of androgen, testosterone, estrogen, and progesterone. Women with a bigger-than-average build often are inclined to participate in sports because of their natural physical advantage. As a result, many people have associated women's participation in sports and strength training with large muscle size.

As the number of females who participate in sports has increased steadily, the myth of strength training in women leading to large increases in muscle size has abated somewhat. For example, per pound of body weight, female gymnasts are among the strongest athletes in the world. These athletes engage regularly in vigorous strength-training programs. Yet, female gymnasts have some of the most well-toned and graceful figures of all women.

Improved body appearance has become the rule rather than the exception for women who participate in strength-training exercises.

Selected Detrimental Effects from Using Anabolic Steroids

- Liver tumors
- Hepatitis
- Hypertension
- Reduction of high-density lipoprotein (HDL) cholesterol
- Elevation of low-density lipoprotein (LDL) cholesterol
- Hyperinsulinism
- Impaired pituitary function
- Impaired thyroid function
- Mood swings
- Aggressive behavior
- Increased irritability
- Acne
- Fluid retention
- Decreased libido
- HIV infection (via injectable steroids)
- Prostate problems (men)
- Testicular atrophy (men)
- Reduced sperm count (men)
- Clitoral enlargement (women)
- Decreased breast size (women)
- Increased body and facial hair (irreversible in women)
- Deepening of the voice (irreversible in women)

Improved body appearance has become the rule rather than the exception for women who participate in strength-training programs. Some of the most attractive female movie stars also train with weights to further improve their personal image.

Nonetheless, you may ask, "If weight training does not masculinize women, why do so many women body builders develop such heavy musculature?" In the sport of bodybuilding, the athletes follow intense training routines consisting of two or more hours of constant weight lifting with short rest intervals between sets. Many bodybuilding training routines call for back-to-back exercises using the same muscle groups. The objective of this type of training is to pump extra blood into the muscles. This additional fluid makes the muscles appear much bigger than they do in a resting condition. Based on the intensity and the length of the training session, the muscles can remain filled with blood, appearing measurably larger for an hour or longer after completing the training session. Performing such routines is a common practice before competitions. Therefore, in real life, these women are not as muscular as they seem when they are participating in a contest.

In the sport of bodybuilding (among others), a big point of controversy is the use of **anabolic steroids** and human growth hormones. These hormones produce detrimental and undesirable side effects, even more so in women (such as hypertension, fluid retention, decreased breast size, deepening of the voice, and whiskers and other atypical body hair growth), which some women deem tolerable. Anabolic steroid use in general—except for medical reasons and when carefully monitored by a physician—can lead to serious health consequences.

Use of anabolic steroids by female body builders and female track-and-field athletes is not uncommon. Athletes use anabolic steroids to remain competitive at the highest level. During the 2004 Olympic Games in Athens, Greece, two women shot putters, including the gold medal winner (later stripped of the medal), were expelled from the

Critical Thinking

What role should strength training have in a fitness program? • Should people be motivated for the health fitness benefits, or should they participate to enhance their body image? • What are your feelings about individuals (male or female) with large body musculature?

Activities of daily living Everyday behaviors that people normally do to function in life (cross the street, carry groceries, lift objects, do laundry, sweep floors).

Sarcopenia Age-related loss of lean body mass, strength, and function.

Metabolism All energy and material transformations that occur within living cells; necessary to sustain life.

Hypertrophy An increase in the size of the cell, as in muscle hypertrophy.

Resting metabolism Amount of energy (expressed in milliliters of oxygen per minute or total calories per day) an individual requires during resting conditions to sustain proper body function.

Anabolic steroids Synthetic versions of the male sex hormone testosterone, which promotes muscle development and hypertrophy.

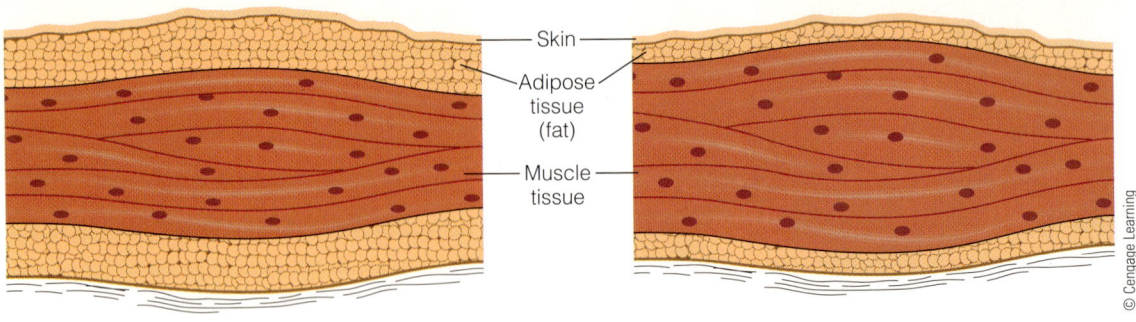

Figure 7.1 Changes in body composition as a result of a combined aerobic and strength-training program.

games for using steroids. Women who take steroids undoubtedly will build heavy musculature, and if they take them long enough, the steroids will produce masculinizing effects.

To prevent steroid use, the International Federation of Bodybuilding instituted a mandatory steroid-testing program for women participating in the Miss Olympia contest. When drugs are not used to promote development, improved body image is the rule rather than the exception among women who participate in bodybuilding, strength training, and sports in general.

Changes in Body Composition A benefit of strength training, accentuated even more when combined with aerobic exercise, is a decrease in adipose or fatty tissue around muscle fibers themselves. This decrease is often greater than the amount of muscle hypertrophy (see Figure 7.1). Therefore, losing inches but not body weight is common.

Because muscle tissue is more dense than fatty tissue (and despite the fact that inches are lost during a combined strength-training and aerobic program), people, especially women, often become discouraged because they cannot see the results readily on the scale. They can offset this discouragement by determining body composition regularly to monitor their changes in percent body fat rather than simply measuring changes in total body weight (see Chapter 4).

7.2 Assessment of Muscular Strength and Endurance

Although muscular strength and endurance are interrelated, they do differ. **Muscular strength** is the ability to exert maximum force against resistance. **Muscular endurance** is the ability of a muscle to exert submaximal force repeatedly over time.

Muscular endurance (also referred to as "localized muscular endurance") depends to a large extent on muscular strength. Weak muscles cannot repeat an action several times or sustain it. Based on these principles, strength tests and training programs have been designed to measure and develop absolute muscular strength, muscular endurance, or a combination of the two.

Muscular strength is usually determined by the maximal amount of resistance (weight)—**one repetition maximum** or **1 RM**—that an individual is able to lift in a single effort. Although this assessment yields a good measure of absolute strength, it does require considerable time, because the 1 RM is determined through trial and error. For example, strength of the chest muscles is frequently measured through the bench press exercise. If an individual has not trained with weights, he may try 100 pounds and lift this resistance easily. After adding 50 pounds, he fails to lift the resistance. Then he decreases resistance by 20 or 30 pounds. Finally, after several trials, the 1 RM is established.

Using this method, a true 1 RM might be difficult to obtain the first time an individual is tested, because fatigue becomes a factor. By the time the 1 RM is established, the person already has made several maximal or near-maximal attempts.

In contrast, muscular endurance typically is established by the number of repetitions an individual can perform against a submaximal resistance or by the length of time a given contraction can be sustained. For example, how many push-ups can an individual do? Or how many times can a 30-pound resistance be lifted? Or how long can a person hold a chin-up?

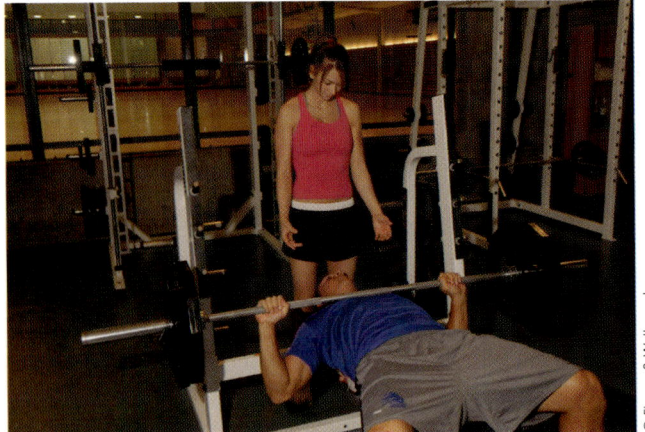

The maximal amount of resistance that an individual is able to lift in one single effort (1 repetition maximum or 1RM) is a measure of absolute strength.

If time is a factor and only one test item can be done, the Hand Grip Strength Test, described in Figure 7.2, is commonly used to assess strength. This test, though, provides only a weak correlation with overall body strength. Two additional strength tests are provided in Figures 7.3 and 7.4. Activity 7.1 also offers you the opportunity to assess your own level of muscular strength or endurance with all three tests. You may take one or more of these tests, according to your time and the facilities available.

In strength testing, several body sites should be assessed, because muscular strength and muscular endurance are both highly specific. A high degree of strength or endurance in one body part does not necessarily indicate similarity in other parts, so no single strength test provides a good assessment of overall body strength. Accordingly, exercises for the strength tests were selected to include the upper body, lower body, and abdominal regions.

Before strength testing, you should become familiar with the procedures for the respective tests. For safety reasons, always take at least one friend with you whenever you train with weights or undertake any type of strength assessment. Also, these are different tests, so to make valid comparisons, you should use the same test for pre- and post-assessments. The following are your options.

Figure 7.2 Procedure for the Hand Grip Strength Test.

1. Adjust the width of the dynamometer* so the middle bones of your fingers rest on the distant end of the dynamometer grip.
2. Use your dominant hand for this test. Place your elbow at a 90° angle and about 2 inches away from the body.
3. Now grip as hard as you can for a few seconds. Do not move any other body part as you perform the test (do not flex or extend the elbow, do not move the elbow away or toward the body, and do not lean forward or backward during the test).
4. Record the dynamometer reading in pounds (if reading is in kilograms, multiply by 2.2046).
5. Three trials are allowed for this test. Use the highest reading for your final test score. Look up your percentile rank for this test in Table 7.1.
6. Based on your percentile rank, obtain the hand grip strength fitness category according to the following guidelines:

Percentile Rank	Fitness Category
≥90	Excellent
70–80	Good
50–60	Average
30–40	Fair
≤20	Poor

*A Lafayette model 78010 dynamometer is recommended for this test (Lafayette Instruments Co., Sagamore and North 9th Street, Lafayette, IN 47903).

Table 7.1 Scoring Table for Hand Grip Strength Test

Percentile Rank	Men	Women
99	153	101
95	145	94
90	141	91
80	139	86
70	132	80
60	124	78
50	122	74
40	114	71
30	110	66
20	100	64
10	91	60
5	76	58

High physical fitness standard
Health fitness standard

© Cengage Learning

Muscular Strength: Hand Grip Strength Test As indicated previously, when time is a factor, the Hand Grip Strength Test can be used to provide a rough estimate of strength. Unlike the next two tests, this one is isometric (involving static contraction, discussed later in the chapter). If the proper grip is used, no finger motion or body movement is visible during the test. The test procedure is given in Figure 7.2, and percentile ranks based on your results are provided in Table 7.1. You can record the results of this test in Activity 7.1.

Changes in strength are more difficult to evaluate with the Hand Grip Strength Test. Most strength-training programs are dynamic in nature (body segments are moved through a range of motion), whereas this test provides an isometric assessment. Further, grip-strength exercises seldom are used in strength training, and increases in strength are specific to the body parts exercised. This test, however, can be used to supplement the following strength tests.

Muscular Endurance Test Three exercises were selected to assess the endurance of the upper body, lower body, and midbody muscle groups (see Figure 7.3). The advantage of the Muscular Endurance Test is that it does not require strength-training equipment—only a stopwatch; a metronome; a bench or gymnasium bleacher that is 16¼ inches high; a cardboard strip that is 3½ inches wide by 30 inches long; and a partner. A percentile

> **Muscular strength** The ability of a muscle to exert maximum force against resistance (e.g., 1 repetition maximum [or 1 RM] on the bench press exercise).
>
> **Muscular endurance** The ability of a muscle to exert submaximal force repeatedly over time.
>
> **One repetition maximum (1 RM)** The maximum amount of resistance an individual is able to lift in a single effort.

The hand grip tests strength.

rank is given for each exercise according to the number of repetitions performed (see Table 7.2). An overall endurance rating can be obtained by totaling the number of points obtained on each exercise. Record the results of this test in Activity 7.1 and Appendix A.

Muscular Strength and Endurance Test In the Muscular Strength and Endurance Test, you will lift a submaximal resistance as many times as possible using the six strength-training exercises listed in Figure 7.4. The resistance for each lift is determined according to selected percentages of body weight shown in Figure 7.4 and Activity 7.1.

With this test, if an individual does only a few repetitions, primarily absolute strength will be measured. For those who are able to do a lot of repetitions, the test will be an indicator of muscular endurance. If you are not familiar with the different lifts, see the illustrations provided at the end of this chapter.

A strength/endurance rating is determined according to the maximum number of repetitions you are able to perform on each exercise. Fixed-resistance strength units are necessary to administer all but the abdominal exercises in this test. (See "Dynamic Training" on pages 246–248 for an explanation of fixed-resistance equipment.)

A percentile rank for each exercise is given based on the number of repetitions performed (see Table 7.3). As with the Muscular Endurance Test, an overall muscular strength/endurance rating is obtained by totaling the number of points obtained on each exercise.

If no fixed-resistance equipment is available, you can still perform the test using different equipment. In that case, though, the percentile rankings and strength fitness categories may not be completely accurate because a certain resistance (e.g., 50 pounds) is seldom the same on two different strength-training machines (e.g., Universal Gym versus Nautilus). The industry has no standard calibration procedure for strength equipment. Consequently, if you lift a certain resistance for a specific exercise (e.g., bench press) on one machine, you may or may not be able to lift the same amount for this exercise on a different machine.

Even though the percentile ranks may not be valid across different equipment, test results can be used to evaluate changes in fitness. For example, you may be able to do 7 repetitions during the initial test, but if you can perform 14 repetitions after 12 weeks of training, that's a measure of improvement. Results of the Muscular Strength and Endurance Test can be recorded in Activity 7.1.

Figure 7.3 Muscular Endurance Test.

Three exercises are conducted on this test: bench jumps, modified dips (men) or modified push-ups (women), and bent-leg curl-ups or abdominal crunches. All exercises should be conducted with the aid of a partner. The correct procedure for performing each exercise is as follows:

Bench jump. Using a bench or gymnasium bleacher 16¼" high, attempt to jump up onto and down off of the bench as many times as possible in 1 minute. If you cannot jump the full minute, you may step up and down. A repetition is counted each time both feet return to the floor.

Modified dip. Men only: Using a bench or gymnasium bleacher, place the hands on the bench with the fingers pointing forward. Have a partner hold your feet in front of you. Bend the hips at approximately 90° (you also may use three sturdy chairs: Put your hands on two chairs placed by the sides of your body and place your feet on the third chair in front of you). Lower your body by flexing the elbows until they reach a 90° angle, then return to the starting position (also see Exercise 6 at the end of this chapter). Perform the repetitions to a two-step cadence (down-up) regulated with a metronome set at 56 beats per minute. Perform as many continuous repetitions as possible. Do not count any more repetitions if you fail to follow the metronome cadence.

Figure 7.3a Bench jump

Figure 7.3b Modified dip

Modified push-up. Women only: Lie down on the floor (face down), bend the knees (feet up in the air), and place the hands on the floor by the shoulders with the fingers pointing forward. The lower body will be supported at the knees (as opposed to the feet) throughout the test (see Figure 7.3c). The chest must touch the floor on each repetition. As with the modified dip exercise (above), perform the repetitions to a two-step cadence (up-down) regulated with a metronome set at 56 beats per minute. Perform as many continuous repetitions as possible. Do not count any more repetitions if you fail to follow the metronome cadence.

Figure 7.3c Modified push-up

Bent-leg curl-up. Lie down on the floor (face up) and bend both legs at the knees at approximately 100°. The feet should be on the floor, and you must hold them in place yourself throughout the test. Cross the arms in front of the chest, each hand on the opposite shoulder. Now raise the head off the floor, placing the chin against the chest. This is the starting and finishing position for each curl-up (see Figure 7.3d). **The back of the head may not come in contact with the floor, the hands cannot be removed from the shoulders, nor may the feet or hips be raised off the floor at any time during the test. The test is terminated if any of these four conditions occur.**

When you curl up, the upper body must come to an upright position before going back down (see Figure 7.3e). The repetitions are performed to a two-step cadence (up-down)

Figure 7.3d Bent-leg curl-up

regulated with the metronome set at 40 beats per minute. For this exercise, you should allow a brief practice period of 5 to 10 seconds to familiarize yourself with the cadence (the *up* movement is initiated with the first beat, then you must wait for the next beat to initiate the *down* movement; one repetition is accomplished every two beats of the metronome). Count as many repetitions as you are able to perform following the proper cadence. The test is also terminated if you fail to maintain the appropriate cadence or if you accomplish 100 repetitions. Have your partner check the angle at the knees throughout the test to make sure to maintain the 100° angle as close as possible.

Figure 7.3e Bent-leg curl-up

Abdominal crunch. This test is recommended only for individuals who are unable to perform the bent-leg curl-up test because of susceptibility to low back injury. Exercise form must be carefully monitored during the test. Several authors and researchers have indicated that proper form during this test is extremely difficult to control. Subjects often slide their bodies, bend their elbows, or shrug their shoulders during the test. Such actions facilitate the performance of the test and misrepresent the actual test results. Biomechanical factors also limit the ability to perform this test. Further, lack of spinal flexibility keeps some individuals from being able to move the full 3½" range of motion. Others are unable to keep their heels on the floor during the test. The validity of this test as an effective measure of abdominal strength or abdominal endurance has also been questioned through research.

Tape a 3½" × 30" strip of cardboard onto the floor. Lie down on the floor in a supine position (face up) with the knees bent at approximately 100°. The feet should be on the floor, and you must hold them in place yourself throughout the test. Straighten out your arms and place them on the floor alongside the trunk with the palms down and the fingers fully extended. The fingertips of both hands should barely touch the closest edge of the cardboard (see Figure 7.3f). Bring the head off the floor until the chin is 1" to 2" away from your chest. Keep the head in this position during the entire test (do not move the head by flexing or extending the neck). You are now ready to begin the test.

Perform the repetitions to a two-step cadence (up-down) regulated with a metronome set at 60 beats per minute. As you curl up, slide the fingers over the cardboard until the fingertips reach the far edge (3½") of the board (see Figure 7.3g), then return to the starting position.

Allow a brief practice period of 5 to 10 seconds

Figure 7.3f Abdominal crunch test

Figure 7.3g Abdominal crunch test

to familiarize yourself with the cadence. Initiate the *up* movement with the first beat and the *down* movement with the next beat. Accomplish one repetition every two beats of the metronome. Count as many repetitions as you are able to perform following the proper cadence. You may not count a repetition if the fingertips fail to reach the distant edge of the cardboard.

Terminate the test if you (a) fail to maintain the appropriate cadence, (b) bend the elbows, (c) shrug the shoulders, (d) slide

(continued)

*Novel Products, Inc. Figure Finder Collection, P.O. Box 408, Rockton, IL 61072-0408. 1-800-323-5143, Fax 815-624-4866.

Figure 7.3 Muscular Endurance Test.

the body, (e) lift heels off the floor, (f) raise the chin off the chest, (g) accomplish 100 repetitions, or (h) no longer can perform the test. Have your partner check the angle at the knees throughout the test to make sure that the 100° angle is maintained as closely as possible.

Figure 7.3h

Figure 7.3i

Abdominal crunch test performed with a Crunch-Ster Curl-Up Tester.

For this test you may also use a Crunch-Ster Curl-Up Tester, available from Novel Products.* An illustration of the test performed with this equipment is provided in Figures 7.3h and 7.3i.

According to the results, look up your percentile rank for each exercise in the far left column of Table 7.2 and determine your muscular endurance fitness category according to the following classification:

Average Score	Fitness Category	Points
≥90	Excellent	5
70–80	Good	4
50–60	Average	3
30–40	Fair	2
≤20	Poor	1

Look up the number of points assigned for each fitness category above. Total the number of points and determine your overall strength endurance fitness category according to the following ratings:

Total Points	Strength Endurance Category
≥13	Excellent
10–12	Good
7–9	Average
4–6	Fair
≤3	Poor

*Novel Products, Inc. Figure Finder Collection, P.O. Box 408, Rockton, IL 61072-0408. 1-800-323-5143, Fax 815-624-4866.

© Cengage Learning

Table 7.2 Muscular Endurance Scoring Table

Percentile Rank	Men				Women			
	Bench Jumps	Modified Dips	Bent-Leg Curl-Ups	Abdominal Crunches	Bench Jumps	Modified Push-Ups	Bent-Leg Curl-Ups	Abdominal Crunches
99	66	54	100	100	58	95	100	100
95	63	50	81	100	54	70	100	100
90	62	38	65	100	52	50	97	69
80	58	32	51	66	48	41	77	49
70	57	30	44	45	44	38	57	37
60	56	27	31	38	42	33	45	34
50	54	26	28	33	39	30	37	31
40	51	23	25	29	38	28	28	27
30	48	20	22	26	36	25	22	24
20	47	17	17	22	32	21	17	21
10	40	11	10	18	28	18	9	15
5	34	7	3	16	26	15	4	0

■ High physical fitness standard   ■ Health fitness standard

© Cengage Learning

Figure 7.4 Muscular Strength and Endurance Test.

1. Familiarize yourself with the six lifts used for this test: lat pull-down, leg extension, bench press, bent-leg curl-up or abdominal crunch,* leg curl, and arm curl. Graphic illustrations for each lift are given at the end of this chapter. For the leg curl exercise, the knees should be flexed to 90°. A description and illustration of the bent-leg curl-up and the abdominal crunch exercises are provided in Figure 7.3. On the leg extension lift, maintain the trunk in an upright position.
2. Determine your body weight in pounds.
3. Determine the amount of resistance to be used on each lift. To obtain this number, multiply your body weight by the percent given below for each lift.

Lift	Percent of Body Weight	
	Men	Women
Lat Pull-Down	.70	.45
Leg Extension	.65	.50
Bench Press	.75	.45
Bent-Leg Curl-Up or Abdominal Crunch*	NA**	NA**
Leg Curl	.32	.25
Arm Curl	.35	.18

*The abdominal crunch exercise should be used only by individuals who suffer or are susceptible to low back pain.
**NA = not applicable—see Figure 7.3.

4. Perform the maximum continuous number of repetitions possible.
5. Based on the number of repetitions performed, look up the percentile rank for each lift in the left column of Table 7.3.
6. The individual strength fitness category is determined according to the following classification:

Percentile Rank	Fitness Category	Points
≥90	Excellent	5
70–80	Good	4
50–60	Average	3
30–40	Fair	2
≤20	Poor	1

7. Look up the number of points assigned for each fitness category under item 6 above. Total the number of points and determine your overall strength fitness category according to the following ratings:

Total Points	Strength Category
≥25	Excellent
19–24	Good
13–18	Average
7–12	Fair
≤6	Poor

8. Record your results in Activity 7.1.

*Novel Products, Inc. Figure Finder Collection, P.O. Box 408, Rockton, IL 61072-0408. 1-800-323-5143, Fax 815-624-4866.

Table 7.3 Muscular Strength and Endurance Scoring Table

Percentile Rank	Men							Women						
	Lat Pull-Down	Leg Extension	Bench Press	Bent-Leg Curl-Up	Abdominal Crunch	Leg Curl	Arm Curl	Lat Pull-Down	Leg Extension	Bench Press	Bent-Leg Curl-Up	Abdominal Crunch	Leg Curl	Arm Curl
99	30	25	26	100	100	24	25	30	25	27	100	100	20	25
95	25	20	21	81	100	20	21	25	20	21	100	100	17	21
90	19	19	19	65	100	19	19	21	18	20	97	69	12	20
80	16	15	16	51	66	15	15	16	13	16	77	49	10	16
70	13	14	13	44	45	13	12	13	11	13	57	37	9	14
60	11	13	11	31	38	11	10	11	10	11	45	34	7	12
50	10	12	10	28	33	10	9	10	9	10	37	31	6	10
40	9	10	7	25	29	8	8	9	8	5	28	27	5	8
30	7	9	5	22	26	6	7	7	7	3	22	24	4	7
20	6	7	3	17	22	4	5	6	5	1	17	21	3	6
10	4	5	1	10	18	3	3	3	3	0	9	15	1	3
5	3	3	0	3	16	1	2	2	1	0	4	0	0	2

High physical fitness standard Health fitness standard

Activity 7.1: Muscular Strength and Endurance Assessment

Name _____ Date _____

Course _____ Section _____ Gender _____ Age _____

I. Hand Grip Strength Test

The instructions for the Hand Grip Strength Test are provided in Figure 7.2, page 237. Perform the test according to the instructions and look up your results in Table 7.1, page 237.

Hand used: _____ Right _____ Left

Reading: _____ lbs.

Fitness category (see Figure 7.2, page 237): _____

II. Muscular Endurance Test

Conduct this test using the guidelines provided in Figure 7.3, pages 239–240, and Table 7.2, page 240. Record your repetitions, fitness category, and points in the spaces provided below.

Exercise	Metronome Cadence	Repetitions	Fitness Category	Points
Bench jumps	none			
Modified dips—men only	56 bpm			
Modified push-ups—women only	56 bpm			
Bent-leg curl-ups	40 bpm			
Abdominal crunches	60 bpm			
			Total Points:	

Overall muscular endurance fitness category (see Figure 7.3, pages 239–240): _____

III. Muscular Strength and Endurance Test

Perform the Muscular Strength and Endurance Test according to the procedure outlined in Figure 7.4, page 241. Record the results, fitness category, and points in the appropriate blanks provided below.

Body weight: _____ lbs.

Lift	Percent of Body Weight (pounds)		Resistance	Repetitions	Fitness Category	Points
	Men	Women				
Lat pull-down	.70	.45				
Leg extension	.65	.50				
Bench press	.75	.45				
Bent-leg curl-up or abdominal crunch	NA*	NA*				
Leg curl	.32	.25				
Arm curl	.35	.18				

*Not applicable—no resistance required. Use test described in Figure 7.3, pages 239–240.

Overall muscular strength fitness category (see Figure 7.4, page 241) ☐

IV. Muscular Strength and Endurance Goals

Indicate the muscular strength/endurance category that you would like to achieve by the end of the term: ☐

Briefly state your feelings about your current strength level and indicate how you are planning to achieve your strength objective:

_____
_____
_____
_____
_____
_____
_____
_____
_____
_____
_____
_____
_____
_____
_____
_____

7.3 Strength-Training Prescription

The capacity of muscle cells to exert force increases and decreases according to the demands placed on the muscular system. If muscle cells are overloaded beyond their normal use, such as in strength-training programs, the cells increase in size (hypertrophy) and strength. If the demands placed on the muscle cells decrease, such as in sedentary living or required rest because of illness or injury, the cells **atrophy** and lose strength. A good level of muscular fitness is important to develop and maintain health and total well-being.

Factors That Affect Muscular Fitness Several physiological factors combine to create muscle contraction and subsequent strength gains: neural stimulation, type of muscle fiber, overload, specificity of training, training volume, and periodization. Basic knowledge of these concepts is important to understand the principles involved in strength development.

Neural Function

Within the neuromuscular system, single **motor neurons** branch and attach to multiple muscle fibers. The motor neuron and the fibers it innervates (supplies with nerves) form a **motor unit**. The number of fibers that a motor neuron can innervate varies from just a few in muscles that require precise control (e.g., eye muscles) to as many as 1,000 or more in large muscles that do not perform refined or precise movements.

Stimulation of a motor neuron causes the muscle fibers to contract maximally or not at all. Variations in the number of fibers innervated and the frequency of their stimulation determine the strength of the muscle contraction. As the number of fibers innervated and frequency of stimulation increase, so does the strength of the muscular contraction.

Neural adaptations are prominent in the early stages of strength training. In novice participants, significant strength increases seen during the first two to three weeks of training are largely related to enhanced neural function by increasing motor neuron stimulation and muscle fiber recruitment (skill acquisition). Long-term strength development is primarily related to increased physiological adaptation within the muscle(s) and to a lesser extent to continued neural adaptations.

Types of Muscle Fiber

The human body has two basic types of muscle fibers: (a) slow-twitch or red fibers and (b) fast-twitch or white fibers. **Slow-twitch fibers** have a greater capacity for aerobic work. **Fast-twitch fibers** have a greater capacity for anaerobic work and produce more overall force. The latter are important for quick and powerful movements commonly used in strength-training activities.

The proportion of slow- and fast-twitch fibers is determined genetically and consequently varies from one person to another. Nevertheless, training increases the functional capacity of both types of fiber, and more specifically, strength training increases their ability to exert force.

During muscular contraction, slow-twitch fibers always are recruited first. As the force and speed of muscle contraction increase, the relative importance of the fast-twitch fibers increases. To activate the fast-twitch fibers, an activity must be intense and powerful.

Overload

Strength gains are achieved in two ways:

1. Through increased ability of individual muscle fibers to generate a stronger contraction
2. By recruiting a greater proportion of the total available fibers for each contraction

These two factors combine in the **overload principle**. The demands placed on the muscle must be increased systematically and progressively over time, and the resistance must be of a magnitude significant enough to cause physiological adaptation. In simpler terms, just like all other organs and systems of the human body, to increase in physical capacity, muscles have to be taxed repeatedly beyond their accustomed loads. Because of this principle, strength training also is called progressive resistance training.

Several procedures can be used to overload in strength training[9]

1. Increasing the intensity (resistance of amount of weight used)
2. Increasing the number of repetitions at the current intensity
3. Increasing or decreasing the speed at which the repetitions are performed
4. Decreasing the rest interval for endurance improvements (with lighter resistances) or lengthening the rest interval for strength and power development (with higher resistances)
5. Increasing the volume (sum of the repetitions performed multiplied by the resistance used)
6. Using any combination of the above

Specificity of Training

Training adaptations are specific to the impetus applied. In strength training, the principle of **specificity of training** holds that for a muscle to increase in strength or endurance, the training program must be specific to obtain the desired effects (see also the discussion on resistance on pages 248–249).

The principle of specificity also applies to activity or sport-specific development and is commonly referred to as **specific adaptation to imposed demand (SAID) training**. The SAID principle implies that if an individual is attempting to improve specific sport skills, the strength-training exercises performed should resemble as closely as possible the movement patterns encountered in that particular activity or sport.

For example, a soccer player who wishes to become stronger and faster would emphasize exercises that will develop leg strength and power. In contrast, an individual recovering from a lower-limb fracture initially exercises to increase strength and stability, and subsequently muscle endurance.

Training Volume

Volume is the sum of all the repetitions performed multiplied by the resistances used during a strength-training session. Volume frequently is used to quantify the amount of work performed in a given training session. For example, an individual who does three sets of six repetitions with 150 pounds has performed a training volume of 2,700 (3 × 6 ×150) for this exercise. The total training volume can be obtained by totaling the volume of all exercises performed.

The volume of training done in a strength-training session can be modified by changing the total number of exercises performed, the number of sets done per exercise, or the number of repetitions performed per set. Athletes typically use high training volumes and low intensities to achieve muscle hypertrophy, and low volumes and high intensities to increase strength and power.

Periodization

The concept of **periodization** (variation) entails systematically altering training variables over time to keep the program challenging and lead to greater strength development. Periodization means cycling one's training objectives (hypertrophy, strength, and endurance), with each phase of the program lasting anywhere from 2 to 12 weeks. Training variables altered include resistance (weight lifted), number of repetitions, number of sets, and/or number of exercises performed.

The periodized training approach is popular among athletes and is frequently used to prevent **overtraining**. Training volume should not increase by more than 5 percent from one phase to the next. Periodization now is popular among fitness participants who wish to achieve maximal strength gains. Over the long run, for intermediate and advanced participants, the periodized approach has been shown to be superior to nonperiodized training (using the same exercises, sets, and repetitions repeatedly).

Three types of periodized training, based on program design and objectives, are commonly used. These are:

- **Classical Periodization.** The classical or linear model is used by individuals seeking maximal strength development. It starts with an initial high volume of training using low resistances. In subsequent cycles, the program gradually switches to a lower volume and higher resistances.
- **Reverse Periodization.** A model used primarily by individuals seeking greater muscular endurance. Also a linear model, it is opposite to the classical model. The resistances are highest at the beginning of training with a low volume, subsequently followed by progressive decreases in resistances and increases in training volume.
- **Undulating Periodization.** This model uses a combination of volumes and resistances within a cycle by alternating in a nonlinear fashion (randomly or systematically) among the muscular fitness components: strength, hypertrophy, power, and endurance. The undulating model compares favorably, and in some cases, it is even superior to the classical and reverse models.

Understanding all five training concepts that affect strength (neural stimulation, muscle fiber types, overload, specificity, and periodization) discussed thus far is required to design an effective strength-training program.

7.4 Principles Involved in Strength Training

Because muscular strength and endurance are important in developing and maintaining overall fitness and well-being, the principles necessary to develop a strength-training program have to be understood, just as in the prescription for cardiorespiratory endurance. These principles are mode, resistance, sets, frequency, and volume of training. The key factor in successful muscular fitness development, however, is the individualization of the program according to these principles and the person's goals, as well as the magnitude of the individual's effort during training itself.

Mode of Training

Two types of training methods are used to improve strength: isometric (static) and dynamic (previously called "isotonic"). In **isometric training**, muscle contractions produce little or no movement, such as pushing or pulling against an immovable object or holding a given position

---

Atrophy Decrease in the size of a cell.

Motor neurons Nerves connecting the central nervous system to the muscle.

Motor unit The combination of a motor neuron and the muscle fibers that neuron innervates.

Slow-twitch fibers Muscle fibers with greater aerobic potential and slow speed of contraction.

Fast-twitch fibers Muscle fibers with greater anaerobic potential and fast speed of contraction.

Overload principle Training concept that the demands placed on a system (cardiorespiratory or muscular) must be increased systematically and progressively over time to cause physiological adaptation (development or improvement).

Specificity of training Principle that training must be done with the specific muscle(s) the person is attempting to improve.

Specific adaptation to imposed demand (SAID) training Training principle stating that, for improvements to occur in a specific activity, the exercises performed during a strength-training program should resemble as closely as possible the movement patterns encountered in that particular activity.

Volume (in strength training) The sum of all repetitions performed multiplied by the resistance used during a training session.

Periodization A training approach that divides the season into cycles using a systematic variation in intensity and volume of training to enhance fitness and performance.

Overtraining An emotional, behavioral, and physical condition marked by increased fatigue, decreased performance, persistent muscle soreness, mood disturbances, and feelings of "staleness" or "burnout" as a result of excessive physical training.

Isometric training Strength-training method referring to a muscle contraction that produces little or no movement, such as pushing or pulling against an immovable object.

against resistance for a given period of time. In dynamic training, the muscle contractions produce movement, such as extending the knees with resistance on the ankles (leg extension). The specificity of training principle applies here, too. To increase isometric versus dynamic strength, an individual must use static instead of dynamic training to achieve the desired results.

Isometric Training

Isometric training does not require much equipment. Because strength gains with isometric training are specific to the angle of muscle contraction, this type of training is beneficial in a sport such as gymnastics, which requires regular static contractions during routines. As presented in Chapter 8, however, isometric training is a critical component of health conditioning programs for the low back (see "Preventing and Rehabilitating Low Back Pain," pages 290–295) and for spinal-stabilization musculature and healthy posture. Selected exercises, in particular core exercises, are recommended as a part of a comprehensive strength-training program.

Dynamic Training

Dynamic training is the most common mode for strength training. The primary advantage is that strength is gained through the full **range of motion**. Most daily activities are dynamic in nature. We are constantly lifting, pushing, and pulling objects, and strength is needed through a complete range of motions. Another advantage is that improvements are measured easily by the amount lifted.

Dynamic training consists of two action phases when an exercise is performed: (1) **concentric** or **positive resistance** and (2) **eccentric** or **negative resistance**. In the concentric phase, the muscle shortens as it contracts to overcome the resistance. In the eccentric phase, the muscle lengthens to overcome the resistance. For example, during a bench press exercise, when the person lifts the resistance from the chest to full-arm extension, the triceps muscle on the back of the upper arm shortens to extend (straighten) the elbow. During the eccentric phase, the same triceps muscle is used to lower the weight during elbow flexion, but the muscle lengthens slowly to avoid dropping the resistance. Both motions work the same muscle against the same resistance.

Eccentric muscle contractions allow us to lower weights in a smooth, gradual, and controlled manner. Without eccentric contractions, weights would be suddenly dropped on the way down. Because the same muscles work when you lift and lower a resistance, always be sure to execute both actions in a controlled manner. Failure to do so diminishes the benefits of the training program and increases the risk for injuries. Eccentric contractions seem to be more effective in producing muscle hypertrophy but result in greater muscle soreness.[10]

Dynamic training programs can be conducted without weights; using exercise bands; and with **free weights**, **fixed-resistance** machines, **variable-resistance** machines, or isokinetic equipment. When you perform dynamic exercises without weights (e.g., pull-ups and push-ups), with free weights, or with fixed-resistance machines, you move a constant resistance through a joint's full range of motion. The greatest resistance that can be lifted equals the maximum weight that can be moved at the weakest angle of the joint. This is because of changes in length of muscle and angle of pull as the joint moves through its range of motion. This type of training is also referred to as **dynamic constant external resistance**, or DCER.

As strength training became more popular, new strength-training machines were developed. This technology brought about **isokinetic training** and variable-resistance training programs, which require special machines equipped with mechanical devices that provide differing amounts of resistance, with the intent of overloading the muscle group maximally through the entire range of motion. A distinction of isokinetic training is that the speed of the muscle contraction is kept constant because the machine provides resistance to match the user's force through the range of motion. The mode of training that an individual selects depends mainly

In isometric training, muscle contraction produces little or no movement.

In dynamic training, muscle contraction produces movement in the respective joint.

Strength-training can be done using free weights.

on the type of equipment available and the specific objective the training program is attempting to accomplish.

The benefits of isokinetic and variable-resistance training are similar to those of the other dynamic training methods. Theoretically, strength gains should be better because maximum resistance is applied at all angles. Research, however, has not shown this type of training to be more effective than other modes of dynamic training.

Free Weights versus Machines in Dynamic Training

The most popular weight-training devices available during the first half of the 20th century were plate-loaded barbells (free weights). Strength-training machines were developed in the middle of the century but did not become popular until the 1970s. With subsequent technological improvements to these machines, a debate arose over which of the two training modalities was better.

Free weights require that the individual balance the resistance through the entire lifting motion. Free weights may provide greater strength development because additional muscles are needed to balance the resistance as it is moved through the range of motion. Strength-training machines, nonetheless, are an excellent training modality for individuals who are either starting strength training for the first time, those who are primarily attempting to maintain strength levels, and for older adults concerned with safety and ease of use. Let's examine the advantages of each system.

Advantages of Free Weights

Following are the advantages of using free weights instead of machines in a strength-training program:

- Cost: Free weights are much less expensive than most exercise machines. On a limited budget, free weights are a better option.
- Variety: A bar and a few plates can be used to perform many exercises to strengthen most muscles in the body.
- Portability: Free weights can be easily moved from one area or station to another.
- Coordination: Free weights require greater muscular coordination that mimics movement requirements of specific tasks.
- Balance: Free weights require that a person bal-

In isokinetic training, the speed of muscle contraction is constant.

> **Range of motion** Entire arc of movement of a given joint.
>
> **Dynamic training** Strength-training method referring to a muscle contraction with movement.
>
> **Concentric** Describes shortening of a muscle during muscle contraction.
>
> **Positive resistance** The lifting, pushing, or concentric phase of a repetition during a strength-training exercise.
>
> **Eccentric** Describes lengthening of a muscle during muscle contraction.
>
> **Negative resistance** The lowering or eccentric phase of a repetition during a strength-training exercise.
>
> **Free weights** Barbells and dumbbells.
>
> **Fixed resistance** Type of exercise in which a constant resistance is moved through a joint's full range of motion (dumbbells, barbells, machines using a constant resistance).
>
> **Variable resistance** Training using special machines equipped with mechanical devices that provide differing amounts of resistance through the range of motion.
>
> **Dynamic constant external resistance (DCER)** See Fixed resistance.
>
> **Isokinetic training** Strength-training method in which the speed of the muscle contraction is kept constant because the equipment (machine) provides an accommodating resistance to match the user's force (maximal) through the range of motion.

ance the weight through the entire range of motion. This feature involves additional support and stabilizing muscles to keep the weight moving properly.
- One size fits all: People of almost all ages can use free weights. A drawback of machines is that individuals who are at the extremes in terms of height or limb length often do not fit into the machines. In particular, small women and adolescents are at a disadvantage.

Advantages of Machines

Strength-training machines have the following advantages over free weights:

- Safety: Machines are safer because spotters are rarely needed to monitor lifting.
- Ease of use: Only a minimal amount of skill is required because the machines guide and control the movement through the entire range of motion.
- Machines are an excellent training option for novice lifters and older adults.
- Selection: A few exercises—such as hip flexion, hip abduction, leg curls, lat pull-downs, and neck exercises—can be performed only with machines.
- Variable resistance: Most machines provide variable resistance. Free weights provide only fixed resistance.
- Isolation: Individual muscles are better isolated with machines because stabilizing muscles are not used to balance the weight during the exercise.
- Time: Exercising with machines requires less time because you can set the resistance quickly by using a selector pin instead of having to manually change dumbbells or weight plates on both sides of a barbell.
- Flexibility: Most machines can provide resistance over a greater range of movement during the exercise, thereby contributing to more flexibility in the joints. For example, a barbell pullover exercise provides resistance over a range of 100 degrees, whereas a weight machine may allow for as much as 260 degrees.
- Rehabilitation: Machines are more useful during injury rehabilitation. A knee injury, for instance, is practically impossible to rehab using free weights, whereas with a weight machine, small loads can be easily selected through a limited range of motion.
- Skill acquisition: Learning a new exercise movement—and performing it correctly—is faster because the machine controls the direction of the movement.

An ideal training program actually incorporates both free weights and machines. You can choose free weights for some exercises and machines for others. Although each modality has pros and cons, muscles do not know whether the source of a resistance is a barbell, a dumbbell, a Universal Gym machine, a Nautilus machine, or a simple cinder block. The most important component that determines the extent of a person's strength development is the quality of the program and the individual's effort during the training program itself—not the type of equipment used. Thus, the general recommendation that early on machines be used, subsequently both machines and free weights can be used by intermediate and advanced participants.

Resistance (Intensity)

Resistance in strength training is the equivalent of intensity in cardiorespiratory exercise prescription. To stimulate strength development, the general recommendation has been to use a resistance of approximately 80 percent of the maximum capacity (1 RM). For example, a person with a 1 RM of 150 pounds should work with about 120 pounds (150 × .80).

The number of repetitions that one can perform at 80 percent of the 1 RM, however, varies among exercises (i.e., bench press, lat pull-down, leg curl; see Table 7.4). Data indicate that the total number of repetitions performed at a certain percentage of the 1 RM depends on the amount of muscle mass involved (bench press versus triceps extension) and whether it is a single- or multi-joint exercise (leg press versus leg curl). In trained and untrained subjects alike, the number of repetitions is greater with larger muscle mass involvement and multi-joint exercises.[11]

Because of the time factor involved in constantly determining the 1 RM on each lift to ensure that the person is indeed working around 80 percent, the accepted rule for many years has been that individuals perform between 8 and 12 repetitions maximum (or 8 to 12 RM zone) for adequate strength gains. For instance, if a person is training with a resistance of 120 pounds and cannot lift it more than 12 times—that is, the person reaches volitional fatigue at or before 12 repetitions—the training stimulus (weight used) is adequate for strength development. It is important to note that volitional fatigue means to the point of muscle fatigue but not muscle failure. Exerting muscles to failure substantially increases the risk of excessive soreness and injury among beginner lifters and older adults. Once the person can lift the resistance more than 12 times, the resistance is in-

Table 7.4 Number of Repetitions Performed at 80 Percent of the One Repetition Maximum (1 RM)

Exercise	Trained		Untrained	
	Men	Women	Men	Women
Leg press	19	22	15	12
Lat pull-down	12	10	10	10
Bench press	12	14	10	10
Leg extension	12	10	9	8
Sit-up*	12	12	8	7
Arm curl	11	7	8	6
Leg curl	7	5	6	6

*Sit-up exercise performed with weighted plates on the chest and feet held in place with an ankle strap.

SOURCE: W. W. K. Hoeger, D. R. Hopkins, S. L. Barette, and D. F. Hale, "Relationship between Repetitions and Selected Percentages of One Repetition Maximum: A Comparison between Untrained and Trained Males and Females," *Journal of Applied Sport Science Research* 4, no. 2 (1990): 47–51.

creased by 5 to 10 pounds and the person again should build up to 12 repetitions. This is referred to as progressive resistance training.

Strength development, however, also can occur when working with less than 80 percent of the 1 RM (60 percent to 80 percent). Although the 8 to 12 RM zone is the most commonly prescribed resistance training zone, benefits do accrue when working with less than 8 RM or greater than 12 RM. Older adults and very deconditioned individuals who are susceptible to musculoskeletal injuries are encouraged to work with 10 to 15 repetitions using moderate resistances (about 50 percent to 60 percent of the 1 RM). If the main objective of the training program is muscular endurance, 15 to 25 repetitions per set are recommended.

In both young and older individuals, all repetitions should be performed at a moderate velocity (about 1 second concentric and 1 second eccentric), as such yields the greatest strength gains. For advanced training, varying training velocity between sets, from very slow to fast, are recommended.

Elite strength and power athletes typically work between 1 and 6 RM, but they often shuffle training (periodized training) with a different number of repetitions and sets for selected periods (weeks) of time. Body builders tend to work with moderate resistance levels (60 to 85 percent of the 1 RM) and perform 8 to 20 repetitions to near fatigue. A foremost objective of bodybuilding is to increase muscle size. Moderate resistance promotes blood flow to the muscles, "pumping up the muscles" (also known as "the pump"), which makes them look much larger than they do in a resting state.

From a general fitness point of view, a moderate resistance of only about 50 percent should be used initially while learning proper form and lifting technique. Following the first two weeks of training, working near a 10-repetition threshold seems to improve overall performance most effectively. We live in a dynamic world in which muscular strength and endurance are both required to lead an enjoyable life. Working around 10 RM produces good results in terms of strength, endurance, and hypertrophy. To maximize training development, advanced participants are encouraged to cycle between 1 and 12 RM.

Sets In strength training, a **set** is the number of repetitions performed for a given exercise. For example, a person lifting 120 pounds eight times has performed one set of eight repetitions ($1 \times 8 \times 120$). For general fitness, the recommendation is two to four sets per exercise (advanced participants often train with up to six sets per exercise) with 2 to 3 minutes rest interval between sets. For a person looking to improve muscular endurance, no more than two sets (of 15 to 25 repetitions each) per exercise are recommended.

When performing multiple sets using the RM zone with the same resistance, if the person truly performs 12 RM to muscle fatigue (or close to it), in subsequent sets fewer RM will be performed (perhaps 10, 9, and 7 RM). Because of the characteristics of muscle fiber, the number of sets the exerciser can do is limited. As the number of sets increases, so does the amount of muscle fatigue and subsequent recovery time.

When time is a factor, and although multiple-set training is most beneficial, single-set programs are still effective, as long as the single set is performed within the RM zone to muscular fatigue. You may also choose to do two sets for multi-joint exercises (bench press, leg press, lat pull-down) and a single RM-zone set for single-joint exercises (arm curl, triceps extension, knee extension).

A recommended program for beginners in their first year of training is one or two light warm-up sets per exercise, using about 50 percent of the 1 RM (no warm-up sets are necessary for subsequent exercises that use the same muscle group), followed by one to four sets to near fatigue per exercise. Maintaining a resistance and effort that will temporarily fatigue the muscle (volitional exhaustion) from the number of repetitions selected in at least one of the sets is crucial to achieve optimal progress. Because of the lower resistances used in body building, four to eight sets can be done for each exercise.

To avoid muscle soreness and stiffness, new participants ought to build up gradually to the three to four sets of maximal repetitions. They can do this by performing only one set of each exercise with a lighter resistance on the first day of training, two sets of each exercise on the second day—the first light and the second with the required resistance to volitional exhaustion. If you choose to do so, you can increase to three sets on the third day—one light and two heavy. After that, a person should be able to perform anywhere from two to four sets as planned.

The time necessary to recover between sets depends mainly on the resistance used during each set. In strength training, the energy to lift heavy weights is derived primarily from the system involving adenosine triphosphate (ATP) and creatine phosphate (CP) or phosphagen (see Chapter 3, "Energy (ATP) Production," page 112). Ten seconds of maximal exercise nearly depletes the CP stores in the exercised muscle(s). These stores are replenished in about three to five minutes of recovery.

Based on this principle, rest intervals between sets vary in length depending on the program goals and are dictated by the amount of resistance used in training. Short rest intervals of less than two minutes are commonly used when one is trying to develop local muscular endurance. Moderate rest intervals of two to four minutes are used for strength development. Long intervals of more than four minutes are used when one is training for power development.[12]

> **Resistance** Amount of weight lifted.
>
> **Set** A fixed number of repetitions; one set of bench presses might be 10 repetitions. Even two-a-day workouts are common. The frequency depends on the amount of resistance, number of sets performed per session, and the person's ability to recover from the previous exercise bout (see Table 7.5). The latter often is dictated by level of conditioning.

Using these guidelines, individuals training for health fitness purposes might allow two minutes of rest between sets. Bodybuilders, who use lower resistances, should rest no more than one minute to maximize the "pumping" effect.

For someone trying to maximize strength gains, the exercise program will be more time-effective if two or three exercises are alternated that require different muscle groups, called **circuit training**. In this way, an individual will not have to wait two to three minutes before proceeding to a new set on a different exercise. For example, the bench press, leg extension, and abdominal curl-up exercises may be combined so that the person can go almost directly from one exercise set to the next.

Men and women alike should observe the guidelines given previously. Many women do not follow them. They erroneously believe that training with low resistances and many repetitions is best to enhance body composition and maximize energy expenditure. Unless a person is seeking to increase muscular endurance for a specific sport-related activity, the use of low resistances and high repetitions is not recommended to achieve optimal strength-fitness goals and maximize long-term energy expenditure.

Frequency In the early stages of training, strength training should be done through a total body workout two to three times a week. Training can be performed more frequently if using a split-body routine, that is, upper body one day and lower body the next. After a maximum strength workout, the trained muscles should be rested at least 2 days (about 48 hours) to allow adequate recovery. If not completely recovered in 2 to 3 days, the person most likely is overtraining and therefore not reaping the full benefits of the program. In that case, the person should do fewer sets of exercises than in the previous workout. A summary of strength-training guidelines for health fitness purposes is provided in Figure 7.5.

To achieve significant strength gains, a minimum of eight weeks of consecutive training is necessary. After an individual has achieved a recommended strength level, from a health fitness standpoint, one to two training session per week will be sufficient to maintain it. Highly trained athletes have to train twice a week to maintain their strength levels.

Frequency of strength training for body builders varies from person to person. Because they use moderate resistance, daily or even two a day workouts are common. The frequency depends on the amount of resistance, number of sets performed per session, and the person's ability to recover from the previous exercise bout (see Table 7.5). The latter often is dictated by level of conditioning.

Exercise Variations Multiple-joint and single-joint exercises are used in strength training. Multiple-joint exercises, such as the squat, bench press, and lat pull-down, require more skill and complex neural responses. Multiple-joint exercises allow you to lift more weight and develop more strength. Single-joint exercises, such as the arm curl or knee extension, are used to target specific muscles for further development. Both are recommended for a comprehensive training program.

Figure 7.5 Strength-training guidelines.

Mode: Select 8 to 10 dynamic strength-training exercises that involve the body's major muscle groups and include opposing muscle groups (chest and upper back, abdomen and lower back, front and back of the legs).

Resistance: Sufficient resistance to perform 8 to 12 repetitions maximum for muscular strength and 15 to 25 repetitions to near fatigue for muscular edurance. Older adults and injury prone individuals should use 10 to 15 repetitions with moderate resistance (50% to 60% of their 1 RM).

Sets: 2 to 4 sets per exercise with 2 to 3 minutes recovery between sets for optimal strength development. Less than 2 minutes per set if exercises are alternated that require different muscle groups (chest and upper back) or between muscular endurance sets.

Frequency: 2 to 3 days per week on nonconsecutive days. More frequent training can be done if different muscle groups are exercised on different days. (Allow at least 48 hours between strength-training sessions of the same muscle group.)

SOURCE: Adapted from American College of Sports Medicine, *ACSM's Guidelines for Exercise Testing and Prescription* (Philadelphia: Wolters Kluwer/Lippincott Williams & Wilkins, 2014).

Many strength-training exercises can be performed bilaterally and unilaterally. Muscle activation differs between the two modes. Unilateral training can enhance selected sport skills, such as single-leg jumping, high jumping, and single-arm throwing. Unilateral training is also used extensively in rehab programs. For example, bilateral concentric knee extension followed by unilateral eccentric knee flexion is strongly recommended for individuals with weak knees and to prevent potential knee problems (see Exercise 28B). Both modes of training are recommended to maximize strength gains.

Table 7.5 Guidelines for Various Strength-Training Programs

Strength-Training Program	Resistance	Sets	Rest Between Sets*	Frequency (workouts per week)**
General fitness	8–12 reps max	2–4	2–3 min	2–3
Muscular endurance	15–25 reps	1–2	1–2 min	2–3
Maximal strength	1–6 reps max	2–5	3 min	2–3
Body building	8–20 reps near max	3–8	up to 1 min	4–12

*Recovery between sets can be decreased by alternating exercises that use different muscle groups.

**Weekly training sessions can be increased by using a split-body routine.

© Cengage Learning

From a health-fitness standpoint, one to two strength-training sessions per week are sufficient to maintain strength.

7.5 Plyometrics

Strength, speed, and explosiveness are all crucial for success in athletics. All three of these factors are enhanced with a progressive resistance-training program, but greater increases in speed and explosiveness are thought to be possible with **plyometric exercise**. The objective is to generate the greatest amount of force in the shortest time. A solid strength base is necessary before attempting plyometric exercises.

Plyometric training is popular in sports that require powerful movements, such as basketball, volleyball, sprinting, jumping, and gymnastics. A typical plyometric exercise involves jumping off and back onto a box, attempting to rebound as quickly as possible on each jump. Box heights are increased progressively from about 12 to 22 inches.

The bounding action attempts to take advantage of the stretch-recoil and stretch reflex characteristics of muscle. The rapid stretch applied to the muscle during contact with the ground is thought to augment muscle contraction, leading to more explosiveness. Plyometrics can be used, too, for strengthening upper body muscles. An example is doing push-ups so that the extension of the arms is forceful enough to drive the hands (and body) completely off the floor during each repetition.

A drawback of plyometric training is its higher risk for injuries compared with conventional modes of progressive resistance training. For instance, the potential for injury in rebound exercise escalates with the increase in box height or the number of repetitions.

Strength Gains A common question by many strength-training participants is: How quickly can strength gains be observed? Strength-training studies have revealed that most of the strength gains are seen in the first 8 weeks of training. The amount of improvement, however, is related to previous training status. Increases of 40 percent are seen in individuals with no previous strength-training experience, 16 percent in previously strength-trained people, and 10 percent in advanced individuals.[13] Using a periodized strength-training program can yield further improvements (also see "Periodization," Chapter 9).

Critical Thinking

Your roommate started a strength-training program last year and has seen good results. He is now strength training on a nearly daily basis and taking performance-enhancing supplements hoping to accelerate results. What are your feelings about his program? • What would you say (and not say) to him?

7.6 Strength-Training Exercises

The strength-training programs introduced on pages 262–278 provide a complete body workout. The major muscles of the human body referred to in the exercises are pointed out in Figure 7.6 and with the exercises themselves at the end of the chapter.

Only a minimum of equipment is required for the first program, Strength-Training Exercises without Weights (exercises 1 through 14). You can conduct this program in your own home. Your body weight is used as the primary resistance for most exercises. A few exercises call for a friend's help or some basic implements from around your house to provide greater resistance.

Strength-Training Exercises with Weights (Exercises 15 through 37) require machines as shown in the accompanying photographs. These exercises can be conducted on either fixed-resistance or variable-resistance equipment. Many of these exercises also can be performed with free weights. The first 13 of these exercises (15 to 27) are recommended to get a complete workout. You can do these exercises as circuit training. If time is a factor, as a minimum perform the first nine (15 through 23) exercises. Exercises 28 to 37 are supplemental or can replace some of the basic 13 (e.g., substitute Exercise 29 or 30 for 15; 31 for 16; 33 for 19; 34 for 24; 35 for 26; 32 for 27). Exercises 38 to 46 are stability ball exercises that can be used to complement your workout. Some of these exercises can also take the place of others that you use to strengthen similar muscle groups.

Selecting different exercises for a given muscle group is recommended between training sessions (e.g., chest press for bench press). No evidence indicates that a given exercise is best for a given muscle group. Changing exercises works the specific muscle group through a different range of motion and may change the difficulty of the exercise. Alternating exercises is also beneficial to avoid the monotony of repeating the same training program each training session.

Dietary Guidelines for Strength Development

Individuals who wish to enhance muscle growth and strength during periods of intense strength training should increase protein to 1.2 to 2.0 grams per kilogram of

> **Circuit training** Alternating exercises by performing them in a sequence of three to six or more.
>
> **Plyometric exercise** Explosive jump training, incorporating speed and strength training to enhance explosiveness.

body weight per day. The selected amount should be based on the volume of the undertaken strength-training program. An additional 500 daily calories are also recommended to optimize muscle mass gain. If protein intake is already in the range of 1.2 to 2.0 grams per kilogram of body weight, the additional 500 calories should come primarily from complex carbohydrates to provide extra nutrients to the body and glucose for the working muscles.

The time of day when carbohydrates and protein are consumed in relation to the strength-training workout also plays a role in promoting muscle growth. Studies suggest that consuming a pre-exercise snack consisting of a combination of carbohydrates and protein is beneficial to muscle development. The carbohydrates supply energy for training, and the availability of amino acids (the building blocks of protein) in the blood during training enhances muscle building. A peanut butter, turkey, or tuna sandwich; milk or yogurt and fruit; or nuts and fruit consumed 30 to 60 minutes before training are excellent choices for a pre-workout snack.

Consuming a carbohydrate/protein snack immediately following strength training and a second snack an hour thereafter further promotes muscle growth and strength development.

Figure 7.6 Major muscles of the human body.

> ## Behavior Modification Planning
>
> ### Healthy Strength Training
>
> - Make a progressive resistance strength-training program a priority in your weekly schedule.
> - Strength train at least once a week; even better, twice a week.
> - Find a facility where you feel comfortable training and where you can get good professional guidance.
> - Learn the proper technique for each exercise.
> - Train with a friend or group of friends.
> - Consume a pre-exercise snack consisting of a combination of carbohydrates and some protein about 30 to minutes before each strength-training session.
> - Use a minimum of 8 to 10 exercises that involve all major muscle groups of your body.
> - Perform at least one set of each exercise to near muscular fatigue.
> - To enhance protein synthesis, consume one post-exercise snack with a 4-to-1 gram ratio of carbohydrates to protein immediately following strength training; and a second snack one hour thereafter.
> - Allow at least 48 hours between strength-training sessions that involve the same muscle groups.
>
> ### Try It
>
> Attend the school's fitness or recreation center and have an instructor or fitness trainer help you design a progressive resistance strength-training program. Train twice a week for the next four weeks. Thereafter, evaluate the results and write down your feelings about the program.

Post-exercise carbohydrates help restore muscle glycogen depleted during training and, in combination with protein, induce an increase in blood insulin and growth hormone levels. These hormones are essential to the muscle-building process.

Muscle fibers also absorb a greater amount of amino acids up to 48 hours following strength training. The first hour, nonetheless, seems to be the most critical. A higher level of circulating amino acids in the bloodstream immediately after training is believed to increase protein synthesis to a greater extent than amino acids made available later in the day. A ratio of 4-to-1 grams of carbohydrates to protein is recommended for a post-exercise snack—for example, a snack containing 40 grams of carbohydrates (160 calories) and 10 grams of protein (40 calories).

Distributing protein intake throughout the day is important to build and maintain lean tissue. Spreading the intake over three meals (25 to 30 grams of high-quality protein per meal) is most effective in keeping people satisfied, build and maintain tissues, and reduce caloric intake the rest of the day.

Core Strength Training The trunk (spine) and pelvis are referred to as the "core" of the body. Core muscles include the abdominal muscles (rectus, transversus, and internal and external obliques), hip muscles (front and back), and spinal muscles (lower and upper back muscles). These muscle groups are responsible for maintaining the stability of the spine and pelvis.

Many of the major muscle groups of the legs, shoulders, and arms attach to the core. A strong core allows a person to perform activities of daily living with greater ease, improve sports performance through a more effective energy transfer from large to small body parts, and decrease the incidence of low back pain. Core strength training also contributes to better posture and balance.

A major objective of core training is to exercise the abdominal and lower back muscles in unison. Furthermore, individuals should spend as much time training the back muscles as they do the abdominal muscles. Besides enhancing stability, core training improves dynamic balance, which is often required during physical activity and participation in sports.

Key core training exercises include the abdominal crunch and bent-leg curl-up, reverse crunch, pelvic tilt, lateral plank, prone plank, leg press, seated back, lat pull-down, back extension, lateral trunk flexion, supine plank, and pelvic clock (Exercises 4, 11, 12, 13, 14, 16, 20, 24, 36, and 37 in this chapter and Exercises 26 and 27 in Chapter 8, respectively). Stability ball exercises 38 through 46 are also used to strengthen the core.

When core training is used in athletic conditioning programs, athletes attempt to mimic the dynamic skills they use in their sport. To do so, they use special equipment such as balance boards, stability balls, and foam pads. Using this equipment allows the athletes to train the core while seeking balance and stability in a sport-specific manner.

> **Core strength training** A program designed to strengthen the abdominal, hip, and spinal muscles (the core of the body).
>
> **Pilates** A training program that uses exercises designed to help strengthen the body's core by developing pelvic stability and abdominal control; exercises are coupled with focused breathing patterns.

Pilates Exercise System

Pilates exercises have become increasingly popular in recent years. Previously, Pilates training was used primarily by dancers, but now this exercise modality is embraced by a large number of fitness participants, rehab patients, models, actors, and even professional athletes. Pilates studios, college courses, and classes at health clubs are available nationwide.

The Pilates training system was originally developed in the 1920s by German physical therapist Joseph Pilates. He designed the exercises to help strengthen the body's core by developing pelvic stability and abdominal control, coupled with focused breathing patterns.

Pilates exercises are performed either on a mat (floor) or with specialized equipment to help increase strength and flexibility of deep postural muscles. The intent is to improve muscle tone and length (a limber body), instead of increasing muscle size (hypertrophy). Pilates mat classes focus on body stability and proper body mechanics. The exercises are performed in a slow, controlled, and precise manner. When performed properly, these exercises require intense concentration. Initially, Pilates training should be conducted under the supervision of certified instructors with extensive Pilates teaching experience.

Fitness goals of Pilates programs include better flexibility, muscle tone, posture, spinal support, body balance, low-back health, sports performance, and mind–body awareness. Individuals with loose or unstable joints benefit from Pilates because the exercises are designed to enhance joint stability. The Pilates program is also used to help lose weight, increase lean tissue, and manage stress. Although Pilates programs are quite popular, more research is required to corroborate the benefits attributed to this training system.

Stability Exercise Balls A stability exercise ball is a large flexible and inflatable ball used for exercises that combines the principles of Pilates with core strength training. Stability exercises are specifically designed to develop abdominal, hip, chest, and spinal muscles by addressing core stabilization while the exerciser maintains a balanced position over the ball. Particular emphasis is placed on correct movement and maintenance of proper body alignment to involve as much of the core as possible. Although the primary objective is core strength and stability, many stability exercises can be performed to strengthen other body areas as well.

Stability exercises are thought to be more effective than similar exercises on the ground. For instance, just sitting on the ball requires the use of stabilizing core muscles (including the rectus abdominis and the external and internal obliques) to keep the body from falling off the ball. Traditional strength-training exercises are primarily for strength and power development and do not contribute as much to body balance.

When performing stability exercises, choose a ball size based on your height. Your thighs should be parallel to the floor when you sit on the ball. A slightly larger ball may be used if you suffer from back problems. Several stability ball exercises are provided on pages 276–278. For best results, have a trained specialist teach you the proper technique and watch your form while you learn the exercises. Individuals who have a weak muscular system, poor balance, or who are older than the age of 65 should perform stability exercises under the supervision of a qualified trainer.

Elastic-Band Resistive Exercise Elastic bands and tubing can also be used for strength training. This type of constant-resistance training has increased in popularity and can be used to supplement traditional strength training as it has shown to help increase strength, mobility, functional ability (particularly in older adults), and to aid in the rehab of many types of injuries. Some of the advantages to using this type of training include low cost, versatility (you can create resistance in almost all angles and directions of the range of motion), use of a large number of exercises to work all joints of the body, and they provide a great way to work out while traveling (exercise bands can be easily packed in a suitcase). This type of resistance training can also add variety to your routine workout.

Elastic-band resistive exercise workouts can be just as challenging as with free weights or machines. Due to the constant resistance provided by the bands or tubing, the training may appear more difficult to some individuals because the resistance is used both during the eccentric and concentric phases of the repetition. Additionally, the bands can be used by beginners and strength-trained individuals. That is because several different tension cords (up to eight bands) are available and all participants can progress through various resistance levels.

At the beginning, it may be a little confusing trying to determine how to use the bands and create the proper loops to grip the bands. The assistance of a training video, an instructor, or a personal trainer is helpful. The bands can be wrapped around a post, a doorknob, or you can stand on them as well for some of the exercises. A few sample exercises with elastic-band resistive exercises are provided in Figure 7.7. Instructional booklets are available for purchase with your elastic band or tubing.

7.7 Exercise Safety Guidelines

As you prepare to design your strength-training program, keep the following guidelines in mind:

- Safety is the most important component in strength training. If you are new to strength training or if you are lifting alone, strength-training machines are the best option for you. Experienced lifters like to use a combination of both free weights and strength-training machines.
- Select exercises that will involve all major muscle groups: chest, shoulders, back, legs, arms, hip, and trunk.
- Select exercises that will strengthen the core. Use controlled movements and start with light-to-moderate re-

sistances. (Later, athletes may use explosive movements with heavier resistances.)

- Never lift weights alone. Always have someone work out with you in case you need a spotter or help with an injury. When you use free weights, one to two spotters are recommended for certain exercises (e.g., bench press, squats, and overhead press).
- Prior to lifting weights, warm up properly by performing a light- to moderate-intensity aerobic activity (5 to 7 minutes) and some gentle stretches for a few minutes.
- Use proper lifting technique for each exercise. The correct lifting technique will involve only those muscles and joints intended for a specific exercise. Involving other muscles and joints to "cheat" during the exercise to complete a repetition or to be able to lift a greater resistance decreases the long-term effectiveness of the exercise and can lead to injury (such as arching the back during the push-up, squat, or bench press exercises). Proper lifting technique also implies performing the exercises in a controlled manner and throughout the entire range of motion. Perform each repetition in a rhythmic manner and at a moderate speed. Avoid fast and jerky movements, and do not throw the entire body into the lifting motion. Do not arch the back when lifting a weight.
- Don't lock your elbows and knee joints while lifting. See that you always leave a slight bend in the elbows and knees when straightening out the legs and arms.
- Maintain proper body balance while lifting. Proper balance involves good posture, a stable body position, and correct seat and arm/leg settings on exercise machines. Loss of balance places undue strain on smaller muscles and leads to injuries because of the heavy resistances suddenly placed on them. In the early stages of a program, first-time lifters often struggle with bar control and balance when using free weights. This problem is overcome quickly with practice following a few training sessions.
- Exercise larger muscle groups (such as those in the chest, back, and legs) before exercising smaller muscle groups (arms, abdominals, ankles, and neck). For example, the bench press exercise works the chest, shoul-

Figure 7.7 Sample elastic-band resistive exercises.

ders, and back of the upper arms (triceps), whereas the triceps extension works the back of the upper arms only.
- Exercise opposing muscle groups for a balanced workout. When you work the chest (bench press), also work the back (rowing torso). If you work the biceps (arm curl), also work the triceps (triceps extension).
- Breathe naturally. Inhale during the eccentric phase (bringing the weight down), and exhale during the concentric phase (lifting or pushing the weight up). Practice proper breathing with lighter weights when you are learning a new exercise.
- Avoid holding your breath while straining to lift a weight. Holding your breath increases the pressure inside the chest and abdominal cavity greatly, making it nearly impossible for the blood in the veins to return to the heart. Although rare, a sudden high intrathoracic pressure may lead to dizziness, blackout, stroke, heart attack, or hernia.
- Based on the program selected, allow adequate recovery time between sets of exercises (see Table 7.5).
- If you experience unusual discomfort or pain, discontinue training. Strength-training exercises should not cause pain while lifting. Stay within a range of motion that is comfortable and as you progress along, you can gradually extend the range. The high tension loads used in strength training can exacerbate potential injuries. Discomfort and pain are signals to stop and determine what's wrong. Be sure to evaluate your condition properly before you continue training.
- Use common sense on days when you feel fatigued or when you are performing sets to complete fatigue. Excessive fatigue affects lifting technique, body balance, muscles involved, and range of motion—all of which increase the risk for injury. Learn to listen to your body and decrease exercise intensity and volume if you are not feeling right. A spotter is recommended when sets are performed to complete fatigue. The spotter's help through the most difficult part of the repetition will relieve undue stress on muscles, ligaments, and tendons—and help ensure that you perform the exercise correctly.
- At the end of each strength-training workout, stretch out for a few minutes to help your muscles return to their normal resting length and to minimize muscle soreness and risk for injury.

7.8 Setting Up Your Own Strength-Training Program

The same pre-exercise guidelines outlined for cardiorespiratory endurance training apply to strength training (see Activity 1.3, "PAR-Q and Health History Questionnaire," on page 36). If you have any concerns about your present health status or ability to participate safely in strength training, consult a physician before you start. Strength training is not advised for people with advanced heart disease.

Before you proceed to write your strength-training program, you should determine your stage of change for this fitness component in Activity 7.2 at the end of the chapter. Next, if you are prepared to do so, and depending on the facilities available, you can choose one of the training programs outlined in this chapter (use Activity 7.2). Once you begin your strength-training program, you may use the form provided in Activity 7.3 to keep a record of your training sessions.

You should base the resistance, number of repetitions, and sets you use with your program on your current strength-fitness level and the amount of time that you have for your strength workout. If you are training for reasons other than general health fitness, review Table 7.5 for a summary of the guidelines.

Activity 7.2: Designing Your Strength Training Program

Name _____ Date _____

Course _____ Section _____ Gender _____ Age _____

I. Stage of Change for Muscular Strength or Endurance
Using Figure 2.5 (page 63) and Table 2.3 (page 62), identify your current stage of change for participation in a muscular strength or muscular endurance program:

[   ]

II. Instructions
Select one of the two strength-training exercise programs. Perform all of the recommended exercises and, with the exception of the abdominal curl-up exercises, determine the resistance required to do approximately 10 repetitions maximum. For "Strength-Training Exercises without Weights," simply indicate the total number of repetitions performed. For the abdominal crunches or curl-up exercises, perform or build up to about 20 repetitions.

1. Strength-Training Exercises without Weights

Exercise	Repetitions
Step-up	
Rowing torso	
Push-up	
Abdominal crunch or bent-leg curl-up	
Leg curl	
Modified dip	
Pull-up or arm curl	
Heel raise	
Leg abduction and adduction	
Reverse crunch	
Pelvic tilt	
Lateral plank	
Prone plank	

2. Strength-Training Exercises with Weights

Exercise	Repetitions	Resistance
Bench press, shoulder press, or chest press (select and circle one)		
Leg press or squat (select one)		
Abdominal crunch or bent-leg curl-up		N/A
Rowing torso		
Arm curl or upright rowing (select one)		
Leg curl or seated leg curl (select one)		
Seated back		
Heel raise		
Lat pull-down or bent-arm pullover (select one)		
Rotary torso		
Triceps extension or dip (select one)		
Leg extension		
Back extension		

III. Your Personalized Strength-Training Program

Once you have performed the strength-training exercises in this lab, and depending on your personal preference (strength versus endurance), design your strength-training program selecting a minimum of 8 to 10 exercises. Indicate the number of sets, repetitions, and approximate resistance that you will use. Also state the days of the week, time, and facility that will be used for this program.

Strength-training days: M ☐ T ☐ W ☐ Th ☐ F ☐ Sa ☐ Su ☐ Time of day: ☐ Facility: ☐

	Exercise	Sets / Reps / Resistance		Exercise	Sets / Reps / Resistance
1.			9.		
2.			10.		
3.			11.		
4.			12.		
5.			13.		
6.			14.		
7.			15.		
8.			16.		

Activity 7.3: Strength-Training Record Form

Name: _____ Date: _____ Course: _____ Section: _____ Gender: _____ Age: _____

Date									
Exercise	St/Reps/Res*	St/Reps/Res*	St/Reps/Res*	St/Reps/Res*	St/Reps/Res*	St/Reps/Res*	St/Reps/Res*	St/Reps/Res*	St/Reps/Res*

*St/Reps/Res = Sets, Repetitions, and Resistance (e.g., 1/6/125 = 1 set of 6 repetitions with 125 pounds)

© Cengage Learning

Name: _____ Date: _____ Course: _____ Section: _____ Gender: _____ Age: _____

Date																	
Exercise	St/Reps/Res*	St/Reps/Res*	St/Reps/Res*	St/Reps/Res*	St/Reps/Res*	St/Reps/Res*	St/Reps/Res*	St/Reps/Res*	St/Reps/Res*	St/Reps/Res*	St/Reps/Res*	St/Reps/Res*	St/Reps/Res*	St/Reps/Res*	St/Reps/Res*	St/Reps/Res*	St/Reps/Res*

*St/Reps/Res = Sets, Repetitions, and Resistance (e.g., 1/6/125 = 1 set of 6 repetitions with 125 pounds)

© Cengage Learning

ASSESS YOUR BEHAVIOR

To access course materials, including companion resources, please visit www.cengagebrain.com.

1. Are your strength levels sufficient to perform tasks of daily living (climbing stairs, carrying a backpack, opening jars, doing housework, mowing the yard) without requiring additional assistance or feeling unusually fatigued?

2. Do you regularly participate in a strength-training program that includes all major muscle groups of the body, and do you perform at least one set of each exercise to near fatigue?

ASSESS YOUR KNOWLEDGE

Evaluate how well you understand the concepts presented in this chapter using the chapter-specific quizzing available in the online materials at www.cengagebrain.com.

1. The ability of a muscle to exert submaximal force repeatedly over time is known as
   a. muscular strength.
   b. plyometric training.
   c. muscular endurance.
   d. isokinetic training.
   e. isometric training.

2. In older adults, each additional pound of muscle tissue increases resting metabolism by
   a. 10 calories.
   b. 17 calories.
   c. 23 calories.
   d. 35 calories.
   e. 50 calories.

3. The Hand Grip Strength Test is an example of
   a. an isometric test.
   b. an isotonic test.
   c. a dynamic test.
   d. an isokinetic test.
   e. a plyometric test.

4. A 70th-percentile rank places an individual in the ___ fitness category.
   a. excellent
   b. good
   c. average
   d. fair
   e. poor

5. During an eccentric muscle contraction,
   a. the muscle shortens as it overcomes the resistance.
   b. there is little or no movement during the contraction.
   c. a joint has to move through the entire range of motion.
   d. the muscle lengthens as it contracts.
   e. the speed is kept constant throughout the range of motion.

6. The training concept stating that the demands placed on a system must be increased systematically and progressively over time to cause physiological adaptation is referred to as
   a. the overload principle.
   b. positive-resistance training.
   c. specificity of training.
   d. variable-resistance training.
   e. progressive resistance.

7. A set in strength training refers to
   a. the starting position for an exercise.
   b. the recovery time required between exercises.
   c. a given number of repetitions.
   d. the starting resistance used in an exercise.
   e. the sequence in which exercises are performed.

8. For health fitness, the recommendation of the American College of Sports Medicine is that a person should perform a maximum of between
   a. 1 and 6 reps.
   b. 4 and 10 reps.
   c. 8 and 12 reps.
   d. 10 and 25 reps.
   e. 20 and 30 reps.

9. Plyometric training frequently is used to help with performance in
   a. gymnastics.
   b. basketball.
   c. volleyball.
   d. sprinting.
   e. all of these sports.

10. The posterior deltoid, rhomboids, and trapezius muscles can be developed with the
    a. bench press.
    b. lat pull-down.
    c. rotary torso.
    d. squat.
    e. rowing torso.

Correct answers can be found at the back of the book.

Strength-Training Exercises without Weights

EXERCISE 1 Step-Up

ACTION Step up and down using a box or chair approximately 12 to 15 inches high (a). Conduct one set using the same leg each time you step up, and then conduct a second set using the other leg. You also could alternate legs on each step-up cycle. You may increase the resistance by holding a child or an object in your arms (b). Hold the child or object close to the body to avoid increased strain in the lower back.

Back Front Back

A

B

MUSCLES DEVELOPED Gluteal muscles, quadriceps, gastrocnemius, and soleus

EXERCISE 2 Rowing Torso

ACTION Raise your arms laterally (abduction) to a horizontal position and bend your elbows to 90°. Have a partner apply enough pressure on your elbows to gradually force your arms forward (horizontal flexion) while you try to resist the pressure. Next, reverse the action, horizontally forcing the arms backward as your partner applies sufficient forward pressure to create resistance.

Back

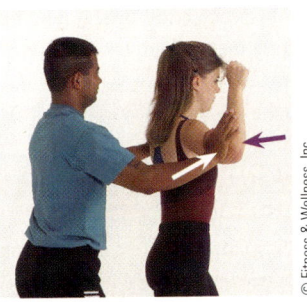

MUSCLES DEVELOPED Posterior deltoid, rhomboids, and trapezius

EXERCISE 3 Push-Up

ACTION Maintaining your body as straight as possible (a), flex the elbows, lowering the body until you almost touch the floor (b), then raise yourself back up to the starting position. If you are unable to perform the push-up as indicated, decrease the resistance by supporting the lower body with the knees rather than the feet (c).

MUSCLES DEVELOPED Triceps, deltoid, pectoralis major, abdominals, and erector spinae

Back

Back

Front

Front

A

B

C

EXERCISE 4
Abdominal Crunch and Bent-Leg Curl-Up

ACTION Start with your head and shoulders off the floor, arms crossed on your chest, and knees slightly bent (a). The greater the flexion of the knee, the more difficult the curl-up. Now curl up to about 30° (abdominal crunch—illustration b) or curl up all the way (abdominal curl-up—illustration c), then return to the starting position without letting the head or shoulders touch the floor or allowing the hips to come off the floor. If you allow the hips to rise off the floor and the head and shoulders to touch the floor, you most likely will "swing up" on the next crunch or curl-up, which minimizes the work of the abdominal muscles. If you cannot curl up with the arms on the chest, place the hands by the side of the hips or even help yourself up by holding on to your thighs (d and e). Do not perform the sit-up exercise with your legs completely extended, because this will strain the lower back.

MUSCLES DEVELOPED Abdominal muscles and hip flexors

Front

NOTE The abdominal curl-up exercise should be used only by individuals of at least average fitness without a history of lower back problems. New participants and those with a history of lower back problems should use the abdominal crunch exercise in its place.

EXERCISE 5 Leg Curl

ACTION Lie on the floor face down. Cross the right ankle over the left heel (a). Apply resistance with your right foot while you bring the left foot up to 90° at the knee joint (b). Apply enough resistance so that the left foot can only be brought up slowly. Repeat the exercise, crossing the left ankle over the right heel.

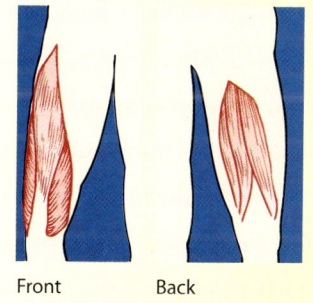
Front   Back

MUSCLES DEVELOPED Hamstrings (and quadriceps)

EXERCISE 6 Modified Dip

ACTION Place your hands on a box or gymnasium bleacher. The feet are supported and held in place by an exercise partner (a). Dip down at least to a 90° angle at the elbow joint (b), and then return to the starting position.

A   B

Back   Front

MUSCLES DEVELOPED Triceps, deltoid, and pectoralis major

EXERCISE 7 Pull Up

ACTION Suspend yourself from a bar with a pronated (thumbs-in) grip (a). Pull your body up until your chin is above the bar (b), then lower the body slowly to the starting position. If you are unable to perform the pull-up as described, have a partner hold your feet to push off and facilitate the movement upward (c and d).

A   B   C   D

Front   Front

MUSCLES DEVELOPED
Biceps, brachioradialis, brachialis, trapezius, and latissimus dorsi

---

EXERCISE 8 Arm Curl

ACTION Using a palms-up grip, start with the arm completely extended and, with the aid of a backpack filled with books as needed (a), curl up as far as possible (b), then return to the initial position. Repeat the exercise with the other arm.

A   B

Front

MUSCLES DEVELOPED
Biceps, brachioradialis, and brachialis

EXERCISE 9 Heel Raise

ACTION From a standing position with feet flat on the floor or at the edge of a step (a), raise and lower your body weight by moving at the ankle joint only (b). For added resistance, have someone else hold your shoulders down as you perform the exercise.

A   B

Back

MUSCLES DEVELOPED
Gastrocnemius and soleus

EXERCISE 10 Leg Abduction and Adduction

ACTION Both participants sit on the floor. The person on the left places the feet on the inside of the other person's feet. Simultaneously, the person on the left presses the legs laterally (to the outside—abduction), while the person on the right presses the legs medially (adduction). Hold the contraction for 5 to 10 seconds. Repeat the exercise at all three angles, and then reverse the pressing sequence: The person on the left places the feet on the outside and presses inward while the person on the right presses outward.

MUSCLES DEVELOPED Hip abductors (rectus femoris, sartori, gluteus medius and minimus) and adductors (pectineus, gracilis, dductor magnus, adductor longus, and adductor brevis)

Back

EXERCISE 11 Reverse Crunch

ACTION Lie on your back with arms to the sides and knees and hips flexed at 90° (a). Now attempt to raise the pelvis off the floor by lifting vertically from the knees and lower legs (b). This is a challenging exercise that may be difficult for beginners to perform.

Front

MUSCLES DEVELOPED Abdominals

A   B

EXERCISE 12 Pelvic Tilt

ACTION Lie flat on the floor with the knees bent at about a 90° angle (a). Tilt the pelvis by tightening the abdominal muscles, flattening your back against the floor, and raising the lower gluteal area ever so slightly off the floor (b). Hold the final position for several seconds.

AREAS STRETCHED Low back muscles and ligaments

AREAS STRENGTHENED Abdominal and gluteal muscles

Front   Back

A

B

EXERCISE 13 Lateral Plank

ACTION Lie on your side with legs bent (a: easier version) or straight (b: harder version) and support the upper body with your arm. Straighten your body by raising the hip off the floor and hold the position for several seconds. Repeat the exercise with the other side of the body.

MUSCLES DEVELOPED Abdominals (obliques and transversus abdominus) and quadratus lumborum (lower back)

Front   Back

A

B

EXERCISE 14
Prone Plank

ACTION Starting in a prone position on a floor mat, balance yourself on the tips of your toes and elbows while attempting to maintain a straight body from heels to shoulders (do not arch the lower back [a]). You can increase the difficulty of this exercise by placing your hands in front of you and straightening the arms (b).

MUSCLES DEVELOPED Anterior and posterior muscle groups of the trunk and pelvis

Front   Back

A

B

Strength-Training Exercises with Weights

EXERCISE 15 Bench (Chest) Press

MUSCLES DEVELOPED Pectoralis major, triceps, and deltoid

MACHINE From a seated position, grasp the bar handles (a) and press forward until the arms are completely extended (b), then return to the original position. Do not arch the back during this exercise.

FREE WEIGHTS Lie on the bench with arms extended and have one or two spotters help you place the barbell directly over your shoulders (a). Lower the weight to your chest (b) and then push it back up until you achieve full extension of the arms. Do not arch the back during this exercise.

Front   Back

A

A   B

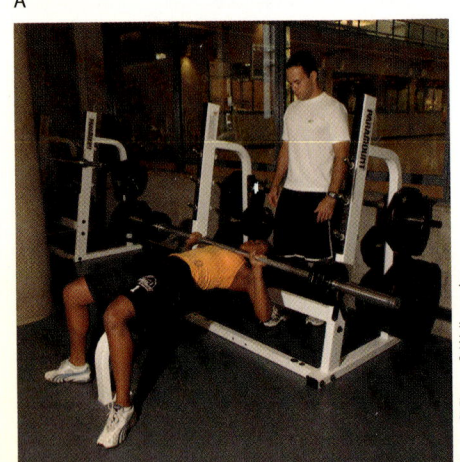
B

EXERCISE 16 Leg Press

ACTION From a sitting position with the knees flexed at about 100° and both feet on the footrest (a), extend the legs fully (b), then return slowly to the starting position.

MUSCLES DEVELOPED Quadriceps and gluteal muscles

Front   Back

A

B

EXERCISE 17 Abdominal Crunch

ACTION Sit in an upright position. Grasp the handles in front of the chest pad and crunch forward. Return slowly to the original position.

MUSCLES DEVELOPED Abdominals

A

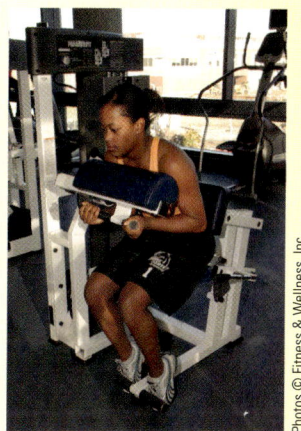
B

EXERCISE 18A Rowing Torso

ACTION Sit in the machine and grasp the handles in front of you (a). Press back as far as possible, drawing the shoulder blades together (b). Return to the original position.

A

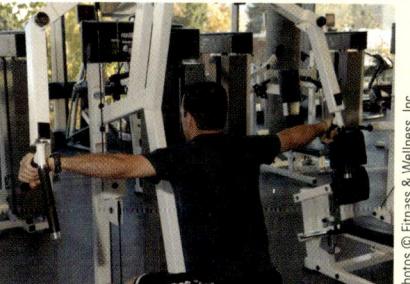
B

Back

MUSCLES DEVELOPED Posterior deltoid, rhomboids, and trapezius

EXERCISE 18B Bent-Over Lateral Raise

ACTION Bend over with your back straight and knees bent at about 5 to 10° (a). Hold one dumbbell in each hand. Raise the dumbbells laterally to about shoulder level (b) and then slowly return them to the starting position.

A

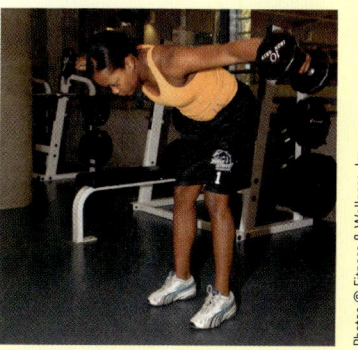
B

EXERCISE 19 Leg Curl

ACTION Lie with the face down on the bench, legs straight, and place the back of the feet under the padded bar (a). Curl up to at least 90° (b), and return to the original position.

MUSCLES DEVELOPED
Hamstrings

Back

A

B

EXERCISE 20 Seated Back

ACTION Sit in the machine with your trunk flexed and the upper back against the shoulder pad. Place the feet under the padded bar and hold on with your hands to the bars on the sides (a). Start the exercise by pressing backward, simultaneously extending the trunk and hip joints (b). Slowly return to the original position.

MUSCLES DEVELOPED Erector spinae and gluteus maximus

Back

A

B

Exercise 21 Calf Press

MACHINE Start with your feet flat on the plate (a). Now extend the ankles by pressing on the plate with the balls of your feet (b).

FREE WEIGHTS In a standing position, place a barbell across the shoulders and upper back. Grip the bar by the shoulders (a). Raise your heels off the floor or step box as far as possible (b) and then slowly return them to the starting position.

A

B

Back

MUSCLES DEVELOPED
Gastrocnemius and soleus

A

B

EXERCISE 22   Leg (Hip) Adduction

ACTION Adjust the pads on the inside of the thighs as far out as the desired range of motion to be accomplished during the exercise (a). Press the legs together until both pads meet at the center (b). Slowly return to the starting position.

MUSCLES DEVELOPED Hip adductors (pectineus, gracilis, adductor magnus, adductor longus, and adductor brevis)

Front

A

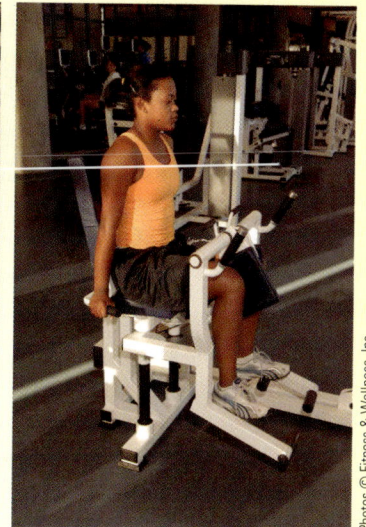
B

EXERCISE 23   Leg (Hip) Abduction

ACTION Place your knees together with the pads directly outside the knees (a). Press the legs laterally out as far as possible (b). Slowly return to the starting position.

MUSCLES DEVELOPED Hip abductors (rectus femoris, sartori, gluteus medius, and minimus)

Front   Back

A

B

EXERCISE 24   Lat Pull-Down

ACTION Starting from a sitting position, hold the exercise bar with a wide grip (a). Pull the bar down in front of you until it reaches the upper chest (b), then return to the starting position.

Back   Front

MUSCLES DEVELOPED Latissimus dorsi, pectoralis major, and biceps

A

B

EXERCISE 25   Rotary Torso

ACTION Stand with your feet slightly apart. Place a barbell across your shoulders and upper back, holding on to the sides of the barbell. Now gently, and in a controlled manner, twist your torso to one side as far as possible and then do so in the opposite direction.

MUSCLES DEVELOPED Internal and external obliques (abdominal muscles)

Front

EXERCISE 26   Triceps Extension

MUSCLES DEVELOPED Triceps

Back

MACHINE Sit in an upright position and grasp the bar behind the shoulders (a). Fully extend the arms (b) and then return to the original position.

A   B

MACHINE Using a palms-down grip, grasp the bar slightly closer than shoulder-width and start with the elbows almost completely bent (a). Extend the arms fully (b), then return to starting position.

A   B

FREE WEIGHTS In a standing position, hold a barbell with both hands overhead and with the arms in full extension (a). Slowly lower the barbell behind your head (b) and then return it to the starting position.

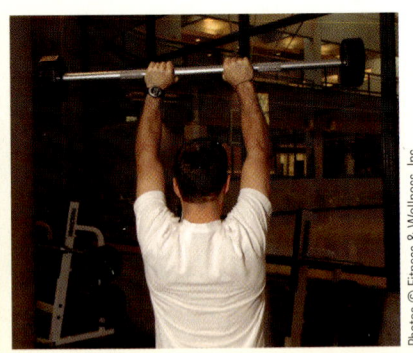
A   B

EXERCISE 27 Arm Curl

A   B

MACHINE Using a supinated (palms-up) grip, start with the arms almost completely extended (a). Curl up as far as possible (b), then return to the starting position.

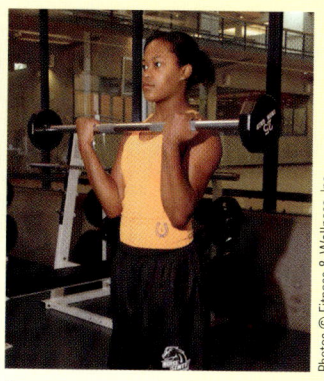

A   B

FREE WEIGHTS Standing upright, hold a barbell in front of you at about shoulder width with arms extended and the hands in a thumbs-out position (supinated grip) (a). Raise the barbell to your shoulders (b) and slowly return it to the starting position.

MUSCLES DEVELOPED Biceps, brachioradialis, and brachialis

Front

EXERCISE 28A
Leg Extension

ACTION Sit in an upright position with the feet under the padded bar and grasp the handles at the sides (a). Extend the legs until they are completely straight (b), then return to the starting position.

MUSCLES DEVELOPED Quadriceps

Front

A   B

EXERCISE 28B Unilateral Eccentric Knee Flexion

ACTION Using a moderate resistance, raise the padded bar by extending both knees (a and b). Next, remove the left foot from the padded bar while holding the bar in place with the right leg (c). Now slowly lower the resistance (padded bar) to about 45° (d). Return the left foot to the padded bar and once again press the bar up to full knee extension. Alternate legs by releasing the right foot next and lower the resistance with the left foot. Repeat the exercise about 10 times with each leg. This exercise is quite helpful to strengthen weak knees and prevent potential future knee problems.

C   D   E

EXERCISE 29 Shoulder Press

Back   Front

MUSCLES DEVELOPED Triceps, deltoid, and pectoralis major

A   B

MACHINE Sit in an upright position and grasp the bar wider than shoulder width (a). Press the bar all the way up until the arms are fully extended (b), then return to the initial position.

A   B

FREE WEIGHTS Place a barbell on your shoulders (a) and press the weight overhead until complete extension of the arms is achieved (b). Return the weight to the original position. Be sure not to arch the back or lean back during this exercise.

EXERCISE 30A Chest Fly

ACTION Start with the arms out to the side, and grasp the handlebars with the arms straight (a). Press the movement arms forward until they are completely in front of you (b). Slowly return to the starting position.

Front

MUSCLES DEVELOPED Pectoralis major and deltoid

A   B

EXERCISE 30B Bent-Arm Fly

ACTION Lie down on your back on a bench and hold a dumbbell in each hand directly overhead (a). Keeping your elbows slightly bent, lower the weights laterally to a horizontal position (b) and then bring them back up to the starting position.

 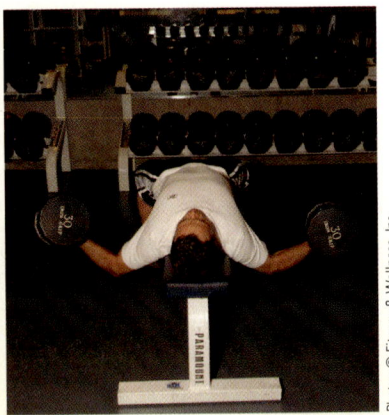

A   B

EXERCISE 31 Squat

MACHINE Place the shoulders under the pads and grasp the handles in front of you (a). Slowly bend the knees to about 120° (b). Return to the starting position.

MUSCLES DEVELOPED Quadriceps, gluteus maximus, and erector spinae

Front   Back   Back

A

B

FREE WEIGHTS From a standing position, and with a spotter to each side, support a barbell over your shoulders and upper back (a). Keeping your head up and back straight, bend at the knees and the hips until you achieve an approximate 120° angle at the knees (b). Return to the starting position. *Do not perform this exercise alone.* If no spotters are available, use a squat rack to ensure that you will not get trapped under a heavy weight.

A

B

EXERCISE 32 Upright Rowing

A

B

MACHINE Start with the arms extended and grip the handles with the palms down (a). Pull all the way up to the chin (b), then return to the starting position.

FREE WEIGHTS Hold a barbell in front of you, with the arms fully extended and hands in a thumbs-in (pronated) grip less than shoulder-width apart (a). Pull the barbell up until it reaches shoulder level (b) and then slowly return it to the starting position.

A

B

Front

Front

Back

MUSCLES DEVELOPED Biceps, brachioradialis, brachialis, deltoid, and trapezius

EXERCISE 33 Seated Leg Curl

ACTION Sit in the unit and place the thigh pad over the upper thighs. With legs extended, place the back of the feet over the lower-leg pad (a). Flex the knees until you reach a 90° to 100° angle (b). Slowly return to the starting position.

A

B

Back

MUSCLES DEVELOPED Hamstrings

EXERCISE 34 Bent-Arm Pullover

ACTION Lie on your back on an exercise bench with your head over the edge of the bench. Hold a barbell over your chest with the hands less than shoulder-width apart (a). Keeping the elbows shoulder-width apart, lower the weight over your head until your shoulders are completely extended (b). Slowly return the weight to the starting position.

A

B

Back   Front

MUSCLES DEVELOPED Latissimus dorsi, pectoral muscles, deltoid, and serratus anterior

EXERCISE 35 Dip

ACTION Start with the elbows flexed (a), then extend the arms fully (b), and return slowly to the initial position.

A

B

Back   Front

MUSCLES DEVELOPED Triceps, deltoid, and pectoralis major

EXERCISE 36 Back Extension

ACTION Place your feet under the ankle pad and the hips over the padded seat. Start with the trunk in a flexed position and the arms crossed over the chest (a). Slowly extend the trunk to a horizontal position (b), hold the extension for 2 to 5 seconds, and then slowly flex (lower) the trunk to the original position.

A

B

MUSCLES DEVELOPED Erector spinae, gluteus maximus, and quadratus lumborum (lower back)

Back

EXERCISE 37   Lateral Trunk Flexion

ACTION Lie sideways on the padded seat with the right foot under the left side of the padded ankle pad (right knee slightly bent) and the left foot stabilized behind the vertical bar. Cross the arms over the abdomen or chest and start with the body in a straight line. Raise (flex) your upper body about 30 to 40° and then slowly return to the starting position.

Front   Back

A

B

MUSCLES DEVELOPED Erector spinae, rectus abdominus, internal and external abdominal obliques, quadratus lumborum, and gluteal muscles

Stability Ball Exercises

EXERCISE 38   The Plank

ACTION Place your knees or feet (increased difficulty) on the ball and raise your body off the floor to a horizontal position. Pull the abdominal muscles in and hold the body in a straight line for 5 to 10 seconds. Repeat the exercise 3 to 5 times.

MUSCLES INVOLVED Abdominals, erector spinae, lower back, hip flexors, gluteal, quadriceps, hamstrings, chest, shoulder, and triceps

EXERCISE 39   Abdominal Crunches

ACTION On your back and with the feet slightly separated, lie with the ball under your back and shoulder blades. Cross the arms over your chest (a). Press your lower back into the ball and crunch up 20° to 30°. Keep your neck and shoulders in line with your trunk (b). Repeat the exercise 10 to 20 times (you may also do an oblique crunch by rotating the ribcage to the opposite hip at the end of the crunch [c]).

MUSCLES INVOLVED Rectus abdominus and internal and external abdominal obliques

A

B

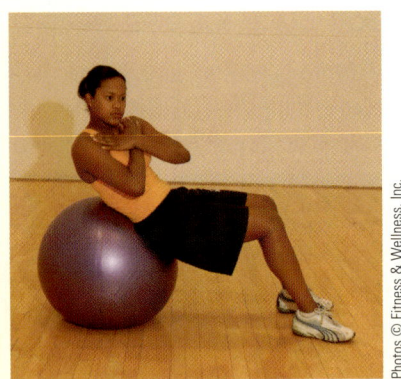
C

Chapter 7 Muscular Fitness: Strength and Endurance 277

EXERCISE 40 Supine Plank

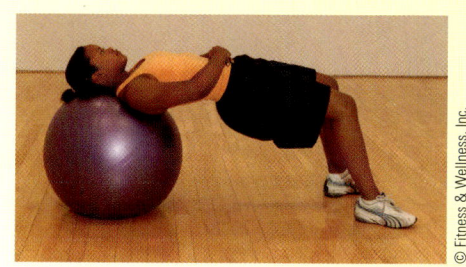

ACTION With the feet slightly separated and knees bent, lie with your neck and upper back on the ball; hands placed on the abdomen. Gently squeeze the gluteal muscles while raising your hips off the floor until the upper legs and trunk reach a straight line. Hold this position for 5 to 10 seconds. Repeat the exercise 3 to 5 times.

MUSCLES INVOLVED Gluteal, abdominals, lower back, hip flexors, quadriceps, and hamstrings

EXERCISE 41 Reverse Supine Plank

ACTION Lie face up on the floor with the heels on the ball. Keeping the abdominal muscles tight, slowly lift the hips off the floor and squeeze the gluteal muscles until the body reaches a straight line. Hold the position for 5 to 10 seconds. Repeat the exercise 3 to 5 times.

MUSCLES INVOLVED Gluteal, abdominals, lower back, erector spinae, hip flexors, quadriceps, and hamstrings

A   B

EXERCISE 42 Push-Ups

ACTION Place the front of your thighs (knees or feet—more difficult) over the ball with the body straight, the arms extended, and the hands under your shoulders. Now bend the elbows and lower the upper body as far as possible. Return to the original position. Repeat the exercise 10 times.

MUSCLES INVOLVED Triceps, chest, shoulder, abdominals, erector spinae, lower back, hip flexors, quadriceps, and hamstrings

EXERCISE 43 Back Extension

ACTION Lie face down with the hips over the ball. Keep the legs straight with the toes on the floor and slightly separated (a). Keep your arms to the sides and extend the trunk until the body reaches a straight position (b). Repeat the exercise 10 times.

MUSCLES INVOLVED Erector spinae, abdominals, and lower back

 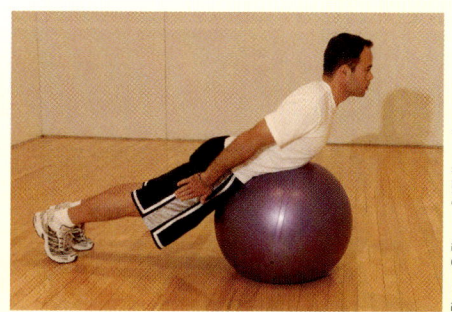

A   B

278 Lifetime Physical Fitness and Wellness

EXERCISE 44 Wall Squat

ACTION Stand upright and position the ball between your lower back and a wall. Place your feet slightly in front of you, about a foot apart (a). Lean into the ball and lower your body by bending the knees until the thighs are parallel to the ground (b) (to avoid excessive strain on the knees, it is not recommended that you go beyond this point). Return to the starting position. Repeat the exercise 10 to 20 times.

MUSCLES INVOLVED Quadriceps, hip flexors, hamstrings, abdominals, erector spinae, lower back, gastrocnemius, and soleus

A

B

EXERCISE 45 Jack Knives

ACTION Lie face down with the hips on the ball and walk forward with your hands until the thighs are over the ball. Keep the arms fully extended, hands on floor, and the body straight (a). Now, pull the ball forward with your legs by bending at the knees and raising your hips while keeping the abdominal muscles tight (b). Repeat the exercise 10 times.

MUSCLES INVOLVED Hip flexors, abdominals, erector spinae, lower back, quadriceps, hamstrings, chest, and shoulder

A

B

EXERCISE 46 Hamstring Roll

ACTION Lie on your back with your knees bent and the heels on the ball. Raise your hips off the floor, while keeping the knees bent (a). Tighten the abdominal muscles and roll the ball out with your feet to extend the legs (b). Now roll the ball back into the original position. Repeat the exercise 10 times.

MUSCLES INVOLVED Hamstrings, abdominals, erector spinae, lower back, hip flexors, quadriceps, and chest

A

B

Muscular Flexibility

8

"Regrettably, most people neglect flexibility training, limiting freedom of movement, physical and mental relaxation, release of muscle tension and soreness, and injury prevention."
—American Council on Exercise (ACE)

Objectives

- **Explain** the importance of muscular flexibility to adequate fitness.
- **Identify** the factors that affect muscular flexibility.
- **Explain** the health-fitness benefits of stretching.
- **Become** familiar with a battery of tests to assess overall body flexibility (Modified Sit-and-Reach Test, Total Body Rotation Test, and Shoulder Rotation Test).
- **Be** able to interpret flexibility test results according to health-fitness and physical-fitness standards.
- **Learn** the principles that govern development of muscular flexibility.
- **List** some exercises that may cause injury.
- **Become** familiar with a program for preventing and rehabilitating low-back pain.
- **Create** your own personal flexibility program.

CENGAGEbrain.com

Visit www.cengagebrain.com to access course materials and companion resources for this text, including quiz questions designed to check your understanding of the chapter contents. See the preface on page ix for more information.

FAQ

Will stretching before exercise prevent injuries?

The research on this subject is controversial. Some data suggest that intense stretching prior to physical activity modestly increases the risk for injuries and leads to a temporary decrease in muscle contraction velocity, strength, and power. Other studies, however, show no changes and even some improvement with intense pre-exercise stretching. The most important factor prior to vigorous exercise is to gradually increase the exercise intensity through mild calisthenics and light- to moderate-intensity aerobic exercise.

To prevent injuries while participating in activities that require flexibility, the American College of Sports Medicine recommends stretching following an appropriate warm-up phase. For activities that do not require much flexibility, you can perform the flexibility program following the aerobic and/or strength-training phase of your training.

Does strength training limit flexibility?

A popular myth is that individuals with large musculature, frequently referred to as "muscle-bound," are inflexible. Data show that strength-training exercises, when performed through a full range of motion, do not limit flexibility. With few exceptions, most strength-training exercises can be performed from complete extension to complete flexion. Body builders and gymnasts, who train heavily with weights, have better than average flexibility.

Will stretching exercises help me lose weight?

The energy (caloric) expenditure of stretching exercises is extremely low. In 30 minutes of aerobic exercise you can easily burn an additional 250 to 300 calories as compared with 30 minutes of stretching. Flexibility exercises help develop overall health-related fitness but do not contribute much to weight loss or weight maintenance.

How much should stretching "hurt" to gain flexibility?

Proper stretching should not cause undue pain. Pain is an indication that you are stretching too aggressively. Stretching exercises should be performed to the point of feeling tightness or mild tension. It is best to decrease the degree of stretch to mild tension and hold the final position for a longer period of time (10 to 30 seconds).

Real Life Story | Maria's Experience

I have suffered from really bad back pain over the last couple years. When I moved out of my parents' house to an apartment with a friend, the only bed I could afford was an old, hand-me-down mattress from my older sister. The mattress was fairly soft and sagged a little, so it did not give good support. I started waking up most mornings with an aching back. I was also not very active. Sometimes when I was studying, I would sit hunched over my computer for hours and hours at a time, and between the stress and the sitting in one position for so long, by the time I went to bed my whole back and shoulders would be in intense pain. I went on this way for a long time, having daily back pain. I just assumed it was something I had to live with. It wasn't until I read the *Lifetime Physical Fitness and Wellness* text for school that I learned about the steps you can take to prevent back pain. I learned that my posture when sitting, standing, and sleeping was mostly incorrect, so I tried to pay attention to fixing it. I got a foot rest for when I sit at my desk, and I started sleeping with a pillow supporting my knees when I lie on my back. I also finally saved enough money to buy a new bed with a firmer mattress, which really helped. But one of the most helpful changes I made was to start being more active and stretching daily. I like to walk briskly for about 30 minutes, and then do a series of stretches. I especially like the way the "trunk rotation" and "cat" stretches make my back feel. After stretching, not only does my back feel better, but I also feel less stressed. Thanks to these efforts, my back pain is almost totally gone. I am so glad I learned that I didn't have to live in pain every day.

PERSONAL PROFILE: My Personal Flexibility Health

I. Can you touch your toes without bending your knees while sitting on the floor? ___ Yes ___ No How about the tips of your fingers behind your back with the preferred upper arm (hand) over your shoulder and the other hand coming up from behind your lower back? ___ Yes ___ No

II. The most important factor that determines range of motion about a joint is the degree of physical activity. ___ Yes ___ No

III. Vigorous stretching conducted prior to participating in athletic events that rely on force and power for peak performance enhances sports performance. ___ Yes ___ No

IV. Back pain can be reduced greatly through aerobic exercise, muscular flexibility exercise, and muscular strength and endurance training. ___ Yes ___ No

V. Have you ever experienced back pain episodes similar to Gina's, and can you explain the probable cause of Maria's pain? ___ Yes ___ No

---

Very few people who exercise take the time to stretch, and only a few of those who stretch, do so properly. When joints are not regularly moved through their entire range of motion, muscles and ligaments shorten in time, and flexibility decreases. Repetitive movement through regular/structured exercise, such as with running, cycling, or aerobics, without proper stretching also causes muscles and ligaments to tighten. Most fitness participants underestimate and overlook the contribution of good muscular flexibility to overall fitness.

Flexibility refers to the achievable range of motion at a joint or group of joints without causing injury. Some muscular/skeletal problems and injuries are thought to be related to a lack of flexibility. In daily life, we often have to make rapid or strenuous movements that we are not accustomed to making. Abruptly forcing a tight muscle beyond its achievable range of motion may lead to injury.

A decline in flexibility can cause poor posture and subsequent aches and pains that lead to limited and painful joint movement. Inordinate tightness is uncomfortable and debilitating. Approximately 80 percent of all low-back problems in the United States stem from improper alignment of the vertebral column and pelvic girdle, a direct result of inflexible and weak muscles. This backache syndrome costs U.S. industry billions of dollars each year in lost productivity, health services, and worker compensation.

8.1 Benefits of Good Flexibility

Improving and maintaining good range of motion in the joints enhances the quality of life. Good flexibility promotes healthy muscles and joints. Improving elasticity of muscles and connective tissue around joints enables greater freedom of movement and the individual's ability to participate in many types of sports and recreational activities. Adequate flexibility also makes activities of daily living such as turning, lifting, and bending much easier to perform. A person must take care, however, not to overstretch joints. Too much flexibility leads to unstable and loose joints, which may increase injury rate, including joint **subluxation** and dislocation.

Excessive sitting and lack of physical activity lead to chronic back pain.

Taking part in a regular **stretching** program increases circulation to the muscle(s) being stretched, prevents low-back and other spinal column problems, improves and maintains good postural alignment, promotes proper and graceful body movement, improves personal appearance and self-image, and helps to develop and maintain motor skills throughout life.

Flexibility exercises have been prescribed successfully to treat **dysmenorrhea**[1] (painful menstruation), general neuromuscular tension (stress), and knots (trigger points) in muscles and fascia. Regular stretching helps decrease the aches and pains caused by psychological stress and contributes to a decrease in anxiety, blood pressure, and breathing

> **Flexibility** The achievable range of motion at a joint or group of joints without causing injury.
>
> **Subluxation** Partial dislocation of a joint.
>
> **Stretching** Moving the joints beyond the accustomed range of motion.
>
> **Dysmenorrhea** Painful menstruation.

rate.[2] Stretching also helps relieve muscle cramps encountered at rest or during participation in exercise.

Mild stretching exercises in conjunction with calisthenics are helpful in warm-up routines to prepare for more vigorous aerobic or strength-training exercises, and in cool-down routines following exercise to facilitate the return to a normal resting state. Fatigued muscles tend to contract to a shorter-than-average resting length, and stretching exercises help fatigued muscles reestablish their normal resting length.

8.2 Flexibility in Older Adults

Similar to muscular strength, good range of motion is critical in older life (see "Exercise and Aging" in Chapter 9). Because of decreased flexibility, older adults lose mobility and may be unable to perform simple daily tasks such as bending forward or turning. Many older adults cannot turn their head or rotate their trunk to look over their shoulder but, rather, must step around 90° to 180° to see behind them. Adequate flexibility is also important in driving. Individuals who lose range of motion with age are unable to look over their shoulder to switch lanes or to parallel park, which increases the risk for automobile accidents.

Physical activity and exercise can be hampered severely by lack of good range of motion. Because of the pain during activity, older people who have tight hip flexors (muscles) cannot jog or walk very far. A vicious circle ensues, because the condition usually worsens with further inactivity. Lack of flexibility also may be a cause of falls and subsequent injury in older adults. A simple stretching program can alleviate or prevent this problem and help people return to an exercise program.

8.3 Factors Affecting Flexibility

The total range of motion around a joint is highly specific and varies from one joint to another (hip, trunk, shoulder), as well as from one individual to the next. Muscular flexibility relates primarily to genetic factors. A regular stretching program helps maintain range of motion about a joint and can help improve it as well. Joint structure (shape of the bones), joint cartilage, ligaments, tendons, muscles, skin, tissue injury, and adipose tissue (fat)—all influence range of motion about a joint. Body temperature, age, and gender also affect flexibility.

The range of motion about a given joint depends mostly on the structure of that joint. Greater range of motion, however, can be attained through plastic and elastic elongation. **Plastic elongation** is the permanent lengthening of soft tissue. Even though joint capsules, ligaments, and tendons are basically nonelastic, they can undergo plastic elongation. This permanent lengthening, accompanied by increased range of motion, is best attained through proper stretching exercises.

Elastic elongation is the temporary lengthening of soft tissue. Muscle tissue has elastic properties and responds to stretching exercises by undergoing elastic or temporary lengthening. Elastic elongation increases extensibility, the ability to stretch the muscles.

Changes in muscle temperature can increase or decrease flexibility. Individuals who warm up properly have better flexibility than people who do not. Cool temperatures have the opposite effect, impeding range of motion. Because of the effects of temperature on muscular flexibility, many people prefer to do their stretching exercises after the aerobic phase of their workout. Aerobic activities raise body temperature, facilitating elastic elongation.

Another factor that influences flexibility is the amount of adipose (fat) tissue in and around joints and muscle tissue. Excess adipose tissue will increase resistance to movement, and the added bulk also hampers joint mobility because of the contact between body surfaces.

On the average, women have better flexibility than men, and they seem to retain this advantage throughout life. Aging does decrease the extensibility of soft tissue, though, resulting in less flexibility in both sexes.

The most significant contributor to lower flexibility is sedentary living. With less physical activity, muscles lose their elasticity and tendons and ligaments tighten and shorten. Inactivity also tends to be accompanied by an increase in adipose tissue, which further decreases the range of motion around a joint. Finally, injury to muscle tissue and tight skin from excessive scar tissue have negative effects on range of motion.

Adequate flexibility helps to develop and maintain sports skill throughout life.

> **Figure 8.1** Procedure for the Modified Sit-and-Reach Test.

To perform this test, you will need the Acuflex I* Sit-and-Reach Flexibility Tester, or you may simply place a yardstick on top of a box 12" high.

1. Warm up properly before the first trial.
2. Remove your shoes for the test. Sit on the floor with the hips, back, and head against a wall, the legs fully extended, and the bottom of the feet against the Acuflex I or sit-and-reach box.
3. Place the hands one on top of the other and reach forward as far as possible without letting the head and back come off the wall (the shoulders may be rounded as much as possible, but neither the head nor the back should come off the wall at this time). The technician then can slide the reach indicator on the Acuflex I (or yardstick) along the top of the box until the end of the indicator touches the participant's fingers. The indicator then must be held firmly in place throughout the rest of the test.

4. Now your head and back can come off the wall. Gradually reach forward three times, the third time stretching forward as far as possible on the indicator (or yardstick) and holding the final position for at least 2 seconds. Be sure that during the test you keep the backs of the knees flat against the floor.
5. Record the final number of inches reached to the nearest half inch.

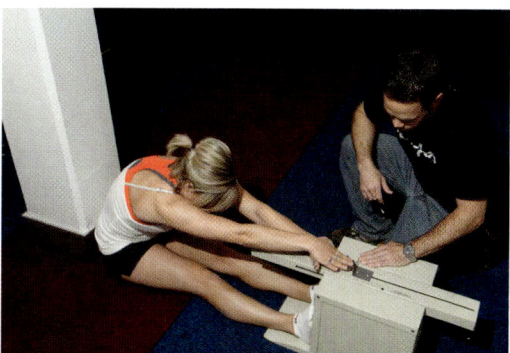
Modified Sit-and-Reach Test.

You are allowed two trials, and an average of the two scores is used as the final test score. The respective percentile ranks and fitness categories for this test are given in Tables 8.1 and 8.4.

*The Acuflex I Flexibility Tester for the Modified Sit-and-Reach Test can be obtained from Figure Finder Collection, Novel Products, P. O. Box 408, Rockton, IL 61072-0480. Phone: 800-323-5143, Fax 815-624-4866.

Determining the starting position for the Modified Sit-and-Reach Test.

8.4 Assessment of Flexibility

Because of the lack of practical flexibility tests, most health and fitness centers rely strictly on the Sit-and-Reach Test as an indicator of flexibility. This test measures flexibility of the hamstring muscles (back of the thigh) and, to a lesser extent, the lower back muscles.

Flexibility is joint specific. This means that a lot of flexibility in one joint does not necessarily indicate that other joints are just as flexible. Therefore, the Total Body Rotation Test and the Shoulder Rotation Test—indicators of the ability to perform everyday movements such as reaching, bending, and turning—are included to determine your flexibility profile.

The Sit-and-Reach Test has been modified from the traditional test to take length of arms and legs into consideration in determining the score (see Figure 8.1). In the original Sit-and-Reach Test, the 15-inch mark of the yardstick used to measure flexibility is always set at the edge of the box where the feet are placed. This does not take into consideration an individual with long arms and/or short legs or one with short arms and/or long legs, or both.[3] All other factors being equal, an individual with longer arms or shorter legs, or both, receives a better rating because of the structural advantage.

The procedures and norms for the flexibility tests are described in Figures 8.1, 8.2, and 8.3 and Tables 8.1, 8.2, and 8.3. The flexibility test results in these three tables are provided in both inches and centimeters (cm). Be sure to use the proper column to read your percentile score based on your test results. For the flexibility profile, you should take all three tests. You will be able to assess your flexibility profile in Activity 8.1. Because of the specificity of flexibility, pinpointing an "ideal" level of flexibility is difficult. Nevertheless, flexibility is important to health and fitness and independent living, so an assessment will give an indication of your current level of flexibility.

Interpreting Flexibility Test Results After obtaining your scores and fitness ratings for each test, you can determine the fitness category for each flexibility test using the guidelines given in Table 8.4. You also should look up the number of points assigned for each fitness category in this table. The overall flexibility fitness category is obtained by totaling the number of points from all three tests and using the ratings

> **Plastic elongation** Permanent lengthening of soft tissue.
>
> **Elastic elongation** Temporary lengthening of soft tissue.

Figure 8.2 Procedure for the Total Body Rotation Test.

An Acuflex II* Total Body Rotation Flexibility Tester or a measuring scale with a sliding panel is needed to administer this test. The Acuflex II or scale is placed on the wall at shoulder height and should be adjustable to accommodate individual differences in height. If you need to build your own scale, use two measuring tapes and glue them above and below the sliding panel centered at the 15" mark. Each tape should be at least 30" long. If no sliding panel is available, simply tape the measuring tapes onto a wall oriented in opposite directions as shown below. A line also must be drawn on the floor and centered with the 15" mark.

1. Warm up properly before beginning this test.
2. Stand with one side toward the wall, an arm's length away from the wall, with the feet straight ahead, slightly separated, and the toes touching the center line drawn on the floor. Hold out the arm away from the wall horizontally from the body, making a fist with the hand. The Acuflex II measuring scale (or tapes) should be shoulder height at this time.
3. Rotate the trunk, the extended arm going backward (always maintaining a horizontal plane) and making contact with the panel, gradually sliding it forward as far as possible. If no panel is available, slide the fist alongside the tapes as far as possible. Hold the final position at least 2 seconds. Position the hand with the little finger side forward during the entire sliding movement. **Proper hand position is crucial. Many people attempt to open the hand, or push with extended fingers, or slide the panel with the knuckles—none of which is acceptable.** During the test the knees can be bent slightly, but **the feet cannot be moved or rotated**—they must be straight forward. The body must be kept as straight (vertical) as possible.
4. Conduct the test on either the right or the left side of the body. Perform two trials on the selected side. Record the farthest point reached, measured to the nearest half inch and held for at least 2 seconds. Use the average of the two trials as the final test score. Refer to Tables 8.2 and 8.4 to determine the percentile rank and flexibility fitness category for this test.

*The Acuflex II Flexibility Tester for the Total Body Rotation Test can be obtained from Figure Finder Collection, Novel Products, P.O. Box 408, Rockton, IL 61072-0408. Phone: 800-323-5143, Fax 815-624-4866.

Acuflex II measuring device for the Total Body Rotation Test.

Homemade measuring device for the Total Body Rotation Test.

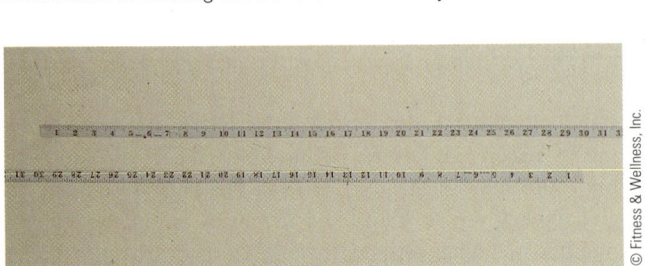
Measuring tapes for the Total Body Rotation Test.

Total Body Rotation Test.

Proper hand position for the Total Body Rotation Test.

Figure 8.3 Procedure for the Shoulder Rotation Test.

This test can be done using the Acuflex III* Flexibility Tester, which consists of a shoulder caliper and a measuring device for shoulder rotation. If this equipment is unavailable, you can construct your own device quite easily. The caliper can be built with three regular yardsticks. Nail and glue two of the yardsticks at one end at a 90° angle, and use the third one as the sliding end of the caliper. Construct the rotation device by placing a 60" measuring tape on an aluminum or wood stick, starting at about 6" or 7" from the end of the stick.

1. Warm up before the test.
2. Using the shoulder caliper, measure the biacromial width to the nearest fourth of an inch (use the top scale on the Acuflex III). Measure biacromial width between the lateral edges of the acromion processes of the shoulders.
3. Place the Acuflex III or homemade device behind the back and use a reverse grip (thumbs out) to hold on to the device. Place the index finger of the right hand next to the zero point of the scale or tape (lower scale on the Acuflex III) and hold it firmly in place throughout the test. Place the left hand on the other end of the measuring device wherever comfortable.
4. Standing straight up and extending both arms to full length, with elbows locked, slowly bring the measuring device over the head until it reaches about forehead level. For subsequent trials, depending on the resistance encountered when rotating the shoulders, move the left grip a half inch to one inch at a time, and repeat the task until you no longer can rotate the shoulders without undue strain or starting to bend the elbows. Always keep the right-hand grip against the zero point of the scale. Measure the last successful trial to the nearest half inch. Take this measurement at the inner edge of the left hand on the side of the little finger.
5. Determine the final score for this test by subtracting the biacromial width from the best score (shortest distance) between both hands on the rotation test. For example, if the best score is 35" and the biacromial width is 15", the final score is 20" (35 − 15 = 20). Using Tables 8.3 and 8.4, determine the percentile rank and flexibility fitness category for this test.

*The Acuflex III Flexibility Tester for the Shoulder Rotation Test can be obtained from Figure Finder Collection, Novel Products, Inc., P. O. Box 408, Rockton, IL 61072-0408. Phone: (800) 323-5143, Fax 815-624-4866.

Measuring biacromial width.

Starting position for the shoulder rotation test (note the reverse grip used for this test).

Shoulder rotation test.

Table 8.1 Percentile Ranks for the Modified Sit-and-Reach Test

	Age Category—Men								Age Category—Women							
Percentile Rank	≤18		19–35		36–49		≥50		Percentile Rank	≤18		19–35		36–49		≥50	
	in.	cm	in.	cm	in.	cm	in.	cm		in.	cm	in.	cm	in.	cm	in.	cm
99	20.8	52.8	20.1	51.1	18.9	48.0	16.2	41.1	99	22.6	57.4	21.0	53.3	19.8	50.3	17.2	43.7
95	19.6	49.8	18.9	48.0	18.2	46.2	15.8	40.1	95	19.5	49.5	19.3	49.0	19.2	48.8	15.7	39.9
90	18.2	46.2	17.2	43.7	16.1	40.9	15.0	38.1	90	18.7	47.5	17.9	45.5	17.4	44.2	15.0	38.1
80	17.8	45.2	17.0	43.2	14.6	37.1	13.3	33.8	80	17.8	45.2	16.7	42.4	16.2	41.1	14.2
70	16.0	40.6	15.8	40.1	13.9	35.3	12.3	31.2	70	16.5	41.9	16.2	41.1	15.2	38.6	13.6	34.5
60	15.2	38.6	15.0	38.1	13.4	34.0	11.5	29.2	60	16.0	40.6	15.8	40.1	14.5	36.8	12.3	31.2
50	14.5	36.8	14.4	36.6	12.6	32.0	10.2	25.9	50	15.2	38.6	14.8	37.6	13.5	34.3	11.1	28.2
40	14.0	35.6	13.5	34.3	11.6	29.5	9.7	24.6	40	14.5	36.8	14.5	36.8	12.8	32.5	10.1	25.7
30	13.4	34.0	13.0	33.0	10.8	27.4	9.3	23.6	30	13.7	34.8	13.7	34.8	12.2	31.0	9.2	23.4
20	11.8	30.0	11.6	29.5	9.9	25.1	8.8	22.4	20	12.6	32.0	12.6	32.0	11.0	27.9	8.3	21.1
10	9.5	24.1	9.2	23.4	8.3	21.1	7.8	19.8	10	11.4	29.0	10.1	25.7	9.7	24.6	7.5	19.0
05	8.4	21.3	7.9	20.1	7.0	17.8	7.2	18.3	05	9.4	23.9	8.1	20.6	8.5	21.6	3.7	9.4
01	7.2	18.3	7.0	17.8	5.1	13.0	4.0	10.2	01	6.5	16.5	2.6	6.6	2.0	5.1	1.5	3.8

High physical fitness standard
Health fitness standard

Table 8.2 Percentile Ranks for the Total Body Rotation Test

	Percentile Rank	Age Category—Left Rotation								Age Category—Right Rotation							
		≤18		19–35		36–49		≥50		≤18		19–35		36–49		≥50	
		in.	cm	in.	cm	in.	cm	in.	cm	in.	cm	in.	cm	in.	cm	in.	cm
Men	99	29.1	73.9	28.0	71.1	26.6	67.6	21.0	53.3	28.2	71.6	27.8	70.6	25.2	64.0	22.2	56.4
	95	26.6	67.6	24.8	63.0	24.5	62.2	20.0	50.8	25.5	64.8	25.6	65.0	23.8	60.5	20.7	52.6
	90	25.0	63.5	23.6	59.9	23.0	58.4	17.7	45.0	24.3	61.7	24.1	61.2	22.5	57.1	19.3	49.0
	80	22.0	55.9	22.0	55.9	21.2	53.8	15.5	39.4	22.7	57.7	22.3	56.6	21.0	53.3	16.3	41.4
	70	20.9	53.1	20.3	51.6	20.4	51.8	14.7	37.3	21.3	54.1	20.7	52.6	18.7	47.5	15.7	39.9
	60	19.9	50.5	19.3	49.0	18.7	47.5	13.9	35.3	19.8	50.3	19.0	48.3	17.3	43.9	14.7	37.3
	50	18.6	47.2	18.0	45.7	16.7	42.4	12.7	32.3	19.0	48.3	17.2	43.7	16.3	41.4	12.3	31.2
	40	17.0	43.2	16.8	42.7	15.3	38.9	11.7	29.7	17.3	43.9	16.3	41.4	14.7	37.3	11.5	29.2
	30	14.9	37.8	15.0	38.1	14.8	37.6	10.3	26.2	15.1	38.4	15.0	38.1	13.3	33.8	10.7	27.2
	20	13.8	35.1	13.3	33.8	13.7	34.8	9.5	24.1	12.9	32.8	13.3	33.8	11.2	28.4	8.7	22.1
	10	10.8	27.4	10.5	26.7	10.8	27.4	4.3	10.9	10.8	27.4	11.3	28.7	8.0	20.3	2.7	6.9
	05	8.5	21.6	8.9	22.6	8.8	22.4	0.3	0.8	8.1	20.6	8.3	21.1	5.5	14.0	0.3	0.8
	01	3.4	8.6	1.7	4.3	5.1	13.0	0.0	0.0	6.6	16.8	2.9	7.4	2.0	5.1	0.0	0.0
Women	99	29.3	74.4	28.6	72.6	27.1	68.8	23.0	58.4	29.6	75.2	29.4	74.7	27.1	68.8	21.7	55.1
	95	26.8	68.1	24.8	63.0	25.3	64.3	21.4	54.4	27.6	70.1	25.3	64.3	25.9	65.8	19.7	50.0
	90	25.5	64.8	23.0	58.4	23.4	59.4	20.5	52.1	25.8	65.5	23.0	58.4	21.3	54.1	19.0	48.3
	80	23.8	60.5	21.5	54.6	20.2	51.3	19.1	48.5	23.7	60.2	20.8	52.8	19.6	49.8	17.9	45.5
	70	21.8	55.4	20.5	52.1	18.6	47.2	17.3	43.9	22.0	55.9	19.3	49.0	17.3	43.9	16.8	42.7
	60	20.5	52.1	19.3	49.0	17.7	45.0	16.0	40.6	20.8	52.8	18.0	45.7	16.5	41.9	15.6	39.6
	50	19.5	49.5	18.0	45.7	16.4	41.7	14.8	37.6	19.5	49.5	17.3	43.9	14.6	37.1	14.0	35.6
	40	18.5	47.0	17.2	43.7	14.8	37.6	13.7	34.8	18.3	46.5	16.0	40.6	13.1	33.3	12.8	32.5
	30	17.1	43.4	15.7	39.9	13.6	34.5	10.0	25.4	16.3	41.4	15.2	38.6	11.7	29.7	8.5	21.6
	20	16.0	40.6	15.2	38.6	11.6	29.5	6.3	16.0	14.5	36.8	14.0	35.6	9.8	24.9	3.9	9.9
	10	12.8	32.5	13.6	34.5	8.5	21.6	3.0	7.6	12.4	31.5	11.1	28.2	6.1	15.5	2.2	5.6
	05	11.1	28.2	7.3	18.5	6.8	17.3	0.7	1.8	10.2	25.9	8.8	22.4	4.0	10.2	1.1	2.8
	01	8.9	22.6	5.3	13.5	4.3	10.9	0.0	0.0	8.9	22.6	3.2	8.1	2.8	7.1	0.0	0.0

High physical fitness standard
Health fitness standard
© Cengage Learning

Table 8.3 Percentile Ranks for the Shoulder Rotation Test

Percentile Rank	Age Category—Men								Percentile Rank	Age Category—Women							
	≤18		19–35		36–49		≥50			≤18		19–35		36–49		≥50	
	in.	cm	in.	cm	in.	cm	in.	cm		in.	cm	in.	cm	in.	cm	in.	cm
99	2.2	5.6	−1.0	−2.5	18.1	46.0	21.5	54.6	99	2.6	6.6	−2.4	−6.1	11.5	29.2	13.1	33.3
95	15.2	38.6	10.4	26.4	20.4	51.8	27.0	68.6	95	8.0	20.3	6.2	15.7	15.4	39.1	16.5	41.9
90	18.5	47.0	15.5	39.4	20.8	52.8	27.9	70.9	90	10.7	27.2	9.7	24.6	16.8	42.7	20.9	53.1
80	20.7	52.6	18.4	46.7	23.3	59.2	28.5	72.4	80	14.5	36.8	14.5	36.8	19.2	48.8	22.5	57.1
70	23.0	58.4	20.5	52.1	24.7	62.7	29.4	74.7	70	16.1	40.9	17.2	43.7	21.5	54.6	24.3	61.7
60	24.2	61.5	22.9	58.2	26.6	67.6	29.9	75.9	60	19.2	48.8	18.7	47.5	23.1	58.7	25.1	63.8
50	25.4	64.5	24.4	62.0	28.0	71.1	30.5	77.5	50	21.0	53.3	20.0	50.8	23.5	59.7	26.2	66.5
40	26.3	66.8	25.7	65.3	30.0	76.2	31.0	78.7	40	22.2	56.4	21.4	54.4	24.4	62.0	28.1	71.4
30	28.2	71.6	27.3	69.3	31.9	81.0	31.7	80.5	30	23.2	58.9	24.0	61.0	25.9	65.8	29.9	75.9
20	30.0	76.2	30.1	76.5	33.3	84.6	33.1	84.1	20	25.0	63.5	25.9	65.8	29.8	75.7	31.5	80.0
10	33.5	85.1	31.8	80.8	36.1	91.7	37.2	94.5	10	27.2	69.1	29.1	73.9	31.1	79.0	33.1	84.1
05	34.7	88.1	33.5	85.1	37.8	96.0	38.7	98.3	05	28.0	71.1	31.3	79.5	33.4	84.8	34.1	86.6
01	40.8	103.6	42.6	108.2	43.0	109.2	44.1	112.0	01	32.5	82.5	37.1	94.2	34.9	88.6	35.4	89.9

High physical fitness standard
Health fitness standard
© Cengage Learning

Table 8.4 Flexibility Fitness Categories According to Percentile Ranks

Percentile Rank	Fitness Category	Points
≥90	Excellent	5
70–80	Good	4
50–60	Average	3
30–40	Fair	2
≤20	Poor	1

© Cengage Learning

Table 8.5 Overall Flexibility Fitness Category

Total Points	Flexibility Category
≥13	Excellent
10–12	Good
7–9	Average
4–6	Fair
≤3	Poor

© Cengage Learning

given in Table 8.5. Record your results in Activity 8.1 and Appendix A.

8.5 Principles of Muscular Flexibility Prescription

Even though genetics play a crucial role in body flexibility, the range of joint mobility can be increased and maintained through a regular stretching program. Because range of motion is highly specific to each body part (ankle, trunk, shoulder), a comprehensive stretching program should include all body parts and follow the basic guidelines for development of flexibility.

The overload and specificity of training principles (discussed in conjunction with strength development in Chapter 7) also apply to the development of muscular flexibility. To increase the total range of motion of a joint, the specific muscles surrounding that joint have to be stretched progressively beyond their accustomed length. The principles of mode, intensity, repetitions, and frequency of exercise can also be applied to flexibility programs.

Modes of Training There are several modes of stretching exercises, and some modes are safer and more effective in terms of helping to increase flexibility:

1. Static (slow-sustained stretching)
2. Passive stretching
3. Ballistic stretching
4. Dynamic stretching
5. Controlled ballistic stretching
6. Proprioceptive neuromuscular facilitation (PNF) stretching

Static Stretching

With **static stretching** or slow-sustained stretching, muscles are lengthened gradually through a joint's complete range of motion and the final position is held for a few seconds. A slow-sustained stretch causes the muscles to relax and thereby achieve greater length. This type of stretch causes little pain and has a low risk for injury. In flexibility-development programs, slow sustained stretching exercises are the most frequently used and recommended.

Passive Stretching

Although similar to static stretching, in **passive stretching** the muscles are relaxed, that is, they are in a passive state, and an external force, provided by another person or apparatus, is applied to increase the range of motion.

Ballistic Stretching

Ballistic stretching requires the impetus of a moving body or body part to force a joint or group of joints beyond the normal range of motion. This type of stretching requires a fast and repetitive bouncing motion to achieve a greater degree of stretch. An example would be repeatedly bouncing down and up to touch the toes. Ballistic stretching is the least recommended form of stretching. Fitness professionals feel that it causes muscle soreness and increases the risk of injuries to muscles and nerves. Limited data, however, are available to corroborate such effects. This form of stretching should never be performed without a previous mild aerobic warm-up.

Dynamic Stretching

Speed of movement, momentum, and active muscular effort are used in **dynamic stretching** to increase the range of motion about a joint or group of joints. Unlike ballistic stretching, it does not require bouncing motions. Exaggerating a kicking action, walking lunges, and arm circles are all examples of dynamic stretching. Research indicates that dynamic stretches are preferable to static stretches before competition because dynamic stretching does not seem to have a negative effect on the athlete's strength and power. Dynamic stretching is beneficial for athletes such as gymnasts, dancers, figure skaters, divers, and hurdlers, whose sports activities require ballistic actions.

Precautions must be taken not to overstretch liga-

> **Static stretching (slow-sustained stretching)** Exercises in which the muscles are lengthened gradually through a joint's complete range of motion.
>
> **Passive stretching** Stretching exercises performed with the aid of an external force applied by either another individual or an external apparatus.
>
> **Ballistic (dynamic) stretching** Stretching exercises performed with jerky, rapid, and bouncy movements.
>
> **Dynamic stretching** Stretching exercises that require speed of movement, momentum, and active muscular effort to help increase the range of motion about a joint or group of joints.

ments with ballistic and dynamic stretching. Ligaments undergo plastic or permanent elongation. If the stretching force cannot be controlled—as often occurs in fast, jerky movements—ligaments can easily be overstretched. This, in turn, leads to excessively loose joints, increasing the risk for injuries.

Controlled Ballistic Stretching
Controlled ballistic stretching, that is, exercises that are performed through slow, gentle, and controlled ballistic movements (instead of jerky, rapid, and bouncy movements) is quite effective in developing flexibility. Properly performed, this type of stretching can be done safely by most individuals.

Proprioceptive Neuromuscular Facilitation
Proprioceptive neuromuscular facilitation (PNF) stretching is based on a "contract-and-relax" method and requires the assistance of another person. The procedure is as follows:

1. The person assisting with the exercise provides initial force by pushing slowly in the direction of the desired stretch. This first stretch does not cover the entire range of motion.
2. The person being stretched then applies force in the opposite direction of the stretch, against the assistant, who tries to hold the initial degree of stretch as close as possible. This results in an isometric contraction at the angle of the stretch.
3. After 5 or 6 seconds of isometric contraction, the person being stretched relaxes the target muscle(s) completely. The assistant then increases the degree of stretch slowly to a greater angle and for the PNF technique the stretch is held for 10 to 30 seconds.
4. If a greater degree of stretch is achievable, the isometric contraction is repeated for another 5 or 6 seconds, after which the degree of stretch is slowly increased again and held for 10 to 30 seconds.

If a progressive degree of stretch is used, steps 1 through 4 can be repeated up to five times. Each isometric contraction is held for about 6 seconds. The progressive stretches are held for 10 seconds, until the last trial, when the final stretched position is held for up to 30 seconds.

Theoretically, with the PNF technique, the isometric contraction helps relax the muscle being stretched, which results in lengthening of the muscle. Some research indicates that PNF stretching yields greater gains in range of motion than the other forms of stretching.[4] Another benefit of PNF is an increase in strength of the muscle(s) being stretched. Research has shown increases in absolute strength and muscular endurance with PNF stretching. These increases are attributed to the isometric contractions performed during PNF. Disadvantages of PNF are (1) more pain, (2) the need for a second person to assist, and (3) the need for more time to conduct each session.

Physiological Response to Stretching Located within skeletal muscles are two sensory organs, also known as proprioceptors: the muscle spindle and the Golgi tendon organ. Their function is to protect muscles from injury during stretching.

Muscle spindles are located within the belly of the muscle, and their primary function is to detect changes in muscle length. If overstretched or stretched too fast, the spindles send messages to the central nervous system, and through a feedback loop, motor neurons are activated and cause muscle contraction to resist muscle stretch. This mechanism is known as the stretch reflex. Muscle spindle action explains why injury rates are higher with ballistic stretching. Fast stretching speeds trigger the stretch reflex and cause muscles to contract and develop tension that can lead to injury.

Golgi tendon organs are located at the point where muscle fibers attach to the muscle tendon. When a muscle generates excessive force, these organs trigger a response opposite to that of the spindles: an inverse stretch reflex action that inhibits the muscle contraction and leads to muscle relaxation. The Golgi tendon organ prevents injury to the muscle by keeping it from generating too much tension while being stretched. This response explains the effectiveness of the PNF technique in increasing joint range of motion. The isometric contraction following the initial stretch triggers the inverse stretch reflex, thus lessening the tension and allowing the muscle to relax. At this point, the muscle tolerates a greater degree of stretch.

Intensity The **intensity,** or degree of stretch, when doing flexibility exercises should be to only a point of mild discomfort or feeling tightness at the end of the range of motion.

A
Isometric phase

B
Stretching phase

Proprioceptive neuromuscular facilitation (PNF) stretching technique: (a) isometric phase (b) stretching phase.

Undue pain does not have to be part of the stretching routine. All stretching should be done to slightly below the pain threshold. As participants reach this point, they should try to relax the muscle being stretched as much as possible. If you feel pain, the load is too high and may cause injury. After completing the stretch, the body part is brought back gradually to the starting point.

> **Critical Thinking**
>
> Carefully consider the relevance of stretching exercises to your personal fitness program. • How much importance do you place on these exercises? • Have some conditions improved through your stretching program, or have certain specific exercises contributed to your health and well-being?

Repetitions The time required for an exercise session for development of flexibility is based on the number of **repetitions** and the length of time each repetition is held in the final stretched position. As a general recommendation, a minimum of 10 minutes of flexibility exercise, including the major muscle and tendon units of the body, should be performed. Two to four repetitions per exercise should be done, holding the final position each time for 10 to 30 seconds.[5,6] The goal is to achieve 60 seconds of total stretching per exercise by adjusting the duration and repetitions. Older adults may derive greater improvements when the final stretched position is held for 30 to 60 seconds.

Data indicate that stretching for 10 to 30 seconds is better to increase range of motion than stretching for shorter periods of time and is just as effective as stretching for longer durations. Individuals who are susceptible to flexibility injuries should limit each stretch to 20 seconds. Pilates exercises are recommended for these individuals, as they increase joint stability (also see Chapter 7, pages 253-254).

Frequency of Exercise Flexibility exercises should be conducted a minimum of two or three days per week, but ideally five to seven days per week. After six to eight weeks of almost daily stretching, flexibility can be maintained with two or three sessions per week, involving the major muscle/tendon groups of the body and doing two to four repetitions for up to a total of 60 seconds for each exercise performed. Figure 8.4 summarizes the guidelines for flexibility development.

Over the years, people who lack adequate flexibility, and those who neglect stretching, can expect to see a decline in functional capacity and become more susceptible to injuries. Regular stretching increases not only range of motion by increasing muscular elongation but also by enhancing a person's level of stretch tolerance.

When to Stretch? Many people do not differentiate a warm-up from stretching. Warming up means starting a workout slowly with walking, cycling, or slow jogging, followed by gentle stretching (not through the entire range of motion). Stretching implies movement of joints through their full range of motion and holding the final degree of stretch according to recommended guidelines.

A warm-up that progressively increases muscle temperature and mimics movement that will occur during training enhances performance. For some activities, gentle stretching is recommended in conjunction with warm-up routines. Before steady activities (walking, jogging, cycling), a warm-up of 3 to 5 minutes is recommended. The recommendation is up to 10 minutes before stop-and-go activities (e.g., racquet sports, basketball, and soccer) and athletic participation in general (e.g., football and gymnastics). Activities that require abrupt changes in direction are more likely to cause muscle strains if they are performed without proper warm-up that includes mild stretching.

Sports-specific/pre-exercise stretching can improve performance in sports that require a greater-than-average range of motion, such as gymnastics, dance, diving, and figure skating. A few studies suggest that intense stretching during warm-up can lead to a temporary short-term (up to 60 minutes) decrease in strength and power. Thus, intense stretching conducted prior to participating in athletic events that rely on force and power for peak performance is not recommended.[7,8] More recent data show that short-duration static stretching combined with dynamic stretching does not elicit performance impairments.[9]

In terms of whether stretching before or after exercise is more effective for preventing injuries, the best time to stretch is controversial. In limited

Figure 8.4 Guidelines for flexibility development.

Mode: Static, dynamic, proprioceptive neuromuscular facilitation (PNF), or controlled ballistic stretching to include all major muscle/tendon groups of the body.
Intensity: To the point of feeling tightness in the stretched area or mild discomfort.
Repetitions: Repeat each exercise 2 to 4 times, holding the final position between 10 and 30 seconds each, with a target of 60 seconds of total stretching for each exercise performed.
Frequency: At least 2 or 3 days per week but ideally 5 to 7 days per week.

SOURCE: Adapted from American College of Sports Medicine, *ACSM's Guidelines for Exercise Testing and Prescription* (Philadelphia: Wolters Kluwer/Lippincott Williams & Wilkins, 2014).

> **Controlled ballistic stretching** Exercises done with slow, short, gentle, and sustained movements.
>
> **Proprioceptive neuromuscular facilitation (PNF)** Mode of stretching that uses reflexes and neuromuscular principles to relax the muscles being stretched.
>
> **Intensity (for flexibility exercises)** Degree of stretch when doing flexibility exercises.
>
> **Repetitions** Number of times a given resistance is performed.

studies on athletic populations, the evidence is unclear. Additional research is necessary to clarify this issue.

In general, unless the activity requires extensive range of motion, a good time to stretch is after an aerobic workout. Higher body temperature in itself helps to increase the joint range of motion. Muscles also are fatigued following exercise, and a fatigued muscle tends to shorten, which can lead to soreness and spasms. Stretching exercises help fatigued muscles reestablish their normal resting length and prevent unnecessary pain.

8.6 Flexibility Exercises

To improve body flexibility, each major muscle group should be subjected to at least one stretching exercise. A complete set of exercises for developing muscular flexibility is presented on pages 300–302.

Although you may not be able to hold a final stretched position with some of these exercises (such as lateral head tilts and arm circles), you still should perform the exercise through the joint's full range of motion. Depending on the number and length of repetitions, a complete workout will last between 15 and 30 minutes.

Contraindicated Exercises Most strength and flexibility exercises are relatively safe to perform, but even safe exercises can be hazardous if they are performed incorrectly. Some exercises may be safe to perform occasionally but, when executed repeatedly, may cause trauma and injury. Pre-existing muscle or joint conditions (old sprains or injuries) can further increase the risk of harm during certain exercises. As you develop your exercise program, you are encouraged to follow the exercise descriptions and guidelines given in this book.

A few exercises, however, are not recommended because of the potential high risk for injury. These exercises sometimes are done in videotaped workouts and some fitness classes. **Contraindicated exercises** may cause harm because of the excessive strain they place on muscles and joints, in particular the spine, lower back, knees, neck, or shoulders.

Illustrations of contraindicated exercises are presented in Figure 8.5. Safe alternative exercises are listed below each contraindicated exercise and are illustrated in the exercises for strength (pages 262–278) and flexibility (pages 300–302). In isolated instances, a qualified physical therapist may select one or a few of the contraindicated exercises to treat a specific injury or disability in a carefully supervised setting. Unless you are specifically instructed to use one of these exercises, it is best that you select safe exercises from this book.

8.7 Preventing and Rehabilitating Low Back Pain

Few people make it through life without having low back pain at some point. An estimated 60 to 80 percent of the population has been afflicted by back pain or injury. Estimates indicate that more than 75 million Americans suffer from chronic back pain. Each year more than $86 billion are spent in the United States to care for back pain, with limited evidence that increased spending really helps people. When it comes to back pain, prevention and treatment through physical exercise is by far the best medicine.

It has been determined that backache syndrome is caused by (a) physical inactivity, (b) poor postural habits and body mechanics, (c) excessive body weight, and/or (d) psychological stress and is preventable more than 80 percent of the time. Data also indicate that back injuries are more common among smokers because it reduces blood flow to the spine—increasing back pain susceptibility.

More than 95 percent of all back pain is related to strain and sprain injuries, and only 1 to 5 percent is related to intervertebral disk damage.[10] Strains affect ligaments, whereas sprains affect muscles and tendons. Usually, back pain is the result of repeated micro-injuries that occur over an extended time (sometimes years) until a certain movement, activity, or excessive overload causes a significant injury to the tissues.[11]

People tend to think of back pain as a problem with the skeleton. Actually, the spine's curvature, alignment, and move-

Most Common Causes of Back Pain

- Physical inactivity
- Lack of flexibility and strength
- Poor body mechanics
- Excessive body weight
- Excessive sitting
- Poor posture
- Stress
- Intervertebral disk degeneration
- Trauma and injury
- Herniated disk (nerve compression)
- Spinal stenosis (nerve compression)
- Arthritis
- Osteoporosis
- Scoliosis
- Pregnancy
- Kidney stones

> **Contraindicated exercises** Exercises that are not recommended because they may cause injury to a person.

Figure 8.5 — Contraindicated exercises. Excessive strain on the spine and knees.

Double-Leg Lift

Upright Double-Leg Lifts

V-Sits

All three of these exercises cause excessive strain on the spine and may harm discs.
Alternatives: Strength Exercises 4 and 17, pages 300 and 303

Standing Toe Touch
Excessive strain on the knee and lower back.
Alternative: Flexibility Exercise 12, page 302

Swan Stretch
Excessive strain on the spine; may harm intervertebral discs.
Alternative: Flexibility Exercise 20, page 303

Cradle
Excessive strain on the spine, knees, and shoulders.
Alternatives: Flexibility Exercises 20 and 8, pages 303 and 301

Full Squat
Excessive strain on the knees.
Alternatives: Flexibility Exercise 8, page 301; Strength Exercises 1, 16, 28A and 28B, pages 300, 302, and 265

Head Rolls
May injure neck discs.
Alternative: Flexibility Exercise 1, page 300

Knee to Chest
(with hands over the shin)
Excessive strain on the knee.
Alternative: Flexibility Exercises 15 and 16, page 302

Sit-Ups with Hands Behind the Head
Excessive strain on the neck.
Alternatives: Strength Exercises 4 and 17, pages 300 and 303

Yoga Plow
Excessive strain on the spine, neck, and shoulders.
Alternatives: Flexibility Exercises 12, 15, 16, 17, and 19, pages 302 and 303

Hurdler Stretch
Excessive strain on the bent knee.
Alternatives: Flexibility Exercises 8 and 12, pages 301 and 302

The Hero
Excessive strain on the knees.
Alternatives: Flexibility Exercises 8 and 14, pages 301 and 302

Windmill
Excessive strain on the spine and knees.
Alternatives: Flexibility Exercises 12 and 19, pages 302 and 303

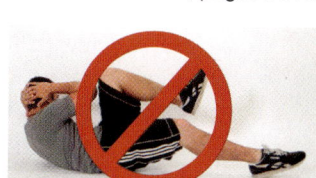

Straight-Leg Sit-Ups

Alternating Bent-Leg Sit-Ups

These exercises strain the lower back.
Alternatives: Strength Exercises 4 and 17, pages 300 and 303

Donkey Kicks
Excessive strain on the back, shoulders, and neck.
Alternatives: Flexibility Exercises 20, 14, and 1, pages 303, 302, and 300

ment are controlled by surrounding muscles. The most common reason for chronic low back pain is a lack of physical activity. In particular, a major contributor to back pain is excessive sitting, which causes back muscles to shorten, stiffen, and become weaker.

Deterioration or weakening of the abdominal and gluteal muscles, along with tightening of the lower back (erector spinae) muscles, brings about an unnatural forward tilt of the pelvis (Figure 8.6). This tilt puts extra pressure on the spinal vertebrae, causing pain in the lower back. Accumulation of fat around the midsection of the body contributes to the forward tilt of the pelvis, which further aggravates the condition.

Low back pain frequently is associated with faulty posture and improper body mechanics, or body positions. Incorrect posture and poor mechanics, such as prolonged static postures, repetitive bending and pushing, twisting a loaded spine, and prolonged (more than an hour) sitting with little movement increase strain on the lower back and many other bones, joints, muscles, and ligaments. Figure 8.7 provides a summary of proper body mechanics that promote back health.

Data recently published in 2013 indicate that between 40 percent and 80 percent of people with long-term back pain due to a herniated or slipped disk may be related to a bacterial infection caused by *Propionibacterium acnes*.[12,13] This infection can lead to swelling and tissue damage in the spine. Long-term (100 days) treatment with antibiotics provided significant relief of pain and disability for up to a year later in most of these patients. Additional clinical studies are still required to confirm these findings, but people who suffer from persistent back pain should request a blood test to check for such a bacterial infection.

In the majority of back injuries, pain is present only with movement and physical activity. According to the National Institutes of Health (NIH), most back pain goes away on its own in a few weeks. A physician should be consulted if any of the following conditions are present:

- Numbness in the legs
- Trouble urinating
- Leg weakness
- Fever
- Unintentional weight loss
- Persistent severe pain even at rest

A physician can rule out any disk damage, arthritis, osteoporosis, slipped vertebrae, spinal stenosis (narrowing of the spinal canal), or other serious condition. For common back pain, your physician may prescribe proper bed rest using several pillows under the knees for leg support (Figure 8.7). This position helps relieve muscle spasms by stretching the muscles involved. Your doctor may also prescribe a muscle relaxant or anti-inflammatory medication (or both) and some type of physical therapy.

In most cases, an x-ray and MRI is not required unless pain lingers for more than four to six weeks. In the early stages of back pain, tight muscles and muscle spasms tend to compress the vertebrae, squeezing the intervertebral disks and revealing apparent disk problems on an x-ray. In these cases, the real problem is the tight muscles and subsequent muscle spasms. A daily physical activity and stretching program helps to decompress the spine, stretch tight muscles, strengthen weak muscles, and increases blood flow (promoting healing) to the back muscles.

Time is often the best treatment approach. Even with severe pain, most people feel better within days or weeks without being treated by health care professionals.[14] Up to 90 percent of people will heal on their own. To relieve symptoms, you may use over-the-counter pain relievers and hot or cold packs. You also should stay active to avoid further weakening of the back muscles. Low-impact activities such as walking, swimming, water aerobics, and cycling are recommended. Once you are pain free in the resting state, you need to start correcting the muscular imbalance by stretching the tight muscles and strengthening the weak ones. Stretching exercises always are performed first.

If there is no indication of disease or injury (such as leg numbness or pain), a herniated disk, or fractures, spinal manipulation by a chiropractor or other health care professional can provide pain relief. Spinal manipulation as a treatment modality for low back pain has been endorsed by the federal Agency for Health Care Policy and Research. The guidelines suggest that spinal manipulation may help to alleviate discomfort and pain during the first few weeks of an acute episode of low-back pain. Generally, benefits are seen in fewer than 10 treatments. People who have had chronic pain for more than 6 months should avoid spinal

Figure 8.6 Incorrect and correct pelvic alignment.

Figure 8.7   Proper Back Care.

Low-back pain is caused by (a) physical inactivity, (b) poor postural habits and body mechanics, (c) excessive body weight, and/or (d) psychological stress. To protect your back and avoid debilitating low-back strain, you need to use proper body mechanics and correct improper body posture. Using appropriate body positions and actions in all daily activities is vital for back health. The following guidelines help avoid unnecessary back strain and protect and support your back.

Correct standing position

To learn the correct standing posture, stand a foot away from a wall and place your upper body completely straight against the wall. You will need to tighten the abdominal and gluteal muscles to do so. Next, walk around for a few minutes holding this same position and at the end return to the wall to evaluate how well you maintained the posture.

Standing, lifting, and carrying positions

Incorrect:		Correct:
	Stand with the aid of a footrest	
	Always bend at the hips and knees	
	Hold and carry objects close to the body	
	Bend at the knees to lean forward	

Correct sitting position

Most people spend many daily hours sitting. Proper sitting and preventing a forward slump is essential for back health. To straighten your back (a) put your head back, (b) pull in your chin toward your chest, (c) tighten your abdominal muscles, and (d) raise your chest. You should always sit in this manner. The following guidelines will also help correct improper sitting throughout the day.

Always use a footrest to keep the knees higher than the hips		Avoid severe rounding of upper back and neck while seated	
Sit close to the pedals when driving		To lean forward, bend at the hips and keep the neck and back as straight as possible	

Bed posture

A firm mattress is recommended for proper back support. Avoid sleeping flat on your back or face down with large pillows for head support. Lying sideways in a fetal position with a small pillow for head support and a small pillow between the knees, or on your back with the knees supported by a larger pillow, is best.

Incorrect:	Correct:

When resting, do it right

When at home resting or relaxing, lie flat on your back with a small pillow under your neck and with pillows under the knees for support. You may also place the lower legs on a chair with your knees bent at 90 degrees. This position is also good to relieve back spasms when suffering from back pain.

When watching TV or sitting on the floor, do so by lying on a straight-back chair covered with a firm pillow and a second large pillow under the knees.

© Cengage Learning 2013

Behavior Modification Planning

Tips to Prevent Low Back Pain

I PLAN TO / I DID IT

- ❏ ❏ Be physically active.
- ❏ ❏ Maintain recommended body weight (excess weight strains the back).
- ❏ ❏ Stretch often using spinal exercises through a functional range of motion.
- ❏ ❏ Regularly strengthen the core of the body using sets of 10 to 12 repetitions to near fatigue with isometric contractions when applicable.
- ❏ ❏ Lift heavy objects by bending at the knees and carry them close to the body. Place one foot forward and keep your knees slightly bent while standing.
- ❏ ❏ Avoid sitting (over 50 minutes) or standing in one position for lengthy periods of time.
- ❏ ❏ Maintain correct posture.
- ❏ ❏ Sleep on your back with a pillow under the knees or on your side with the knees drawn up and a small pillow between the knees.
- ❏ ❏ Try out different mattresses of firm consistency before selecting a mattress.
- ❏ ❏ Warm up properly using mild stretches before engaging in physical activity.
- ❏ ❏ Practice adequate stress management techniques.
- ❏ ❏ Don't smoke (it reduces blood flow to the spine—increasing back pain risk).

Try It

In your class notebook, record how many of these actions are a regular part of your healthy low-back program. If you are not using all of them, what is necessary to incorporate these behaviors into your lifestyle?

---

manipulation until they have been thoroughly examined by a physician.

Back pain is considered chronic if it persists longer than three months. Surgery is seldom the best option, as it often weakens the spine. Scar tissue and surgical alterations also decrease the success rate of a subsequent surgery. Only about 10 percent of people with chronic pain are candidates for surgery. If surgery is recommended, always seek a second opinion. And consider all other options. In many cases, pushing beyond the pain and participating in aggressive physical therapy ("exercise boot camps" for back pain) aimed at strengthening the muscles that support the spine are what's needed to overcome the condition. Data from the Physician's Neck & Back Clinic in Minneapolis showed that only 3 in 38 patients recommended for surgery needed such on completion of a 10-week aggressive physical therapy program.[15]

Back pain can be reduced greatly through aerobic exercise, muscular flexibility exercise, and muscular strength and endurance training that includes specific exercises to strengthen the spine-stabilizing muscles. Exercise requires effort by the patient, and it may create discomfort initially, but exercise promotes circulation, healing, muscle size, and muscle strength and endurance. Many patients abstain from aggressive physical therapy because they are unwilling to commit the time required for the program.

In terms of alleviating back pain, *exercise is medicine*, but it needs to be the right type of exercise. Aerobic exercise is beneficial because it helps decrease body fat and psychological stress. During an episode of back pain, however, people often avoid activity and cope by getting more rest. Rest is recommended if the pain is associated with a herniated disk, but if your physician rules out a serious problem, exercise is a better choice of treatment. Exercise helps restore physical function, and individuals who start and maintain an aerobic exercise program have back pain less frequently. Individuals who exercise also are less likely to require surgery or other invasive treatments.

Regular stretching exercises that help the hip and trunk go through a functional range of motion, rather than increasing the range of motion, are recommended. That is, for proper back care, stretching exercises should not be performed to the extreme range of motion. Individuals with a greater spinal range of motion also have a higher incidence of back injury. Spinal stability, instead of mobility, is desirable for back health.[16]

Yoga exercises are particularly beneficial to enhance flexibility, and **Iyegar yoga** in particular, has been shown to relieve chronic low back pain.[17] In fact yoga may help relieve chronic back pain better than conventional medicine. Following 24 weeks of biweekly classes, yoga participants had greater improvement in functional disability along with a decrease in pain intensity and low-back-pain–related depression. These benefits were still present six months after the end of class participation.

A strengthening program for a healthy back should be conducted around the endurance threshold—15 or more repetitions to near fatigue. Muscular endurance of the muscles that support the spine is more important than absolute strength because these muscles perform their work during the course of an entire day.

> **Critical Thinking**
>
> Consider your own low-back health. • Have you ever had episodes of low-back pain? • If so, how long did it take you to recover, and what helped you recover from this condition?

Several exercises for preventing and rehabilitating the backache syndrome are given on pages 290–295. These exercises can be done twice or more daily when a person has back pain. Under normal circumstances, doing these exercises three or four times a week is enough to prevent the syndrome. Using some of the additional core exercises listed in Chapter 7 ("Core Strength Training," page 253) will further enhance your low back management program. A strong core musculature is critical for spine and back health and will reduce or completely eliminate pain flare-ups. Back pain recurs more often in people who rely solely on medication, compared with people who use both medication and exercise therapy to recover.[18]

Effects of Posture

Good posture enhances personal appearance, self-image, improves balance and endurance, protects against misalignment-related pains and aches, prevents falls, projects self-confidence and self-assurance, and enhances your overall sense of well-being.[19] The relationship between different body parts is the essence of posture.

Poor posture strains muscles and ligaments and becomes a risk factor for musculoskeletal problems of the neck, shoulders, and lower back. Incorrect posture also strains hips and knees. Faulty posture and weak and inelastic muscles are also a leading cause of chronic low-back problems.

Adequate body mechanics also aid in reducing chronic low-back pain. Proper body mechanics means using correct positions in all the activities of daily life, including sleeping, sitting, standing, walking, driving, working, and exercising. Because of the high incidence of low back pain, illustrations of proper body mechanics and a series of corrective and preventive exercises are shown in Figure 8.7 and Activity 8.2. Besides engaging in the recommended exercises you need to continually strive to maintain good posture. As posture improves, you frequently become motivated to change other aspects, such as muscular strength and flexibility and decreasing body fat.

Effects of Stress

Psychological stress, too, may lead to back pain.[20] The brain is "hardwired" to the back muscles. Excessive stress causes muscles to contract. Frequent tightening of the back muscles can throw the back out of alignment and constrict blood vessels that supply oxygen and nutrients to the back. Chronic stress also increases the release of hormones that have been linked to muscle and tendon injuries. Furthermore, people under stress tend to forget proper body mechanics, placing themselves at unnecessary risk for injury. If you are undergoing excessive stress and back pain at the same time, proper stress management (see Chapter 12) should be a part of your comprehensive back-care program.

Proper Body Mechanics for Back Care

The following guidelines should be incorporated into daily living to maintain a healthy, strong back and prevent the backache syndrome:

1. Incorporate stretching and strengthening exercises into your regular exercise program (see exercises 17 through 34 at the end of this chapter).
2. Always use proper lifting techniques in strength training. Do not compromise proper technique to lift more weight.
3. Perform the pelvic tilt exercise (tightening the abdominal and gluteal muscles while flattening the lower back; see exercise 12, Chapter 7, page 265) not only during your exercise session but throughout the day while standing, sitting, or lying down.
4. Always lift objects, regardless of weight, by bending at the hips and knees. Never bend from the waist only.
5. Do not lift heavy objects higher than your waist.
6. Carry all objects close to your body, never away from the body.
7. Do not suddenly overload your back muscles. Always ask for help if an object is heavier than you can comfortably lift or carry. Exercise caution when opening windows and doors.
8. Avoid sudden bodily torques, twists, or movements.
9. Always keep your head and neck in a straight line over your spine.
10. Follow proper mechanics when standing, sitting, resting, and sleeping (see Figure 8.7).
11. When resting, do it right (see Figure 8.7).
12. When in doubt, if significant back pain persists for several days, or back pain is severe, do not hesitate to see your doctor.

Personal Flexibility and Low-Back Conditioning Program

Activity 8.2 allows you to develop your own flexibility and low-back conditioning programs. Some of the exercises that help increase spinal stability and muscular strength endurance require isometric contractions. The recommendation calls for these contractions to be held for 2 to 20 seconds. The length of the hold will depend on your current fitness level and the difficulty of each exercise. For most exercises, you may start with a 2- to 5-second hold. Over the course of several weeks, you can increase the length of the hold up to 20 seconds.

> **Iyegar yoga** Form of yoga that aims to develop flexibility, strength, balance, and stamina using props (belts, blocks, blankets, and chairs) to aid in the correct performance of asanas, or yoga postures.

Activity 8.1: Muscular Flexibility Assessment

Name _____ Date _____

Course _____ Section _____ Gender _____ Age _____

Test	Score	Fitness Category	Point
Modified Sit-and-Reach			
Total Body Rotation ☐ Right ☐ Left			
Shoulder Rotation			

Total Points: ____

Overall Flexibility Category: ____

Activity 8.2: Flexibility Development and Low Back Conditioning Programs

Name _____ Date _____

Course _____ Section _____ Gender _____ Age _____

I. Stage of Change for Flexibility Training
Using Figure 2.5 (page 63) and Table 2.3 (page 62), identify your current stage of change for participation in a muscular stretching program.

II. Instruction
Perform all of the recommended flexibility exercises given on pages 300–302. Use a combination of slow-sustained and proprioceptive neuromuscular facilitation stretching techniques. Indicate the technique(s) used for each exercise and, where applicable, the number of repetitions performed and the length of time that the final degree of stretch was held.

Stretching Exercises

Exercise	Stretching Technique	Repetitions	Length of Final Stretch
Lateral head tilt			NA*
Arm circles			NA
Side stretch			
Body rotation			
Chest stretch			
Shoulder hyperextension stretch			
Shoulder rotation stretch			NA
Quad stretch			
Heel cord stretch			
Adductor stretch			
Sitting adductor stretch			
Sit-and-reach stretch			
Triceps stretch			

*Not Applicable

Stretching Schedule (Indicate days, time, and place where you will stretch):

Flexibility-training days: M ☐ T ☐ W ☐ Th ☐ F ☐ Sa ☐ Su ☐   Time of day: ☐   Place: ☐

Low Back Conditioning Program

Perform all of the recommended exercises for the prevention and rehabilitation of low back pain given on pages 303–304. Indicate the number of repetitions performed for each exercise.

Flexibility Exercises	Repetitions	Strength/Endurance Exercises	Repetitions	Seconds Held
Hip flexor stretch		Pelvic tilt		
Single-knee-to-chest stretch		The cat		
Double-knee-to-chest stretch		Abdominal crunch or abdominal curl-up		
Upper and lower back stretch		Reverse crunch		
Sit-and-reach stretch		Supine bridge		
Gluteal stretch		Pelvic clock		
Back extension stretch		Lateral bridge		
Trunk rotation and lower back stretch		Prone bridge		
		Leg press		
		Seated back		
		Lat pull-down		
		Back extension		

Proper Body Mechanics

Perform the following tasks using the proper body mechanics given in Figure 8.7 (page 293). Check off each item as you perform the task:

☐ Standing (carriage) position
☐ Sitting position
☐ Bed posture
☐ Resting position for tired and painful back
☐ Lifting an object

Proper Body Mechanics for Back Care

According to the guidelines provided in this chapter and in Figure 8.7 (page 293), indicate below actions that you need to work on to improve posture and body mechanics and prevent low back pain.

ASSESS YOUR BEHAVIOR

CENGAGEbrain To access course materials, including companion resources, please visit www.cengagebrain.com.

1. Do you give flexibility exercises the same priority in your fitness program as you do aerobic and strength training?
2. Are stretching exercises a part of your fitness program at least two times per week?
3. Do you include exercises to strengthen and enhance body alignment in your regular strength and flexibility program?

ASSESS YOUR KNOWLEDGE

Evaluate how well you understand the concepts presented in this chapter using the chapter-specific quizzing available in the online materials at www.cengagebrain.com.

1. Muscular flexibility is defined as
   a. the capacity of joints and muscles to work in a synchronized manner.
   b. the achievable range of motion at a joint or group of joints without causing injury.
   c. the capability of muscles to stretch beyond their normal resting length without injury to the muscles.
   d. the capacity of muscles to return to their proper length following the application of a stretching force.
   e. the limitations placed on muscles as the joints move through their normal planes.

2. Good flexibility
   a. promotes healthy muscles and joints.
   b. decreases the risk of injury.
   c. improves posture.
   d. decreases the risk of chronic back pain.
   e. All are correct choices.

3. Plastic elongation is a term used in reference to
   a. permanent lengthening of soft tissue.
   b. increased flexibility achieved through dynamic stretching.
   c. temporary elongation of muscles.
   d. the ability of a muscle to achieve a complete degree of stretch.
   e. lengthening of a muscle against resistance.

4. The most significant contributors to loss of flexibility are
   a. sedentary living and lack of physical activity.
   b. weight and power training.
   c. age and injury.
   d. muscular strength and endurance.
   e. excessive body fat and low lean tissue.

5. Which of the following is *not* a mode of stretching?
   a. proprioceptive neuromuscular facilitation
   b. elastic elongation
   c. ballistic stretching
   d. slow-sustained stretching
   e. All are modes of stretching.

6. PNF can help increase
   a. muscular strength.
   b. muscular flexibility.
   c. muscular endurance.
   d. range of motion.
   e. All are correct choices.

7. When performing stretching exercises, the degree of stretch should be
   a. through the entire arc of movement.
   b. to about 80 percent of capacity.
   c. to mild tension at the end of the range of motion.
   d. applied until the muscle(s) start shaking.
   e. progressively increased until the desired stretch is attained.

8. When stretching, the final stretch should be held for
   a. 1 to 10 seconds.
   b. 15 to 60 seconds.
   c. 30 to 90 seconds.
   d. 1 to 3 minutes.
   e. as long as the person is able to sustain the stretch.

9. Low-back pain is associated primarily with
   a. physical inactivity.
   b. faulty posture.
   c. excessive body weight.
   d. improper body mechanics.
   e. All are correct choices.

10. The following exercise helps stretch the lower back and hamstring muscles:
    a. adductor stretch.
    b. cat stretch.
    c. back extension stretch.
    d. single-knee-to-chest stretch.
    e. quad stretch.

Correct answers can be found at the back of the book.

Flexibility Exercises

EXERCISE 1 Neck Stretches

ACTION Gently tilt the head laterally (a). You may increase the degree of stretch by gently pulling with one hand (b). You may also stretch the neck by raising your head toward the ceiling (c—do not extend your head backward; look straight forward). You may also turn your head 30° and gradually bring the head forward until you feel an adequate stretch in the muscles on the back of the neck (d). The degree of stretch can again be increased by gently pulling forward with the hand (e). Perform the exercises on both the right and left sides. Repeat each exercise several times, and hold the final stretched position for several seconds.

AREAS STRETCHED Neck flexors and extensors; ligaments of the cervical spine

EXERCISE 2 Arm Circles

ACTION Gently circle your arms all the way around. Conduct the exercise in both directions.

AREAS STRETCHED
Shoulder muscles and ligaments

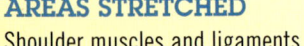

EXERCISE 3 Side Stretch

ACTION Stand straight up, feet separated to shoulder-width, and place your hands on your waist. Now move the upper body to one side and hold the final stretch for a few seconds. Repeat on the other side.

AREAS STRETCHED Muscles and ligaments in the pelvic region

EXERCISE 4 Body Rotation

ACTION Place your arms slightly away from the body and rotate the trunk as far as possible, holding the final position for several seconds. Conduct the exercise for both the right and left sides of the body. You also can perform this exercise by standing about two feet away from the wall (back toward the wall) and then rotating the trunk, placing the hands against the wall.

AREAS STRETCHED Hip, abdominal, chest, back, neck, and shoulder muscles; hip and spinal ligaments

EXERCISE 5 Chest Stretch

ACTION Place your hands on the shoulders of your partner, who in turn will push you down by your shoulders. Hold the final position for a few seconds.

AREAS STRETCHED Chest (pectoral) muscles and shoulder ligaments

EXERCISE 6 Shoulder Hyperextension

ACTION Have a partner grasp your arms from behind by the wrists and slowly push them upward. Hold the final position for a few seconds.

AREAS STRETCHED Deltoid and pectoral muscles; ligaments of the shoulder joint

EXERCISE 7 Shoulder Rotation Stretch

ACTION With the aid of surgical tubing or an aluminum or wood stick, place the tubing or stick behind your back and grasp the two ends using a reverse (thumbs-out) grip. Slowly bring the tubing or stick over your head, keeping the elbows straight. Repeat several times (bring the hands closer together for additional stretch).

AREAS STRETCHED Deltoid, latissimus dorsi, and pectoral muscles; shoulder ligaments

EXERCISE 8 Quad Stretch

ACTION Lie on your side and move one foot back by flexing the knee. Grasp the front of the ankle and pull the ankle toward the gluteal region. Hold for several seconds. Repeat with the other leg.

AREAS STRETCHED Quadriceps muscle; knee and ankle ligaments

EXERCISE 9 Heel Cord Stretch

ACTION Stand against the wall or at the edge of a step and stretch the heel downward, alternating legs. Hold the stretched position for a few seconds.

AREAS STRETCHED Heel cord (Achilles tendon); gastrocnemius and soleus muscles

EXERCISE 10 Adductor Stretch

ACTION Stand with your feet about twice shoulder-width apart and place your hands slightly above the knees. Flex one knee and slowly go down as far as possible, holding the final position for a few seconds. Repeat with the other leg.

AREAS STRETCHED Hip adductor muscles

EXERCISE 11 Sitting Adductor Stretch

ACTION Sit on the floor and bring your feet in close to you, allowing the soles of the feet to touch each other. Now place your forearms (or elbows) on the inner part of the thigh and push the legs downward, holding the final stretch for several seconds.

AREAS STRETCHED Hip adductor muscles

EXERCISE 12 Sit-and-Reach Stretch

ACTION Sit on the floor with legs together and gradually reach forward as far as possible. Hold the final position for a few seconds. This exercise also may be performed with the legs separated, reaching to each side as well as to the middle.

AREAS STRETCHED Hamstrings and lower back muscles; lumbar spine ligaments

EXERCISE 13 Triceps Stretch

ACTION Place the right hand behind your neck. Grasp the right arm above the elbow with the left hand. Gently pull the elbow backward. Repeat the exercise with the opposite arm.

AREAS STRETCHED Back of upper arm (triceps muscle); shoulder joint

NOTE Exercises 14 through 21 and 23 are also flexibility exercises and can be added to your stretching program.

EXERCISE 14 Hip Flexor Stretch

ACTION Kneel down on an exercise mat or a soft surface, or place a towel under your knees. Raise the left knee off the floor and place the left foot about 3 feet in front of you. Place your left hand over your left knee and the right hand over the back of the right hip. Keeping the lower back flat, slowly move forward and downward as you apply gentle pressure over the right hip. Repeat the exercise with the opposite leg forward.

AREAS STRETCHED Flexor muscles in front of the hip joint

EXERCISE 15 Single-Knee-to-Chest Stretch

ACTION Lie down flat on the floor. Bend one leg at approximately 100° and gradually pull the opposite leg toward your chest. Hold the final stretch for a few seconds. Switch legs and repeat the exercise.

AREAS STRETCHED Lower back and hamstring muscles; lumbar spine ligaments

EXERCISE 16 Double-Knee-to-Chest Stretch

ACTION Lie flat on the floor and then curl up slowly into a fetal position. Hold for a few seconds.

AREAS STRETCHED Upper and lower back and hamstring muscles; spinal ligaments

Exercises for the Prevention and Rehabilitation of Low Back Pain

EXERCISE 17 Upper and Lower Back Stretch

ACTION Sit on the floor and bring your feet in close to you, allowing the soles of the feet to touch each other. Holding on to your feet, bring your head and upper chest gently toward your feet.

AREAS STRETCHED Upper and lower back muscles and ligaments

EXERCISE 18 Sit-and-Reach Stretch
(see Exercise 12 on page 302)

EXERCISE 19 Gluteal Stretch

ACTION Lie on the floor, bend the right leg, and place your right ankle slightly above the left knee. Grasp behind the left thigh with both hands and gently pull the leg toward the chest. Repeat the exercise with the opposite leg.

AREAS STRETCHED Buttock area (gluteal muscles)

EXERCISE 20 Back Extension Stretch

ACTION Lie face down on the floor with the elbows by the chest, forearms on the floor, and the hands beneath the chin. Gently raise the trunk by extending the elbows until you reach an approximate 90° angle at the elbow joint. Be sure the forearms remain in contact with the floor at all times. Do not extend the back beyond this point. Hyperextension of the lower back may lead to or aggravate an existing back problem. Hold the stretched position for about 10 seconds.

AREAS STRETCHED Abdominal region

ADDITIONAL BENEFITS Restore lower back curvature

EXERCISE 21 Trunk Rotation Stretch

ACTION Sit on the floor and bend the left leg, placing the left foot on the outside of the right knee. Place the right elbow on the left knee and push against it. At the same time, try to rotate the trunk to the left (counterclockwise). Hold the final position for a few seconds. Repeat the exercise with the other side.

AREAS STRETCHED Lateral side of the hip and thigh; trunk and lower back

EXERCISE 22 Pelvic Tilt

(see Exercise 12 in Chapter 7, page 265) This is perhaps the most important exercise for the care of the lower back. It should be included as a part of your daily exercise routine and should be performed several times throughout the day when pain in the lower back is present as a result of muscle imbalance.

EXERCISE 23 The Cat

ACTION Kneel on the floor and place your hands in front of you (on the floor) about shoulder-width apart. Relax the trunk and lower back (a). Now arch the spine and pull in your abdomen as far as you can and hold this position for a few seconds (b). Repeat the exercise 4 to 5 times.

AREAS STRETCHED Low-back muscles and ligaments

AREAS STRENGTHENED Abdominal and gluteal muscles

EXERCISE 24 Abdominal Crunch or Abdominal Curl-up

(see Exercise 4 in Chapter 7, page 263) It is important that you do not stabilize your feet when performing either of these exercises, because doing so decreases the work of the abdominal muscles. Also, remember not to "swing up" but, rather, to curl up as you perform these exercises.

EXERCISE 25 Reverse Crunch

(see Exercise 11 in Chapter 7, page 265)

EXERCISE 26 Supine Bridge

ACTION Lie face up on the floor with the knees bent at about 120°. Do a pelvic tilt (exercise 12 in Chapter 7, page 265) and maintain the pelvic tilt while you raise the hips off the floor until the upper body and upper legs are in a straight line. Hold this position for several seconds.

AREAS STRENGTHENED Gluteal and abdominal flexor muscles

EXERCISE 27 Pelvic Clock

ACTION Lie face up on the floor with the knees bent at about 120°. Fully extend the hips as in the supine bridge (exercise 26). Now progressively rotate the hips in a clockwise manner (2 o'clock, 4 o'clock, 6 o'clock, 8 o'clock, 10 o'clock, and 12 o'clock), holding each position in an isometric contraction for about 1 second. Repeat the exercise counterclockwise.

AREAS STRENGTHENED Gluteal, abdominal, and hip flexor muscles

EXERCISE 28 Lateral Bridge
(see Exercise 13 in Chapter 7, page 265)

EXERCISE 29 Prone Bridge
(see Exercise 14 in Chapter 7, page 266)

EXERCISE 30 Leg Press
(see Exercise 16 in Chapter 7, page 267)

EXERCISE 31 Seated Back
(see Exercise 20 in Chapter 7, page 268)

EXERCISE 32 Lat Pull-Down
(see Exercise 24 in Chapter 7, page 269)

EXERCISE 33 Back Extension
(see Exercise 36 in Chapter 7, page 275)

EXERCISE 34 Lateral Trunk Flexion
(see Exercise 37 in Chapter 7, page 276)

Comprehensive Fitness Programming

9

"To give anything less than your best is to sacrifice the gift."
—Steve Prefontaine

Objectives

- **Identify** popular cardiorespiratory activities and their specific benefits.
- **Identify** worldwide fitness trends
- **Dispel** common misconceptions related to physical fitness and wellness.
- **Become** aware of safety considerations for exercising.
- **Learn** concepts for preventing and treating injuries.
- **Describe** the relationship between fitness and aging.
- **Be able** to write a comprehensive fitness program.

CENGAGEbrain.com
Visit **www.cengagebrain.com** to access course materials and companion resources for this text, including quiz questions designed to check your understanding of the chapter contents. See the preface on page ix for more information.

What is the best fitness activity?

No single physical activity, sport, or exercise contributes to the development of overall fitness (see Chapter 6, Table 6.9, page 223). Most people who exercise pick and adhere to a single mode, such as walking, swimming, or jogging. Many activities will contribute to cardiorespiratory development. The extent of contribution to other fitness components, though, varies among the activities. For total fitness, aerobic activities should be supplemented with strength and flexibility programs. Cross-training—that is, selecting different activities for fitness development and maintenance (jogging, water aerobics, spinning)—adds enjoyment to the program, decreases the risk of incurring injuries from overuse, and keeps exercise from becoming monotonous.

Is it best not to eat before exercise?

Despite popular belief, research indicates that eating some food, liquid or solid, prior to physical activity provides energy and nutrients that improve endurance and exercise performance. Of course, how long before exercise, how much food, and what type of food you eat depends on the intensity of exercise and your stomach's tolerance to pre-exercise food. The primary fuel for exercise is provided by carbohydrates, which the body converts to glucose and stores as glycogen. Some protein along with carbohydrates is also recommended (see next question).

Aim to consume 1 gram of carbohydrate per kilogram of body weight (.5 gram of carbohydrate per pound of body weight) one hour prior to exercise. For high-intensity aerobic activities, sports drinks consumed 30 to 60 minutes prior to exercise are best because they are rapidly absorbed by the body. Solid foods (granola bars, energy bars, bagel, sugar wafers, crackers) or semi-liquid solid foods (yogurt, gelatin, pudding) are acceptable for light-intensity aerobic exercise or strength training. Even a snack consumed a few minutes before exercise will help you, as long as you exercise longer than 30 minutes. Through trial and error you will need to learn which sport snacks best suit your stomach without interfering with exercise performance.

Are there specific nutrient requirements for optimal development and recovery following exercise?

Carbohydrates with some protein appear to be best. A combination of these nutrients is recommended prior to and immediately following high-intensity aerobic or strength-training exercise. A small snack or a sports drink containing protein 30 to 60 minutes before intense exercise is beneficial. Intense exercise causes microtears in muscle tissue, and the presence of amino acids (the building blocks of proteins) in the blood contributes to the healing process and subsequent development and strengthening of the muscle fibers. Post-exercise protein consumption along with carbohydrates also accelerates glycogen replenishment in the body after intense or prolonged exercise. Thus, carbohydrates provide energy for exercise and replenishment of glycogen stores after exercise, whereas protein optimizes muscle repair, growth, glycogen replenishment, and recovery following exercise. Although muscles absorb a greater amount of amino acids up to 48 hours following intense exercise, consumption of the carbohydrate/protein snack immediately following intense exercise, and an hour thereafter, appear to be most beneficial. Aim for a ratio of 4:1 grams of carbohydrates to protein. For example, you may consume a snack that contains 40 grams of carbohydrates (160 calories) and 10 grams of protein (40 calories). To optimize development, make sure that you consume some protein with snacks or meals for the next 48 hours as well. Examples of good recovery foods include milk and cereal, a tuna fish sandwich, a peanut butter and jelly sandwich, and pasta with turkey meat sauce. Commercial sports drinks and snacks with a 4:1 ratio are now also readily available.

What is high-intensity interval training (HIIT)?

HIIT is primarily an aerobic training program that had been used mainly by athletes, but has now become popular among fitness participants seeking better, faster, and more effective development. Following an appropriate warm-up, HIIT includes high- to very high-intensity intervals that are interspersed with a low-to-moderate intensity recovery phase. Typically, a 1:3, 1:2, or 1:1 work-to-recovery ratio is used: The more intense the interval, the longer the recovery period. Research indicates that additional health and fitness benefits are reaped as the intensity of exercise increases. HIIT produces the greatest improvements in aerobic capacity (VO_{2max}) and increases the capability to exercise at a higher percentage of that capacity (anaerobic threshold), thus allowing the participant to burn more calories during the exercise session. The data also show that HIIT increases the capacity for fat oxidation during exercise. Although the fuel used during high-intensity intervals is primarily glucose (carbohydrates), molecular changes occur in the muscles that increase the body's capability for fatty acid oxidation (fat burning). Furthermore, following light- to moderate-intensity aerobic activity, resting metabolism returns to normal in about 90 minutes. Depending on the volume of training (intensity and number of intervals performed), with HIIT it takes 24 to 72 hours for the body to return to its "normal" resting metabolic rate. Thus, a greater amount of calories (primarily from fat) are burned up to three days following HIIT. While the extra calories burned during the recovery phase of HIIT sessions can make a difference in the long run, keep in mind that the most significant factor are the number of calories actually burned during the HIIT session. The extra calories burned during recovery do help, but do not compare to those used in training.

Real Life Story | Oliver's Experience

As a kid, I always hated gym class. I was not very coordinated and I couldn't hit the ball very far in baseball or score in basketball. I always seemed to be one of the last ones picked for any team. So I told myself I was not meant for sports, and avoided them as much as possible. However, when I got to college, I was feeling out of shape and wanted to find a fun way to get some exercise. I remembered that as a kid I had been pretty good at ping-pong, and that I had sometimes beaten my friends when we would race short distances on foot. So I thought that even though I wasn't the greatest athlete on the whole, that I might have fair speed and agility. Then I searched for a sport that would make use of those advantages, and I decided to try tennis. I took a tennis class, and worked at improving my skills. I made some friends in class that I continue to play with regularly. After a fair amount of practice, I eventually became a halfway decent tennis player! Learning to do well at this one sport has helped me get in better shape and actually develop the confidence to try other athletic activities, like mountain biking and ultimate Frisbee. I learned that just because I didn't excel at the first few sports I tried, that doesn't mean that I was totally lacking in athletic ability. I am happy that I am able to experience the fun of competing in a sport, and sometimes even winning!

PERSONAL PROFILE: Your Lifetime Physical Fitness Program

I. What is the most efficient type (mode) of exercise that contributes to good health and contributes to lifetime weight management? Can you explain and justify your answer?

II. Can you name three benefits of cross-training?

III. Have you ever participated in a HIIT program? If so, how did you feel at the end of each training session, and what results did you obtain?

IV. Is it better to get fit before playing sports or play sports to get fit? Can you elaborate?

V. What is your take-home message from Oliver's experience, and how may it influence your personal fitness program?

One of the fun aspects of exercise is that you can choose from many different activities to promote fitness. While energy expenditure varies among activities and your intensity of effort, the most important factor to promote health and lifetime weight maintenance is regular participation. Select one or a combination of activities for your program. The choice should be based on personal enjoyment, convenience, and availability. An element of fun and social support from family and friends that are willing to join your program greatly enhance exercise compliance. Set short-term and long-term SMART goals and reward yourself for goals met. To increase motivation, regularly look for fun challenges, such as participating in a walkathon, 5K, swim meet, bike race, extended hike, or sports league (soccer, basketball, volleyball, or tennis). The time is now to take advantage of the myriad benefits derived through physical activity and exercise by making physical activity a priority in your daily lifestyle.

9.1 Choices of Aerobic Activities

A summary of the most popular adult physical activities in the United States is presented in Figure 9.1. To facilitate your choice of activities, a discussion of traditional exercise modalities and new trends in fitness activities follows next in this chapter. The discussion focuses on the characteristics of the activities along with benefits, requirements, and safety recommendations for some of the activities.

Traditional Fitness Activities As you select your activities, keep in mind that exercise sessions should be convenient. To enjoy exercise, be sure to select a time when you will not be rushed. A nearby location is recommended. People do not enjoy driving across town to get to the gym, health club, track, or pool. If parking is a problem, you may get discouraged quickly and quit. All of these factors are used as excuses not to stick to an exercise program.

Walking The most natural, easiest, safest, and least expensive form of aerobic exercise is walking. Walking at speeds of four miles per hour or faster improves cardiorespiratory fitness. From a health-fitness viewpoint, a regular walking program can prolong life significantly (see the discussion of cardiovascular disease in Chapter 10). Although walking takes longer than jogging, the caloric cost of brisk walking is only about 10 percent lower than jogging the same distance.

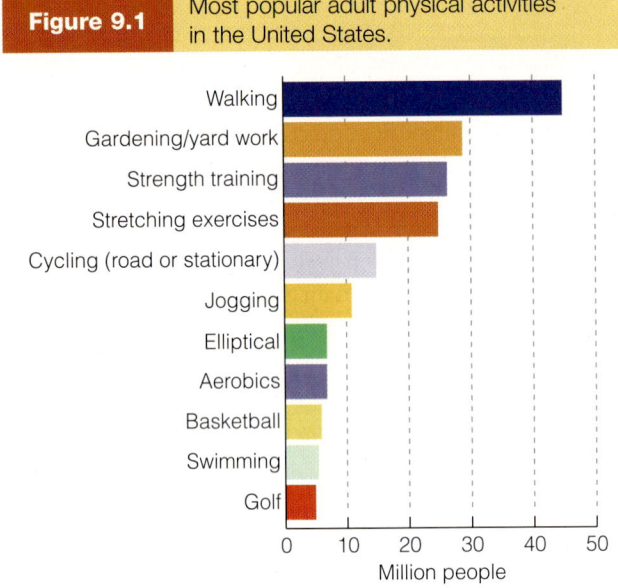

Figure 9.1 Most popular adult physical activities in the United States.

SOURCE: Adapted from the Centers for Disease Control and Prevention, Atlanta, 2013.

Walking is perhaps the best activity to start a conditioning program for the cardiorespiratory system. Inactive people should start with one-mile walks four or five times per week. Walk times can be increased gradually by five minutes each week. Following three to four weeks of conditioning, a person should be able to walk two miles at a four-mile-per-hour pace, five times per week. Greater aerobic benefits accrue from walking longer and swinging the arms faster than normal. Light hand weights, a backpack (four to six pounds), or walking poles add to the intensity of walking. Because of the additional load on the cardiorespiratory system, extra weights or loads are not recommended for people who have cardiovascular disease.

Walking in water (chest-deep level) is another excellent form of aerobic activity, particularly for people with leg and back problems. Because of the buoyancy that water provides, individuals submerged in water to armpit level weigh only about 10 to 20 percent of their weight outside the water. The resistance the water creates as a person walks in the pool makes the intensity quite high, providing an excellent cardiorespiratory workout.

Jogging Next to walking, jogging it is one of the most accessible forms of exercise. A person can find places to jog almost everywhere. The lone requirement to prevent injuries is a good pair of jogging shoes.

Jogging three to five times a week is one of the fastest ways to improve cardiorespiratory fitness. The risk of injury, however, especially in beginners, is greater with jogging than walking. For proper conditioning, jogging programs should start with 1 to 2 weeks of walking. As fitness improves, walking and jogging can be combined, gradually increasing the jogging segment until it composes the full 20 to 30 minutes.

A word of caution when it comes to jogging: The risk of injury increases greatly as speed (running instead of jogging) and mileage go up. Jogging approximately 15 miles per week is sufficient to reach an excellent level of cardiorespiratory fitness.

A good pair of shoes is a must for joggers. Many foot, knee, and leg problems originate from improperly fitting or worn-out shoes. A good pair of shoes should offer good lateral stability and not lean to either side when placed on a flat surface. The shoe also should bend at the ball of the foot, not at midfoot. Worn-out shoes should be replaced. If you suddenly have problems, check your shoes first. It may be time for a new pair.

For safety reasons, joggers should stay away from high-speed roads, not wear headphones, and always run (or walk) against the traffic so that they will be able to see all oncoming traffic. At night, reflective clothing or fluorescent material should be worn on different parts of the body. Carrying a flashlight is even better, because motorists can see the light from a greater distance than they can see the reflective material.

An alternative form of jogging, especially for injured people, those with chronic back problems, and overweight individuals, is deep-water running. This entails running in place while treading water and is almost as strenuous as jogging on land. The running motions used on land are accentuated by pumping the arms and legs hard through the full range of motion. The participant usually wears a flotation vest to help maintain the body in an upright position. Many elite athletes train in water to lessen the wear and tear on the body caused by long-distance running. These athletes have been able to maintain high oxygen uptake values through rigorous water running programs.

Strength Training Thoroughly discussed in Chapter 7, strength training is one of the strongest trends in worldwide fitness. More adults are embracing strength training to enhance muscular fitness, health, functional capacity, and use it to either complement their aerobic conditioning, or in some instances as their primary mode of exercise. Worldwide, fitness participants strength train to further develop or maintain muscular strength and endurance in mid-life and throughout the aging process.

Hiking Hiking is an excellent activity for the entire family, especially during the summer and on summer vacations. Many people feel guilty if they are unable to continue their exercise routine during vacations. The intensity of hiking over uneven terrain is greater than walking. An 8-hour hike can burn as many calories as a 20-mile walk or jog.

Another benefit of hiking is the relaxing effects of beautiful scenery. This is an ideal activity for highly stressed people who live near woods and hills. A rough day at the office can be forgotten quickly in the peacefulness and beauty of the outdoors.

Aerobics Aerobics is a very popular fitness activity for women in the United States. Routines consist of a combination of stepping, walking, jogging, skipping, kicking, and arm-swinging movements performed to music. It is a fun way to exercise and promote cardiorespiratory development at the same time.

High-impact aerobics (HIA) was the original form of aerobics. The movements exert a great amount of vertical force on the feet as they contact the floor. Proper leg conditioning through other forms of weight-bearing aerobic exercises (brisk walking and jogging), as well as strength training, are recommended prior to participating in high-impact aerobics.

High-impact aerobics is an intense activity, and it produces the highest rate of aerobics injuries due to the constant impact of the feet on firm surfaces. As a result, several alternative forms of aerobics have been developed.

In **low-impact aerobics** (LIA) the impact is less because one foot always remains in contact with the floor. The recommended exercise intensity is therefore more difficult to maintain than HIA. To help elevate the exercise heart rate, all arm movements and weight-bearing actions that lower the center of gravity should be accentuated. Sustained movement throughout the program is also crucial to keep the heart rate in the target cardiorespiratory zone.

Step aerobics (SA) is an activity in which participants step up and down from a bench that ranges in height from 2 to 10 inches. SA is viewed as a high-intensity but low-impact activity. The intensity is controlled easily by the height of the bench. Aerobic benches or plates, commercially available, can be stacked together safely to adjust the height of the steps. Beginners are encouraged to use the lowest step height and then advance gradually to a higher bench to decrease the risk of injury. Even though one foot is always in contact with the floor or bench during step aerobics, this activity is not recommended for individuals with ankle, knee, or hip problems.

Other forms of aerobics include a combination of HIA and LIA, as well as moderate-impact aerobics (MIA). The latter incorporates **plyometric training**, a type of training frequently used by jumpers (high, long, and triple jumpers) and athletes in sports that require quick jumping ability, such as basketball and gymnastics. With moderate-impact aerobics, one foot is in contact with the ground most of the time. Plyometric training participants, however, focus on quick, forceful recovery from all lower-body flexion actions. This is done by extending the hip, knee, and ankle joints quickly without allowing the foot (or feet) to leave the ground. These quick movements make the exercise intensity of moderate-impact aerobics quite high.

Swimming Swimming is another excellent form of aerobic exercise because it requires the use of almost all of the major muscle groups in the body, thereby providing a good training stimulus for the heart and lungs. Swimming is a great exercise option for individuals who cannot jog or walk for extended periods.

Compared with other activities, the risk of injuries from swimming is low. The aquatic medium helps to support the body, taking pressure off bones and joints in the lower extremities and the back.

Maximal heart rates during swimming are approximately 10 to 13 beats per minute (bpm) lower than during running. The horizontal position of the body is thought to aid blood flow distribution throughout the body, decreasing the demand on the cardiorespiratory system. Cool water temperatures and direct contact with the water seem to help dissipate body heat more efficiently, further decreasing the strain on the heart.

Some exercise specialists recommend that this difference in maximal heart rate (10 to 13 bpm) be subtracted prior to determining cardiorespiratory training intensities. For example, the estimated maximal swimming heart rate for a 20-year-old would be approximately 180 bpm [$207 - (.7 \times 20) - 13$]. Studies are inconclusive as to whether this decrease in heart rate in water also occurs at submaximal intensities less than 70 percent of maximal heart rate.

To produce better training benefits during swimming, the swimmer should minimize gliding periods such as those in the breaststroke and side stroke. Achieving proper training intensities with these strokes is difficult. The front crawl is recommended for better aerobic results.

Overweight individuals need to swim fast enough to achieve an adequate training intensity. Ex-

An 8-hour hike can burn as many calories as a 20-mile walk or jog.

> **Aerobics** A series of exercise routines performed to music.
>
> **High-impact aerobics** Exercises incorporating movements in which both feet are off the ground at the same time momentarily.
>
> **Low-impact aerobics** Exercises in which at least one foot is in contact with the ground or floor at all times.
>
> **Step aerobics** A form of exercise that combines stepping up and down from a bench with arm movements.
>
> **Plyometric training** A form of aerobic exercise that requires forceful jumps or springing off the ground immediately after landing from a previous jump.

cessive body fat makes the body more buoyant, and often the tendency is to just float along. This may be good for reducing stress and relaxing, but it does not greatly increase caloric expenditure to aid with weight loss. Walking or jogging in waist- or armpit-deep water are better choices for overweight individuals who cannot walk or jog on land for very long. If swimming is your main mode of exercise, however, pay particular attention not to overeat following exercise as cold-water swimming has been shown to stimulate appetite.

Swimming participants also need to remember the principle of specificity of training, which dictates that cardiorespiratory improvements cannot be measured adequately with a land-based walk/jog test. Most of the work with swimming is done by the upper body musculature. Although the heart's ability to pump more blood improves significantly with any type of aerobic activity, the primary increase in the cells' ability to utilize oxygen (VO_2 or oxygen uptake) with swimming occurs in the upper body and not the lower extremities. Therefore, fitness improvements with swimming are best measured through a swim test.

Water Aerobics Water aerobics is a form of exercise that is fun and safe for people of all ages. Besides developing fitness, it provides an opportunity for socialization and fun in a comfortable and refreshing setting.

Water aerobics incorporates a combination of rhythmic arm and leg actions performed in a vertical position while submerged in waist- to armpit-deep water. The vigorous limb movements against the water's resistance during water aerobics provide the training stimuli for cardiorespiratory development.

Water aerobics offers fitness, fun, and safety to people of all ages.

The popularity of water aerobics as an exercise modality is based on several factors:

1. Water buoyancy reduces weight-bearing stress on joints and thereby lessens the risk for injuries.
2. Water aerobics is a more feasible type of exercise for overweight individuals and those with arthritic conditions who may not be able to participate in land-based weight-bearing activities such as walking, jogging, and aerobics.
3. Water aerobics is an excellent exercise modality to improve functional fitness in older adults (see section titled "Exercise and Aging" later in this chapter).
4. Heat dissipation in water is beneficial to obese participants, who seem to undergo a higher heat strain than average-weight individuals.
5. Water aerobics is available to swimmers and nonswimmers alike.

The exercises used during water aerobics are designed to elevate the heart rate, which contributes to cardiorespiratory development. In addition, the aquatic medium provides increased resistance for strength improvement with virtually no impact. Because of this resistance to movement, strength gains with water aerobics seem to be better than with land-based aerobic activities.

Another benefit is the reduction of pain and fear of injuries common to many people who initiate exercise programs. Water aerobics provides a relatively safe environment for injury-free participation in exercise. The cushioned environment of the water allows patients recovering from leg and back injuries, individuals with joint problems, injured athletes, pregnant women, and obese people to benefit from water aerobics.

As observed with swimming, maximal heart rates achieved during water aerobics are lower than during running. The difference between water aerobics and running is about 10 bpm. Further, research comparing physiologic differences between self-paced treadmill running and self-paced water aerobics exercise showed that even though individuals worked at a lower heart rate in water (163 bpm versus 152 bpm—the equivalent of 85 and 79 percent of maximal heart rate on land, respectively), oxygen uptake level was the same for both exercise modalities (32.4 versus 32.5 mL/kg/min—both 69 percent of land VO_{2max}).[1] Healthy people, nonetheless, can sustain land-based exercise intensities during a water aerobics workout and experience similar fitness benefits than during land aerobics.[2]

Cycling Most people learn cycling in their youth. Because it is a nonweight-bearing activity, cycling is a good exercise modality for people with lower-body or lower-back injuries. Cycling helps to develop the cardiorespiratory system as well as muscular fitness (strength and endurance) in the lower extremities.

As a nonweight-bearing activity, raising the heart rate to the proper training intensity is more difficult with cycling. As the amount of muscle mass involved during aerobic exercise decreases, so does the demand placed on the cardiorespiratory system. The thigh muscles do most of the work in cycling, making it harder to achieve and maintain a high cardiorespiratory training intensity.

Maintaining a continuous pedaling motion and eliminating coasting periods help the participant achieve a faster heart rate. Exercising for longer periods also helps to compensate for the lower heart rate intensity during cycling. Comparing cycling with jogging, similar aerobic benefits take roughly three times the distance at twice the speed of jogging. Cycling, however, puts less stress on muscles and joints than jogging does, making the former a good exercise modality for people who cannot jog or walk for extended periods of time.

The height of the bike seat should be adjusted so that the knee is flexed at about 30 degrees when the foot is at the bottom of the pedaling cycle. The body should not sway from side to side as the person rides. The cycling cadence also is important for maximal efficiency. Bike tension or gears should be set at a moderate level so that the rider can achieve about 60 to 100 revolutions per minute.

Safety is a key issue in road cycling. More than a million bicycle injuries occur each year. Proper equipment and common sense are necessary. A well-designed and well-maintained bike is easier to maneuver. Toe clips are recommended to keep feet from sliding and to maintain equal upward and downward force on the pedals.

Skill is important in road cycling. Cyclists must be in control of the bicycle at all times. They have to be able to maneuver the bike in traffic, maintain balance at slow speeds, switch gears, apply the brakes, watch for pedestrians and stoplights, and ride through congested areas. Stationary cycling, in contrast, does not require special skills. Nearly everyone can do it.

Bike riders must follow the same rules as motorists. Many accidents happen because cyclists run traffic lights and stop signs. Some further suggestions are as follows:

- Select the right bike. Frame size is important. The size is determined by standing flat-footed while straddling the bike. On regular bikes, a one- to two-inch clearance should exist between the groin and the top tube of the frame. For mountain bikes, the clearance should be about three inches. The recommended height of the handlebars is about one inch below the top of the seat. Upright handlebars can also be used by individuals with neck or back problems. Hard/narrow seats on racing bikes tend to be especially uncomfortable for women. To avoid saddle soreness, use wider and more cushioned seats such as gel-filled saddles.
- Use bike hand signals to let the traffic around you know of your intended actions.
- Don't ride side by side with another rider.
- Be aware of turning vehicles and cars backing out of alleys and parking lots; always yield to motorists in these situations.
- Be on the lookout for storm drains, railroad tracks, and cattle guards, which can cause unpleasant surprises. Front wheels can get caught and riders may be thrown from the bike if not crossed at the proper angle (preferably 90 degrees).
- Wear a good helmet, certified by the Snell Memorial Foundation or the American Society for Testing Materials (ASTM). Serious accidents and even deaths have been prevented by use of helmets. Fashion, aesthetics, comfort, or price should not be a factor when selecting and using a helmet for road cycling. Health and life are too precious to give up because of vanity and thriftiness.
- Wear appropriate clothes and shoes. Clothing should be bright, very visible, lightweight, and not restrict movement. Cycling shorts are recommended to prevent skin irritation. For greater comfort, the shorts have extra padding sewn into the seat and crotch areas. They do not tend to wrinkle and they wick away perspiration from the skin. Shorts should be long enough to keep the skin from rubbing against the seat. Experienced cyclists also wear special shoes with a cleat that snaps directly onto the pedal. Take extra warm clothing in a backpack during the winter months in case you have a breakdown and have to walk a long distance for assistance.
- Watch out for ice when it's cold outside. If there is ice on car windows, there will be ice on the road. Be especially careful on bridges as they tend to have ice even when the roads are dry.
- Use the brightest bicycle lights you can when riding in the dark and always keep the batteries well charged. For additional safety, wear reflectors on the upper torso, arms, and legs. Moving bright objects are easier to see by passing motorists. And stay on streets that have good lighting and plenty of room on the side of the road, even if that means riding an extra few minutes to get to your destination.
- Take a cell phone if you have one, and let someone else know where you are going and when to expect you back.

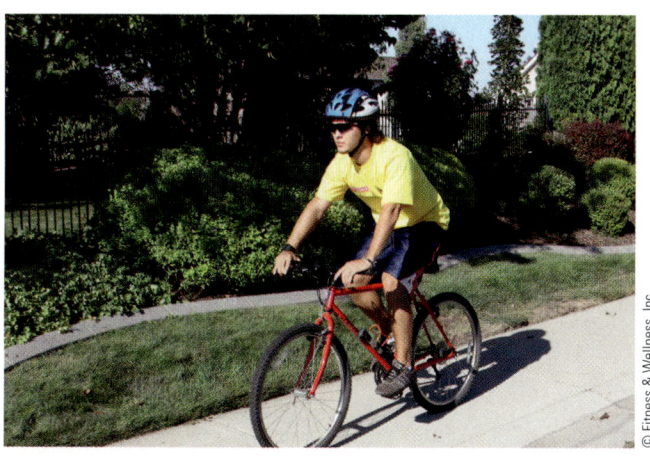

Skill is required for safety and enjoyment of road cycling.

If you decide to try stationary cycling, before buying a stationary bike, be sure to try the activity for a few days. If you enjoy it, you may want to purchase one. Invest with caution. If you opt to buy a lower-priced model, you may be disappointed. Good stationary bikes have comfortable seats, are stable, and provide a smooth and uniform pedaling motion. A sticky bike that is hard to pedal leads to discouragement and ends up stored in the corner of a basement.

Cross-Training Cross-training combines two or more activities in an exercise program. This type of training is designed to enhance fitness, provide needed rest to tired muscles, decrease injuries, and eliminate the monotony and burnout of single-activity programs. Cross-training may combine aerobic and nonaerobic activities such as moderate jogging, speed training, and strength training.

Cross-training can produce better workouts than a single activity. For example, jogging develops the lower body and swimming builds the upper body. Rowing contributes to upper-body development and cycling builds the legs. Combining activities such as these provides good overall conditioning and at the same time helps to improve or maintain fitness. Cross-training also offers an opportunity to develop new skills and have fun with different activities.

Speed training is often coupled with cross-training. Faster performance times in aerobic activities (running, cycling) are generated with speed or **interval training**. People who want to improve their running times often run shorter intervals at faster speeds than the actual racing pace. For example, a person wanting to run a 6-minute mile may run four 440-yard intervals at a speed of 1 minute and 20 seconds per interval. A 440-yard walk/jog can become a recovery interval between fast runs.

Strength training is also used commonly with cross-training. It helps to condition muscles, tendons, and ligaments. Improved strength enhances overall performance in many activities and sports. For example, although road cyclists in one study who trained with weights showed no improvement in aerobic capacity, the cyclists had a 33-percent improvement in riding time to exhaustion when exercising at 75 percent of their maximal capacity.[3]

Cross-Country Skiing Many consider cross-country skiing to be the ultimate aerobic exercise because it requires vigorous lower and upper body movements. The large amount of muscle mass involved in cross-country skiing makes the intensity of the activity high, yet it places little strain on muscles and joints. One of the highest maximal oxygen uptakes ever measured (85 mL/kg/min) was found in an elite cross-country skier.

In addition to being an excellent aerobic activity, cross-country skiing is soothing. Skiing through the beauty of the snow-covered countryside can be highly enjoyable. Although the need for snow is an obvious limitation, simulation equipment for year-round cross-country training is available at many sporting goods stores.

Some skill is necessary to be proficient at cross-country skiing. Poorly skilled individuals are not able to elevate their heart rate enough to cause adequate aerobic development. Individuals contemplating this activity should seek out instruction to fully enjoy and reap the rewards of cross-country skiing.

Rowing Rowing is a low-impact activity that provides a complete body workout. It mobilizes most major muscle groups, including those in the arms, legs, hips, abdomen, trunk, and shoulders. Rowing is a good form of aerobic exercise and, because of the nature of the activity (constant pushing and pulling against resistance), also promotes total strength development.

To accommodate different fitness levels, workloads can be regulated on most rowing machines. Stationary rowing, however, is not among the most popular forms of aerobic exercise. Similar to stationary bicycles, people should try the activity for a few weeks before purchasing a unit.

Elliptical Training/Stair Climbing If sustained for at least 20 minutes, elliptical training and stair climbing are very efficient forms of aerobic exercise. Precisely because of the high intensity of stair climbing, many people stay away from stairs and instead take escalators and elevators. Many

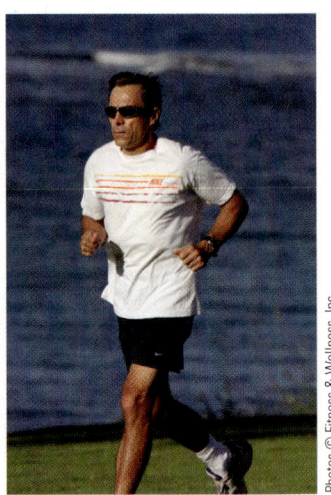

Cross-training enhances fitness, decreases the rate of injuries, and eliminates the monotony of single-activity programs.

people dislike living in two-story homes because they have to climb the stairs frequently.

Elliptical training and stair climbing are relatively safe exercise modalities. Because the feet never leave the climbing surface, they are considered low-impact activities. Joints and ligaments are not strained during climbing. The intensity of exercise is controlled easily, because the equipment can be programmed to regulate the workload.

Racquet Sports In racquet sports such as tennis, racquetball, squash, and badminton, the aerobic benefits are dictated by players' skill, intensity of the game, and how long a given game lasts. Skill is necessary to participate effectively in these sports and also is crucial to sustain continuous play. Frequent pauses during play do not allow people to maintain the heart rate in the appropriate target zone to stimulate cardiorespiratory development.

Many people who participate in racquet sports do so for enjoyment, social fulfillment, and relaxation. For cardiorespiratory fitness development, these people supplement the sport with other forms of aerobic exercise such as jogging, cycling, or swimming.

If a racquet sport is the main form of aerobic exercise, participants need to try to run hard, fast, and as constantly as possible during play. They should not have to spend much time retrieving balls (or, in badminton, the bird or shuttlecock). Similar to low-impact aerobics, all movements should be accentuated by reaching out and bending more than usual, for better cardiorespiratory development.

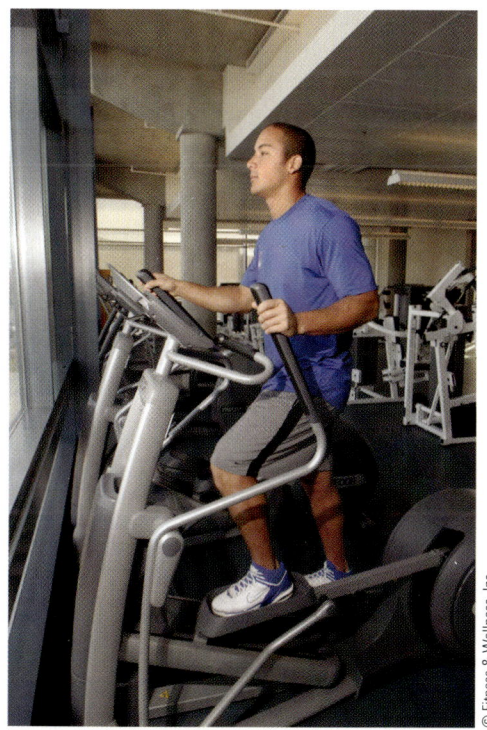

Elliptical training provides a rigorous low-impact aerobic workout.

Yoga Yoga consists of a system of exercises designed to help align the musculoskeletal system and develop flexibility, muscular fitness, and balance. Yoga is also used as a relaxation technique for stress management. The exercises involve a combination of postures (known as "asanas") along with diaphragmatic breathing, relaxation, and mediation techniques. Different forms of yoga exist, including Anuara, Ashtanga, Bikram, Integral, Iyengar, Kripalu, Kundalini, and Sivananda, Viny, Yogalates, and Yogarobics yoga.

> **Critical Thinking**
>
> Sports participation is a good predictor of adherence to exercise later in life. • What previous experiences have you had with participation in sports? • Were these experiences positive? • What effect do they have on your current physical activity patterns?

9.2 New Fitness Trends

Life in the 21st century requires that we participate in physical activities that promote and maintain fitness, health, and wellness. As people search for proven programs, fitness trends emerge to achieve these goals. Some of the activity trends have been with us and continue to evolve to gain popularity among participants, whereas others have been recently developed and gained approval among fitness enthusiasts. According to the American College of Sports Medicine's Worldwide Survey of Fitness Trends in 2013, among the newest fitness activities the following trends have emerged:

High-Intensity Interval Training (HIIT) HIIT is a challenging training program, mostly aerobic, that involves high- to very high-intensity (80 to 90 percent of maximal capacity) intervals, each followed by a low- to moderate-intensity recovery interval. Usually a 1:3 or less work-to-recovery ratio is used. HIIT provides greater health and fitness benefits than traditional lower-intensity programs. Fitness enthusiasts like HIIT because higher fitness and weight loss goals are reached with this type of training (as long as caloric intake is carefully monitored and not increased following training).

Stability Exercise Balls Stability exercise balls enhance stability, balance, and muscular strength. The emphasis is on correct movements and maintenance of proper body alignment while involving the core as much as possible. Additional exercises can be performed to strengthen other body areas. Fur-

> **Cross-training** A combination of aerobic activities that contribute to overall fitness.
>
> **Interval training** A system of exercise wherein a short period of intense effort is followed by a specified recovery period according to a prescribed ratio; for instance, a 1:3 work-to-recovery ratio.

ther information on Stability Exercise Balls and sample exercises are provided in Chapter 7, pages 276–278).

Core Training The "core" of the body consists of the muscles that stabilize the trunk (spine) and pelvis. Core training emphasizes conditioning of all the muscles around the abdomen, pelvis, lower back, and hips. These muscles enhance body stability, activities of daily living, sport performance, and support the lower back. Core conditioning often incorporates the use of stability balls, foam rollers, and wobble boards, among other pieces of equipment. Further information on Core Strength Training is provided in Chapter 7 (page 253).

Fitness Boot Camp A new vigorous-intensity outdoor/indoor group exercise program that combines traditional calisthenics, running, interval training, bodyweight training (using exercises such as push-ups, lunges, pull-ups, burpees, squats), plyometrics (see Chapter 7, page 251) and competitive games to develop cardiorespiratory fitness, muscular fitness, muscular flexibility, and lose body fat. This program is based on military style–training and also aims at developing camaraderie and team effort. The program (camp) typically lasts 4 to 8 weeks. Fitness boot camps are challenging, but the group dynamic helps to motivate participants.

Bodyweight Training Bodyweight training has been around as a strength-training modality for centuries, but fitness enthusiasts are now embracing the concept as they seek to "return to basics." Bodyweight training participants' use their own body weight as resistance to develop fitness. Bodyweight exercises are ideal for individuals interested in fitness but do not have access to equipment or facilities. Because body weight provides the only source of resistance, a training session can be conducted anywhere. Exercise examples include pull-ups, push-ups, modified dips, curl-ups, step-ups, prone and lateral planks, and pelvic tilts. Some of these exercises are provided in the Strength-Training Exercises without Weights (Bodyweight Training) section on pages 262-266. As discussed next under "*Circuit training*," bodyweight training can be used to develop both cardiorespiratory endurance and muscular fitness.

Circuit Training Circuit training has also been around for decades. It was often used to condition elite athletes and military personnel in the middle of the 20th century. Circuit training involves a combination of 6 to 12 aerobic and bodyweight-training (strength) exercises performed in rapid sequence one after the other, with very limited rest between exercise stations. Each exercise is performed for a given period of time (10–30 seconds) or by a specified number of repetitions (10–20 repetitions), typically interspaced by short rest periods of 10 to 30 seconds between exercises. Early on, you may use a moderate intensity (less time or repetitions per exercise) and allow longer rest (30 seconds) between exercises. Over the course of several weeks, you can gradually increase the intensity (time and/or repetitions) and decrease the rest interval between exercises. The exercise-sequence is set in an order that allows for opposing muscle groups to alternate between exercise stations. For instance, push-ups can be followed by step-ups, and abdominal crunches. For best results, all major muscle groups of the body should be used in each circuit.

Because of the high intensity and limited rest intervals used with this type of training, the exercise modality is often referred to as high-intensity circuit training, or HICT.[4] The combination of high-intensity aerobic and bodyweight-strength training, with limited rest between exercises, can elicit similar of greater health and fitness benefits in a much shorter period of time than the traditional 20- to 60-minute sessions. A HICT session involving 12 different exercises can be performed in less than 10 minutes per circuit. One to three

When properly designed and implemented, a person's own body weight can be used to derive both cardiorespiratory endurance and muscular fitness benefits.

circuits with two to three minutes rest between circuits can be performed per training session. When time is of the essence and a traditional training session is not realistic, a HICT session is recommended.

Functional Fitness Functional fitness involves primarily weight-bearing exercises to develop balance, coordination, good posture, muscular fitness, and muscular flexibility to enhance the person's ability to perform activities of daily living (walking, climbing stairs, lifting, bending) with ease and with minimal risk for injuries. The program goal is to "train people for real life," rather than a specific fitness component or a given event. Functional fitness training often requires use of fitness equipment such as stability balls, foam blocks, and balancing cushions.

Zumba Zumba is a dance fitness program that was created in Colombia by Alberto "Beto" Perez in the mid 1990s. Following great popularity in Colombia, the Zumba program was brought to the United States in 1999. The program is now offered globally and classes are offered at most health fitness clubs in the United States. Zumba combines Latin and international music (cumbia, salsa, merengue, reggaeton, tango, and rock and roll among others) with dance to develop fitness and make exercise fun. The Zumba motto has become "Ditch the workout, join the party!" Several types of Zumba have been developed, including traditional Zumba, Zumba Gold, Zumba Toning, Aqua Zumba, Zumbatomic, and Zumba Marumba.

9.3 Specific Exercise Considerations

In addition to the exercise-related issues already discussed in this book, many other concerns require clarification or are somewhat controversial. Let's examine some of these issues.

1. Do people get a "physical high" during aerobic exercise?

   During vigorous exercise, **endorphins** are released from the pituitary gland in the brain. Endorphins can create feelings of euphoria and natural well-being. Higher levels of endorphins often result from aerobic endurance activities and may remain elevated for as long as 30 to 60 minutes after exercise. Many experts believe that these higher levels explain the physical high that some people get during and after prolonged exercise.

   Endorphin levels also have been shown to increase during pregnancy and childbirth. Endorphins act as painkillers. The higher levels could explain a woman's greater tolerance for the pain and discomfort of natural childbirth and her pleasant feelings shortly after the baby's birth. Several reports have indicated that well-conditioned women have shorter and easier labor. These women may attain higher endorphin levels during delivery, making childbirth less traumatic than it is for untrained women.

2. Can people with asthma exercise?

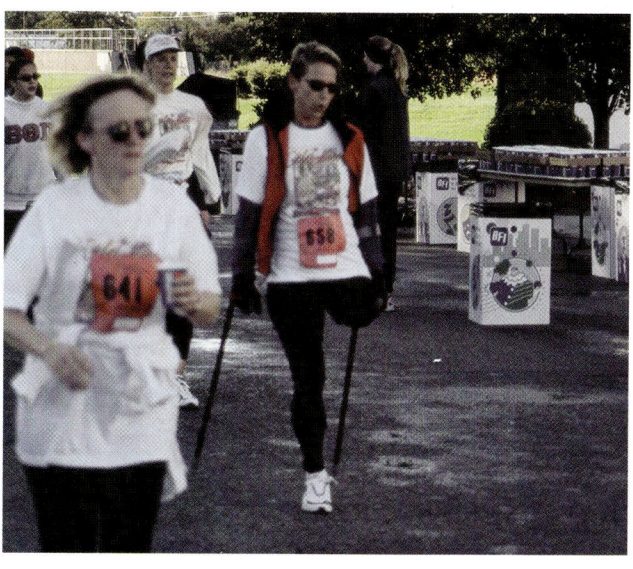

Physically challenged people can participate in and derive health and fitness benefits from a high-intensity exercise program.

   Asthma, a condition that causes difficult breathing, is characterized by coughing, wheezing, and shortness of breath induced by narrowing of the airway passages because of contraction (bronchospasm) of the airway muscles, swelling of the mucous membrane, and excessive secretion of mucus. In a few people, asthma can be triggered by exercise itself, particularly in cool and dry environments. This condition is referred to as exercise-induced asthma (EIA).

   People with asthma need to obtain proper medication from a physician prior to initiating an exercise program. A regular program is best, because random exercise bouts are more likely to trigger asthma attacks. In the initial stages of exercise, an intermittent program (with frequent rest periods during the exercise session) is recommended. Gradual warm-up and cool-down are essential to reduce the risk of an acute attack. Furthermore, exercising in warm and humid conditions (such as swimming) is better because it helps to moisten the airways and thereby minimizes the asthmatic response. For land-based activities (such as walking and aerobics), drinking water before, during, and after exercise helps to keep the airways moist, decreasing the risk of an attack. During the winter months, wearing an exercise mask is recommended to increase the warmth and humidity of inhaled air. People with asthma should not exercise alone and should always carry their medication with them during workouts.

3. What types of activities are recommended for people with arthritis?

> **Endorphins** Morphine-like substances released from the pituitary gland (in the brain) during prolonged aerobic exercise; thought to induce feelings of euphoria and natural well-being.

Individuals who have arthritis should participate in a combined stretching, aerobic, and strength-training program. The participant should do mild stretching prior to aerobic exercise to relax tight muscles. A regular flexibility program following aerobic exercise is encouraged to help maintain good joint mobility. During the aerobic portion of the exercise program, individuals with arthritis should avoid high-impact activities because these may cause greater trauma to arthritic joints. Low-impact activities such as swimming, water aerobics, and cycling are recommended. A complete strength-training program also is recommended, with special emphasis on exercises that will support the arthritic joint(s). As with any other program, individuals with arthritis should start with light-intensity or resistance exercises and build up gradually to a higher fitness level.

4. What precautions should people with diabetes take with respect to exercise?

There are approximately 27 million people with diabetes in the United States, with more than 1 million new cases being diagnosed each year. Estimates also indicate that 60 million Americans have prediabetes. At the current rate, one in three children born in the United States will develop the disease. Type 2 diabetes has been linked to premature mortality and morbidity from cardiovascular disease and to kidney and nerve disease, blindness, and amputation.

There are two types of diabetes: type 1, or insulin-dependent diabetes mellitus (IDDM); and type 2, or noninsulin-dependent diabetes mellitus (NIDDM). In type 1, an autoimmune-related disease found primarily in young people, the pancreas produces little or no insulin. Like everyone else, people with type 1 diabetes benefit from physical activity, but it does not prevent or cure the disease.

Physical activity helps in the prevention and treatment of type 2 diabetes. With type 2, the pancreas may not produce enough insulin or the cells may become insulin resistant, thereby keeping glucose from entering the cell. Type 2 accounts for more than 90 percent of all cases of diabetes, and it occurs mainly in overweight people. (A more thorough discussion of the types of diabetes is given in Chapter 10, pages 259–260.)

If you have diabetes, consult your physician before you start exercising. You may not be able to begin until the diabetes is under control. Never exercise alone, and always wear a bracelet that identifies your condition. If you take insulin, the amount and timing of each dose may have to be regulated with your physician. If you inject insulin, do so over a muscle that won't be exercised, then wait an hour before exercising.

Both types of diabetes improve with exercise, although the results are more notable in patients with type 2 diabetes. Exercise usually lowers blood sugar and helps the body use food more effectively. The extent to which the blood glucose level can be controlled in overweight people with NIDDM seems to be related directly to how long and how hard a person exercises. Normal or near-normal blood glucose levels can be achieved through a proper exercise program.

As with any fitness program, the exercise must be done regularly to be effective against diabetes. The benefits of a single exercise bout on blood glucose are highest between 12 and 24 hours following exercise. These benefits are completely lost within 72 hours after exercise. Thus, regular participation is crucial to derive ongoing benefits. In terms of fitness, all diabetic patients can achieve higher fitness levels, including reductions in weight, blood pressure, and total cholesterol and triglycerides.

The biggest concern for people with diabetes is exercise-induced hypoglycemia during, following, or even a day after the exercise session. Common symptoms of hypoglycemia include weakness, confusion, shakiness, anxiousness, tiredness, hunger, increased perspiration, headaches, and even loss of consciousness. Physical activity increases insulin sensitivity and muscle glucose uptake, thus lowering blood glucose, an effect that may last several hours after exercise. With enhanced insulin sensitivity, a unit of insulin lowers blood glucose to a much greater extent during and following exercise than under nonexercise conditions. Typically, the longer and more intense the exercise bout, the greater the effect on insulin sensitivity.

Both aerobic exercise and strength training are recommended for individuals with type 2 diabetes. According to the American College of Sports Medicine and the American Diabetes Association,[5] patients with type 2 diabetes should adhere to the following guidelines to make their exercise program safe and derive the most benefit:

Aerobic Exercise

- Intensity. Exercise at a moderate intensity (40 to 60 percent VO_{2max}). Additional benefits, however, are gained through a vigorous-intensity program. The research indicates better blood glucose control by increasing intensity rather that exercise volume. Start your program with 10 to 15 minutes per session, on at least 3 nonconsecutive days, but preferably exercise 5 days per week.
- Duration. Aerobic activity duration should be no less than 150 minutes per week or the equivalent of 30 minutes per day at least 5 days per week. As a minimum, each aerobic exercise bout should be at least 10 minutes long and spread throughout the week. Diabetic individuals with a weight problem should build up daily physical activity to 60 minutes per session.
- Mode. Any type of aerobic activity or preferably a combination of aerobic activities that involves large muscle groups and increases oxygen uptake (VO_2) is recommended. Choose activities that you enjoy doing, and stay with them. As you select your activities, be aware of your

condition. For example, if you have lost sensation in your feet, swimming or stationary cycling is better than walking or jogging to minimize the risk for injury.
- Frequency. Exercise aerobically at least three times per week and do not allow more than two consecutive days between exercise sessions. Five days per week are strongly encouraged.
- Rate of progression. A gradual increase in exercise to at least 150 weekly minutes in both intensity and volume (duration and frequency) is strongly encouraged. Progression up to 7 hours per week (420 minutes) has been reported by individuals who have successfully been able to maintain a substantial amount of weight loss.

Strength Training

- Resistance (intensity). For optimal insulin action, resistance training should be conducted between 50 and 80 percent of the maximal capacity (1 RM) for each exercise, either on free weights or resistance machines.
- Sets. A minimum of one set performed to near fatigue of 5 to 10 exercises involving the body's major muscle groups (upper body, core, and lower body). Initially, each set should consist of 10 to 15 repetitions maximum (RM).
- Frequency. A minimum of twice per week, but preferably three times per week on nonconsecutive days.
- Rate of Progression. Progression of intensity, sets, and frequency (in that order) are recommended. Type 2 diabetics are encouraged to gradually increase the resistance and aim to work with 8 to 10 RM. Next, sets can progressively be increased up to four sets per exercise. Finally, frequency may be increased from twice weekly to three times per week.

Additional Exercise Guidelines

- Check your blood glucose levels before and after exercise. Do not exercise if your blood glucose is greater than 300 mg/dL or fasting blood glucose is greater than 250 mg/dL and you have ketones in your urine. If your blood glucose is less than 100 mg/dL, eat a small carbohydrate snack before exercise.
- If you are on insulin or diabetes medication, monitor your blood glucose regularly and check it at least twice within 30 minutes of starting exercise.
- Schedule your exercise one to three hours after a meal, and avoid exercise when your insulin is peaking. If you are going to exercise one to two hours following a meal, you may have to reduce your insulin or blood glucose-reducing medication.
- To prevent hypoglycemia, consume between .15 and .20 gram of carbohydrates per pound of body weight for each hour of moderate-intensity activity. This amount, however, should be adjusted based on your blood glucose monitoring. Up to .25 gram of carbohydrates per pound of body weight may be required for vigorous exercise. Your goal should be to regulate carbohydrate intake and medication dosage so as to maintain blood glucose level between 100 and 200 mg/dL. With physical activity and exercise, you will probably need to reduce your insulin or oral medication, increase carbohydrate consumption, or both.
- Be ready to treat low blood sugar with a fast-acting source of sugar, such as juice, raisins, or other source recommended by your doctor.
- If you feel that a reaction is about to occur, discontinue exercise immediately. Check your blood glucose level and treat the condition as needed.
- When you exercise outdoors, always do so with someone who knows what to do in a diabetes-related emergency.
- Stay well hydrated. Dehydration can have a negative effect on blood glucose, heart function, and performance. Consume adequate amounts of fluids before and after exercise. Drink about 8 ounces of water before you start each exercise session. If you are going to exercise for longer than an hour, drink 8 ounces (one cup) of a 6 to 8 percent carbohydrate sports drink every 15 to 20 minutes.

People with type 1 diabetes should ingest 15 to 30 grams of carbohydrates during each 30 minutes of intense exercise and follow it with a carbohydrate snack after exercise.

In addition, strength training twice per week using 8 to 10 exercises with a minimum of one set of 10 to 15 repetitions to near fatigue is recommended for individuals with diabetes. A complete description of strength-training programs is provided in Chapter 7.

1. Is exercise safe during pregnancy?

    Exercise is beneficial during pregnancy. According to the American College of Obstetricians and Gynecologists (ACOG), in the absence of contraindications, healthy pregnant women are encouraged to participate in regular, moderate-intensity physical activities to continue to derive health benefits during pregnancy.[6] Pregnant women, however, should consult their physicians to ensure that they have no contraindications to exercise during pregnancy. Overall, women who are physically active either before or during pregnancy are better able to maintain weight gain within the recommended range, and as compared to inactive women, they do not deliver large babies. They also have a lower risk for pregnancy-associated diabetes and high blood pressure.

    As a general rule, healthy pregnant women can also accumulate 30 minutes of moderate-intensity physical activity on most, if not all, days of the week (a minimum of 150 minutes per week). Physical activity strengthens the body and helps prepare for the challenges of labor and childbirth.

    The average labor and delivery lasts 10 to 12 hours. In most cases, labor and delivery are highly intense, with repeated muscular contractions interspersed with short rest periods. Proper conditioning will better pre-

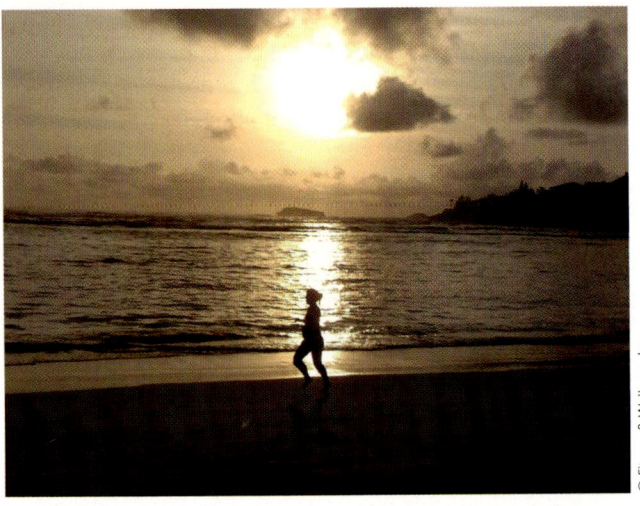

Light- to moderate-intensity exercise is recommended throughout pregnancy.

pare the body for childbirth. Moderate exercise during pregnancy also helps to prevent back pain and excessive weight gain, and it speeds recovery following childbirth.

The most common recommendations for exercise during pregnancy for healthy pregnant women with no additional risk factors are as follows:

- Don't start a new or more rigorous exercise program without proper medical clearance.
- Accumulate 30 minutes of moderate-intensity physical activities on most days of the week.
- Instead of using heart rate to monitor intensity, exercise at an intensity level between "low" and "somewhat hard," using the physical activity perceived exertion (H-PAPE) scale in Chapter 6, Figure 6.9 (see page 219).
- Gradually switch from weight-bearing and high-impact activities, such as jogging and aerobics, to nonweight-bearing/lower-impact activities, such as walking, stationary cycling, swimming, and water aerobics. The latter activities minimize the risk of injury and may allow exercise to continue throughout pregnancy.
- Avoid exercising at an altitude above 6,000 feet (1,800 meters), as well as scuba diving, because either may compromise the availability of oxygen to the fetus.
- Women who are accustomed to strenuous exercise may continue in the early stages of pregnancy but should gradually decrease the amount, intensity, and exercise mode as pregnancy advances. (Most healthy pregnant women, however, slow down during the first few weeks of pregnancy until morning sickness and fatigue subside.)
- Pay attention to the body's signals of discomfort and distress, and never exercise to exhaustion. When fatigued, slow down or take a day off. Do not stop exercising altogether unless you experience any of the contraindications for exercise listed.
- To prevent fetal injury, avoid activities that involve potential contact or loss of balance or that cause even mild trauma to the abdomen. Examples of these activities are basketball, soccer, volleyball, Nordic or water skiing, ice skating, road cycling, horseback riding, and motorcycle riding.
- During pregnancy, don't exercise for weight loss purposes.
- Get proper nourishment (pregnancy requires between 150 and 300 extra calories per day), and eat a small snack or drink some juice 20 to 30 minutes prior to exercise.
- Prevent dehydration by drinking a cup of fluid 20 to 30 minutes before exercise, and drink 1 cup of liquid every 15 to 20 minutes during exercise.
- During the first 3 months in particular, don't exercise in the heat. Wear clothing that allows for proper dissipation of heat. A body temperature above 102.6°F (39.2°C) can harm the fetus.
- After the first trimester, avoid exercises that require lying on the back. This position can block blood flow to the uterus and the baby.
- Perform stretching exercises gently because hormonal changes during pregnancy increase the laxity of muscles and connective tissue. Although these changes facilitate delivery, they also make women more susceptible to injuries during exercise.

2. Does exercise help relieve dysmenorrhea?

Although exercise has not been shown to either cure or aggravate **dysmenorrhea**, it has been shown to relieve menstrual cramps because it improves circulation to the uterus. Less severe menstrual cramps also could be caused by higher levels of endorphins produced during prolonged physical activity, which may

Contraindications to Exercise during Pregnancy

Stop exercise and seek medical advice if you experience any of the following symptoms:

- Unusual pain or discomfort, especially in the chest or abdominal area
- Cramping, primarily in the pelvic or lower back areas
- Muscle weakness, excessive fatigue, or shortness of breath
- Abnormally high heart rate or a pounding (palpitations) heart rate
- Decreased fetal movement
- Insufficient weight gain
- Amniotic fluid leakage
- Nausea, dizziness, or headaches
- Persistent uterine contractions
- Vaginal bleeding or rupture of the membranes
- Swelling of ankles, calves, hands, or face

counteract pain. Particularly, stretching exercises of the muscles in the pelvic region seem to reduce and prevent painful menstruation that is not the result of disease.[7]

3. Does participation in exercise hinder menstruation?

Although, on the average, women have a lower physical capacity during menstruation, medical surveys at the Olympic Games have shown that women have broken Olympic and world records at all stages of the menstrual cycle. Menstruation should not keep a woman from exercising, and it will not necessarily have a negative impact on performance.

In some instances, highly trained athletes develop **amenorrhea** during training and competition. This condition is seen most often in extremely lean women who also engage in sports that require strenuous physical effort over a sustained period of time. It is by no means irreversible. At present, we do not know whether the condition is caused by physical or emotional stress related to high-intensity training, excessively low body fat, an energy deficit (low caloric intake) over long periods of time, or other factors.

4. Does exercise offset the detrimental effects of cigarette smoking?

Physical exercise often motivates a person to stop smoking, but it does not offset any ill effects of smoking. Smoking greatly decreases the ability of the blood to transport oxygen to working muscles.

Oxygen is carried in the circulatory system by hemoglobin, the iron-containing pigment of the red blood cells. Carbon monoxide, a by-product of cigarette smoke, has 210 to 250 times greater affinity for hemoglobin over oxygen. Consequently, carbon monoxide combines much faster with hemoglobin, decreasing the oxygen-carrying capacity of the blood.

Chronic smoking also increases airway resistance, requiring the respiratory muscles to work much harder and consume more oxygen just to ventilate a given amount of air. If a person quits smoking, exercise does help increase the functional capacity of the pulmonary system.

A regular exercise program seems to be a powerful incentive to quit smoking. A random survey of 1,250 runners conducted at the 6.2-mile Peachtree Road Race in Atlanta provided impressive results. The survey indicated that of the men and women who smoked cigarettes when they started running, 81 percent and 75 percent, respectively, had quit before the date of the race.

5. How long should a person wait after a meal before exercising strenuously?

The length of time to wait before exercising after a meal depends on the amount of food eaten. On the average, after a regular meal, you should wait about two hours before participating in strenuous physical activity. But a walk or some other light physical activity is fine following a meal, as it helps burn extra calories and may help the body metabolize fats more efficiently.

6. What type of clothing should I wear when I exercise?

The type of clothing worn during exercise is important. In general, clothing should fit comfortably and allow free movement of the various body parts. Select clothing according to air temperature, humidity, and exercise intensity. Avoid nylon and rubberized materials and tight clothes that interfere with the cooling mechanism of the human body or obstruct normal blood flow. Choose fabrics made of polypropylene, Capilene, Thermax, or any synthetic that draws (wicks) moisture away from the skin, enhancing evaporation and cooling of the body. It's also important to consider exercise intensity, because the harder a person exercises, the more heat the body produces.

When exercising in the heat, avoid the hottest time of the day, between 11:00 a.m. and 5:00 p.m. Surfaces such as asphalt, concrete, and artificial turf absorb heat, which then radiates to the body. Therefore, these surfaces are not recommended. (Also see the discussion about heat and humidity in the section "Why Is Exercising in Hot and Humid Conditions Unsafe?")

Only a minimal amount of clothing is necessary during exercise in the heat, to allow for maximal evaporation. Clothing should be lightweight, light-colored, loose-fitting, airy, and absorbent. Examples of commercially available products that can be used during exercise in the heat are CoolMax and Nike's Dri-FIT. Double-layer acrylic socks are more absorbent than cotton and help prevent blistering and chafing of the feet. A straw-type hat can be worn to protect the eyes and head from the sun. (Clothing for exercise in the cold is discussed in the "What Precautions Must a Person Take When Exercising in the Cold?" section, page 321.)

For decades, a good pair of shoes has been recommended by most professionals to prevent injuries to lower limbs. Shoes manufactured specifically for the choice of activity have been encouraged. Shoes should have good stability, motion control, and comfortable fit. Purchase shoes in the middle of or later in the day when feet have expanded and might be one half size larger. For increased breathability, shoes with nylon or mesh uppers are recommended. Salespeople at reputable athletic shoe stores can help you select a good shoe that fits your needs.

More recently, a trend has emerged toward barefoot running. For most of human history, people ran either barefoot or with minimal shoes. As in walking, the modern running shoe with its bulky padded heel cushion allows runners to land on the heel and roll forward toward the ball of the foot. The impact-collision force while running is often more than three times the person's bodyweight. Researchers have observed that joggers and runners who

---

Dysmenorrhea Painful menstruation.
Amenorrhea Cessation of regular menstrual flow.

don't wear shoes, or who use minimal footwear, land on the front (ball) or middle of the foot. This motion induces them to flex the ankle as contact is made with the ground, resulting in smaller impact forces than ankle-strike runners. Such running mechanics are thought to decrease impact-related repetitive stress injuries.

Some experts believe that both the spring in the arch of the foot and the Achilles tendon diminish ground-impact forces. A good illustration is to compare the impact forces generated by landing a jump on the heels versus on the toes.

Shoeless-running proponents believe that wearing cushioned shoes with arch supports alters natural foot-landing actions, weakening muscles and ligaments and rendering feet, ankles, and knees more susceptible to injuries. They recommend wearing a flexible shoe without a heel cushion or arch support. This recommendation has led to the development of barefoot running "shoes." These shoes feature a thin, abrasion-resistant stretch nylon with breathable mesh upper material that wraps around the entire foot to keep rocks and dirt out. At present, the verdict is still out. Data are insufficient to support either recommendation (shoe versus shoeless running). Research is being conducted to determine the best type of footwear to use with repetitive-impact activities. If you decide to give shoeless running a try, be sure to make a gradual transition into the minimal footwear; otherwise, you may end up with a challenging or severe injury (including foot fractures).

7. What time of the day is best for exercise?

You can do intense exercise almost any time of the day, with the exception of about two hours following a heavy meal or the midday and early afternoon hours on hot, humid days. Moderate exercise seems to be beneficial shortly after a meal because exercise enhances the **thermogenic response**. A walk shortly after a meal burns more calories than a walk several hours after a meal.

Many people enjoy exercising early in the morning because it gives them a boost to start the day. People who exercise in the morning also seem to stick with it more than others, because the chances of putting off the exercise session for other reasons are minimized. Some prefer the lunch hour for weight-control reasons. By exercising at noon, they do not eat as big a lunch, which helps keep down the daily caloric intake. Highly stressed people seem to like the evening hours because of the relaxing effects of exercise.

8. Why is exercising in hot and humid conditions unsafe?

When a person exercises, only 20 to 30 percent of the energy the body produces is used for mechanical work or movement. The rest of the energy (60 to 70 percent) is converted into heat. If this heat cannot be dissipated properly because the weather is too hot or the relative humidity is too high, body temperature increases, and in extreme cases, it can result in death.

The specific heat of body tissue (the heat required to raise the temperature of the body by 1°C) is .38 calorie per pound of body weight (.38 cal/lb). This indicates that if no body heat is dissipated, a 150-pound person has to burn only 57 calories (150 × .38) to increase total body temperature by 1°C. If this person were to conduct an exercise session requiring 300 calories (e.g., running about 3 miles) without any dissipation of heat, the inner body temperature would increase by 5.3°C (300 ÷ 57), which is the equivalent of going from 98.6°F to 108.1°F.

This example illustrates clearly the need for caution when exercising in hot or humid weather. If the relative humidity is too high, body heat cannot be lost through evaporation because the atmosphere already is saturated with water vapor. In one instance, a football casualty occurred when the temperature was only 64°F, but the relative humidity was 100 percent. People must be cautious when air temperature is greater than 90°F and the relative humidity is greater than 60 percent.

The ACSM recommends avoiding strenuous physical activity when the readings of a wet-bulb globe thermometer exceed 82.4°F. With this type of thermometer, the wet bulb is cooled by evaporation, and on dry days it shows a lower temperature than the regular (dry) thermometer. On humid days, the cooling effect is less because of less evaporation; hence, the difference between the wet and dry readings is not as great.

Following are descriptions of, and first-aid measures for, the three major signs of heat illness:

- **Heat cramps.** Symptoms include cramps; spasms; and muscle twitching in the legs, arms, and abdomen. To relieve heat cramps, stop exercising, get out of the heat, massage the painful area, stretch slowly, and drink plenty of fluids (water, fruit drinks, or electrolyte beverages).
- **Heat exhaustion.** Symptoms include fainting, dizziness, profuse sweating, cold and clammy skin, weakness, headache, and a rapid, weak pulse. If you incur any of these symptoms, stop and find a cool place to rest. If conscious, drink cool water. Do not give water to an unconscious person. Loosen or remove clothing and rub your body with a cool, wet towel or apply ice packs. Place yourself in a supine position with the legs elevated 8 to 12 inches. If you are not fully recovered in 30 minutes, seek immediate medical attention.
- **Heat stroke.** Symptoms include serious disorientation; warm, dry skin; no sweating; rapid, full pulse; vomiting; diarrhea; unconsciousness; and high body temperature. As the body temperature climbs, unexplained anxiety sets in. When the body temperature reaches 104°F to 105°F, the individual may feel a cold sensation in the trunk of the body, goose bumps, nausea, throbbing in the temples, and numbness in the extremities. Most people become incoherent after this stage.
- When body temperature reaches 105°F to 107°F, disorientation, loss of fine-motor control, and muscular weakness set in. If the temperature exceeds 106°F, serious neurological injury and death may be imminent.

Symptoms of Heat Illness

If any of these symptoms occur, stop physical activity, get out of the sun, and start drinking fluids.

- Decreased perspiration
- Cramping
- Weakness
- Flushed skin
- Throbbing head
- Nausea/vomiting
- Diarrhea
- Numbness in the extremities
- Blurred vision
- Unsteadiness
- Disorientation
- Incoherency

Fluid and carbohydrate replacement are essential when exercising in the heat or for a prolonged period.

Heat stroke requires immediate emergency medical attention. Request help and get out of the sun and into a cool, humidity-controlled environment. While you are waiting to be taken to the hospital emergency room, you should be placed in a semi-seated position, and your body should be sprayed with cool water and rubbed with cool towels. If possible, cold packs should be placed in areas that receive an abundant blood supply, such as the head, neck, armpits, and groin. Fluids should not be given if you are unconscious. In any case of heat-related illness, if the person refuses water, vomits, or starts to lose consciousness, an ambulance should be summoned immediately. Proper initial treatment of heat stroke is vital.

9. What should a person do to replace fluids lost during prolonged aerobic exercise?

   The main objective of fluid replacement during prolonged aerobic exercise is to maintain the blood volume so circulation and sweating can continue at normal levels. Adequate water replacement is the most important factor in preventing heat disorders. Drinking about 6 to 8 ounces of cool water every 15 to 20 minutes during exercise is recommended to prevent dehydration. Cold fluids seem to be absorbed more rapidly from the stomach.

   Other relevant points follow:

- Drinking commercially prepared sports drinks is recommended when exercise will be strenuous and carried out for more than an hour. For exercise lasting less than an hour, water is just as effective in replacing lost fluid. The sports drinks you select may be based on your personal preference. Try different drinks at 6 to 8 percent glucose concentration to see which drink you tolerate best and suits your tastes as well.
- Commercial fluid-replacement solutions (such as Powerade® and Gatorade®) contain about 6 to 8 percent glucose, which seems to be optimal for fluid absorption and performance. Sugar does not become available to the muscles until about 30 minutes after consumption of a glucose solution.
- Drinks high in fructose or with a glucose concentration greater than eight percent are not recommended because they slow water absorption during exercise in the heat.
- Most sodas (both cola and noncola) contain between 10 and 12 percent glucose, which is too high for proper rehydration during exercise in the heat.
- Do not overhydrate with just water during a very or ultralong-distance event, as such can lead to hyponatremia (see also "Hyponatremia" in Chapter 3, page 114) or low sodium concentration in the blood. When water loss through sweat during prolonged exercise is replaced by water alone, blood sodium is diluted to the point where it creates serious health problems, including seizures and coma in severe cases.

10. What precautions must a person take when exercising in the cold?

    When exercising in the cold, the two factors to consider are frostbite and **hypothermia**.

> **Thermogenic response** Amount of energy required to digest food.
>
> **Heat cramps** Muscle spasms caused by heat-induced changes in electrolyte balance in muscle cells.
>
> **Heat exhaustion** Heat-related fatigue.
>
> **Heat stroke** Emergency situation resulting from the body being subjected to high atmospheric temperatures.
>
> **Hypothermia** A breakdown in the body's ability to generate heat; a drop in body temperature below 95°F.

In contrast to hot and humid conditions, cold weather usually does not threaten health because clothing can be selected for heat conservation, and exercise itself increases the production of body heat.

Most people actually overdress for exercise in the cold. Because exercise increases body temperature, a moderate workout on a cold day makes a person feel that the temperature is 20 to 30 degrees warmer than it actually is. Overdressing for exercise can make the clothes damp from excessive perspiration. The risk for hypothermia increases when a person is wet or after exercise stops, when the person is not moving around sufficiently to increase (or maintain) body heat.

Initial warning signs of hypothermia include shivering, losing coordination, and having difficulty speaking. With a continued drop in body temperature, shivering stops, the muscles weaken and stiffen, and the person feels elated or intoxicated and eventually loses consciousness. To prevent hypothermia, use common sense, dress properly, and be aware of environmental conditions.

The popular belief that exercising in cold temperatures (32°F and lower) freezes the lungs is false, because the air is warmed properly in the air passages before it reaches the lungs. Cold is not what poses a threat; wind velocity is what increases the chill factor most.

For example, exercising at a temperature of 25°F with adequate clothing is not too cold to exercise, but if the wind is blowing at 25 miles per hour, the chill factor makes it feel like the temperature is 15°F. The rate of heat loss depends on the action of the wind on the body's surface. There is an insulating layer of warm air on the body's skin. Moving air disrupts this warm layer and allows cooler air to replace the warm air on the body's surface. The faster the wind speed, the quicker the surface cools. This effect is even worse if a person is wet and exhausted. When the weather is windy, the individual should exercise (jog or cycle) against the wind on the way out and with the wind upon returning.

Even though the lungs are under no risk when you exercise in the cold, your face, head, hands, and feet should be protected because they are subject to frostbite. Watch for signs of frostbite: numbness and discoloration. In cold temperatures, as much as half of the body's heat can be lost through an unprotected head and neck. A wool or synthetic cap, hood, or hat will help to hold in body heat. Mittens are better than gloves, because they keep the fingers together so that the surface area from which to lose heat is less. Inner linings of synthetic material to wick moisture away from the skin are recommended. Avoid cotton next to the skin, because once cotton gets wet, whether from perspiration, rain, or snow, it loses its insulating properties.

Wearing several layers of lightweight clothing is preferable to wearing one single, thick layer because warm air is trapped between layers of clothes, enabling greater heat conservation. As body temperature increases, you can remove layers as necessary.

The first layer of clothes should wick moisture away from the skin. Polypropylene, Capilene, and Thermax are recommended materials. Next, a layer of wool, Dacron, or polyester fleece insulates well even when wet. Lycra tights or sweatpants help protect the legs. The outer layer should be waterproof, wind resistant, and breathable. A synthetic material such as Gore-Tex is best, so moisture can still escape from the body. A ski mask or face mask helps protect the face. In extremely cold conditions, exposed skin, such as the nose, cheeks, and around the eyes, can be insulated with petroleum jelly.

For lengthy or long-distance workouts (cross-country skiing or long runs), take a small backpack to carry the clothing you removed. You also can carry extra warm and dry clothes in case you stop exercising away from shelter. If you remain outdoors following exercise, added clothing and continuous body movement are essential to maintain body temperature and avoid hypothermia.

11. Can I exercise when I have a cold or the flu?

The most important consideration is to use common sense and pay attention to your symptoms. Usually, you may continue to exercise if your symptoms include a runny nose, sneezing, or a scratchy throat. But, if your symptoms include fever, muscle ache, vomiting, diarrhea, or a hacking cough, you should avoid exercise. After an illness, be sure to ease back gradually into your program. Do not attempt to return at the same intensity and duration that you were used to prior to your illness.

9.4 Exercise-Related Injuries

To enjoy and maintain physical fitness, preventing injury during a conditioning program is essential. Exercise-related injuries, nonetheless, are common in individuals who participate in exercise programs. Surveys indicate that more than half of all new participants incur injuries during the first 6 months of the conditioning program.

The four most common causes of injuries are:

1. High-impact activities
2. Rapid conditioning programs (doing too much too quickly)
3. Improper shoes or training surfaces
4. Anatomical predisposition (i.e., body propensity)

High-impact activities and a significant increase in quantity, intensity, or duration of activities are by far the most common causes of injuries. The body requires time to adapt to more intense activities. Most of these injuries can be prevented through a more gradual and correct conditioning (low-impact) program.

Softer training surfaces, such as artificial turf, grass, or dirt, produce less trauma than wood, asphalt, or concrete.

Table 9.1 Reference Guide for Exercise-Related Problems

Injury	Signs/Symptoms	Treatment*
Bruise (contusion)	Pain, swelling, discoloration	Cold application, compression, rest
Dislocations/fracture	Pain, swelling, deformity	Splinting, cold application, seek medical attention
Heat cramp	Cramps, spasms, and muscle twitching in the legs, arms, and abdomen	Stop activity, get out of the heat, stretch, massage the painful area, drink plenty of fluids
Heat exhaustion	Fainting, profuse sweating, cold/clammy skin, weak/rapid pulse, weakness, headache	Stop activity, rest in a cool place, loosen clothing, rub body with cool/wet towel, drink plenty of fluids, stay out of heat for 2–3 days
Heat stroke	Hot/dry skin, no sweating, serious disorientation, rapid/full pulse, vomiting, diarrhea, unconsciousness, high body temperature	Seek immediate medical attention, request help and get out of the sun, bathe in cold water/spray with cold water/rub body with cold towels, drink plenty of cold fluids
Joint sprains	Pain, tenderness, swelling, loss of use, discoloration	Cold application, compression, elevation, rest; heat after 36–48 hours (if no further swelling)
Muscle cramps	Pain, spasm	Stretch muscle(s), use mild exercises for involved area
Muscle soreness and stiffness	Tenderness, pain	Mild stretching, low-intensity exercise, warm bath
Muscle strains	Pain, tenderness, swelling, loss of use	Cold application, compression, elevation, rest; heat after 36–48 hours (if no further swelling)
Shin splints	Pain, tenderness	Cold application prior to and following any physical activity, rest; heat (if no activity is carried out)
Side stitch	Pain on the side of the abdomen below the rib cage	Decrease level of physical activity or stop altogether, gradually increase level of fitness
Tendinitis	Pain, tenderness, loss of use	Rest, cold application, heat after 48 hours

*Cold should be applied 3 to 5 times a day for 15 minutes. Heat can be applied 3 times a day for 15 to 20 minutes.

© Cengage Learning

Because few people have perfect body alignment, injuries associated with overtraining may occur eventually. In case of injury, proper treatment can avert a lengthy recovery process. A summary of common exercise-related injuries and how to manage them follows.

Acute Sports Injuries The best treatment always has been prevention. If an activity causes unusual discomfort or chronic irritation, you need to treat the cause by decreasing the intensity, switching activities, substituting equipment, or upgrading clothing (such as buying proper-fitting shoes).

In cases of acute injury, the standard treatment is rest, cold application, compression or splinting (or both), and elevation of the affected body part. This is commonly referred to as **RICE**:

R = rest
I = ice (cold) application
C = compression
E = elevation

Cold should be applied 3 to 5 times a day for 15 minutes at a time during the first 36 to 48 hours, by submerging the injured area in cold water, using an ice bag, or applying ice massage to the affected part. An elastic bandage or wrap can be used for compression. Elevating the body part decreases blood flow (and therefore swelling) in that body part.

The purpose of these treatment modalities is to minimize swelling in the area and thus hasten recovery time. After the first 36 to 48 hours, heat can be used if the injury shows no further swelling or inflammation. If you have doubts as to the nature or seriousness of the injury (such as suspected fracture), you should seek a medical evaluation.

Obvious deformities (exhibited by fractures, dislocations, or partial dislocations, as examples) call for splinting, cold application with an ice bag, and medical attention. Do not try to reset any of these conditions by yourself, because you could further damage muscles, ligaments, and nerves. Treatment of these injuries should always be left to specialized medical personnel. A quick reference guide for the signs or symptoms and treatment of exercise-related problems is provided in Table 9.1.

Muscle Soreness and Stiffness Individuals who begin an exercise program or participate after a long layoff from exercise often develop muscle soreness and stiffness. The acute soreness that sets in the first few hours after exercise is thought to be related to general fatigue of the exercised muscles.

Delayed muscle soreness that appears several hours after exercise (usually about 12 hours later) and lasts 2 to 4 days may be related to actual microtears in muscle tissue, muscle spasms that increase fluid retention (stimulating the pain nerve endings), and overstretching or tearing of connective tissue in and around muscles and joints.

Mild stretching before and adequate stretching after exercise help

> **RICE** An acronym used to describe the standard treatment procedure for acute sports injuries: rest, ice (cold application), compression, and elevation.

to prevent soreness and stiffness. Gradually progressing into an exercise program is important, too. A person should not attempt to do too much too quickly. To relieve pain, mild stretching, light-intensity exercise to stimulate blood flow, and a warm bath are recommended.

Exercise Intolerance When starting an exercise program, participants should stay within safe limits. The best method to determine whether you are exercising too strenuously is to check your heart rate and make sure that it does not exceed the limits of your target zone. Exercising above this target zone may not be safe for unconditioned or high-risk individuals. You do not have to exercise beyond your target zone to gain the desired cardiorespiratory benefits.

Several physical signs will tell you when you are exceeding your functional limitations—that is, experiencing **exercise intolerance**. Signs of intolerance include rapid or irregular heart rate, difficult breathing, nausea, vomiting, lightheadedness, headache, dizziness, unusually flushed or pale skin, extreme weakness, lack of energy, shakiness, sore muscles, cramps, and tightness in the chest. Learn to listen to your body. If you notice any of these symptoms, seek medical attention before continuing your exercise program.

Recovery heart rate is another indicator of overexertion. To a certain extent, recovery heart rate is related to fitness level. The higher your cardiorespiratory fitness level, the faster your heart rate will decrease following exercise. As a rule, heart rate should be below 120 bpm 5 minutes into recovery. If your heart rate is above 120, you most likely have overexerted yourself or possibly could have some other cardiac abnormality. If you lower the intensity or the duration of exercise, or both, and you still have a fast heart rate 5 minutes into recovery, you should consult your physician.

Side Stitch Side stitch is a cramp-like pain in the ribcage that can develop in the early stages of participation in exercise. It occurs primarily in unconditioned beginners and in trained individuals when they exercise at higher intensities than usual. As one's physical condition improves, this condition tends to disappear unless training is intensified.

The exact cause is unknown. Some experts suggest that it could relate to a lack of blood flow to the respiratory muscles during strenuous physical exertion. Some people encounter side stitch during downhill running. If you experience side stitch during exercise, slow down. If it persists, stop altogether. Lying down on your back and gently bringing both knees to the chest and holding that position for 30 to 60 seconds also helps.

Some people get side stitch if they drink juice or eat anything shortly before exercise. Drinking only water one to two hours prior to exercise sometimes prevents side stitch. Other individuals have problems with commercially available sports drinks during vigorous-intensity exercise. Unless carbohydrate replacement is crucial to complete a long-distance event (more than 60 minutes, such as road cycling, a marathon, or a triathlon), drink cool water for fluid replacement or try a different carbohydrate solution.

Shin Splints Shin splints, one of the most common injuries to the lower limbs, usually results from one or more of the following: (a) lack of proper and gradual conditioning, (b) doing physical activities on hard surfaces (wooden floors, hard tracks, cement, or asphalt), (c) fallen arches, (d) chronic overuse, (e) muscle fatigue, (f) faulty posture, (g) improper shoes, or (h) participating in weight-bearing activities when excessively overweight.

To manage shin splints:

1. Remove or reduce the cause (exercise on softer surfaces, wear better shoes or arch supports, or completely stop exercise until the shin splints heal).
2. Do stretching exercises before and after physical activity.
3. Use ice massage for 10 to 20 minutes before and after exercise.
4. Apply active heat (whirlpool and hot baths) for 15 minutes, 2 to 3 times a day.
5. Use supportive taping during physical activity (a qualified athletic trainer can teach you the proper taping technique).

Muscle Cramps Muscle cramps are caused by the body's depletion of essential electrolytes or a breakdown in the coordination between opposing muscle groups. If you have a muscle cramp, you should first attempt to stretch the muscles involved. In the case of the calf muscle, for example, pull your toes up toward the knees. After stretching the muscle, rub it down gently, and, finally, do some mild exercises requiring the use of that muscle.

In pregnant and lactating women, muscle cramps often are related to a lack of calcium. If women get cramps during these times, calcium supplements usually relieve the problem. Tight clothing also can cause cramps by decreasing blood flow to active muscle tissue.

9.5 Exercise and Aging

The elderly constitute the fastest-growing segment of the population. The number of Americans aged 65 and older increased from 3.1 million in 1900 (4.1 percent of the population) to about 40 million (13 percent) in 2010. By the year 2030, more than 72 million people, or 20 percent of the U.S. population, are expected to be older than 65.

The main objectives of fitness programs for older adults should be to help them improve their functional status and contribute to healthy aging. This implies the ability to maintain independent living status and to avoid disability. Older adults are encouraged to participate in programs that will help develop cardiorespiratory endurance, muscular strength and endurance, muscular flexibility, agility, balance, and motor coordination.

Physical Training in the Older Adult Regular participation in physical activity provides both physical and psychological benefits to older adults. In particular, regular physical activity decreases the risk for cardiovascular disease, stroke, hypertension, type 2 diabetes, osteoporosis, obesity, colon cancer, breast cancer, cognitive impairment, anxiety, and depression.[8] Physical activity also improves self-confidence and self-esteem. Furthermore, both cardiorespiratory endurance and strength training help to increase functional capacity, improve overall health status, and increase life expectancy. Strength training also decreases the rate at which strength and muscle mass are lost.

The trainability of older men and women alike and the effectiveness of physical activity in enhancing health have been demonstrated in research. Older adults who increase their physical activity experience significant changes in cardiorespiratory endurance, strength, and flexibility. The extent of the changes depends on their initial fitness level and the types of activities they select for their training (walking, cycling, strength training, and so on).

Improvements in maximal oxygen uptake in older adults are similar to those of younger people, although older people seem to require a longer training period to achieve these changes. Declines in maximal oxygen uptake average about 1 percent per year between ages 25 and 75. A slower rate of decline is seen in people who maintain a lifetime aerobic exercise program.

Results of research on the effects of aging on the cardiorespiratory system of male exercisers versus nonexercisers showed that the maximal oxygen uptake of regular exercisers was almost twice that of the nonexercisers (see Table 9.2).[9] The study revealed a decline in maximal oxygen uptake between ages 50 and 68 of only 13 percent in the active group, compared with 41 percent in the inactive group. These changes indicate that about one-third of the loss in maximal oxygen uptake results from aging, and two-thirds of the loss comes from inactivity. Blood pressure, heart rate, and body weight also were remarkably better in the exercising group. Aerobic training seems to decrease high blood pressure in older patients at the same rate as in young hypertensive people.

In terms of aging, muscle strength declines by 10 to 20 percent between ages 20 and 50; but between ages 50 and 70,

Table 9.2 Effects of Physical Activity and Inactivity on Older Men

	Exercisers	Nonexercisers
Age (yr)	68.0	69.8
Weight (lb)	160.3	186.3
Resting heart rate (bpm)	55.8	66.0
Maximal heart rate (bpm)	157.0	146.0
Heart rate reserve* (bpm)	101.2	80.0
Blood pressure (mm Hg)	120/78	150/90
Maximal oxygen uptake (mL/kg/min)	38.6	20.3

*Heart rate reserve = maximal heart rate − resting heart rate.

Data from F. W. Kash, J. L. Boyer, S. P. Van Camp, L. S. Verity, and J. P. Wallace, "The Effect of Physical Activity on Aerobic Power in Older Men (A Longitudinal Study)," *The Physician and Sports Medicine* 18, no. 4 (1990): 73-83.

it drops by another 25 to 30 percent. Through strength training, frail adults in their 80s or 90s can double or triple their strength in just a few months. The amount of muscle hypertrophy achieved, however, decreases with age. Strength gains close to 200 percent have been found in previously inactive adults over age 90.[10] In fact, research has shown that regular strength training improves balance, gait, speed, **functional independence**, morale, depression symptoms, and energy intake.[11] Strength-trained older adults are 30 percent to 50 percent stronger than their sedentary counterparts.

Although muscle flexibility drops by about 5 percent per decade of life, 10 minutes of stretching every other day can prevent most of this loss as a person ages. Improved flexibility also enhances mobility skills. The latter promotes independence because it helps older adults successfully perform activities of daily living.

In terms of body composition, lean body mass typically declines by 2 to 3 percent per decade starting at age 30. Muscle mass starts to decrease at age 40 and accelerates after age 65, with the legs losing muscle mass at a faster rate. Sedentary adults gain about 20 pounds of body weight between ages 18 and 55. As a result, body fat continues to increase through adult life, with a greater tendency toward visceral fat accumulation (especially in men), leading to further increase in risk for chronic disease. Regular aerobic activity and strength training have been shown to help older adults properly manage body weight and significantly reduce visceral fat.

Older adults who wish to initiate an exercise program are strongly encour-

Older adults who exercise enjoy better health, functional capacity, and quality of life than physically inactive adults.

> **Exercise intolerance** Inability to function during exercise because of excessive fatigue or extreme feelings of discomfort.
>
> **Side stitch** A sharp pain in the side of the abdomen.
>
> **Shin splints** Injury to the lower leg characterized by pain and irritation in the shin region of the leg.
>
> **Functional independence** Ability to carry out activities of daily living without assistance from other individuals.

aged to have a complete medical evaluation. Recommended activities for older adults include calisthenics, walking, jogging, swimming, cycling, and water aerobics. Strength training is particularly important for bone health in the absence of weight bearing aerobic activities.

Older people should avoid isometric and very high-intensity strength-training exercises (see Chapter 7). Activities that require all-out effort or that require participants to hold their breath tend to lessen blood flow to the heart, cause a significant increase in blood pressure, and increase the load placed on the heart. Older adults should participate in activities that require continuous and rhythmic muscular activity (about 40 to 60 percent of heart rate reserve). These activities do not cause large increases in blood pressure or overload the heart.

9.6 Preparing for Sports Participation[12]

To enhance your participation in sports, keep in mind that in most cases it is better to get fit before playing sports rather than playing sports to get fit. A good preseason training program will help make the season more enjoyable and prevent exercise-related injuries.

Properly conditioned individuals can participate safely in sports and enjoy the activities to their fullest with few or no limitations. Unfortunately, sports injuries are often the result of poor fitness and a lack of sport-specific conditioning. Many injuries occur when fatigue sets in following overexertion by unconditioned individuals.

Base Fitness Conditioning Preactivity screening that includes a health history (see "See PAR-Q and Health History Questionnaire," page 36) and/or a medical evaluation appropriate to your sport selection is recommended. Once cleared for exercise, start by building a base of general athletic fitness that includes the four health-related fitness components: cardiorespiratory fitness, muscular fitness, flexibility, and recommended body composition. The base fitness conditioning program should last a minimum of six weeks.

As explained in Chapter 6, for cardiorespiratory fitness select an activity that you enjoy (such as walking, jogging, cycling, step aerobics, cross-country skiing, elliptical training) and train three to five times per week at a minimum of 20 minutes of continuous activity per session. Exercise between 60 percent and 80 percent intensity for adequate conditioning. You should feel as though you are training "somewhat hard" to "hard" at these intensity levels.

Strength (resistance) training helps maintain and increase muscular strength and endurance. Following the guidelines provided in Chapter 7, select 10 to 12 exercises that involve the major muscle groups and train 2 or 3 times per week on nonconsecutive days. Select a resistance (weight) that allows you to do 8 to 12 repetitions to near fatigue (8 to 12 RM [repetition maximum] zone based on your fitness goals—see Chapter 7). That is, the resistance will be heavy enough so that when you perform one set of an exercise, you will not be able to do more than the predetermined number of repetitions at that weight. Begin your program slowly and perform between one and three sets of each exercise. Recommended exercises include the bench press, lat pull-down, leg press, leg curl, triceps extension, arm curl, rowing torso, heel raise, abdominal crunch, and back extension.

Flexibility is important in sports participation to enhance the range of motion in the joints. Using the guidelines from Chapter 8, schedule flexibility training two or three days per week. Perform each stretching exercise 4 times, and hold each stretch for 15 to 30 seconds. Examples of stretching exercises include the side body stretch, body rotation, chest stretch, shoulder stretch, sit-and-reach stretch, adductor stretch, quad stretch, heel cord stretch, and knee-to-chest stretch.

In terms of body composition, excess body fat hinders sports performance and increases the risk for injuries. Depending on the nature of the activity, fitness goals for body composition range from 12 percent to 20 percent body fat for men and 17 percent to 25 percent for most women.

Sport-Specific Conditioning Once you have achieved the general fitness base, continue with the program but make adjustments to add sport-specific training. This training should match the sport's requirements for aerobic/anaerobic capabilities, muscular strength and endurance, and range of motion.

During the sport-specific training, about half of your aerobic/anaerobic training should involve the same muscles used during your sport. Ideally, allocate 4 weeks of sport-specific training before you start participating in the sport. Then continue the sport-specific training on a more limited basis throughout the season. Depending on the nature of the sport (aerobic versus anaerobic), once the season starts, sports participation itself can take the place of some or all of your aerobic workouts.

The next step is to look at the demands of the sport. For example, soccer, bicycle racing, cross-country skiing, and snowshoeing are aerobic activities, whereas basketball, racquetball, alpine skiing, snowboarding, and ice hockey are stop-and-go sports that require a combination of aerobic and anaerobic activity. Consequently, aerobic training may be appropriate for cross-country skiing, but it will do little to prepare your muscles for the high-intensity requirements of combined aerobic and anaerobic sports.

High-intensity interval training (HIIT), performed twice per week, is added to the program at this time. HIIT allows you to break up your workout into smaller segments so that you can perform a greater training volume at a higher exercise intensity. HIIT has been shown to help improve both aerobic and anaerobic fitness at a much faster rate.

Four training variables impact HIIT. The acronym DIRT is frequently used to denote these variables[13]:

D = Distance of each speed interval
I = Interval or length of recovery between speed intervals

R = Repetitions or number of speed intervals to be performed
T = Time of each speed interval

Using these four variables, a person can practically design an unlimited number of HIIT sessions.

The intervals consist of a 1:4 to a 1:1 work-to-recovery ratio. The more intense the speed interval, the longer the required recovery interval. For aerobic intervals (lasting longer than 3 minutes), 1:2, 1:1, or even lower ratios are used. For intense anaerobic speed intervals (30 seconds to 3 minutes), recovery intervals that last two to four times as long (1:2 to 1:4) as the work period are required.

A 1:3 ratio, for example, indicates that you'll work at a fairly high intensity for, say, 30 seconds and then spend 90 seconds on light- to moderate-intensity recovery. Be sure to keep moving during the recovery phase. Perform 4 or 5 intervals at first, and then gradually progress to 10 intervals. As your fitness improves, you can lengthen the high-intensity proportion of the intervals progressively to 1 minute and/or decrease the total recovery time.

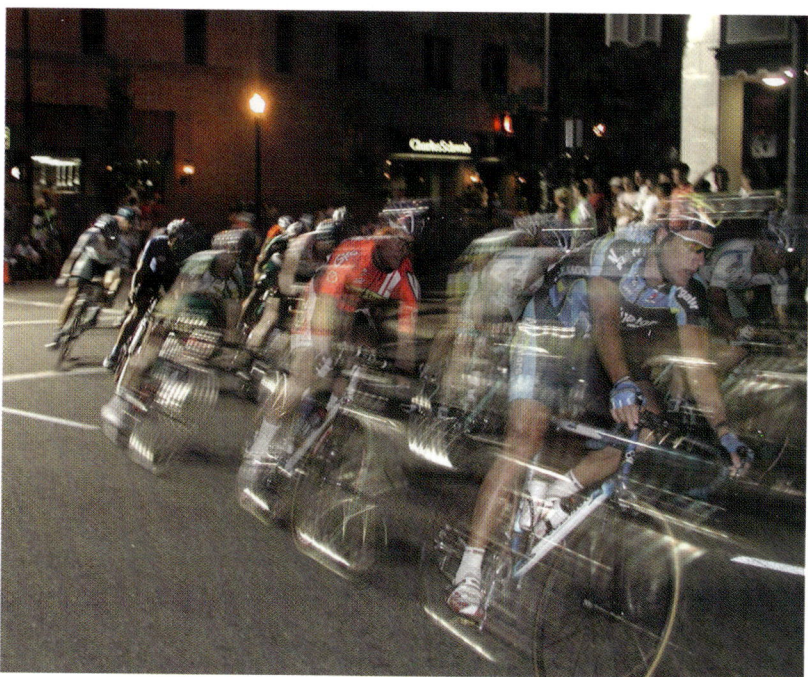

High-intensity interval training promotes fitness, enhances energy expenditure and weight loss, and augments health benefits.

For aerobic sports, HIIT at least once per week improves performance. Most commonly done at a 1:2 or lower work-to-recovery ratio, you also can do a 5- to 10-minute aerobic work interval followed by 1 to 2 minutes of recovery, but the intensity of these longer intervals should not be as high, and only three to five intervals are recommended. Note that the HIIT workouts are not performed in addition to the regular aerobic workouts but, instead, take the place of one of these workouts.

Consider sport-specific strength requirements as well. Look at the primary muscles used in your sport, and make sure your choice of exercises works those muscles. Try to perform your strength training through a range of motion similar to those used in your sport. Aerobic/anaerobic sports require greater strength; during the season, the recommendation is 3 sets of 8 to 12 repetitions to near fatigue, 2 or 3 times per week. For aerobic endurance sports, the recommendation is a minimum of one set of 8 to 12 repetitions to near fatigue, once or twice per week during the season.

Stop-and-go sports (basketball, racquetball, soccer) require greater strength than pure endurance sports (triathlon, long-distance running, cross-country skiing). For example, recreational participants during the sport-specific training phase for stop-and-go sports perform 3 sets of 8 to 12 repetitions to near fatigue, 2 to 3 times per week. Competitive athletes and those desiring greater strength gains typically conduct 3 to 5 sets of 4 to 12 repetitions to near fatigue three times per week.

For some winter sports, such as alpine skiing and snowboarding, gravity supplies most of the propulsion, and the body acts as a shock absorber. Muscles in the hips, knees, and trunk are used to control the forces on the body and equipment. Multi-joint exercises, such as the leg press, squats, and lunges, are suggested for these activities.

Before the season starts, make sure that your equipment is in proper working condition. For example, alpine skiers' bindings should be cleaned and adjusted properly so that they will release as needed. This is one of the most important things you can do to help prevent knee injuries. A good pair of bindings is cheaper than knee surgery.

The first few times you participate in the sport of your choice, go easy, practice technique, and do not continue once you are fatigued. Gradually increase the length and intensity of your workouts. Consider taking a lesson to have someone watch your technique and help correct flaws early in the season. Even Olympic athletes have coaches watching them. Proper conditioning allows for a more enjoyable and healthier season.

Overtraining Rest is important in any fitness conditioning program. Although the term **overtraining** is associated most frequently with athletic performance, it applies just as well to fitness participants. We all know that hard work im-

> **High-intensity interval training (HIIT)** Training program that involves high- to very high-intensity (80 to 90 percent of maximal capacity) intervals, each followed by a low-to-moderate intensity recovery interval. Usually 1:3 or lower work-to-recovery ratio is used.
>
> **Overtraining** An emotional, behavioral, and physical condition marked by increased fatigue, decreased performance, persistent muscle soreness, mood disturbances, and feelings of "staleness" or "burnout" as a result of excessive physical training.

Sample High-Intensity Interval Training (HIIT) Programs

The following are sample HIIT programs that you can use. For intensity levels, you should use the Physical Activity Perceived Exertion Scale (H-PAPE) in Figure 6.9, page 219. Prior to HIIT, be sure to have a sound general aerobic (cardiorespiratory) fitness base—that is, at least 6 weeks of aerobic training, 5 times per week for 20 to 60 minutes per session. Once you are ready for HIIT, always have a proper 5- to 10-minute aerobic warm-up prior to the first high-intensity interval. Also, in all cases, follow up the final high-intensity interval with a 5- to 10-minute cool-down phase. You can use the same exercise modality (running, cycling, elliptical training, stair climbing, or swimming) for your entire HIIT, or you may use a combination of these activities with some of the following programs, if such is feasible at your facility. Do not perform back-to-back HIIT on consecutive days. Preferably, depending on the intensity and volume of training, allow 2 to 3 days between HIIT sessions.

Five-minute very hard-intensity aerobic intervals: Exercise at a very hard rate (90 percent of maximal capacity) for 5 minutes, followed by 5 to 10 minutes of recovery at a light to moderate intensity. Start with one interval and work up to three by the third to fifth training session. Initially, use a 1:2 work-to-recovery ratio. Gradually decrease the recovery to a 1:1 ratio or even less.

Step-wise intensity interval training: Using 3- to 5-minute intervals, start at a light-intensity rate of perceived exertion and then progressively step up to the very hard-intensity level (light, moderate, somewhat hard, vigorous, hard, and very hard). Start with 3-minute intervals, and as you become more fit, increase to 5 minutes each. As time allows and you develop greater fitness, you can add a step-down approach by progressively stepping down to hard, vigorous, somewhat hard, moderate, and light.

Fartlek training: Fartlek training was developed in 1937 by Swedish coach Gösta Holmér. The word "fartlek" means "speed play" in Swedish. It is an unstructured form of interval training where intensity (speed) and distance of each interval is varied as the participant wishes. There is no set structure and the individual alternates the intensity (from somewhat hard to very hard) and length of each speed interval, along with the recovery intervals (light to moderate) and length thereof. Total duration of fartlek training is between 20 and 60 minutes.

Tempo training: Although no formal intervals are conducted with tempo training, the intensity of training qualifies it as a HIIT program. Following an appropriate warm-up, tempo runs involve continuous training between vigorous (70%) and hard (80%) for 20 to 60 minutes at a time.

All-out or supramaximal interval training: All-out interval training involves 10 to 20 supramaximal or sprint intervals lasting 30 to 60 seconds each. Depending on the level of conditioning and the length of the speed interval, 2 to 5 minutes recovery at a light to moderate level are allowed.

Cardio/resistance training program: You may use a combination of aerobic and resistance training for your HIIT. Following a brief aerobic and strength-training warm-up, select about eight resistance-training exercises that you can alternate with treadmill running, cycling, elliptical training, or rowing. Perform one set of 8 to 20 RM (based on personal preference) on each exercise followed by 90 seconds of aerobic work after each set. You can pace the aerobic intensity according to the preceding strength-training set. For example, you may choose a light intensity aerobic interval following a 10 RM for the leg press exercise and a vigorous aerobic interval after a 10 RM arm-curl set. Allow no greater recovery time (2 to 5 seconds) between exercise modes than what it takes to walk from the strength-training exercise to the aerobic station (and vice versa).

---

proves fitness and performance. Hard training without adequate recovery, however, breaks down the body and leads to loss of fitness.

Physiological improvements in fitness and conditioning programs occur during the rest periods following training. As a rule, a hard day of training must be followed by a day of light training. Equally, a few weeks of increased training **volume** are to be followed by a few days of light recovery work. During these recovery periods, body systems strengthen and compensate for the training load, leading to a higher level of fitness. If proper recovery is not built into the training routine, overtraining occurs. Decreased performance, staleness, and injury are frequently seen with overtraining. Thus, to obtain optimal results, training regimens are altered during different phases of the year.

Periodization Periodization is a training approach that uses a systematic variation in intensity and volume to enhance fitness and performance. This model was designed around the premise that the body becomes stronger as a result of training, but if similar workouts are constantly repeated, the body tires and enters a state of staleness and fatigue.

Periodization is used most frequently for athletic conditioning. Because athletes cannot maintain peak fitness during

Behavior Modification Planning

Common Signs and Symptoms of Overtraining

- Decreased fitness
- Decreased sports performance
- Increased fatigue
- Loss of concentration
- Staleness and burnout
- Loss of competitive drive
- Increased resting and exercise heart rate
- Decreased appetite
- Loss of body weight
- Altered sleep patterns
- Decreased sex drive
- Generalized body aches and pains
- Increased susceptibility to illness and injury
- Mood disturbances
- Depression

Try It

If following several weeks or months of hard training you experience some of these symptoms, you need to substantially decrease training volume and intensity for a week or two. This recovery phase will allow the body to recover, strengthen, and prepare for the next training phase. In your Behavior Change Tracker or your Online Journal, modify your training program to allow a light week of training following each five to eight weeks of hard exercise training.

---

an entire season, most athletes seeking peak performance use a periodized training approach. Studies have documented that greater improvements in fitness are achieved by using a variety of training loads. Using the same program and attempting to increase volume and intensity over a prolonged time will be manifested in overtraining.

The periodization training system involves three cycles:

1. Macrocycles
2. Mesocycles
3. Microcycles

These cycles vary in length depending on the requirements of the sport. Typically, the overall training period (season or year) is referred to as a macrocycle. For athletes who need to peak twice a year, such as cross-country and track runners, two macrocycles can be developed within the year.

Macrocycles are divided into smaller weekly or monthly training phases known as mesocycles. A typical season, for example, is divided into the following mesocycles: base fitness conditioning (off-season), preseason or sport-specific conditioning, competition, peak performance, and transition (active recovery from sport-specific training and competition). In turn, mesocycles are divided into smaller weekly or daily microcycles. During microcycles, training follows the general objective of the mesocycle, but the workouts are altered to avoid boredom and fatigue.

The concept behind periodizing can be used in both aerobic and anaerobic sports. In the case of a long-distance runner, for instance, training can start with a general strength-conditioning program and cardiorespiratory endurance cross-training (jogging, cycling, swimming) during the off-season. In preseason, the volume of strength training is decreased, and the total weekly running mileage, at moderate intensities, is progressively increased. During the competitive season, the athlete maintains a limited strength-training program but now increases the intensity of the runs while decreasing the total weekly mileage. During the peaking phase, volume (miles) of training is reduced even further, while the intensity is maintained at a high level. At the end of the season, a short transition period of two to four weeks, involving light- to moderate-intensity activities other than running and lifting weights, is recommended.

Periodization is frequently used for development of muscular strength, progressively cycling through the various components (hypertrophy, strength, and power) of strength training. Research indicates that varying the volume and intensity over time is more effective for long-term progression than either single- or multiple-set programs with no variations. Training volume and intensity are typically increased only for large muscle/multi-joint lifts (e.g., bench press, squats, and lat pulldowns). Single-joint lifts (triceps extension, biceps curls, hamstring curls) usually remain in the range of three sets of 8 to 12 repetitions.

A sample sequence—one macrocycle—of periodized training is provided in

Volume (of training) The total amount of training performed in a given work period (day, week, month, or season).

Periodization A training approach that divides the season into three cycles (macrocycles, mesocycles, and microcycles) using a systematic variation in intensity and volume of training to enhance fitness and performance and to contribute to overall fitness.

Table 9.3. The program starts with high volume and light intensity. During subsequent mesocycles (divided among the objectives of hypertrophy, strength, and power), the volume is decreased, and the intensity (resistance) increases. Following each mesocycle, the recommendation is up to seven days of very light training. This brief resting period allows the body to fully recuperate, preventing overtraining and risk for injury. Other models of periodization are available, but the example provided is the most commonly used.

For aerobic endurance sports, 1 to 3 sets of 8 to 12 repetitions to near fatigue performed once or twice a week is recommended. Although strength training does not enhance maximal oxygen uptake, and strength requirements are not as high with endurance sports, data indicate that strength training does help the individual sustain submaximal exercise for longer periods of time.

In recent years, the practice of altering or cycling workouts has become popular among fitness participants. Research indicates that periodization is not limited to athletes but has been used successfully by fitness enthusiasts who are preparing for special events such as a 10K run, a triathlon, or a bike race and by those who are simply aiming for higher fitness. Altering training is also recommended for people who progressed nicely in the initial weeks of a fitness program but now feel "stale" and "stagnant." Studies indicate that even among general fitness participants, systematically altering volume and intensity of training is most effective for progress in long-term fitness. Because training phases change continually during a macrocycle, periodization breaks the staleness and the monotony of repeated workouts.

For the nonathlete, a periodization program does not have to account for every detail of the sport. You can periodize workouts by altering mesocycles every two to eight weeks. You can use different exercises, change the number of sets and repetitions, vary the speed of the repetitions, alter recovery time between sets, and even cross-train.

Periodization is not for everyone. People who are starting an exercise program, who enjoy a set routine, or who are satisfied with their fitness routine and fitness level do not need to periodize. For new participants, the goal is to start and adhere to exercise long enough to adopt the exercise behavior.

9.7 Personal Fitness Programming: An Example

Now that you understand the principles of fitness assessment and exercise prescription given in Chapters 6 through 8 and this chapter, you can review this program to cross-check and improve the design of your own fitness program. Let's look at an example.

Mary is 20 years old and 5 feet 6 inches tall. She participated in organized sports on and off throughout high school. During the last 2 years, however, she has participated only minimally in physical activity. She was not taught the principles for exercise prescription and has not participated in regular exercise to improve and maintain the various health-related components of fitness.

Mary became interested in fitness and contemplated signing up for a fitness and wellness course. As she was preparing her class schedule for the semester, she noted a "Lifetime Fitness and Wellness" course. In registering for the course, Mary anticipated some type of structured aerobic exercise. She knew that good fitness was important to health and weight management, but she didn't quite know how to plan and implement a program.

Once the new course started, she and her classmates received the "Stages of Change Questionnaire." Mary learned that she was in the Preparation stage for cardiorespiratory endurance, the Precontemplation stage for muscular fitness, the Maintenance stage for flexibility, and the Preparation stage for body composition (see the discussion of the Transtheoretical model in Chapter 2, pages 55–58). Various fitness assessments determined that her cardiorespiratory endurance level was fair, her muscular strength and endurance were poor, her flexibility was good, and her percent body fat was 25 (Moderate category).

Table 9.3 Periodization Program for Strength

	One Macrocycle			
	Mesocycle 1* Hypertrophy	Mesocycle 2* Strength & Hypertrophy	Mesocycle 3* Strength & Power	Mesocycle 4* Peak Performance
Sets per exercise	3–5	3–5	3–5	1–3
Repetitions	8–12	6–9	1–5	1–3
Intensity (resistance)	Low	Moderate	High	Very high
Volume	High	Moderate	Low	Very low
Weeks (microcycles)	6–8	4–6	3–5	1–2

*Each mesocycle is followed by several days of light training.

> **Critical Thinking**
>
> In your own experience with personal fitness programs throughout the years, what factors have motivated you and helped you the most to stay with a program? • What factors have kept you from being physically active and what can you do to change these factors?

Cardiorespiratory Endurance At the beginning of the semester, the instructor informed the students that the course would require self-monitored participation in activities outside the regularly scheduled class hours. Thus, Mary was in the Preparation stage for cardiorespiratory endurance. She knew she would be starting exercise in the next couple of weeks.

While in this Preparation stage, Mary chose three processes of change to help her implement her program (see Chapter 2, Table 2.1, page 56). She thought she could adopt an aerobic exercise program (Positive Outlook process of change) and set a realistic goal to reach the "Good" category for cardiorespiratory endurance by the end of the semester (Goal Setting). By staying in this course, she committed to go through with exercise (Commitment). She prepared a 12-week Personalized Cardiorespiratory Exercise Prescription, wrote down her goal, signed the prescription (now a contract), and shared the program with her instructor and roommates.

As her exercise modalities, Mary selected walking/jogging and aerobics. Initially she walked/jogged twice a week and did aerobics once a week. By the 10th week of the program, she was jogging three times per week and participating in aerobics twice a week. She also selected Self-Monitoring, Self-Reevaluation, and Countering as techniques of change (see Chapter 2, Table 2.2, page 62). Using the exercise log in Activity 6.5 in Chapter 6 (page 226), she monitored her exercise program. At the end of six weeks, she scheduled a follow-up cardiorespiratory assessment test (Self-Reevaluation process of change), and she replaced her evening television hour with aerobic training (Countering).

Mary also decided to increase her daily physical activity. She chose to walk 10 minutes to and from school, take the stairs instead of elevators whenever possible, and add 5-minute walks every hour during study time. On Saturdays, she cleaned her apartment and went to a school-sponsored dance at night. On Sundays, she opted to walk to and from church and took a 30-minute leisurely walk after the dinner meal. Mary now was fully in the Action stage of change for cardiorespiratory endurance.

Muscular Fitness (Strength and Endurance)
After Mary had started her fitness and wellness course, she wasn't yet convinced that she wanted to strength train. Still, she contemplated strength training because a small part of her grade depended on it. When she read the information on the effect of lean body mass on basal metabolic rate and weight maintenance (Consciousness-Raising process of change), she thought that perhaps it would be good to add strength training to her program. She also was contemplating the long-term consequences of loss of lean body mass, its effect on her personal appearance, and the potential for decreased independence and quality of life (Emotional Arousal process of change).

Mary visited her course instructor for additional guidance. Following this meeting, Mary committed herself to strength-train. While yet in the Preparation stage, she outlined a 10-week periodized training program (see Figure 9.2) and opted to aim for the "Good" strength category by the end of the program.

Because this was the first time Mary had lifted weights, the course instructor introduced her to two other students who were already lifting (Helping Relationships process of change). She also monitored her program with the form provided in Chapter 7, Activity 7.3. Mary promised herself a movie and dinner out if she completed the first 5 weeks of strength training, and a new blouse if she made it through 10 weeks (Rewards process and technique for change).

Muscular Flexibility Good flexibility is not a problem for Mary because she regularly stretched 15 to 30 minutes while watching the evening news on television. She had developed this habit during the last 2 years of high school to maintain flexibility as a member of the dance-drill team (Environment Control—as a team member, she needed good flexibility).

Because Mary had been stretching regularly for more than 3 years, she was in the Maintenance stage for flexibility. The flexibility fitness tests revealed that she had good flexibility. These results allowed her to pursue her stretching program because she thought that she would be excellent for this fitness component (Self-Evaluation process of change).

To gain greater improvements in flexibility, Mary chose slow-sustained stretching and proprioceptive neuromuscular facilitation (PNF). She would need help to carry out the PNF technique. She spoke to one of her lifting classmates; together they decided to allocate 20 minutes at the end of strength training to stretching (Helping Relationships process of change), and they chose the sequence of exercises presented in Chapter 8, Activity 8.1 (Consciousness-Raising and Goal Setting).

Body Composition One of the motivational factors to enroll in a fitness course was Mary's desire to learn how to better manage her weight. She had gained a few pounds since entering college. To prevent further weight gain, she thought that it was time to learn sound principles for weight management (Behavior Analysis process of change). She was in the Preparation stage of change because she was planning to start a diet and exercise program but wasn't sure how to get it done. All Mary needed was a little consciousness-raising to get her into the Action stage.

With the knowledge she had now gained, Mary planned her program. At 25 percent body fat and 140 pounds, she decided to aim for 23 percent body fat so she would be in the "Good" category for body composition (Goal Setting). This meant that she would have to lose about 4 pounds (see Chapter 4, Activity 4.1).

Mary's daily estimated energy requirement was about 2,027 calories (see Chapter 5, Table 5.3). Mary also figured out that she was expending an additional 400 calories per day through her newly adopted exercise program and increased level of daily physical activity. Thus, her total daily energy intake would be around 2,427 calories (2,027 + 400).

To lose weight, Mary could decrease her caloric intake by 700 calories per day (body weight × 5) (see Chapter 5, Activity 5.1), yielding a target daily intake of 1,727 calories. By decreasing the intake by 700 calories daily, Mary should achieve her target weight in about 20 days (4 pounds of fat × 3,500 calories per pound of fat ÷ 700 fewer calories per day = 20 days). Mary picked the 1,800-calorie diet and eliminated one daily serving of grains (80 calories) to avoid exceeding her target 1,727 daily calorie intake.

The processes of change that will help Mary in the Action stage for weight management are Goal Setting, Countering (exercising instead of watching television), Monitoring, Environment Control, and Rewards. To monitor her daily caloric intake, Mary uses the 1,800-calorie diet plan in Chapter 5, Activity 5.3. To further exert control over her environment, she gave away all of her junk food. She determined that she would not eat out while on the diet, and she bought only low-to-moderate-fat/complex carbohydrate foods during the 3 weeks. As her reward, she achieved her target body weight of 136 pounds.

You Can Get It Done Once they understand the proper exercise, nutrition, and behavior modification guidelines, people find that implementing a fitness lifestyle program is not as difficult as they thought. With adequate preparation and a personal behavioral analysis, you are now ready to design, implement, evaluate, and adhere to a lifetime fitness program that can enhance your functional capacity and zest for life.

Using the concepts provided thus far in this book and the exercise prescription principles that you have learned, you should now update your personal fitness program in Activity 9.1. You also have an opportunity to revise your current stage of change, fitness category for each health-related component of physical fitness, and number of daily steps taken. You have the tools—the rest is up to you!

Figure 9.2 Sample starting muscular strength and endurance periodization program.

	Learning Lifting Technique	Muscular Strength	Muscular Endurance	Muscular Strength
Sets per exercise	1–2	2	2	3
Repetitions	10	12	18–20	8–12 (RM)
Intensity (resistance)	Very low	Moderate	Low	High
Volume	Low	Moderate	Moderate	High
Sessions per week	2	2	2	3
Weeks	2	3	2	3

Selected exercises: Bench press, leg press, leg curl, lat pull-down, rowing torso, rotary torso, seated back, and abdominal crunch.

Training days: ☐ M ☑ T ☐ W ☐ Th ☑ F ☐ S ☐ S

Training time: 3:00 PM

Signature: *Mary Johnson*

Goal: Good   Date: 1/12/2014

ASSESS YOUR BEHAVIOR

CENGAGE brain To access course materials, including companion resources, please visit www.cengagebrain.com.

1. Do you participate in recreational sports as a means to further improve your fitness and add enjoyment to training?
2. Have you been able to meet your cardiorespiratory endurance, muscular strength, muscular flexibility, and recommended body composition goals?
3. Are you able to incorporate a variety of activities into your fitness program, and do you vary exercise intensity and duration from time to time in your training?

ASSESS YOUR KNOWLEDGE

Evaluate how well you understand the concepts presented in this chapter using the chapter-specific quizzing available in the online materials at www.cengagebrain.com.

1. Using a combination of aerobic activities to develop overall fitness is known as
   a. health-related fitness.
   b. circuit training.
   c. plyometric exercises.
   d. cross-training.
   e. skill-related fitness.

2. Maximal heart rate achieved during water-based exercise (swimming and water aerobics) as compared to land-based running is
   a. about 10 bpm lower.
   b. some 13 bpm higher.
   c. about the same.
   d. determined by the person's fitness level.
   e. higher in men and lower in women.

3. To help elevate the exercise heart rate during low-impact aerobics, a person should
   a. include jumping exercises during the routine.
   b. accentuate all arm movements.
   c. allow both feet to leave the ground momentarily.
   d. add bench stepping to the routine.
   e. None of the choices is correct.

4. Diabetics should
   a. not exercise alone.
   b. wear a bracelet that identifies their condition.
   c. exercise at a light-to-moderate intensity.
   d. check blood glucose levels before and after exercise.
   e. follow all four guidelines above.

5. During pregnancy a woman should
   a. accumulate 30 minutes of moderate-intensity activity on most days of the week.
   b. exercise between "low" and "somewhat hard."
   c. avoid exercising at an altitude above 6,000 feet.
   d. All of the above choices are correct.
   e. None of the choices is correct.

6. During exercise in the heat, drinking about a cup of cool water every ___ minutes seems to be ideal to prevent dehydration.
   a. 5
   b. 15 to 20
   c. 30
   d. 30 to 45
   e. 60

7. One of the most common causes of activity-related injuries is
   a. high impact.
   b. low level of fitness.
   c. exercising without stretching.
   d. improper warm-up.
   e. All choices cause about an equal number of injuries.

8. Improvements in maximal oxygen uptake in older adults (as compared with younger adults) as a result of cardiorespiratory endurance training are
   a. lower.
   b. higher.
   c. difficult to determine.
   d. nonexistent.
   e. similar.

9. To participate in sports, it is recommended that you have
   a. base fitness and sport-specific conditioning.
   b. at least a good rating on skill fitness.
   c. good-to-excellent agility.
   d. basic speed.
   e. All of the above.

10. Periodization is a training approach that
    a. uses a systematic variation in intensity and volume.
    b. helps enhance fitness and performance.
    c. is commonly used by athletes.
    d. helps prevent staleness and overtraining.
    e. All are correct choices.

Correct answers can be found at the back of the book.

Activity 9.1: Personal Fitness Plan

Name _____ Date _____
Course _____ Section _____ Gender _____ Age _____

Instructions
Update your personal fitness plan according to the ACSM guidelines provided in Chapters 6–8 and define your stage of change according to the stages of change model in Chapter 2. Also, reevaluate your fitness goals and write down your new goal to achieve by the end of the term. This activity should be carried out as a homework assignment to be completed over the next seven days.

I. Exercise Clearance
Is it safe for you to participate in an exercise program?   ☐ Yes   ☐ No

II. Fitness Evaluation

Component	Current		Fitness Category Goal		
	Test Results	Fitness Category	Training Frequency per Week	Stage of Change	Fitness Goal
Cardiorespiratory endurance					
Muscular fitness (strength and endurance)					
Muscular flexibility					
Body composition			NA		

III. Cardiorespiratory Endurance

Outline your cardiorespiratory endurance program according to ACSM guidelines. Include intensity, frequency, duration, aerobic activities, time of day for training, facility where you will perform the training, and reward for accomplishing your goal.

IV. Muscular Fitness (Strength and Endurance)

Using ACSM guidelines, outline your muscular fitness (strength and endurance) training program. List the exercises used, sets and repetitions, amount of resistance to be used, frequency per week, training facility, and reward for accomplishing your goal.

V. Muscular Flexibility

Design your flexibility training program to include the selected exercises, technique used, number of repetitions for each exercise, length of final hold, site for training, and reward for accomplishing your goal.

VI. Recreational Activities

List any other sports or recreational activities in which you participate and include how often and how long you participate. Indicate also the primary reason for participation in these activities (physical activity, fitness, competition, skill development, recreation, stress management) and your future goals for these activities.

VII. Daily Physical Activity

Indicate the efforts that you are making to increase daily physical activity, your feelings about your choice of activities, and what future goals you have regarding daily physical activities.

Total number of daily steps: _____

VIII. Body Composition and Fitness Benefits

List all of the activities in which you participate regularly and rate the respective contribution to body composition and other fitness components. Use the following rating scale: 1 = low, 2 = fair, 3 = average, 4 = good, and 5 = excellent.

Activity	Body Composition	Cardiorespiratory	Musc. Fitness	Musc. Flexibility
Example: Jogging	5	5	2	1

IX. Contract

I hereby commit to carry out the above described fitness plan and complete my goals by _____.

Upon completion of all my fitness goals I will present my results to _____ and will reward myself with _____.

_____ _____
My signature   Date

_____ _____
Witness signature Date

Preventing Cardiovascular Disease

10

"Exercise can be used as a vaccine to prevent disease and a medication to treat disease. If there were a drug with the same benefits as exercise, it would instantly be the standard of care."
—Robert Sallis

Objectives

- **Define** cardiovascular disease and coronary heart disease.
- **Explain** the importance of a healthy lifestyle in preventing cardiovascular disease.
- **Become** familiar with the major risk factors that lead to the development of coronary heart disease, including physical inactivity, an abnormal cholesterol profile, hypertension, homocysteine, C-reactive protein, diabetes, and smoking.
- **Assess** your own risk for developing coronary heart disease.
- **Outline** a comprehensive program for reducing the risk for coronary heart disease and managing the overall risk for cardiovascular disease.
- **Determine** your risk for heart disease.

CENGAGEbrain.com
Visit **www.cengagebrain.com** to access course materials and companion resources for this text, including quiz questions designed to check your understanding of the chapter contents. See the preface on page ix for more information.

As a young college student, why should I have to worry about heart disease?

Young people should not think that heart disease will not affect them. The process begins early in life, as shown in American soldiers who died during the Korean and Vietnam conflicts. Autopsies conducted on soldiers killed at 22 years of age and younger revealed that approximately 70 percent had early stages of atherosclerosis. Other studies found elevated blood cholesterol levels in children as young as 10 years old. Overall risk factor management and positive lifestyle habits are the best ways to prevent disease. The choices you make today will affect your health and well-being in middle age and later.

Trans fats have been debated extensively lately. What foods are most likely to contain trans fats?

With extensive media coverage of their possible harmfulness, the amount of trans fats in foods is decreasing significantly. According to the Centers for Disease Control (CDC), trans fats have decreased by about 60 percent in the last decade, primarily because of its removal from processed foods. Although good news, many foods still contain significant amounts. Trans fats are found primarily in fried foods such as French fries, doughnuts, and apple fritters, but they are also found in baked foods, including pastries, biscuits, crackers, pie crusts, and pizza crust. Stick margarine and shortenings also contain trans fats.

Trans fats increase the risk for heart disease and stroke not only by increasing low-density lipoprotein (LDL, or "bad") cholesterol but also by decreasing cardioprotective high-density lipoprotein (HDL, or "good") cholesterol. To decrease consumption of trans fats, always read the food label for trans fat content and look for "hydrogenated fat/oil" or "partially hydrogenated fat/oil" (i.e., trans fats) on the list of ingredients. The Food and Drug Administration (FDA) does not require food companies to list trans fat content on the label if it is less than .5 gram per serving. The American Heart Association recommends that on average we consume less than 2 grams per day of trans fat. Four servings of a product that contains .49 gram of partially hydrogenated oil, not listed on the food label, provide almost the entire daily allowance of trans fats.

Is resveratrol the "super" nutrient that prevents heart disease?

Resveratrol is a compound found naturally in plant foods, particularly in red and purple grapes (and thus red wine), Japanese knotweed, peanuts, deep blue/red/purple berries, some juices, and soy. The nutrient is believed to provide many health benefits, including a decreased risk for heart disease. Most of the research, however, has been conducted in animal studies, and there is no definite evidence for health benefits in humans. The media has capitalized on the idea that red wine is good for the heart because of its resveratrol content. There may be other nutrients found in red wine that either alone or in synergy with resveratrol provide benefits. Also, the amount of resveratrol obtained in red wine, juice, or other natural foods is too low in comparison to the therapeutic dose used in the research studies. It is practically impossible, if not foolish, to drink the amount of red wine necessary to approach the therapeutic dose used in the animal studies. More research in humans is clearly needed before definitive claims can be made.

Is chocolate heart healthy?

Chocolate is heart healthy because of its content of cocoa antioxidant polyphenol compounds called flavonoids. Chocolate helps lower the risk for heart attacks, strokes, and even type 2 diabetes. Some of the ingredients in chocolate help reduce LDL (bad) cholesterol, increase blood flow to the brain, improve blood sugar absorption and insulin sensitivity, discourage blood clots, and increase nitric oxide levels. Nitric oxide helps relax and dilate arteries and keep them flexible, lowering blood pressure slightly in hypertensive and prehypertensive individuals. Even modest reductions in blood pressure (two to three points on both systolic and diastolic pressure scales) significantly lower coronary artery disease and stroke mortality.

Dark chocolate has a much higher concentration of flavonoids than milk chocolate, while white chocolate has none. Flavonoids enhance activity of special proteins called sterol regulatory element-binding proteins (SREBPs), which are involved in cholesterol metabolism. Activated SREBPs bind to genes on DNA that increase a protein called apolipoprotein A1 in the liver, which is the major protein component of the "good" HDL cholesterol. Flavonoids also decrease liver production of another protein, apolipoprotein B, which is the major protein component of the "bad" LDL cholesterol and increase activity of LDL receptors that induce more cholesterol for removal from the bloodstream. Flavonoids may also fight atherosclerosis (plaque buildup) in the arteries by decreasing the amount of oxidized LDL cholesterol, a major contributor to atherosclerosis.

Dark chocolate with at least 70 percent cocoa content provides the healthiest compounds. The darker the chocolate, the less room for sugar. Milk chocolate contains about twice as much sugar as the darkest chocolate. And although chocolate has saturated fat, it is primarily stearic acid, which has a neutral effect on cholesterol. Unfortunately, the chocolate Americans love most is loaded with sugar, fat, and calories. Do not consume chocolate made with palm, coconut, hydrogenated, or partially hydrogenated oils, and avoid chewy, caramel, marshmallow, or cream-covered chocolates.

High-quality dark chocolate is not a food to be eaten liberally, but it's a health food to be enjoyed in moderation. Keep in mind that chocolate is calorie dense. Eat too much of any type of chocolate, and you will gain weight. Overweightness and obesity are major health problems, with corresponding negative effects on morbidity and mortality. As little as .25 ounce of daily dark chocolate has been shown to provide health benefits. The equivalent of one (26 calories, .6 ounce) to two daily dark-chocolate Hershey's Kisses is all that is needed. Unsweetened cocoa powder with skim or fat-free milk and a touch of sweetener is an even better choice. Chocolate should be viewed as a treat—not a health food. Fruits and vegetables are still better sources of flavonoids.

Real Life Story | Peter's Experience

My father died at the age of 42 of a heart attack. One of my grandfathers also died from heart disease in his fifties. It was a great tragedy for my family to lose my dad and grandpa at such early ages, but it never occurred to me that this was something that could happen to me. However, last year at the age of 25 I found myself weighing almost 240 pounds on a 6-foot frame. I loved high fat foods like bacon, cheese, and especially baked goods such as muffins or donuts. I have now learned these foods are high in saturated fats, trans fats, and processed carbohydrates. Eating this way caused me to carry a "spare tire" of extra weight around my middle. I knew my habits weren't healthy, but I didn't give it a lot of thought because I figured, "I'm still young. I can start eating healthier when I get older." However, when I went to see my doctor, I learned that my cholesterol was high: 220. This was a wake-up call for me and I realized that if I didn't change things I could be heading down the same path that led to the deaths of my father and grandfather. I immediately started an exercise program of walking or biking four to five days a week. I drastically cut down on high-fat foods, most red meats, and refined sugars. I started trying to get 25 grams or more of fiber a day, eating whole grains, fruits, and vegetables. At first the new diet tasted very boring to me, but after a while I developed a taste for healthy foods. I also limited my portion sizes. Over the course of a little over a year, I lost 60 pounds. People I hadn't seen for a while sometimes didn't recognize me at first! When I went back to my doctor recently, I learned that my cholesterol had dropped to 182. I feel like I have given myself and my heart a whole new lease on life.

PERSONAL PROFILE: My Cardiovascular Risk Profile

I. Do you try to incorporate as much physical activity as possible and avoid excessive sitting on a daily basis?
___ Yes ___ No

II. Does your diet have ample amounts of grains, fruits, and vegetables, and do you limit the intake of red meats, whole milk products, simple carbohydrates, refined sugars, and processed foods in your diet? ___ Yes ___ No

III. Are you aware of the most significant risk factors that lead to coronary heart disease and the factors that you have control over by the way you choose to live your life?
___ Yes ___ No

IV. Have you ever had a blood lipid analysis test done and what do the results tell you about your current lifestyle, genetics, and potential risk for cardiovascular disease?
___ Yes ___ No

V. Are you familiar with the effects of low-grade inflammation on heart disease and lifestyle factors that increase C-reactive protein levels? ___ Yes ___ No

10.1 Prevalence of Cardiovascular Disease

About 30 percent of all deaths in the United States are attributable to **cardiovascular disease** (CVD), the most prevalent degenerative condition in the United States.[1] Half of all American adults presently have at least one of three leading **risk factors** for cardiovascular disease: uncontrolled high cholesterol, hypertension, or cigarette smoking; and more than a third of the adult population has some form of heart and blood vessel disease. According to the Centers for Disease Control and Prevention (CDC), about 60 percent of deaths from heart disease are sudden and unexpected, with no previous symptoms of the disease. Almost half of these deaths occur outside of the hospital, most likely because the individuals failed to recognize early warning symptoms of a heart attack.

Some examples of CVD are coronary heart disease, stroke, **peripheral vascular disease**, congenital heart disease, rheumatic heart disease, atherosclerosis, high blood pressure, and congestive heart failure. According to CDC estimates, if all deaths from major CVDs were eliminated, life expectancy in the United States would increase by about 7 years.

The American Heart Association estimates the cost of heart and blood vessel disease in the United States at $312.6 billion per year. About 1 million people have new or recurrent heart attacks each year, and more than 40 percent of them will die as a result. More than half of these deaths occur within 1 hour of the onset of symptoms, before the person reaches the hospital.

10.2 Stroke

When CVDs are separated by categories, **stroke** becomes the third leading cause of death in the United States, accounting for approximately 129,000 deaths each year. About 800,000 new or recurrent strokes are reported each year, and of these, more than a third of these people are left with permanent disabilities. About 20 percent of those who survive require institutional care.

Stroke is the most significant contributor to mental and physical disability in the United States, yet it does not draw the same attention as coronary heart disease, high blood pressure, diabetes, or cancer. Similar to those for coronary heart disease, most risk factors for stroke are preventable. Table 10.1 lists the major risk factors; the first four factors are beyond a person's control, whereas the latter seven are fully manageable.

Although heart and blood vessel disease is still the number-one health problem in the United States, the incidence declined by 45 percent between 1960 and 2010 (see Figure 10.1), in large part because of health education. People now are aware of the risk factors for CVD and are changing their lifestyle to lower their potential risk for these diseases.

Table 10.1 Stroke Risk Factors

Unchangeable factors
Age: Increased risk after age 55
Gender: Higher risk in men
Race: African Americans are at greater risk
Family history

Manageable factors
Tobacco use: Stop!
Blood pressure: Maintain in normal range
Diet: Decrease fat and sodium consumption and increase intake of potassium, fruits, and vegetables
Activity level: Increase frequency and intensity
Weight: Maintain within recommended range
Cholesterol: Maintain normal levels
Diabetes: Prevent or manage condition

Figure 10.1 Incidence of cardiovascular disease in the United States for selected years: 1900–2010.

SOURCE: Centers for Disease Control and Prevention, Atlanta.

10.3 Coronary Heart Disease

The heart and the coronary arteries are illustrated in Figure 10.2. The major form of CVD is **coronary heart disease (CHD)**, in which fatty deposits, primarily cholesterol, narrow the arteries that supply the heart muscle with oxygen and nutrients. Narrowing of the coronary arteries diminishes the blood supply to the heart muscle, which can precipitate a heart attack.

CHD is the single leading cause of death in the United States, accounting for about 20 percent of all deaths and approximately half of all deaths from CVD. Approximately 80 percent of deaths from CHD in people younger than age 65 occur during the first heart attack. CHD is the leading cause of sudden cardiac deaths. The risk of death is also greater in the least-educated segment of the population. Each year, more than 500,000 coronary bypass operations and more

Chapter 10 Preventing Cardiovascular Disease

Figure 10.2 The heart and its blood vessels.

Normal healthy heart

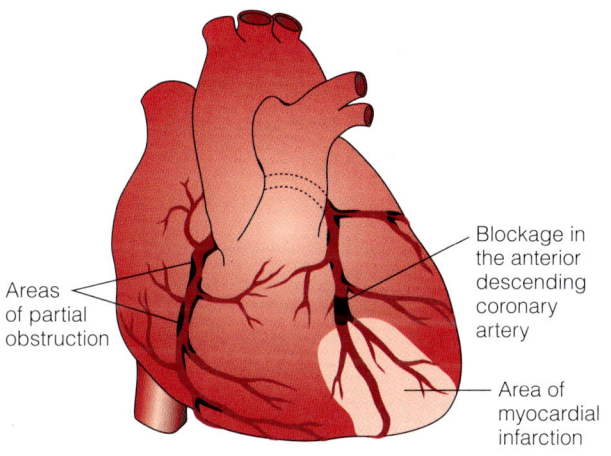

Myocardial infarction (heart attack) as a result of acute reduction in blood flow through the anterior descending coronary artery

Signs of Heart Attack and Stroke

Any or all of the following signs may occur during a heart attack or a stroke. If you experience any of these and they last longer than a few minutes, call 911 and seek medical attention immediately. Failure to do so may cause irreparable damage and even result in death.

Warning Signs of a Heart Attack

- Chest pain, discomfort, pressure, or squeezing that lasts for several minutes. These feelings may go away and return later.
- Pain or discomfort in the shoulders, neck, or arms or between the shoulder blades.
- Chest discomfort with shortness of breath, lightheadedness, cold sweats, nausea and/or vomiting, a feeling of indigestion, sudden fatigue or weakness, fainting, or sense of impending doom.

Warning Signs of Stroke

- Sudden weakness or numbness of the face, arm, or leg—particularly on one side of the body
- Sudden severe headache
- Sudden confusion, dizziness, or difficulty with speech and understanding
- Sudden difficulty walking; loss of balance or coordination
- Sudden visual difficulty

than 1 million coronary **angioplasty** procedures are performed in the United States.

Coronary Heart Disease Risk Profile Although genetic inheritance plays a role in CHD, the most important determinant is personal lifestyle. Most of the major risk factors for CHD are preventable and reversible. CHD risk factor analyses are administered to evaluate the impact of a person's lifestyle and genetic endowment as potential contributors to the development of coronary disease. The specific objectives of a CHD risk factor analysis follow:

- Screen individuals who may be at high risk for the disease
- Educate people regarding the leading risk factors for developing CHD
- Implement programs aimed at reducing the risks
- Use the analysis as a starting point from which to compare changes induced by the intervention program

Leading Risk Factors for CHD The leading risk factors contributing to CHD are listed in Table 10.2. A self-assessment of risk factors for CHD is given in Activity 10.1. This analysis can be done even if you have little or no medical information about your cardiovascular health. The guidelines for zero risk are outlined for each factor, mak-

> **Cardiovascular disease (CVD)** The array of conditions that affect the heart and the blood vessels.
>
> **Risk factors** Lifestyle and genetic variables that may lead to disease.
>
> **Peripheral vascular disease** Narrowing of the peripheral blood vessels.
>
> **Stroke** Condition in which a blood vessel that feeds the brain ruptures or is clogged, leading to blood flow disruption to the brain.
>
> **Coronary heart disease (CHD)** Condition in which the arteries that supply the heart muscle with oxygen and nutrients are narrowed by fatty deposits, such as cholesterol and triglycerides.
>
> **Angioplasty** A procedure in which a balloon-tipped catheter is inserted, then inflated, to widen the inner lumen of the artery.

Table 10.2 Weighting System for CHD Risk Factors

Risk Factor	Maximal Risk Points
Unhealthy diet	14
Physical inactivity	8
Smoking	8
Body mass index	8
Hypertension	8
Personal history of heart disease	8
Abnormal heart function	8
Diabetes	6
Family history of heart disease	6
Age	4
Tension and stress	3

© Cengage Learning

ing this self-analysis a valuable tool for managing risk factors for CHD.

To provide a meaningful score for CHD risk, a weighting system was developed to show the impact of each risk factor on developing the disease (see Table 10.2 and Activity 10.1). This system is based on current research and on the work done at leading preventive medical facilities in the United States. The most significant risk factors are given the heaviest numerical weight.

Based on actual test results, a person receives a score anywhere from zero to the maximum number of points for each factor. When the risk points from all of the risk factors are totaled, the final number is used to place an individual in one of five overall risk categories for potential development of CHD (see Activity 10.1).

Regular physical activity helps to control most of the major risk factors that lead to heart disease.

Healthy Lifestyle Cuts Risk of Sudden Cardiac Death

Sudden cardiac death (SCD) is caused by a sudden and unexpected loss of heart function. It is the largest cause of natural death in the United States, responsible for more than 300,000 adult deaths each year, or about half of all heart disease deaths. SCD occurs when the heart's electrical system does not function properly and suddenly becomes very irregular. The heart can beat dangerously fast causing the ventricles to flutter or quiver, and blood is not delivered to the body. The greatest concern is the lack of blood flow to the brain during the initial few minutes that causes a person to lose consciousness. Death is almost always imminent unless the person receives immediate emergency treatment. SCD can also take place during an attack itself, as the heart muscle is damaged because it does not receive sufficient oxygen-rich blood.

Research conducted on more than 81,000 women tracked during 26 years showed that adherence to a low-risk lifestyle significantly decreases the risk of SCD. The low-risk lifestyle included the following factors:

- Not smoking
- Being physically active for at least 30 minutes a day
- Not being overweight or obese
- Eating a diet rich in fruits, vegetables, whole grains, nuts, beans, fish, and with considerably more monounsaturated than saturated fat; moderate use of alcohol; and low intake of red and processed meats

The authors concluded that a low-risk lifestyle could prevent as much as 81 percent of the yearly SCDs in the United States.

Source: S. E. Chiuve, "Adherence to a Low-Risk, Healthy Lifestyle and Risk of Sudden Cardiac Death Among Women," *Journal of the American Medical Association* 306 (2011): 62-69.

The "Very Low" CHD risk category designates the group at lowest risk for developing heart disease based on age and gender. "Low" CHD suggests that even though people in this category are taking good care of their cardiovascular health, they can improve it (unless all of the risk points come from age and family history). "Moderate" CHD risk means that the person can definitely improve his or her lifestyle to lower the risk for disease, or medical treatment may be required. A score in the "High" or "Very High" CHD risk category points to a strong probability of developing heart disease within the next few years and calls for immediate implementation of a personal risk-reduction program, including professional medical, nutritional, and physical activity intervention.

The leading risk factors for CHD are discussed next, along with the general recommendations for risk reduction.

Activity 10.1: Self-Assessment Coronary Heart Disease Risk Factor Analysis

Name _____ Date _____

Course _____ Section _____ Gender _____ Age _____

I. Instructions

The disease process for cardiovascular disease starts early in life, primarily as a result of poor lifestyle habits. Studies have shown beginning stages of atherosclerosis and elevated blood lipids in children as young as 10 years old. Consequently, the purpose of this activity is to establish a baseline CHD risk profile and to point out the "zero-risk" level for each coronary risk factor.

			Score
1. Physical Activity	Do you get 30 or more minutes of moderate-intensity physical activity: Fewer than 3 times per week....................8 Between 3 and 4 times per week....................3 5 or more times per week....................0		
2. Abnormal Heart Function	Do you ever feel your heart beat irregularly, skipping beats, fluttering, or palpitating....................2–8		
3. Diet (use the highest score if all apply)	Does your regular diet include: 1 or more daily servings of red meat; 7 or more eggs/week; daily butter, cheese, whole milk, refined carbohydrates, alcohol, processed foods; and frequent grilling or cooking meat and poultry at high temperatures....................10–14 3 to 6 servings of red meat/week; 1% or 2% milk; some cheese, refined carbohydrates, processed foods, and alcohol; some whole grains, fruits, vegetables, and cold-water fish....................4–10 Red meat fewer than 2 times/week; skim milk and skim milk products; limited refined carbohydrates, processed foods, and alcohol; ample daily amounts of whole-grain products, fruits, and vegetables; cold-water fish at least 2 times/week....................0–3		
4. Diabetes	Are you pre-diabetic....................3 Are you diabetic....................6		
5. Blood Pressure Add scores for both readings (e.g., 144/88 score = 4)	Systolic <120....................(0) 121–139....................(1) 140–159....................(3) ≥160....................(4)	Diastolic <80....................(0) 0 81–89....................(1) 1–2 90–99....................(3) 3–6 ≥100....................(4) 4–8	
6. Body Mass Index (BMI)	≤25.0....................0 25.0–29.99....................2 30.0–39.99....................4 ≥40.0....................8		

© Cengage Learning

7. Smoking	Lifetime non-smoker 0	Smoke 1–9 cigarettes/day 3
	Ex-smoker more than 1 year 0	Smoke 10–19 cigarettes/day 4
	Ex-smoker less than 1 year 1	Smoke 20–29 cigarettes/day 5
	Non-smoker, but live or work in	Smoke 30–39 cigarettes/day 6
	smoking environment 2	Smoke 40 or more cigarettes/day 8
	Pipe or cigar smoker, or chew	
	tobacco... 3	
8. Tension and Stress Are you:	Sometimes tense............................... 1 Often tense .... 2 Always tense 3	
9. Personal History	Have you ever had a heart attack, stroke, coronary disease, or any known heart problem:	
	During the last year 8	2–5 years ago 3
	1–2 years ago 5	More than 5 years ago 2
10. Family History	Have any of your blood relatives (parents, uncles, brothers, sisters, grandparents) suffered from cardiovascular disease:	
	One or more before age 51 6	One or more after age 60.................. 2
	One or more between 51 and 60....... 4	None had cardiovascular disease...... 0
11. Age	29 or younger.................................... 0	
	30–39.. 1	
	40–49 2	
	50–59 3	
	≥60 4	

How to Score

Total Risk Score:

Risk Category	Total Risk Score
Very Low	5 or fewer points
Low	Between 6 and 15 points
Moderate	Between 16 and 25 points
High	Between 26 and 35 points
Very High	36 or more points

II. Stage of Change for Cardiovascular Disease Prevention

Using Figure 2.5 (page 63) and Table 2.3 (page 62), identify your current stage of change for participation in a cardiovascular disease risk-reduction program:

III.
In a few sentences, using a separate sheet of paper, discuss your family and personal risk for cardiovascular disease. Also, discuss lifestyle changes that you have already implemented in this course, as well as additional changes that you can make to decrease your own risk for cardiovascular disease.

IV. Physical Activity Rating

Number of daily steps at the beginning of the term: Current number of daily steps:

Current physical activity rating (use Table 1.2, page 12):

> **Critical Thinking**
>
> What do you think of your own risk for diseases of the cardiovascular system? • Is this something you need to concern yourself with at this point in your life? • Why or why not?

Physical Inactivity Physical inactivity is responsible for low levels of cardiorespiratory endurance (the ability of the heart, lungs, and blood vessels to deliver enough oxygen to the cells to meet the demands of prolonged physical activity). The level of cardiorespiratory endurance (or fitness) is given most commonly by the maximal amount of oxygen (in milliliters) that every kilogram (2.2 pounds) of body weight is able to utilize per minute of physical activity (mL/kg/min). As maximal oxygen uptake (VO_{2max}) increases, so does efficiency of the cardiorespiratory system. Improving cardiorespiratory endurance through aerobic exercise and daily physical activity greatly reduces the overall risk for heart disease.

For habitually sedentary people, sudden heavy-duty physical activity, such as shoveling snow or strenuous yard work, can trigger a cardiovascular event. The research shows that unaccustomed physical exertion increases the risk for a cardiovascular incident 50- to 100-fold.

Although specific recommendations can be followed to improve each risk factor, daily physical activity and a regular aerobic exercise program help to control most of the major risk factors that lead to heart disease. Physical activity and aerobic exercise will:

- Increase cardiorespiratory endurance
- Decrease and control blood pressure
- Reduce body fat
- Lower blood lipids (cholesterol and triglycerides)
- Improve HDL cholesterol
- Prevent and help control diabetes
- Decrease low-grade (hidden) inflammation in the body
- Increase and maintain good heart function, sometimes improving certain electrocardiogram abnormalities
- Motivate toward smoking cessation
- Alleviate tension and stress
- Counteract a personal history of heart disease

Data from the research summarized in Figure 1.11 in Chapter 1 clearly show the tie between physical activity and mortality, regardless of age and other risk factors. A higher level of physical fitness benefits even those who exhibit other risk factors, such as high blood pressure and serum cholesterol, cigarette smoking, and a family history of heart disease. In most cases, less fit people in the study without these risk factors had higher death rates than highly fit people with these same risk factors.

The findings show that the higher the level of cardiorespiratory fitness, the longer the life, but the largest drop in premature death is seen between the "unfit" and the "moderately fit" groups. Even small improvements in cardiorespiratory endurance greatly decrease the risk for cardiovascular mortality.

Most adults who engage in a moderate exercise program can attain these fitness levels easily. A 2-mile walk in 30 to 40 minutes, 5 to 7 days a week, is adequate to decrease risk.

Subsequent research published in the *New England Journal of Medicine* substantiated the importance of exercise in preventing CHD.[2] The benefits to previously inactive adults of starting a moderate to vigorous physical activity program were as important as quitting smoking, managing blood pressure, or controlling cholesterol. In relative risk for death from CHD, the increase in physical activity led to the same decrease as giving up cigarette smoking.

The scientific data are quite clear that moderate-intensity physical activity provides substantial benefits in terms of overall cardiovascular risk reduction. The exact amount of aerobic exercise required to decrease the risk for cardiovascular disease is difficult to establish and most likely varies due to genetics, age, gender, body composition, health status, and personal lifestyle, among other factors. What may be sufficient for a low-risk individual may not be enough for someone else with disease risk factors. For example, an apparently healthy individual at recommended body weight may not need more than 30 daily minutes of accumulated moderate-intensity physical activity. Another person with a weight problem and other risk factors such as high blood pressure, cholesterol abnormalities, and borderline high blood sugar may need a much greater amount of activity to counteract these risk factors.

Although research may never indicate the exact amount of aerobic exercise required to lower the risk for cardiovascular disease, pioneer research in this area conducted in the 1980s showed that expending 2,000 calories per week as a result of physical activity yielded the lowest risk for cardiovascular disease among a group of almost 17,000 Harvard alumni. Expending 2,000 calories per week represents about 300 calories per daily exercise session or the equivalent of jogging 3 miles in 30 minutes or walking 3 miles in about 45 minutes.

When feasible, scientific studies indicate that vigorous-intensity activity is preferable because of greater improvements in aerobic fitness, blood pressure, glucose control, and a larger reduction in CHD risk.[3] A note of caution: Do not engage in vigorous exercise without proper clearance and a minimum of six weeks of proper conditioning through moderate-intensity activity.

A comprehensive and systematic research review of the effects of physical activity on all-cause mortality was published in 2011. The research included 80 studies that involved more than 1.3 million people. The review concluded that physical activity prolongs life and that premature death risk decreased the most as activity time increased with vigorous exercise.[4] Each weekly hour of light, moderate, or vigorous activity decreased mortality rates by 4, 6, and 9 percent, respectively. Furthermore, for every 1,000 weekly calories expanded through exercise, the mortality rate decreased by 11 percent.

In terms of life expectancy, 2012 research involving 654,827 individuals looking at leisure time physical activity of moderate to vigorous intensity and their effects on mortality, the results indicated that higher levels of physical activity are associated with greater gains in life expectancy. People at the highest level of physical activity gained 4.5 years in life expectancy and being active and normal weight (BMI of 18.5 to 24.9) yielded a gain of 7.2 years of life as compared to being inactive and obese.[5]

Also, try to minimize total daily sitting time. Research data indicate that excessive daily sitting (at a desk, commuting to and from work, eating meals, and watching television) increases the risk for cardiovascular disease, obesity, some chronic disorders, and premature mortality. The risk is increased even among people who meet the 30 minutes of moderate-intensity physical activity on most days of the week but still spend a large part of the day sitting. If your job (as most nowadays do) requires that a large portion of the day be spent in a sitting position, at least make yourself get up and take frequent breaks. Small creative lifestyle changes make a difference, such as always answering the phone standing; walking to the office next door instead of texting, e-mailing, IMing, or using the phone; and using stairs instead of elevators and escalators. When watching television, make it a point to get up and walk around during each commercial break. Even better, do dips at the edge of the couch or stand up and sit down 20 times to strengthen your thigh muscles.

While aerobically fit individuals have a lower incidence of cardiovascular disease, regular physical activity and aerobic exercise by themselves do not guarantee a lifetime free of cardiovascular problems. Poor lifestyle habits—such as smoking, eating too many fatty/salty/sweet foods, being overweight, and having high stress levels—increase cardiovascular risk, and their effects will not be eliminated completely through an active lifestyle.

Overall management of risk factors is the best guideline to lower the risk for CVD. Still, aerobic exercise is one of the most important factors in preventing and reducing cardiovascular problems. Based on the overwhelming amount of scientific data in this area, evidence of the benefits of aerobic exercise in reducing heart disease is far too impressive to be ignored. Low fitness is more dangerous than obesity, smoking, high cholesterol, or diabetes. The basic principles for cardiorespiratory exercise are given in Chapter 6.

As more research studies are conducted, the addition of strength training is increasingly recommended for good heart function. The American Heart Association (AHA) recommends strength training even for individuals who have had a heart attack or have high blood pressure, as long as they strength-train under a physician's advice. Strength training helps control body weight and blood sugar and lowers cholesterol and blood pressure.

Abnormal Electrocardiograms The **electrocardiogram (ECG or EKG)** is a valuable measure of the heart's function. The ECG provides a record of the electrical impulses that stimulate the heart to contract (see Figure 10.3). In reading an ECG, doctors interpret five general areas: heart rate, heart rhythm, axis of the heart, enlargement or hypertrophy of the heart, and myocardial infarction.

During a standard 12-lead ECG, 10 electrodes are placed on the person's chest. From these 10 electrodes, 12 tracings,

Figure 10.3 Normal electrocardiogram.

P wave = atrial depolarization
QRS complex = ventricular depolarization
T wave = ventricular repolarization

or "leads," of the electrical impulses as they travel through the heart muscle, or **myocardium**, are studied from 12 different positions. By looking at ECG tracings, medical professionals can identify abnormalities in heart functioning (see Figure 10.4). Based on the findings, the ECG may be interpreted as normal, equivocal, or abnormal. An ECG will not always identify problems, so a normal tracing is not an absolute guarantee. Conversely, an abnormal tracing does not necessarily signal a serious condition.

ECGs are taken at rest, during the stress of exercise, and during recovery. A **stress electrocardiogram** is also known as a "graded exercise stress test" or a "maximal exercise tolerance test." Similar to a high-speed test on a car, a stress ECG reveals the tolerance of the heart to increased physical activity. It is a much better test than a resting ECG to discover CHD.

Stress ECGs also are used to assess cardiorespiratory fitness levels, to screen individuals for preventive and cardiac rehabilitation programs, to detect abnormal blood pressure response during exercise, and to establish actual or functional maximal heart rate for exercise prescription. The recovery ECG is another important diagnostic tool to monitor the return of the heart's activity to normal conditions.

Figure 10.4 Abnormal electrocardiogram showing a depressed S–T segment.

S–T segment

Chapter 10 Preventing Cardiovascular Disease 349

Exercise tolerance test with 12-lead electrocardiographic monitoring (an exercise stress ECG).

pectoris, do not start until the arteries are about 75 percent blocked. In many cases, the first symptom is sudden death.

The recommendation of the National Cholesterol Education Program (NCEP) is to keep total cholesterol levels less than 200 mg/dL. Cholesterol levels between 200 and 239 mg/dL are borderline high, and levels of 240 mg/dL and greater indicate high risk for disease (see Table 10.3). The risk for heart attack increases 2 percent for every 1 percent increase in total cholesterol.[6] About one-half of U.S. adults have total cholesterol values of 200 mg/dL or greater.

Preventive medicine practitioners often recommend a range between 160 and 180 mg/dL as best for total cholesterol. Furthermore, in the Framingham Heart Study (a 60-year ongoing project in the community of Framingham, Massachusetts), not a single individual with a total cholesterol level of 150 mg/dL or less has had a heart attack.

As important as it is, total cholesterol is not the best predictor for cardiovascular risk. Many heart attacks occur in people with only slightly elevated total cholesterol. More significant is the way in which cholesterol is carried in the bloodstream. Cholesterol is transported primarily in the form of LDL and HDL.

LDL ("bad") cholesterol tends to release cholesterol, which then may penetrate the lining of the arteries and speed the process of atherosclerosis. The

Not every adult who wishes to start or continue an exercise program needs a stress ECG. No set of guidelines can cover all cases when a stress electrocardiogram is recommended prior to exercise participation. The test, however, is recommended for individuals who are at high risk or are known to have cardiovascular, pulmonary, renal, or metabolic disease. Moreover, people feeling unusually winded in response to normal exertion, unexplained fatigue, or chest pain, should have the test done.

At times, the stress ECG has been questioned as a reliable predictor of CHD. Nevertheless, it remains the most practical, inexpensive, noninvasive procedure available to diagnose latent (undiagnosed/unknown) CHD. The test is accurate in diagnosing CHD about 65 percent of the time. The sensitivity of the test increases along with the severity of the disease, and more accurate results are seen in people who are at high risk for CVD.

Abnormal Cholesterol Profile Cholesterol receives much attention because of its direct relationship to heart disease. **Blood lipids** (cholesterol and triglycerides) are carried in the bloodstream by protein molecules of **HDLs**, **LDLs**, **very low density lipoproteins (VLDLs)**, and **chylomicrons**. An increased risk for CHD has been established in individuals with high total cholesterol, high LDL cholesterol, and low HDL cholesterol.

An abnormal cholesterol profile contributes to **atherosclerosis**, the buildup of fatty tissue in the walls of the arteries (Figure 10.5). As the plaque builds up, it blocks the blood vessels that supply the myocardium with oxygen and nutrients (the coronary arteries), and these obstructions can trigger a **myocardial infarction**, or heart attack.

Unfortunately, the heart disguises its problems quite well, and typical symptoms of heart disease, such as **angina**

Electrocardiogram (ECG or EKG) A recording of the electrical activity of the heart.

Myocardium Heart muscle.

Stress electrocardiogram An exercise test during which the workload is increased gradually until the individual reaches maximal fatigue, with blood pressure and 12-lead electrocardiographic monitoring throughout the test.

Cholesterol A waxy substance, technically a steroid alcohol, found only in animal fats and oil; used in making cell membranes, as a building block for some hormones, in the fatty sheath around nerve fibers, and other necessary substances.

Blood lipids (fat) Cholesterol and triglycerides.

High-density lipoproteins (HDLs) Cholesterol-transporting molecules in the blood ("good" cholesterol) that help clear cholesterol from the blood.

Low-density lipoproteins (LDLs) Cholesterol-transporting molecules in the blood ("bad" cholesterol) that tend to increase blood cholesterol.

Very low density lipoproteins (VLDLs) Triglyceride, cholesterol, and phospholipid-transporting molecules in the blood.

Chylomicrons Triglyceride-transporting molecules.

Atherosclerosis Fatty/cholesterol deposits in the walls of the arteries leading to formation of plaque.

Myocardial infarction Heart attack; damage to or death of an area of the heart muscle as a result of an obstructed artery to that area.

Angina pectoris Chest pain associated with coronary heart disease.

Figure 10.5 Comparison of a normal healthy artery (A) and diseased arteries (B and C).

The Atherosclerotic Process

NCEP guidelines given in Table 10.3 state that an LDL cholesterol value less than 100 mg/dL is optimal.

Even when more LDL cholesterol is present than the cells can use, cholesterol seems not to cause a problem until it is oxidized by free radicals (see discussion under "Antioxidants" in Chapter 3, pages 105–106). After cholesterol is oxidized, white blood cells invade the arterial wall, take up the cholesterol, and clog the arteries.

LDL cholesterol particles are of two types: large, or pattern A; and small, or pattern B. Small particles are thought to pass through the inner lining of the coronary arteries more readily, thereby increasing the risk for a heart attack. A predominance of small particles can lead to a sixfold increase in the risk for CHD.

A genetic variation of LDL cholesterol, known as lipoprotein-a or Lp(a), is also noteworthy because a high level of these particles promotes blood clots and earlier development of atherosclerosis. It is thought that certain substances in the arterial wall interact with Lp(a) and lead to premature formation of plaque. About 10 percent of the population has elevated levels of Lp(a). Only medications help decrease Lp(a), and drug options should be discussed with a physician.

Intermediate-density lipoprotein (IDL) is also of concern because these mid-sized particles are more likely to cause atherosclerosis than a similar amount of LDL cholesterol. For individuals at risk for heart disease, a comprehensive blood lipid profile that includes total cholesterol, HDL cholesterol, LDL cholesterol, Lp(a), IDL, and size pattern (A and B) is recommended.

In a process known as **reverse cholesterol transport**, HDLs act as "scavengers," removing cholesterol from the body and preventing plaque from forming in the arteries. The strength of HDL is in the protein molecules found in its coating. When HDL comes in contact with cholesterol-filled cells, these protein molecules attach to the cells and take their cholesterol.

The more HDL ("good") cholesterol, the better. HDL cholesterol offers some protection against heart disease. A low level of HDL cholesterol is one of the strongest predictors of CHD at all levels of total cholesterol, including levels less than 200 mg/dL. Data suggest that for every 1 mg/dL increase in HDL cholesterol, the risk for CHD drops up to 3 percent in men and 5 percent in women.[7] The recommended HDL cholesterol values to minimize the risk for CHD are at least 40 mg/dL. HDL cholesterol levels greater than 60 mg/dL help to lower the risk for CHD.

Fourteen subgroups of HDL particles have been identified, falling into HDL2 and HDL3 categories. HDL2 are larger particles that carry cholesterol from the arterial wall to the liver for disposal. These particles also have antioxidant and anti-inflammatory effects. In particular, the subgroup HDL2b seems to be most significant because they appear to remove approximately 80 percent of the LDL cholesterol. The HDL3 particles also transports cholesterol out of the arterial wall but may not

Table 10.3 Cholesterol Guidelines

	Amount	Rating
Total Cholesterol	<200 mg/dL	Desirable
	200–239 mg/dL	Borderline high
	≥240 mg/dL	High risk
LDL Cholesterol	<100 mg/dL	Optimal
	100–129 mg/dL	Near or greater than optimal
	130–159 mg/dL	Borderline high
	160–189 mg/dL	High
	≥190 mg/dL	Very high
HDL Cholesterol	<40 mg/dL	Low (high risk)
	≥60 mg/dL	High (low risk)

From National Cholesterol Education Program.

Table 10.4 Cholesterol and Saturated Fat Content of Selected Foods

Food	Serving Size	Cholesterol (mg)	Sat. Fat (gr)
Avocado	1/8 med.	—	3.2
Bacon	2 slices	30	2.7
Beans (all types)	any	—	—
Beef—lean, fat trimmed off	3 oz	75	6.0
Beef heart (cooked)	3 oz	150	1.6
Beef liver (cooked)	3 oz	255	1.3
Butter	1 tsp	12	0.4
Caviar	1 oz	85	—
Cheese			
American	2 oz	54	11.2
Cheddar	2 oz	60	12.0
Cottage (1% fat)	1 cup	10	0.4
Cottage (4% fat)	1 cup	31	6.0
Cream	2 oz	62	6.0
Muenster	2 oz	54	10.8
Parmesan	2 oz	38	9.3
Swiss	2 oz	52	10.0
Chicken (no skin)	3 oz	45	0.4
Chicken liver	3 oz	472	1.1
Chicken thigh, wing	3 oz	69	3.3
Egg (yolk)	1 lrg	218	1.6
Frankfurter	2	90	11.2
Fruits	any	—	—
Grains (all types)	any	—	—
Halibut, flounder	3 oz	43	0.7
Ice cream	½ cup	27	4.4
Lamb	3 oz	60	7.2
Lard	1 tsp	5	1.9
Lobster	3 oz	170	0.5
Margarine (all vegetable)	1 tsp	—	0.7
Mayonnaise	1 tbsp	10	2.1
Milk			
Skim	1 cup	5	0.3
Low fat (2%)	1 cup	18	2.9
Whole	1 cup	34	5.1
Nuts	1 oz	—	1.0
Oysters	3 oz	42	—
Salmon	3 oz	30	0.8
Scallops	3 oz	29	—
Sherbet	½ cup	7	1.2
Shrimp	3 oz	128	0.1
Trout	3 oz	45	2.1
Tuna (canned–drained)	3 oz	55	—
Turkey dark meat	3 oz	60	0.6
Turkey light meat	3 oz	50	0.4
Vegetables			
(except avocado)	any	—	—

© Cengage Learning

be as effective as HDL2. HDL3, however, seems to protect against cholesterol oxidation that results in atherosclerosis.

For the most part, HDL cholesterol is determined genetically. Generally, women have higher levels than men. Because the female sex hormone estrogen tends to raise HDL, premenopausal women have a much lower incidence of heart disease. African American children and adult men have higher HDL values than Caucasians. HDL cholesterol also decreases with age.

Increasing HDL cholesterol improves the cholesterol profile and lessens the risk for CHD. Habitual aerobic exercise, a diet high in omega-3 fatty acids, weight loss, nonsmoking, and modest alcohol intake help raise HDL cholesterol. Drug therapy may also promote higher HDL cholesterol levels. Niacin helps convert HDL3 to HDL2.

Improved HDL cholesterol is clearly related to a regular aerobic exercise program (preferably high intensity, or greater than 6 metabolic equivalents [METs], for at least 20 minutes three times per week—see Chapter 6). Individual responses to aerobic exercise differ, but generally, the more you exercise, the higher your HDL cholesterol level.

Counteracting Cholesterol

The average adult in the United States consumes between 400 and 600 mg of cholesterol daily. The body, however, manufactures more than that. Saturated and trans fats (trans fatty acids) raise cholesterol levels more than anything else in the diet. These fats produce approximately 1,000 mg of cholesterol per day. Because of individual differences, some people can have a higher-than-normal intake of saturated and trans fats and still maintain normal levels. Others, who have a lower intake, can have abnormally high levels.

Saturated fats are found mostly in meats and dairy products and seldom in foods of plant origin (see Table 10.4). Poultry and fish contain less saturated fat than beef does, but should be eaten in moderation (about 3 to 6 ounces per day—see Chapter 3). In a 10-year study of more than 500,000 men and women older than the age of 50, those who ate the most red meat (an average of 4.5 ounces per day), had a much higher risk of dying from heart disease and cancer.[8] Of those who ate the most red meat, men had a 31 percent higher risk of dying during the study period, whereas women had a 50 percent higher risk of dying from heart disease during this time. Cancer risk was about 20 percent higher among men and women who consumed the most red meat.

Unsaturated fats are mainly of plant origin and cannot be converted to cholesterol. Omega-3-rich fish meals (found in salmon, tuna, and mackerel) also help lower **triglycerides** and increase HDL cholesterol.[9] Because of the cardioprotective ben-

> **Reverse cholesterol transport** A process in which HDL molecules attract cholesterol and carry it to the liver, where it is changed to bile and eventually excreted in the stool.
>
> **Triglycerides** Fats formed by glycerol and three fatty acids; also called free fatty acids.

Habitual aerobic exercise helps increase HDL cholesterol ("good" cholesterol).

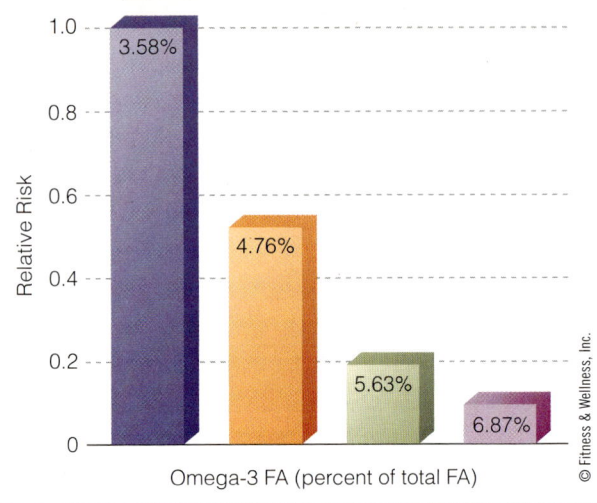

Omega-3 FA (percent of total FA)

efits of omega-3 fatty acids, the American Heart Association recommends eating oily fish at least twice per week. As illustrated in Figure 10.6, baseline blood levels of omega-3 fatty acids are inversely related to the risk of sudden cardiac death.[10] Individuals in the highest quartile of omega-3 fatty acids (mean = 6.87 of total fatty acids) have a 90-percent reduction in sudden cardiac death risk as compared with those in the lowest quartile (mean = 3.58 of total fatty acids).

The antioxidant effect of vitamins C and E may provide benefits. Data suggest that a single unstable free radical (an oxygen compound produced during metabolism—see Chapter 3) can damage LDL particles, accelerating the atherosclerotic process. Vitamin C may inactivate free radicals and slow the oxidation of LDL cholesterol. Vitamin E may protect LDL from oxidation, preventing heart disease, but studies suggest that it does not seem to be helpful in reversing damage once it has taken place.

Trans Fats

Foods that contain trans fatty acids, hydrogenated fat, or partially hydrogenated vegetable oil should be avoided. Studies indicate that these foods elevate LDL cholesterol as much as saturated fats do, but even worse, they lower HDL cholesterol. Trans fats also increase triglycerides. These changes contribute not only to heart disease, but also to gallstone formation. Trans fats are found primarily in **processed foods**.

Food companies have used trans fats because they are inexpensive to produce, easy to use, last a long time, and add taste and texture to food. Restaurants and fast-food chains choose oils with trans fats because they can be used repeatedly in commercial fryers.

Hydrogen frequently is added to monounsaturated and polyunsaturated fats to increase shelf life and to solidify them so that they are more spreadable. Hydrogenation can change the position of hydrogen atoms along the carbon chain, transforming the fat into a trans fatty acid. Margarine and spreads, chips, commercially produced crackers and cookies, and fast foods often contain trans fatty acids. Small amounts of trans fats are also found naturally in some meats, dairy products, and other animal-based foods.

The AHA has issued dietary guidelines for trans fat intake, recommending that people limit trans fat intake to less than 1 percent of the total daily caloric intake.[11] This amount represents about 1.5 grams of trans fats a day for a 1,500 calorie diet, 2 grams for 2,000 calories, and 3 grams for 3,000 calories. Because the FDA now requires that all food labels list the trans fat content, you can keep better track of your daily trans fat intake by paying attention to food labels. Additional information on trans fats is found under the "Trans Fatty Acids" section in Chapter 3 (see page 80).

The FDA allows food manufacturers to label any product that has less than half a gram of trans fat per serving as zero. Be aware that if you eat three or four servings of a particular food near a half a gram of trans fat, you may be getting your maximum daily allowance (1 gram per 1,000 calories of daily caloric intake). Thus, you are encouraged to look at the list of ingredients and search for the words "partially hydrogenated" as an indicator of hidden trans fats.

The labels "partially hydrogenated" and "trans fatty acids" indicate that the product carries a health risk just as high as that of saturated fat. Now that trans fats are listed on food labels, companies are looking to reformulate their products to reduce or eliminate these fats. Some products that once had a high trans fat content now have none. As a consumer, you are encouraged to check food labels often to obtain cur-

Table 10.5 Average Trans Fat Content of Selected Foods*

Food Item	Amount	Grams
Fats/Oils		
Margarine, stick	1 tbsp	2.0
Margarine, tub	1 tbsp	0.5
Butter	1 tbsp	0.3
Shortening	1 tbsp	4.0
Mayonnaise	1 tbsp	0.0
Snacks		
Oreo cookies	3	2.5
Chips Ahoy Chocolate Chip cookies	3	1.5
Ritz crackers	5	1.5
Flavorite Honey Maid Grahams	8 sections	1.5
Fig Newtons	2	1.0
Potato chips	2 oz	3.0
Cake, pound	1 slice (3 oz)	4.5
Candy bar	1	3.0
Fast Foods		
Dunkin' Donuts Apple Fritter	1	2.5
Krispy Kreme Apple Fritter	1	7.0
Krispy Kreme Doughnut, glazed	1	4.0
McDonald's Biscuit	1	5.0
McDonald's Cinnamon Roll	1	4.5
McDonald's Baked Apple Pie	1	4.0
McDonald's Chicken McNuggets	10 pieces	2.5
Burger King French Toast Sticks	5 pieces	4.5
Burger King Chicken Tenders	5 pieces	2.5
Burger King Big Fish Sandwich	1	1.5
KFC Extra Crispy Breast	6 oz	4.5
KFC Breast, original recipe	6 oz	2.5
French fries	1 med (4 oz)	5.0
Taco Bell, Taco	1	0.5
Taco Bell, Taco Supreme	1	1.0
Taco Bell, Burrito	1	2.0
Taco Bell, Burrito Supreme, beef	1	2.0

NOTE: Trans fat intake should be limited to no more than 1 percent of total daily caloric intake or the equivalent of 1 gram per 1,000 calories of energy intake.

*Trans fat content in food items may decrease significantly in the near future as food manufacturers are looking to lower the amount in their products because of FDA regulations that require trans fats to be listed on food labels. Trans fat content also varies between different brands based on food formulation and ingredients. Check food labels regularly to obtain current information.

© Cengage Learning

rent information. Table 10.5 lists the average trans fat content of some foods. These values may vary among brands according to food formulation and ingredients and may change in the near future as manufacturers alter food formulations to decrease or eliminate trans fat content.

Lowering LDL Cholesterol

LDL cholesterol levels higher than ideal can be lowered through dietary changes, by losing body fat, by taking medication, and by participating in a regular aerobic exercise program. Research has shown a higher relative risk of mortality in unfit individuals with low cholesterol than fit people with high cholesterol. The lowest mortality rate, of course, is seen in fit people with low total cholesterol levels.

In terms of dietary modifications, a diet lower in saturated fat, trans fats, and cholesterol and high in fiber is recommended. Saturated fat should be replaced with polyunsaturated and monounsaturated fats because the latter tend to decrease LDL cholesterol and increase HDL cholesterol (see the discussion of "Simple Fats" in Chapter 3, pages 79–82). Total saturated fat intake should be less than 7 percent of the total daily caloric intake, preferably much lower while on a cholesterol-lowering diet. Trans fat intake should be less than 1 percent of daily caloric intake. Exercise is important because dietary manipulation by itself is not as effective in lowering LDL cholesterol as a combination of diet plus aerobic exercise.

Furthermore, "moderate" fat–intake diets (25 to 35 percent of total caloric intake) are better for heart health (as long as most of it is unsaturated fats) than are low-fat diets or highly refined carbohydrate diets. As you increase the intake of unsaturated fats, be sure to substitute these for some other less healthy foods (red meat, sausages, hamburgers, organ meats, butter, margarines, whole-milk products, etc.); otherwise, weight gain will ensue. Excessive carbohydrate intake, especially refined carbohydrates, raises triglycerides, and as triglycerides go up, HDL cholesterol typically decreases.

Total saturated fat intake should be less than 7 percent of the total daily caloric intake and preferably much lower while on a cholesterol-lowering diet. Trans fat intake should be less than 1 percent of the daily caloric intake. Exercise is important because dietary manipulation by itself is not as effective in lowering LDL cholesterol as a combination of diet plus aerobic exercise.

To lower LDL cholesterol significantly, total daily fiber intake must be in the range of 25 to 38 grams per day (see "Fiber" in Chapter 3), and total fat consumption can be in the range of 30 percent of total daily caloric intake—as long as most of the fat is unsaturated fat and the average cholesterol consumption is less than 200 mg. Increasing consumption of cholesterol-lowering foods such as plant sterols (added to some spreads and salad dressings), soy protein, nuts (walnuts, almonds, macadamia nuts, peanuts, pecans, pistachio nuts), vegetables, fruits, whole grains, and foods high in soluble fiber (oats, legumes, and barley), further accelerates the rate of LDL cholesterol reduction. Keep in mind that as you add some of these foods to your diet, you have to take other less healthy foods out.

Among people in the United States, the average fiber intake is less than 15 grams per day. Fiber, in particular the soluble type, has been shown to lower cholesterol. Soluble fiber dissolves in water and forms a gel-like substance that encloses food parti-

> **Processed foods** A food which has been chemically altered from its natural state through additives such as flavors, flavor enhancers, colors, binders, preservatives, stabilizers, emulsifiers, fillers, and so on, or which has been manufactured through combination or other methods.

Behavior Modification Planning

Blood Chemistry Test Guidelines

People who have never had a blood chemistry test should do so to establish a baseline for future reference. The blood test should include total cholesterol, LDL cholesterol, HDL cholesterol, triglycerides, and blood glucose.

Following an initial normal baseline test no later than age 20, for a person who adheres to the recommended dietary and exercise guidelines, a blood analysis at least every 5 years prior to age 40 should suffice. Thereafter, a blood lipid test is recommended every year, in conjunction with a regular preventive medicine physical examination.

A single baseline test is not necessarily a valid measure. Cholesterol levels vary from month to month and sometimes even from day to day. If the initial test reveals cholesterol abnormalities, the test should be repeated within a few weeks to confirm the results.

Try It

Blood chemistry tests are available at many wellness centers on college campuses for less than $25 for a comprehensive test that includes total cholesterol, LDL cholesterol, HDL cholesterol, triglycerides, and blood glucose levels. Have you had your blood test done, and are you aware of your blood lipid profile?

❏ I PLAN TO ❏ I DID IT

---

cles. This property helps bind and excrete fats from the body. Soluble fibers also bind intestinal bile acids that could be recycled into additional cholesterol. Soluble fibers are found primarily in oats, fruits, barley, legumes, and psyllium.

Psyllium, a grain that is added to some multigrain breakfast cereals, also helps lower LDL cholesterol. As little as 3 daily grams of psyllium can lower LDL cholesterol by 20 percent. Commercially available fiber supplements that contain psyllium (such as Metamucil) can be used to increase soluble fiber intake. Three tablespoons daily will add about 10 grams of soluble fiber to the diet.

The incidence of heart disease is very low in populations in which daily fiber intake exceeds 30 grams per day. Further, a Harvard University Medical School study of 43,000 middle-aged men who were followed for more than 6 years showed that increasing fiber intake to 30 daily grams resulted in a 41 percent reduction in heart attacks.[12]

When attempting to lower LDL cholesterol, moderate fat consumption is still encouraged. A drawback of very low-fat diets (less than 25 percent fat) is that they tend to lower HDL cholesterol and increase triglycerides. If HDL cholesterol is already low, monounsaturated and polyunsaturated fats should be added to the diet. Examples of food items that are high in monounsaturated fats and polyunsaturated fats are nuts and olive, canola, corn, and soybean oils. The table of nutritive values in Appendix A can be used to determine food items that are high in monounsaturated and polyunsaturated fats (see also Figure 3.9, page 95).

The NCEP guidelines for people who are trying to decrease LDL cholesterol allow for a diet with up to 35 percent of calories from fat, including 10 percent from polyunsaturated fats and 20 percent from monounsaturated fats.[13] If you are attempting to lower LDL cholesterol, saturated fats should be kept to an absolute minimum.

Margarines and salad dressings that contain stanol ester, a plant-derived compound that interferes with cholesterol absorption in the intestine, are now also on the market. Over the course of several weeks, daily intake of about 3 grams of margarine or 6 tablespoons of salad dressing containing stanol ester lowers LDL cholesterol by 14 percent. Dietary guidelines to lower LDL cholesterol levels are provided in the accompanying box.

The best prescription for controlling blood lipids is the combination of a healthy diet, a sound aerobic exercise program, and weight control. If this does not work, a physician can recommend appropriate drug therapies based on a blood test to analyze the various subcategories of lipoproteins.

The NCEP guidelines recommend that people consider drug therapy if, after 6 months on a diet low in cholesterol and trans fat and saturated fat, cholesterol remains unacceptably high. An unacceptable level is an LDL cholesterol greater than 190 mg/dL for individuals with fewer than two risk factors and no signs of heart disease. For individuals with more than two risk factors and with a history of heart disease, LDL cholesterol greater than 160 mg/dL is unacceptable.

Saturated Fat Replacement in the Diet

Although for years we have known that saturated fat raises LDL cholesterol, a 2010 review of 21 observational research studies involving almost 350,000 people failed to prove a significant association between saturated fat intake and risk of CHD, stroke, or CVD.[14] Researchers are focusing on the foods consumed in the American diet that have replaced saturated fat.

Once people learned that saturated fats were unhealthy, instead of consuming more fruits, vegetables, legumes, and grains, many increased consumption of "low-fat" simple carbohydrates and refined sugars (low-fat varieties of breads, rolls, cereals, cookies, ice cream, cakes, and desserts). Although low in fat, simple carbohydrates and refined sugars are high in calories that lead to weight gain. The data show that exchanging refined carbohydrates for saturated fat exacerbates blood lipid

Behavior Modification Planning

Dietary Guidelines to Lower LDL Cholesterol

I PLAN TO / I DID IT

Minimize the use of simple and refined carbohydrates (including sugars) and processed foods.

- ❑ ❑ Consume between 25 and 38 grams of fiber daily, including a minimum of 10 grams of soluble fiber (good sources are oats, fruits, barley, legumes, and psyllium).
- ❑ ❑ Increase consumption of vegetables, fruits, whole grains, and beans.
- ❑ ❑ Do not consume more than 200 mg of dietary cholesterol a day.
- ❑ ❑ Consume red meats (3 ounces per serving) fewer than 3 times per week and no organ meats (such as liver and kidneys).
- ❑ ❑ Do not eat commercially baked foods.
- ❑ ❑ Avoid foods that contain trans fatty acids, hydrogenated fat, or partially hydrogenated vegetable oil.
- ❑ ❑ Increase intake of omega-3 fatty acids (see Chapter 3) by eating two to three meals of omega-3-rich fish per week.
- ❑ ❑ Consume 25 grams of soy protein a day.
- ❑ ❑ Drink low-fat milk (1 percent or less fat, preferably) and use low-fat dairy products.
- ❑ ❑ Do not use coconut oil, palm oil, or cocoa butter.
- ❑ ❑ Limit egg consumption to fewer than three eggs per week (this is for people with high cholesterol only; others may safely consume an egg on most days of the week).
- ❑ ❑ Use margarines and salad dressings that contain stanol ester instead of butter and regular margarine.
- ❑ ❑ Bake, broil, grill, poach, or steam food instead of frying.
- ❑ ❑ Refrigerate cooked meat before adding to other dishes. Remove fat hardened in the refrigerator before mixing the meat with other foods.
- ❑ ❑ Avoid fatty sauces made with butter, cream, or cheese.
- ❑ ❑ Maintain recommended body weight.

Try It

Dietary guidelines for health and wellness were thoroughly discussed in Chapter 3, "Nutrition for Wellness." How have your dietary habits changed since studying these guidelines, and how well do they support the recommendations to lower LDL cholesterol?

As long as the number of servings and caloric intake are not increased, substituting unsaturated fat/cholesterol-free/trans fat–free products for calorie dense, high-fat/saturated fat products and simple carbohydrate/refined sugar products in the diet significantly decreases the risk for disease.

Table 10.6 Triglycerides Guidelines

Amount	Rating
<150 mg/dL	Desirable
150–199 mg/dL	Borderline-high
200–499 mg/dL	High
≥500 mg/dL	Very high

SOURCE: National Heart, Lung and Blood Institute.

problems, including a higher LDL cholesterol, a reduction in HDL cholesterol, and higher triglycerides.

Experts instead recommend replacing saturated fat with monounsaturated and polyunsaturated fats. The latter are preferable because they provide greater cardioprotective benefits.[15] The recommendation is not to limit fat consumption in the diet to an absolute minimum, but to maintain total fat intake around 25 to 35 percent of total calories, with a primary shift toward polyunsaturated fats. To do so, choose fish, nuts, seeds, and vegetable oils that are liquid at room temperature (with the exception of tropical oils including coconut, palm, and palm kernel oils).

At present, it is unknown whether the cardioprotective benefits are the result of limiting saturated fat intake or increasing polyunsaturated fat consumption. Another 2010 review found that consumption of polyunsaturated fat in place of saturated fat reduced the incidence of heart attacks and cardiac deaths.[16] Thus, moderate fat intake (not low fat), along with decreased refined carbohydrates and decreased caloric intake in most cases, is encouraged. The issue merits further research involving clinical trials (rather than observational studies) before clear answers can be obtained.

Elevated Triglycerides Triglycerides, also known as free fatty acids, make up most of the fat in our diet and most of the fat that circulates in the blood. In combination with cholesterol, triglycerides speed up formation of plaque in the arteries. Triglycerides are carried in the bloodstream primarily by VLDLs and chylomicrons. Triglycerides per se don't end up in the atherosclerotic plaque. Chylomicrons are broken down in the blood into fatty acids and remnant free cholesterol-rich particles. Fatty acids are stored in muscle or adipose tissue (fat) and scavenger cells that do contribute to atherosclerosis then take up the remnant particles.

Although they are found in poultry skin, lunch meats, and shellfish, these fatty acids are manufactured mainly in the liver from refined sugars, starches, and alcohol. High intake of alcohol and sugars (honey and fruit juices included) significantly raises triglyceride levels.

To lower triglycerides, avoid pastries, candies, soft drinks, fruit juices, white bread, pasta, and alcohol. In addition, cutting down on overall fat consumption, quitting smoking, reducing weight (if overweight), and doing aerobic exercise are helpful measures. Omega-3 fatty acids also help, but doses higher than those found in fish are required. The American Heart Association recommends two to four daily grams of fish oil under a physician's supervision.

The desirable blood triglyceride level is less than 150 mg/dL (see Table 10.6). For people with cardiovascular problems, this level should be less than 100 mg/dL. Levels greater than 1,000 mg/dL pose an immediate risk for potentially fatal sudden inflammation of the pancreas.

LDL Phenotype B

Some people consistently have slightly elevated triglyceride levels (greater than 140 mg/dL) and HDL cholesterol levels less than 35 mg/dL. About 80 percent of these people have a genetic condition called LDL phenotype B. Although the blood lipids may not be notably high, these people are at higher risk for atherosclerosis and CHD.

> **Critical Thinking**
>
> Are you aware of your blood lipid profile? • If not, what is keeping you from getting a blood chemistry test? • What are the benefits of having it done now rather than later in life?

Cholesterol-Lowering Medications

Effective medications are available to treat elevated cholesterol and triglycerides. Most notable among them are the statins group (Lipitor®, Mevacor®, Pravachol®, Lescol®, and Zocor®), which can lower cholesterol by up to 60 percent in 2 to 3 months. Statins slow down cholesterol production and increase the liver's ability to remove blood cholesterol. They also decrease triglycerides and produce a small increase in HDL levels. The drug Tricor® is commonly used to lower triglycerides.

In general, it is better to lower LDL cholesterol without medication, because drugs often cause undesirable side effects. Many people with heart disease must take cholesterol-lowering medication, but medication is best combined with lifestyle changes to augment the cholesterol-lowering effect. For example, when Zocor was taken alone over 3 months, LDL cholesterol decreased by 30 percent; but when a Mediterranean diet was adopted in combination with Zocor therapy, LDL cholesterol decreased by 41 percent.[17] In 2012, the FDA added safety alerts to the prescribing information of statins. Although rare among the millions of people who take these medications, the adverse effects include memory loss, cognitive impairment like forgetfulness and confusion, higher blood sugar levels that may lead to a diagnosis of diabetes, and muscle pain. Anyone starting treatment with statin drugs should be aware of these side effects.

Other drugs effective in reducing LDL cholesterol are bile acid sequestrans, which bind the cholesterol found in bile acids. Cholesterol subsequently is excreted in the stools. These drugs often are used in combination with statin drugs.

High dosages (1.5 to 3 grams per day) of nicotinic acid or niacin (a B vitamin) also help lower LDL cholesterol, Lp(a), and triglycerides and increase HDL cholesterol (change HDL3 to HDL2). Niacin in combination with some of the aforementioned drugs also exerts positive effects on IDL and pattern size. A fourth group of drugs, known as fibrates, is used primarily to lower triglycerides.

Elevated Homocysteine Clinical data indicating that many heart attack and stroke victims have normal cholesterol levels have led researchers to look for other risk factors that may contribute to atherosclerosis. Although it is not a blood lipid, one of these factors is a high concentration of the amino acid **homocysteine** in the blood. It is thought to enhance the formation of plaque and the subsequent blockage of arteries.

The body uses homocysteine to help build proteins and carry out cellular metabolism. It is an intermediate amino acid in the interconversion of two other amino acids—methionine and cysteine. This interconversion requires the B vitamin folate (folic acid) and vitamins B_6 and B_{12}. Typically, homocysteine is metabolized rapidly, so it does not accumulate in the blood or damage the arteries. Still, many people have high blood levels of homocysteine. This might result from either a genetic inability to metabolize homocysteine or a deficiency in the vitamins required for its conversion.

Homocysteine typically is measured in micromoles per liter (μmol/L). Guidelines to interpret homocysteine levels are provided in Table 10.7. A 10-year follow-up study of people with high homocysteine levels showed that those individuals with a level above 14.25 μmol/L had almost twice the risk of stroke compared with individuals whose level was less than 9.25 μmol/L.[18] Homocysteine accumulation is theorized to be toxic because it may:

1. Cause damage to the inner lining of the arteries (the initial step in the process of atherosclerosis)
2. Stimulate the proliferation of cells that contribute to plaque formation
3. Encourage clotting, which could completely obstruct an artery and lead to a heart attack or stroke

Keeping homocysteine from accumulating in the blood seems to be as simple as eating the recommended daily servings of vegetables, fruits, grains, and some meat and legumes. Five servings of fruits and vegetables daily can provide sufficient levels of folate and vitamin B_6 to remove and clear homocysteine from the blood. Vitamin B_{12} is found primarily in animal flesh and animal products. Vitamin B_{12} deficiency is rarely a problem because 1 cup of milk or an egg provides the daily requirement. The body also recycles most of this vitamin; therefore, a deficiency takes years to develop. People who consume five servings of fruits and vegetables daily are unlikely to derive extra benefits from a vitamin-B-complex supplement.

Increasing evidence that folate can prevent heart attacks has led to the recommendation that people consume 400 micrograms (mcg) per day—obtainable from five daily servings of fruits and vegetables. Unfortunately, estimates indicate that more than 80 percent of Americans do not get 400 mcg of folate per day. (Adequate folate intake also is critical for women of childbearing age to prevent birth defects.)

Inflammation In addition to homocysteine, scientists are looking at chronic inflammation as a major risk factor for heart attacks. Low-grade inflammation can occur in a variety of places throughout the body. For years it has been known that inflammation plays a role in CHD and that inflammation hidden deep in the body is a common trigger of heart attacks, even when cholesterol levels are normal or low and arterial plaque is minimal.

To evaluate ongoing inflammation in the body, physicians have turned to **C-reactive protein (CRP)**, a protein produced in the liver whose levels in the blood increase with injury or irritation (inflammation) anywhere in the body. Physical inactivity, smoking, excessive body weight, a diet high in saturated fat, chronic stress, periodontal disease, and infections can all cause inflammation.

Ample amounts of fruits and vegetables provide the necessary nutrients to keep homocysteine from causing heart disease or stroke.

Individuals with elevated CRP are more prone to cardiovascular events, even in the absence of elevated LDL cholesterol. The evidence shows that CRP blood levels elevate years before a first heart attack or stroke, and that individuals with elevated CRP have twice the risk of a heart attack. The risk of a heart attack is even higher in people with both elevated CRP and cholesterol, resulting in an almost ninefold increase in risk (see Figure 10.7).

Because high CRP levels might be a better predictor of future heart attacks than high cholesterol alone, a test known as high-sensitivity CRP (hs-CRP), which measures inflammation in the blood vessels, has been approved by the FDA. The term "high sensitivity" was derived from the test's capability to detect small amounts of CRP in the blood.

Results of the hs-CRP test provide a good measure of the probability of plaque

Table 10.7 Homocysteine Guidelines

Level (μmol/L)	Rating
<9.0	Desirable
9–12	Mild elevation
13–15	Elevated
>15	Extreme elevation

Adapted from K. S. McCully, "What You Must Know Now About Homocysteine," *Bottom Line/Health* 18 (January 2004): 7–9.

> **Homocysteine** An amino acid that, when allowed to accumulate in the blood, may lead to plaque formation and blockage of arteries.
>
> **C-reactive protein (CRP)** A protein whose blood levels increase with inflammation, at times hidden deep in the body; elevation of this protein is an indicator of potential cardiovascular events.

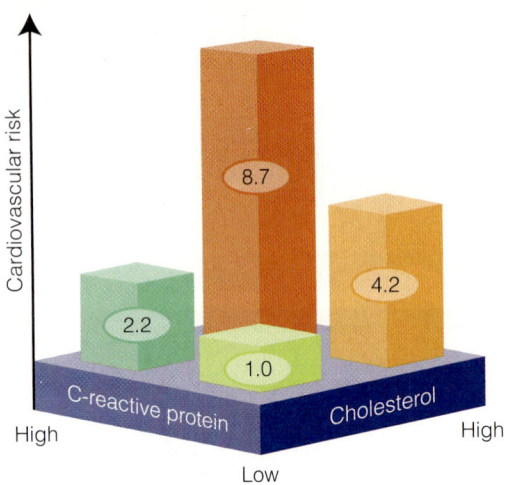

Figure 10.7 Relationships between C-reactive protein, cholesterol, and risk of cardiovascular disease.

SOURCE: Adapted from P. Libby, P. M. Ridker, and A. Masen, "Inflammation and Atherosclerosis," *Circulation* 105 (2002):1135-1143.

Table 10.8 High-Sensitivity CRP Guidelines

Amount	Rating
<1 mg/L	Low risk
1–3 mg/L	Average risk
>3 mg/L	High risk

SOURCE: T. A. Pearson et al., "Markers of Inflammation and Cardiovascular Disease," *Circulation* 107 (2003): 499-511.

rupturing within the arterial wall. The two main types of plaque are soft and hard. Soft plaque is the most likely to rupture. Ruptured plaque releases clots into the bloodstream that can lead to a heart attack or a stroke. Other evidence has linked high CRP levels to high blood pressure and colon cancer.

Excessive intake of alcohol also increases CRP. Evidence further indicates that high-fat fast food increases CRP levels for several hours following the meal. And cooking meat and poultry at high temperatures creates damaged proteins called advanced glycosylation end products (AGEs), which trigger inflammation. Several studies have also indicated that high intake of omega-6 fatty acids causes inflammation (also see Chapter 3, page 80). The current American diet is too high in omega-6 foods. Obesity increases inflammation. With weight loss, CRP levels decrease proportional to the amount of fat lost.

An hs-CRP test is relatively inexpensive, and it is highly recommended for individuals at risk for heart attack. A level greater than 2 mg/L appears to be a better predictor of a heart attack than an LDL cholesterol level greater than 130 mg/dL. General guidelines for hs-CRP levels are given in Table 10.8.

A weakness of the hs-CRP test is that it does not detect differences between acute and chronic inflammation, and results may not be stable from day to day. An acute inflammation, for example, could be the result of a pulled muscle or a passing cold. It is chronic inflammation that increases heart disease risk. Thus, a new test that specifically detects chronic inflammation, lipoprotein phospholipase A2 (PAL2), may soon replace the hs-CRP test.

CRP levels decrease with statin drugs, which also lower cholesterol and reduce inflammation. A 2008 study on 17,802 apparently healthy men and women with LDL cholesterol less than 130 mg/dL, but CRP levels greater 2.0 mg/L showed that a daily dose of the statin drug Crestor® reduced LDL cholesterol by 50 percent, CRP by 37 percent, and the risk of heart attack, stroke, and death by 54 percent, 48 percent, and 47 percent, respectively.[19] The results were so impressive that researchers stopped the trial halfway through the study.

Exercise, weight loss, proper nutrition, and quitting smoking are helpful in reducing CRP. Omega-3 fatty acids inhibit proteins that cause inflammation. Aspirin therapy also helps by controlling inflammation.

Diabetes Diabetes mellitus is a condition in which blood glucose is unable to enter the cells because the pancreas totally stops producing **insulin**, the pancreas does not produce enough to meet the body's needs, or the cells develop **insulin resistance**. The role of insulin is to "unlock" the cells and escort glucose into the cell.

Estimates indicate that more than 27 million adults and children in the United States are affected by diabetes. Between 1980 and 2003, the prevalence of diabetes more than doubled. By the year 2020, diabetes and prediabetes are projected to account for 10 percent of total health care spending, with an estimated yearly cost of $500 billion. At the present rate of escalation, the Centers for Disease Control and Prevention predict that by 2050 one of every three Americans will have diabetes.

The incidence of CVD and death in the diabetic population is quite high. Two of three people with diabetes will die from CVD. People with chronically elevated blood glucose levels may have problems metabolizing fats, which can make them more susceptible to atherosclerosis, coronary heart disease, heart attacks, high blood pressure, and stroke. People with diabetes also have lower HDL cholesterol and higher triglyceride levels.

Further, chronic high blood sugar can lead to stroke, nerve damage, vision loss, kidney damage, sexual dysfunction, and decreased immune function (making the individual more susceptible to infections). Compared with those who do not have diabetes, diabetic patients are 4 times more likely to become blind and 20 times more likely to develop kidney failure. Nerve damage in the lower extremities decreases the person's awareness of injury and infection, and a small, untreated sore can result in severe infection and gangrene, which can even lead to an amputation.

An 8-hour fasting blood glucose level greater than 125 mg/dL on two separate tests confirms a diagnosis of diabetes (see Table 10.9). A level of 126 or higher should be brought to the attention of a physician.

Table 10.9 Blood Glucose Guidelines

Amount	Rating
≤100 mg/dL	Normal
101–125 mg/dL	Prediabetes
≥126 mg/dL	Diabetes*

*Confirmed by two tests on different days.
© Cengage Learning

Regular physical activity increases insulin sensitivity and decreases the risk for diabetes.

Types of Diabetes

Diabetes is of two types: **type 1**, or insulin-dependent diabetes mellitus (IDDM), and **type 2**, or non–insulin-dependent diabetes mellitus (NIDDM). Type 1 also has been called "juvenile diabetes," because it is found mainly in young people. With type 1, the pancreas produces little or no insulin. With type 2, either the pancreas does not produce sufficient insulin, or it produces adequate amounts but the cells become insulin-resistant, thereby keeping glucose from entering the cell. Type 2 accounts for 90 to 95 percent of all cases of diabetes.

Presently, more than 1 in 10 American adults have diabetes. Although diabetes has a genetic predisposition, 60 to 80 percent of type 2 diabetes is related closely to overeating, obesity, and lack of physical activity. Type 2 diabetes, once limited primarily to overweight adults, now accounts for almost half of the new cases diagnosed in children. According to the CDC, one in three children born in the United States today will develop diabetes.

More than 80 percent of all people with type 2 diabetes are overweight or have a history of excessive weight. In most cases, this condition can be corrected through regular exercise, a special diet, and weight loss.

Aerobic exercise helps prevent type 2 diabetes. The protective effect is even greater in those with risk factors such as obesity, high blood pressure, and family propensity. The preventive effect is attributed to less body fat and to better sugar and fat metabolism resulting from the regular exercise program. At 3,500 calories of energy expenditure per week through exercise, the risk is cut in half versus that of a sedentary lifestyle.

Both moderate- and vigorous-intensity physical activity are associated with increased insulin sensitivity and decreased risk for diabetes. The key to increase and maintain proper insulin sensitivity is regularity of the exercise program. Failing to maintain habitual physical activity voids these benefits. Thus, a simple aerobic exercise program (walking, cycling, or swimming four or five times per week) often is prescribed because it increases the body's sensitivity to insulin. Exercise guidelines for diabetic patients are discussed in detail in Chapter 9.

In fact, accumulating evidence indicates that increasing physical activity, losing excess weight, and improving nutrition is more effective to control diabetes and lower CVD risk than relying on drugs to manage the disease.[20] Furthermore, research suggests that diabetic patients are worse off when medications are used to decrease blood sugar levels and blood pressure to *normal or below normal* levels. Accordingly, diabetic patients are strongly encouraged to adopt healthy lifestyle factors even if glucose levels are controlled with medication. Medications are recommended for diabetic patients with a systolic blood pressure greater than 140 mm Hg, but it is only necessary to drive it down to about 130 mm Hg.

A diet high in complex carbohydrates (unrefined whole grains and whole foods) and water-soluble fibers (found in fruits, vegetables, oats, beans, and psyllium), low in saturated fat, low in sugar, and a small amount of lean protein with meals is helpful in treating diabetes. Weight loss, even if only a 5 to 10 percent reduction in weight, can make a notable difference in controlling blood sugar. These lifestyle changes (proper nutrition, physical activity, and weight loss) often allow diabetic patients to normalize their blood sugar level without the use of medication.

Finally, evidence also suggests that consumption of low-fat dairy products lowers the risk for type 2

Diabetes mellitus A disease in which the body doesn't produce or utilize insulin properly.

Insulin A hormone secreted by the pancreas; essential for proper metabolism of blood glucose (sugar) and maintenance of blood glucose level.

Insulin resistance Inability of the cells to respond appropriately to insulin.

Type 1 diabetes Insulin-dependent diabetes mellitus (IDDM), a condition in which the pancreas produces little or no insulin; also known as juvenile diabetes.

Type 2 diabetes Non–insulin-dependent diabetes mellitus (NIDDM), a condition in which insulin is not processed properly; also known as adult-onset diabetes.

diabetes. Research on more than 41,000 men showed that those who consumed the most dairy products had a 23 percent lower incidence of the disease. Furthermore, each additional daily serving of dairy products was associated with a 9 percent decrease in type 2 diabetes risk.[21]

Glycemic Index

Although complex carbohydrates are recommended in the diet, people with diabetes need to pay careful attention to the glycemic index (explained in Chapter 5 and detailed in Table 5.1, page 156). Refined and starchy foods (small-particle carbohydrates, which are quickly digested) rank high in the glycemic index, whereas grains, fruits, and vegetables are low-glycemic foods.

Foods high in the glycemic index cause a rapid increase in blood sugar. A diet that includes many high-glycemic foods increases the risk for CVD in people with high insulin resistance and **glucose intolerance**. Combining a moderate amount of high-glycemic foods with low-glycemic foods or with some fat and protein, however, can bring down the average index.

Hemoglobin A$_{1c}$ Test

Individuals who have high blood glucose levels should consult a physician to decide on the best treatment. They also might obtain information about the hemoglobin A$_{1c}$ test (also called HbA$_{1c}$), which measures the amount of glucose that has been in a person's blood over the last 3 months. Blood glucose can become attached to hemoglobin in the red blood cells. Once attached, it remains there for the life of the red blood cell, which is about 3 months. The higher the blood glucose, the higher is the concentration of glucose in the red blood cells. Results of this test are given in percentages.

The HbA$_{1c}$ goal for diabetic patients is to keep it less than 7 percent. At this level and below, diabetic patients have a lower risk of developing diabetes-related problems of the eyes, kidneys, and nerves. Because the test tells a person how well blood glucose has been controlled over the last 3 months, a change in treatment is almost always recommended if the HbA$_{1c}$ results are greater than 8 percent. All people with type 2 diabetes should have an HbA$_{1c}$ test twice per year.

Metabolic Syndrome As the cells resist the actions of insulin, the pancreas releases even more insulin in an attempt to keep blood glucose from rising. A chronic rise in insulin seems to trigger a series of abnormalities referred to as the **metabolic syndrome**. These abnormal conditions include abdominal obesity, elevated blood pressure, high blood glucose, low HDL cholesterol, high triglycerides, and an increased blood-clotting mechanism. All of these conditions increase the risk for CHD and other diabetes-related conditions (blindness, infection, nerve damage, kidney failure). Approximately 50 million Americans are afflicted with this condition.

People with metabolic syndrome have an abnormal insulin response to carbohydrates, in particular high-glycemic foods. Research on metabolic syndrome indicates that a low-fat, high-carbohydrate diet may not be the best for preventing CHD and actually could increase the risk for the disease in individuals with high insulin resistance and glucose intolerance. It might be best for these people to distribute daily caloric intake so that 45 percent of the calories are derived from carbohydrates (primarily low-glycemic carbohydrates), 40 percent from fat, and 15 percent from protein.[22] Of the 40 percent fat calories, most of the fat should come from mono-

---

Behavior Modification Planning

Guidelines to Prevent and Manage Type 2 Diabetes

Experts agree that the following healthy lifestyle strategies are effective in type 2 diabetes management:

I PLAN TO / **I DID IT**

- ❑ ❑ Follow an overall healthful dietary pattern that includes
- ❑ ❑ A minimum of five daily servings of fruits and vegetables
  - At least three daily servings of whole grains
  - Consumption of at least two 3-oz servings of fatty fish per week
  - A few small portions of nuts each week
  - Skim milk and low-fat dairy products in your daily diet
- ❑ ❑ Maintain recommended body weight
- ❑ ❑ Increase daily physical activity (to at least 30 minutes of daily moderate-intensity activity and strength training two to three times per week)

Try It

Review your Behavior Change Plan and your Online Journal or class notebook. Are you following these guidelines? Are there changes you need to make to your Behavior Change Plan to bring yourself into closer compliance?

and poly-unsaturated fats and less than 7 percent from saturated fat.

Individuals with metabolic syndrome also benefit from weight loss (if overweight), exercise, and smoking cessation. Insulin resistance drops by about 40 percent in overweight people who lose 20 pounds. A total of 45 minutes of daily aerobic exercise enhances insulin efficiency by 25 percent. Quitting smoking also decreases insulin resistance.

Hypertension Some 60,000 miles of blood vessels run through the human body. As the heart forces the blood through these vessels, the fluid is under pressure. **Blood pressure** is measured in milliliters of mercury (mm Hg), usually expressed in two numbers—**systolic blood pressure** is the higher number, and **diastolic blood pressure** is the lower number. Ideal blood pressure is 120/80 or less.

Standards

Statistical evidence indicates that damage to the arteries starts at blood pressures above 120/80. The risk for CVD doubles with each increment of 20/10, starting with a blood pressure of 115/75.[23] All blood pressures greater than 140/90 are considered to be **hypertension** (see Table 10.10). Blood pressures ranging from 120/80 to 139/89 are referred to as prehypertension.

Based on estimates, approximately 1 in every 3 adults, or 77.9 million American adults, is hypertensive. The incidence is higher among African Americans—in fact, it is among the highest in the world. Approximately 30 percent and 20 percent of all deaths in African American men and women, respectively, may be caused by high blood pressure.

Although the threshold for hypertension has been set at 140/90, many experts believe that the lower the blood pressure, the better. Even if the pressure is around 90/50, as long as that person does not have any symptoms of **hypotension**, he or she need not be concerned. Typical symptoms of hypotension are dizziness, lightheadedness, and fainting.

Blood pressure also may fluctuate during a regular day. Many factors affect blood pressure, and one single reading may not be a true indicator of the real pressure. For example, physical activity and stress increase blood pressure, and rest and relaxation decrease blood pressure. Consequently, several measurements should be taken before diagnosing high pressure.

Incidence and Pathology

Currently, more than 60,000 Americans die each year as a direct result of high blood pressure. Hypertension, however, is a contributing factor to many other ailments, and it has been linked to as many 350,000 annual deaths from all causes. The dramatic increase in hypertension seems to be linked to the growing obesity epidemic and the aging of the U.S. population. Unless appropriate, healthy lifestyle strategies are implemented, people who do not have high blood pressure at age 55 have a 90 percent chance of developing it at some point in their lives.

Hypertension has been referred to as "the silent killer." It does not hurt, it does not make you feel sick, and unless you check it, years may go by before you even realize you

Table 10.10 Blood Pressure Guidelines (expressed in mm Hg)

Rating	Systolic	Diastolic
Normal	<120	<80
Prehypertension	121–139	81–89
Stage 1 hypertension	140–159	90–99
Stage 2 hypertension	≥160	≥100

SOURCE: National High Blood Pressure Education Program.

Glucose intolerance A condition characterized by slightly elevated blood glucose levels.

Metabolic syndrome An array of metabolic abnormalities that contribute to the development of atherosclerosis triggered by insulin resistance. These conditions include low HDL cholesterol, high triglycerides, high blood pressure, and an increased blood-clotting mechanism.

Blood pressure A measure of the force exerted against the walls of the vessels by the blood flowing through them.

Systolic blood pressure Pressure exerted by blood against walls of arteries during forceful contraction (systole) of the heart; higher of the two numbers in blood pressure readings.

Diastolic blood pressure Pressure exerted by blood against walls of arteries during relaxation phase (diastole) of the heart; lower of the two numbers in blood pressure readings.

Hypertension Chronically elevated blood pressure.

Hypotension Low blood pressure.

Diagnosis of Metabolic Syndrome

Risk Factor	Defining Level
Blood pressure	≥135/85 mm Hg
Fasting blood glucose	≥100 mg/dL
Abdominal obesity (waist circumference)	
Men	≥40 inches
Women	≥35 inches
Triglycerides	≥150 mg/dL
HDL cholesterol	
Men	<40 inches
Women	<50 inches

have a problem. High blood pressure is a risk factor for CHD, congestive heart failure, stroke, kidney failure, and osteoporosis.

All inner walls of arteries are lined by a layer of smooth endothelial cells. Blood lipids cannot penetrate the healthy lining and start to build up on the walls unless the cells are damaged. High blood pressure is thought to be a leading contributor to destruction of this lining. As blood pressure rises, so does the risk for atherosclerosis. The higher the pressure, the greater is the damage to the arterial wall, making the vessels susceptible to fat deposits, especially if serum cholesterol is also high. Blockage of the coronary vessels decreases blood supply to the heart muscle and can lead to heart attacks. When brain arteries are involved, a stroke may follow.

A clear example of the connection between high blood pressure and atherosclerosis can be seen by comparing blood vessels in the human body. Even when atherosclerosis is present throughout major arteries, fatty plaques rarely are seen in the pulmonary artery, which goes from the right part of the heart to the lungs. The pressure in this artery normally is less than 40 mm Hg, and at such a low pressure, significant deposits do not occur. This is one of the reasons that people with low blood pressure have a lower incidence of CVD.

Constantly elevated blood pressure also causes the heart to work much harder. At first the heart does well, but in time this continual strain produces an enlarged heart, followed by congestive heart failure. Furthermore, high blood pressure damages blood vessels to the kidneys and eyes, which can result in kidney failure and loss of vision.

Treatment

Of all hypertension, 90 percent has no definite cause. Called "essential hypertension," it is treatable. Aerobic exercise, weight reduction, a low-salt/low-fat and high-potassium/high-calcium diet, lower alcohol and caffeine intake, smoking cessation, stress management, and antihypertensive medication all have been used effectively to treat essential hypertension.

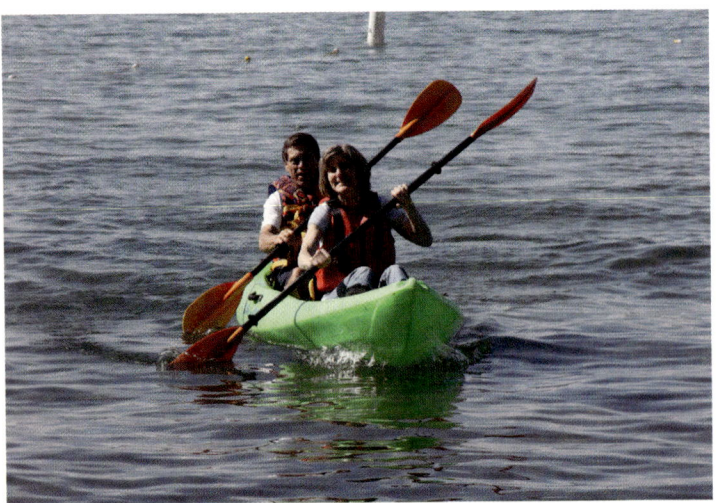

Lifetime physical activity helps maintain healthy blood pressure.

The remaining 10 percent of hypertensive cases are caused by pathological conditions, such as narrowing of the kidney arteries, glomerulonephritis (a kidney disease), tumors of the adrenal glands, and narrowing of the aortic artery. With this type of hypertension, the pathological cause has to be treated before the blood pressure problem can be corrected.

Antihypertensive medicines often are the first choice of treatment, but they produce many side effects. These include lethargy, sleepiness, sexual difficulties, higher blood cholesterol and glucose levels, lower potassium levels, and elevated uric acid levels. A physician may end up treating these side effects as much as the hypertension itself. Because of the many side effects, about half of the patients stop taking the medication within the first year of treatment.

Another factor contributing to elevated blood pressure is too much sodium in the diet. (Salt, or sodium chloride, contains approximately 40 percent sodium.) With a high sodium intake, the body retains more water, which increases the blood volume and, in turn, drives up the pressure. High intake of potassium seems to regulate water retention and lower the pressure slightly. According to the Institute of Medicine of the National Academy of Sciences, we need to consume at least 4,700 mg of potassium per day. Most Americans get only half that amount. Foods high in potassium include vegetables (especially leafy green), citrus fruit, dairy products, fish, beans, and nuts.

> ### Critical Thinking
> Do you know what your most recent blood pressure reading was, and did you know at the time what the numbers meant?
> • How would you react if your doctor were to instruct you to take blood pressure medication?

Although sodium is essential for normal body functions, the body can function with as little as 200 mg, or a tenth of a teaspoon, daily. Even under strenuous conditions in jobs and sports that incite heavy perspiration, the amount of sodium required is seldom more than 3,000 mg per day. Yet, sodium intake in the typical U.S. diet is about 4,000 mg per day.[24] The upper limit (UL) of sodium intake has been set at 2,300 mg per day and the 2010 Dietary Guidelines for Americans recommend a daily sodium intake of less than 2,300 mg. Adults older than 51, African Americans, and all individuals with high blood pressure, diabetes, and chronic kidney disease are encouraged to keep daily intake less than 1,500 mg. Among Americans, about 95 percent of men and 75 percent of women exceed these guidelines.

Salt-sensitive people, even in the absence of high blood pressure, are encouraged to decrease sodium intake because they have death rates similar to people with hypertension. The American Heart Association has issued guidelines calling for everyone to reduce daily sodium intake to less than 1,500 mg. Estimates indicate that if Americans were to follow these guidelines, heart attacks and strokes would decrease by 155,000 cases each year.

Two recent studies corroborate previous concerns. First, a review of 13 sodium consumption-related studies shows that decreasing sodium intake by about 2,000 mg per day is associated with a 23 percent and 17 percent reduction in the risk of strokes and CVD, respectively.[25] A second large study projected that reducing sodium intake by 1,200 mg per day, would prevent as many as 92,000 deaths a year in the United States.[26] To either prevent or postpone the onset of hypertension and to help some hypertensives control their blood pressure, we should consume even less sodium than previously recommended.[27] Lower sodium intake may also reduce the risk of left ventricular hypertrophy, congestive heart failure, gastric cancer, end-stage kidney disease, osteoporosis, and bloating. Research data support the notion that daily sodium intake should be reduced as much as possible.

Where does all the sodium come from? Part of the answer is given in Table 10.11. (The list in Table 10.11 does not include salt added at the table.) Most of the sodium that people consume comes from processed foods, over whose ingredients the consumer has no control. Prepackaged, canned, and frozen foods are often loaded with added salt. Among the worst offenders are soups, spaghetti sauces, lunch meats, pickled foods, soy sauce, salad dressings, cheeses, and crackers.

As a consumer you need to always read food labels and pick only those items which are low in sodium content. When eating out, request that your dish be prepared with less salt. Some restaurant dishes contain up to 6,000 mg of sodium per serving. You will do best by downsizing your portion (taking the rest home), sharing the dish with someone else, or trying to find the lower-sodium dishes. You can also retrain your taste buds to enjoy food with less salt.

When treating high blood pressure (unless it is extremely high), before recommending medication, many sports medicine physicians suggest a combination of aerobic exercise, weight loss, and less sodium in the diet. In most instances, this treatment brings blood pressure under control.

The relative risk for mortality based on blood pressure and fitness levels is similar to that of physical fitness and cholesterol. In men and women alike, the relative risk for early mortality is lower in fit people with high systolic blood pressure (140 mm Hg or greater) than in unfit people with a healthy systolic blood pressure (120 mm Hg or less).

The link between hypertension and obesity seems to be quite strong. Blood volume increases with excess body fat, and each additional pound of fat requires an estimated extra mile of blood vessels to feed this tissue. Furthermore, blood capillaries are constricted by the adipose tissues because these vessels run through them. As a result, the heart muscle must work harder to pump the blood through a longer, constricted network of blood vessels.

Regular physical activity plays a large role in managing blood pressure. On the average, fit individuals have lower

Table 10.11 Sodium and Potassium Levels of Selected Foods

Food	Serving Size	Sodium (mg)	Potassium (mg)
Apple	1 med	1	182
Asparagus	1 cup	2	330
Avocado	½	4	680
Banana	1 med	1	440
Beans			
Kidney (canned)	½ cup	436	330
Lima (cooked)	½ cup	2	478
Pinto (cooked)	½ cup	2	398
Refried (canned)	½ cup	377	336
Bologna	3 oz	1,107	133
Bouillon cube	1	960	4
Cantaloupe	¼	17	341
Carrot (raw)	1	34	225
Cheese			
American	2 oz	614	93
Cheddar	2 oz	342	56
Muenster	2 oz	356	77
Parmesan	2 oz	1,056	53
Chicken (light meat)	6 oz	108	700
Frankfurter	1	627	136
Haddock	6 oz	300	594
Ham (honey/smoked)	2 oz	495	91
Hamburger (reg)	1	500	321
Marinara pasta sauce	½ cup	527	406
Milk (skim)	1 cup	126	406
Nuts			
Brazil	1 nut	1	120
Walnuts	½ cup	1	327
Orange	1 med	1	263
Peach	1 med	2	308
Pickle (dill)	2 oz	550	26
Pizza (cheese—14" diam.)	1/8	456	85
Potato	1 med	6	763
Salami	3 oz	1,047	170
Salmon (baked)	4 oz	75	424
Salmon (canned)	6 oz	198	756
Salt	1 tsp	2,132	0
Soups			
Chicken noodle	1 cup	979	55
Cream of mushroom	1 cup	955	98
Vegetable beef	1 cup	1,046	162
Soy sauce	1 tsp	1,123	22
Spaghetti (tomato sauce and cheese)	6 oz	648	276
Spinach (cooked, fresh)	1 cup	126	838
Strawberries	1 cup	1	244
Tomato (raw)	1 med	3	444
Tomato juice	1 cup	680	430
Tuna (drained)	3 oz	38	255
Whopper with cheese	1	1,432	534

© Cengage Learning

Table 10.12 Effects of Long-Term (14–18 years) Aerobic Exercise on Resting Blood Pressure

	Initial	Final
Exercise Group		
Age	44.6	68.0
Blood Pressure	120/79	120/78
Nonexercise Group		
Age	51.6	69.7
Blood Pressure	135/85	150/90

NOTE: The aerobic exercise program consisted of an average four training sessions per week, each 66 minutes long, at about 76 percent of heart rate reserve.

Based on data from F. W. Kash, J. L. Boyer, S. P. Van Camp, L. S. Verity, and J. P. Wallace, "The Effect of Physical Activity on Aerobic Power in Older Men (A Longitudinal Study)," *The Physician and Sports Medicine* 18, no. 4 (1990): 73-83.

blood pressure than unfit people. Aerobic exercise of moderate intensity supplemented by strength training is recommended for individuals with high blood pressure.[28]

Comprehensive reviews of the effects of aerobic exercise on blood pressure have found that in general, an individual can expect exercise-induced reductions of approximately 4 to 5 mm Hg in resting systolic blood pressure and 3 to 4 mm Hg in resting diastolic blood pressure.[29] Although these reductions do not seem large, a decrease of about 5 mm Hg in resting diastolic blood pressure has been associated with a 40 percent decrease in the risk for stroke and a 15 percent reduction in the risk for CHD.[30] Even in the absence of any decrease in resting blood pressure, hypertensive individuals who exercise have a lower risk for all-cause mortality compared with hypertensive/sedentary individuals. Research data also show that exercise, not weight loss, is the major contributor to the lower blood pressure of exercisers. If they discontinue aerobic exercise, they do not maintain these changes.

Another extensive review of research studies on the effects of at least 4 weeks of strength training on resting blood pressure yielded similar results.[31] Both systolic and diastolic blood pressures decreased by an average of 3 mm Hg. Participants in these studies, however, were primarily individuals with normal blood pressure. Of greater significance, the results showed that strength training did not cause an increase in resting blood pressure. More research remains to be done on hypertensive subjects.

The effects of long-term participation in exercise are apparently much more remarkable. An 18-year follow-up study on exercising and nonexercising subjects showed much lower blood pressures in the active group.[32] The exercise group had an average resting blood pressure of 120/78 compared with 150/90 for the nonexercise group (see Table 10.12).

Aerobic exercise programs for hypertensive patients should be of moderate intensity. Training at 40 to 60 percent

Behavior Modification Planning

Guidelines to Stop Hypertension

I PLAN TO / I DID IT

- ❏ ❏ Participate in a moderate-intensity aerobic exercise program (50% intensity) for 30 to 45 minutes 5 to 7 times per week.
- ❏ ❏ Participate in a moderate-resistance strength-training program (use 12 to 15 repetitions to near-fatigue on each set) 2 times per week (seek your physician's approval and advice for this program).
- ❏ ❏ Lose weight if you are heavier than recommended body weight.
- ❏ ❏ Limit sodium intake to less than 1,500 mg/day.
- ❏ ❏ Do not smoke cigarettes or use tobacco in any other form.
- ❏ ❏ Practice stress management.
- ❏ ❏ Do not consume more than two alcoholic beverages a day if you are a man or one if you are a woman.
- ❏ ❏ Consume more potassium-rich foods.
- ❏ ❏ Follow the Dietary Approach to Stop Hypertension (DASH) diet:

Food Group	Servings
Whole grains	7–8 per day
Fruits and vegetables	8–10 per day
Low-fat or fat-free dairy foods	2–3 per day
Meat, poultry, or fish*	2 or less per day
Beans, peas, nuts, or seeds	4–5 per week
Fats and oils	2–3 servings per day
Snacks and sweets	4–5 per week

*Less than 3 ounces per serving

© Cengage Learning 2013

Try It

In your Online Journal or class notebook, make a comparison of the goals of the DASH diet and Dietary Guidelines for Americans. How do they differ?

intensity seems to have the same effect as training at 70 percent in lowering blood pressure. High-intensity training (greater than 70 percent) in hypertensive patients may not lower the blood pressure as much as moderate-intensity exercise. Even so, a person may be better off being highly fit and having high blood pressure than being unfit and having low blood pressure. The death rates for unfit individuals with low systolic blood pressure are much higher than for highly fit people with high systolic blood pressure. Strength training for hypertensive individuals calls for a minimum of one set of 10 to 15 repetitions that elicit a "somewhat hard" perceived exertion rating, using 8 to 10 multiple-joint exercises two or three times per week.

Most important is a preventive approach. Keeping blood pressure under control is easier than trying to bring it down once it is high. Regardless of your blood pressure history, high or low, you should have it checked routinely. To keep your blood pressure as low as possible, exercise regularly, lose excess weight, eat less salt and sodium-containing foods, do not smoke, practice stress management, do not consume more than two alcoholic beverages a day if you are a man, or one if you are a woman, and consume more potassium-rich foods such as potatoes, bananas, orange juice, cantaloupe, tomatoes, and beans (see the box "Guidelines to Stop Hypertension" on page 364). An alcoholic drink is defined as 5 ounces of wine, 12 ounces of beer, or 1.5 ounces of 80-proof liquor. The Dietary Approach to Stop Hypertension (DASH)—which emphasizes fruits, vegetables, grains, and dairy products—lowers systolic blood pressure by 11 points and diastolic pressure by 5.5 points.[33]

Those who are taking medication for hypertension should not stop without the approval of the prescribing physician. If it is not treated properly, high blood pressure can kill. By combining medication with the other treatments, one might eventually reduce or eliminate the need for drug therapy.

Excessive Body Fat Excessive body fat is an independent risk factor for CHD, but disease risk may actually be augmented by other risk factors that usually accompany excessive body fat. Risk factors such as high blood lipids, hypertension, and diabetes typically are seen in conjunction with obesity. All of these risk factors usually improve with increased physical activity.

Attaining recommended body composition helps to improve several CHD risk factors and also helps to reach a better state of health and wellness. While data indicates that a 10 percent weight loss results in significant improvements in CHD risk factors, some studies have even shown reduction in chronic disease risk factors with only a 2 to 3 percent weight loss.[34]

For years we have known that where people store fat affects risk for disease. People who store body fat in the abdominal area as opposed to in the hips and thighs are at higher risk for disease. Furthermore, when abdominal fat is stored primarily around internal organs (visceral fat—also see Figure 4.7, page 140), disease risk is greater than when abdominal fat is stored subcutaneously or retroperitoneally.

The best approach to prevent increases in visceral fat is through regular exercise. Data on men and women who were followed for 6 months showed no visceral fat gains in groups that either walked (178 min/week) or jogged (120 min/week) an average of 12 miles per week.[35] A sedentary group in this same study actually gained 8.6 percent visceral fat during the 6 months, while a 20-mile-per-week jogging group (173 min/week) lost 7 percent visceral fat. Thus, it appears that 30 minutes of vigorous exercise 6 times per week is best to properly manage visceral fat. Of significant concern, just 6 months of inactivity further increased visceral fat and the concomitant increase in disease risk.

Data published in 2009 on 21,094 men followed for more than 20 years indicated that an elevated BMI (greater than 25) was associated with an increased risk of heart failure.[36] Furthermore, the data showed that as BMI increased in both active and inactive men, so did the risk for heart failure. The increased risk for heart failure improved proportionally with increased BMI or decreased physical activity (see Table 10.13).

If you have a weight problem and want to get down to recommended weight, you must:

1. Increase daily physical activity up to 90 minutes a day, including aerobic and strength-training programs
2. Follow a diet lower in fat, refined sugars, and processed foods, and high in complex carbohydrates and fiber
3. Reduce total caloric intake moderately while getting the necessary nutrients to sustain normal body functions.

A comprehensive weight reduction and weight control program is discussed in detail in Chapter 5.

Cigarette Smoking More than 57 million people in the United States smoke cigarettes. Smoking is the single largest preventable cause of illness and premature death in the United States. It has been linked to CVD, cancer, bronchitis, emphysema, and peptic ulcers. In relation to coronary disease, smoking speeds the process of atherosclerosis and carries a threefold increase in the risk of sudden death after a myocardial infarction.

Table 10.13 Relationship between Body Weight, Physical Activity, and Heart Failure Risk

Body Weight and Activity Status	Percent Risk Increase*
Lean** and inactive	19
Overweight and active	49
Overweight and inactive	78
Obese and active	168
Obese and inactive	293

*As compared with lean and active men.
**Lean = BMI ≤ 25, Overweight = BMI >25 and <30, Obese = BMI ≥30.
SOURCE: S. Kenchaiah et al., "Body Mass Index and Vigorous Physical Activity and the Risk of Heart Failure Among Men," *Circulation* 119 (2009): 44–52.

According to estimates, about 20 percent of all deaths from CVD are attributable to smoking. Smoking prompts the release of nicotine and another 1,200 toxic compounds into the bloodstream. Similar to hypertension, many of these substances are destructive to the inner membrane that protects the walls of the arteries. Once the lining is damaged, cholesterol and triglycerides can be deposited readily in the arterial wall. As the plaque builds up, it obstructs blood flow through the arteries.

Furthermore, smoking encourages the formation of blood clots, which can completely block an artery already narrowed by atherosclerosis. In addition, carbon monoxide, a byproduct of cigarette smoke, decreases the blood's oxygen-carrying capacity. A combination of obstructed arteries, less oxygen, and nicotine in the heart muscle heightens the risk for a serious heart problem.

Smoking also increases heart rate, raises blood pressure, and irritates the heart, which can trigger fatal cardiac **arrhythmias**. Another harmful effect is a decrease in HDL cholesterol, the "good" type that helps control blood lipids. Smoking actually presents a much greater risk of death from heart disease than from lung disease.

Pipe and cigar smoking and tobacco chewing also increase the risk for heart disease. Even if the tobacco user inhales no smoke, he or she absorbs toxic substances through the membranes of the mouth, and these end up in the bloodstream. Individuals who use tobacco in any of these three forms also have a much greater risk for cancer of the oral cavity.

The risks for both CVD and cancer start to decrease the moment a person quits smoking. One year after quitting, the risk for CHD decreases by half, and within 15 years, the relative risk of dying from CVD and cancer approaches that of a lifetime nonsmoker. A more thorough discussion of the harmful effects of cigarette smoking, the benefits of quitting, and a complete program for quitting are detailed in Chapter 13.

Tension and Stress Tension and stress have become part of contemporary life. Everyone has to deal daily with goals, deadlines, responsibilities, and pressures. Almost everything in life (whether positive or negative) can be a source of stress. What creates the health hazard is not the stressor itself but, rather, the individual's response to it.

The human body responds to stress by producing more **catecholamines**, which prepare the body for quick physical action—often called "fight-or-flight." These hormones increase heart rate, blood pressure, and blood glucose levels, enabling the person to take action. If the person actually fights or flees, the higher levels of catecholamines are metabolized and the body can return to a normal state. If, however, a person is under constant stress and unable to take action (as in the death of a close relative or friend, loss of a job, trouble at work, or financial insecurity), the catecholamines remain elevated in the bloodstream.

People who are not able to relax place a constant low-level strain on the cardiovascular system that could manifest itself as heart disease. Higher levels of the hormones epinephrine and cortisol in highly stressed people may raise blood pressure, elevate blood glucose levels, and increase cholesterol by 20 to 50

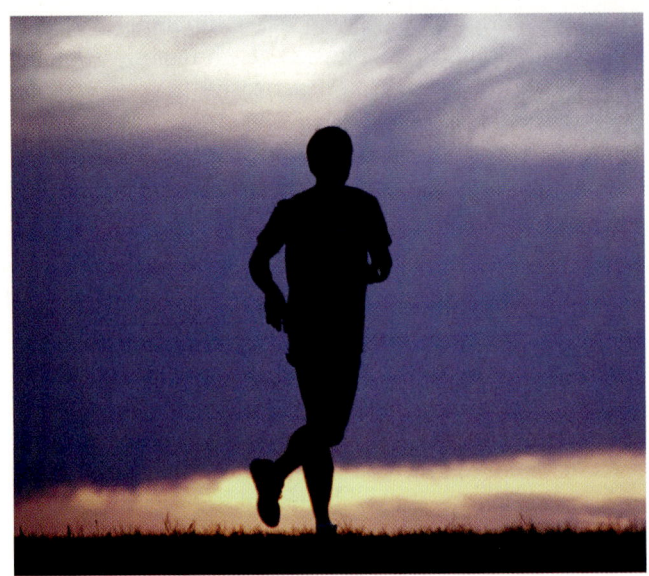

Physical activity is one of the best ways to relieve stress.

percent.[37] Chronic stress also causes an increase of the brain chemical neuropeptide Y that promotes storage of visceral fat, further increasing the risk for type 2 diabetes, heart disease, some cancers, and body-wide inflammation. In addition, when a person is in a stressful situation, the coronary arteries that feed the heart muscle constrict, reducing the oxygen supply to the heart. If the blood vessels are largely blocked by atherosclerosis, arrhythmias, or even a heart attack may follow. The research indicates that people who feel too much stress too often significantly increase their risk for a deadly heart attack.

A little known fact is that the risk of sudden cardiac death is twice as high on Mondays, most likely because of the stress of having to go back to work after the weekend. Heart attacks are also more common in the morning because cortisol levels and stress hormones are highest, on average, at that time of the day.

Anger and hostility also contribute to heart disease by increasing heart rate, blood pressure, blood glucose, cholesterol, and interleukin-6 (a marker for arterial inflammation). Extreme anger may trigger angina, arrhythmias, blood vessel constriction, and increase blood cloths. The risk for a heart attack is two to nine times higher following an outburst of anger.[38] Depression and isolation have also been linked to higher death rates from heart disease.

Weight gain is often the end result of excessive stress. That is because most people tend to eat more when distressed and the choice is typically "comfort foods" that are calorie dense and promote weight gain with the subsequent increased risk for cardiovascular disease.

Individuals who are under a lot of stress and do not cope well with stress need to take measures to counteract the effects of stress in their lives. One way is to identify the sources of stress and learn how to cope with them. People need to take control of themselves, examine and act on the things that are most important in their lives, and ignore less meaningful details.

Physical activity is one of the best ways to relieve stress. When a person takes part in physical activity, the body metabolizes excess catecholamines and is able to return to a normal state. Exercise also steps up muscular activity, which contributes to muscular relaxation after completing the physical activity.

Many executives in large cities are choosing the evening hours for their physical activity programs, stopping after work at the health or fitness club. In doing this, they are able to "burn up" the excess tension accumulated during the day and enjoy the evening hours. This has proved to be one of the best stress management techniques. More information on stress management techniques is presented in Chapter 12.

Personal and Family History Individuals who have had cardiovascular problems are at higher risk than those who have never had a problem. People with this history should control other risk factors as much as they can. Many of the risk factors are reversible, so this will greatly decrease the risk for future problems. The more time that passes after the occurrence of the cardiovascular problem, the lower the risk for recurrence.

A genetic predisposition to heart disease has been demonstrated clearly. All other factors being equal, a person with blood relatives who now have or did have heart disease runs a greater risk than someone with no such history. Premature CHD is defined as a heart attack before age 55 in a close male relative or before age 65 in a close female relative. The younger the age at which the relative incurred the cardiovascular incident, the greater is the risk for the disease.

In some cases, there is no way of knowing whether the heart problem resulted from a person's genetic predisposition or simply poor lifestyle habits. A person may have been physically inactive, been overweight, smoked, and had bad dietary habits—all of which contributed to a heart attack. Regardless, blood relatives fall in the "family history" category. Because we have no reliable way to differentiate all the factors contributing to CVD, a person with a family history should watch all other factors closely and maintain the lowest risk level possible. In addition, the person should have a blood chemistry analysis annually to make sure the body is handling blood lipids properly.

Age Age is a risk factor because of the higher incidence of heart disease as people get older. This tendency may be induced partly by other factors stemming from changes in lifestyle as we get older—less physical activity, poorer nutrition, obesity, and so on. Young people should not think they are exempt from heart disease, though. The process begins early in life. Autopsies conducted on American soldiers killed at age 22 and younger revealed that approximately 70 percent had early stages of atherosclerosis. Other studies found elevated blood cholesterol levels in children as young as 10 years old.

Although the aging process cannot be stopped, it certainly can be slowed. Physiological age versus chronological age is important in preventing disease. An individual in his 60s or older can have the body of a 30-year-old. And a 30-year-old is often in such poor condition and health that he almost seems to have the body of a 60-year-old. The best ways to slow the natural aging process are to engage in risk factor management and positive lifestyle habits.

Other Risk Factors for Coronary Heart Disease Additional evidence points to a few other factors that may be linked to coronary heart disease. One of these factors is gum disease. The oral bacteria that build up with dental plaque can enter the bloodstream and contribute to inflammation, formation of blood vessel plaque, blood clotting, and thus increase the risk for heart attack. Data on women who have periodontal disease indicate that these women also have higher blood levels of CRP and lower HDL cholesterol. Daily flossing, using an electric toothbrush, scraping the tongue, and irrigating the gums with water are all preventive measures that will help protect you from gum disease.

Another factor that has been linked to CVD is loud snoring. People who snore heavily may suffer from sleep apnea, a sleep disorder in which the throat closes for a brief moment, causing breathing to stop. Individuals who snore heavily may triple their risk of a heart attack and quadruple the risk of a stroke.

Sudden emotional-related increases in heart rate often also trigger heart problems.[39] For example, the risk of a heart attack is highest on the day and the first few weeks after receiving unexpected bad news. Sports fans who get overly excited about their team can experience a twofold or higher increase in heart rate. A person with a resting heart rate of 80 to 90 bpm can easily reach near or maximal heart rate in these situations. Heart attacks occur in these cases because the unconditioned heart is unable to sustain the sudden/drastic increase in heart rate.

An extramarital affair can also contribute to a cardiac event. Data indicates that 80 percent of post-sex heart attack deaths occur in people following sex in a hotel room with someone other than their spouse. Researchers believe that such encounters lead to higher levels of arousal, resulting in a sudden and sustained heart rate that an unconditioned heart is unable to tolerate.

Low birth weight, considered to be less than 5.5 pounds, also has been linked to heart disease, hypertension, and diabetes. Individuals with low birth weight should bring this information to the attention of their personal physician and regularly monitor the risk factors for CHD.

Aspirin therapy is recommended to prevent heart disease. For individuals at moderate risk or higher, an aspirin dosage of about 81 mg per day (the equivalent of a baby aspirin) can prevent or dissolve clots that cause heart attack or stroke. With such daily use, the incidence of nonfatal heart attack decreases by about a third.

> **Arrhythmias** Irregular heart rhythms.
> **Catecholamines** "Fight-or-flight" hormones, including epinephrine and norepinephrine.

Behavior Modification Planning

American Heart Association Diet and Lifestyle Goals for Cardiovascular Risk Reduction

I PLAN TO / I DID IT

- ❏ ❏ Consume an overall healthy diet.
- ❏ ❏ Aim for a healthy body weight.
- ❏ ❏ Aim for recommended levels of LDL cholesterol, HDL cholesterol, and triglycerides.
- ❏ ❏ Aim for a normal blood pressure.
- ❏ ❏ Aim for normal blood glucose levels.
- ❏ ❏ Be physically active.
- ❏ ❏ Avoid use of and exposure to tobacco products.

Try It

To significantly offset the risk of cardiovascular disease, you need to aim for all of these goals. You are now aware of the necessary lifestyle and dietary guidelines to do so. In your Online Journal or class notebook, outline the lifestyle changes that are required for you to meet the above goals.

10.4 Cardiovascular Risk Reduction

Most of the risk factors are reversible and preventable. Having a family history of heart disease and some of the other risk factors because of neglect in lifestyle does not mean you are doomed. A healthier lifestyle—free of cardiovascular problems—is something over which you have extensive control. Be persistent! Willpower and commitment are required to develop patterns that eventually will turn into healthy habits and contribute to your total well-being and longevity.

ASSESS YOUR BEHAVIOR

CENGAGEbrain.com To access course materials, including companion resources, please visit www.cengagebrain.com.

1. Do you make a conscious effort to increase daily physical activity, and are you able to accumulate at least 30 minutes of moderate-intensity activity a minimum of 5 days per week?
2. Is your diet fundamentally low in saturated fat, trans fats, refined carbohydrates, processed foods; and do you meet the daily suggested amounts of fruits, vegetables, and fiber?
3. Have you recently had your blood pressure measured, and established your blood lipid profile? Do you know what the results mean, and are you aware of strategies to manage them effectively?

ASSESS YOUR KNOWLEDGE

Evaluate how well you understand the concepts presented in this chapter using the chapter-specific quiz available in the online materials at www.cengagebrain.com.

1. Coronary heart disease
   a. is the single leading cause of death in the United States.
   b. is the leading cause of sudden cardiac deaths.
   c. is a condition in which the arteries that supply the heart muscle with oxygen and nutrients are narrowed by fatty deposits.
   d. accounts for approximately 20 percent of all deaths in the United States.
   e. All of the above are correct.

2. The incidence of cardiovascular disease during the past 40 years in the United States has
   a. increased.
   b. decreased.
   c. remained constant.
   d. increased in some years and decreased in others.
   e. fluctuated according to medical technology.

3. Regular aerobic activity helps
   a. lower LDL cholesterol.
   b. lower HDL cholesterol.
   c. increase triglycerides.
   d. decrease insulin sensitivity.
   e. All of the above.

4. The risk of heart disease increases with
   a. high LDL cholesterol.
   b. low HDL cholesterol.
   c. high concentration of homocysteine.
   d. high levels of CRP.
   e. All of the above factors.

5. An optimal level of LDL cholesterol is
   a. between 200 and 239 mg/dL.
   b. about 200 mg/dL.
   c. between 150 and 200 mg/dL.
   d. between 100 and 150 mg/dL.
   e. less than 100 mg/dL.

6. As a part of a CHD prevention program, saturated fat intake should be kept less than
   a. 35 percent.
   b. 30 percent.
   c. 22 percent.
   d. 15 percent.
   e. 7 percent.

7. Statin drugs
   a. increase the liver's ability to remove blood cholesterol.
   b. decrease LDL cholesterol.
   c. slow cholesterol production.
   d. help reduce inflammation.
   e. accomplish all of the above.

8. Type 2 diabetes is related closely to
   a. overeating.
   b. obesity.
   c. lack of physical activity.
   d. insulin resistance.
   e. All of the above factors.

9. Metabolic syndrome is related to
   a. low HDL cholesterol.
   b. high triglycerides.
   c. increased blood-clotting mechanism.
   d. an abnormal insulin response to carbohydrates.
   e. All of the above.

10. Comprehensive reviews on the effects of aerobic exercise on blood pressure found that in general, an individual can expect exercise-induced reductions of approximately
    a. 3 to 5 mm Hg.
    b. 5 to 10 mm Hg.
    c. 10 to 15 mm Hg.
    d. more than 15 mm Hg.
    e. There is no significant change in blood pressure with exercise.

Correct answers can be found at the back of the book.

Cancer Prevention

"Our science looks at a substance-by-substance exposure and doesn't take into account the multitude of exposures we experience in daily life. If we did, it might change our risk paradigm. The potential risks associated with extremely low-level exposure may be underestimated or missed entirely."
—Heather Logan

Objectives

- **Define** cancer and understand how it starts and spreads.
- **Cite** guidelines for preventing cancer.
- **Delineate** the major risk factors that lead to specific types of cancer.
- **Assess** the risk for developing certain types of cancer.
- **Learn** everyday lifestyle strategies that you can use immediately to decrease overall cancer risk.

CENGAGEbrain.com

Visit www.cengagebrain.com to access course materials and companion resources for this text, including quiz questions designed to check your understanding of the chapter contents. See the preface on page ix for more information.

Can a healthy diet reduce cancer risk?

Much research is currently under way to examine the effects of foods in preventing and fighting off cancer. There is strong scientific evidence that a healthy diet and maintenance of recommended body weight reduce cancer risk. The current state of knowledge, however, cannot indicate that a certain dietary pattern will absolutely reduce your cancer risk. Years of research will be required to unravel most of this knowledge. Moreover, science may never be able to provide conclusive evidence that a certain diet will prevent cancer in most cases. Many of the foods that are currently recommended in a cancer-prevention diet, nonetheless, are similar to those encouraged to decrease disease risk and enhance health and overall well-being. If you are truly adhering to healthy dietary guidelines (see the Behavior Modification Planning box on page 377), you are most likely eating the right foods to decrease your cancer risk.

Does regular physical activity affect cancer risk?

Regular physical activity has been shown to decrease the risk for developing certain types of cancer, in particular cancers of the colon, breast, endometrium, and prostate gland. Research shows that as little as 15 minutes of vigorous exercise three times per week decreases breast cancer risk by up to 40 percent in persons of all races and ethnicities. Other research suggests that strength training at least twice per week cuts the risk of dying from cancer in men up to 40 percent. Physical activity also prevents type 2 diabetes and obesity. The latter have been linked to colon, pancreatic, gallbladder, ovarian, thyroid, cervical, and possibly other types of cancers. The American Cancer Society recommends that you aim for at least 30 minutes of moderate to vigorous physical activity five or more days per week, although 60 to 90 minutes of intentional activity are preferable. For most non-tobacco users, a healthy dietary pattern and regular physical activity are the two most significant lifestyle behaviors that reduce cancer risk.

Does aspirin therapy protect against cancer?

A 2011 study published in the journal *The Lancet* indicated that a regular daily dose of aspirin may decrease cancer risk up to 58 percent in some cases (esophageal cancer) and reduced total cancer deaths by 34 percent after 5 years. Even 15 years later, death rates were still lower by 20 percent among aspirin users with the biggest drop in cancer deaths seen in esophageal, colorectal, lung, and prostate cancers. Low-dose therapy (75 to 81 mg) was as effective as a larger dose. It is believed that aspirin inhibits the effects of enzymes (COX-2) that promote potential cancer-causing cell damage. Aspirin also decreases low-grade inflammation, thought to play a role in cancer development and growth. Aspirin therapy, however, is not recommended for healthy people because of the small risk of gastrointestinal (GI) bleeding and ulcers. About 50,000 yearly deaths in the United States are attributed to GI bleeding caused partially by aspirin and other nonsteroidal anti-inflammatory drug (NSAID) use. Aspirin therapy damage to the GI tract may not cause any noticeable symptoms and a fecal occult blood test may be necessary to detect possible bleeding. Hemorrhagic strokes have also been linked to low-dose aspirin therapy. If you are at high risk for cancer (and cardiovascular disease), you are encouraged to talk to your doctor before starting aspirin therapy. If you take aspirin, do so with warm water as such helps dissolve the tablet faster, making it less likely to cause serious bleeding.

Real Life Story | Joan's Experience

I was never really that concerned with cancer risk. You hear a lot about how various things cause cancer until it gets to the point where it seems like almost everything causes cancer and it is unavoidable. However, when I took lifetime wellness last year, learning about the key lifestyle factors that decrease cancer risk really motivated me. I liked learning about the positive things someone can do, rather than just the negative things that cause cancer. Also, the lifestyle factors were mostly simple and straightforward things to do. I actually hung the page from the book with the list of behaviors by my desk as any easy way to remember. After that, I started being more regular about going to the gym, keeping track of whether I was getting enough fiber, and eating a large variety of fruits and vegetables, particularly cruciferous vegetables in salads. I also started drinking cold green tea. It is very good and refreshing. It was fun to try some of the foods that are known to have protective properties. I never ate soy before, but I tried soy milk and liked it. I also really enjoy eating blueberries, which are very good for you. I wear sunblock when I know that I will be out in the sun for longer than 15 minutes. I don't smoke, and I avoid secondhand smoke at all costs. I feel happy that I am now doing my best to lessen my chances of getting cancer. All the behaviors that help with that are simple things that make me feel good anyway!

PERSONAL PROFILE: Personal Cancer Prevention Program

I. Do you have a family history of cancer? ___ Yes ___ No

II. What role do nutrition and exercise play in your personal cancer prevention program?

III. List lifestyle factors that you are aware of increase cancer risk.

IV. List environmental contaminants that may cause cancer.

V. Is tanning and personal appearance worth the potential risk of developing skin cancer? ___ Yes ___ No

VI. Are you familiar with cancer prevention self-exams and warning signals to look for in a cancer prevention program? ___ Yes ___ No

---

Under normal conditions, the 100 trillion cells in the human body reproduce themselves in an orderly way. Cell growth (cell reproduction) takes place to repair and replace old, worn-out tissue. Cell growth is controlled by **deoxyribonucleic acid (DNA)** and **ribonucleic acid (RNA),** found in the nucleus of each cell. When nuclei lose their ability to regulate and control cell growth, cell division is disrupted and mutant cells can develop (see Figure 11.1). Some of these cells might grow uncontrollably and abnormally, forming a mass of tissue called a tumor, which can be either **benign** or **malignant.** Benign tumors do not invade other tissues. Although they can interfere with normal bodily functions, they rarely cause death. A malignant tumor is a **cancer.** More than 100 types of cancer can develop in any tissue or organ of the human body.

The process of cancer actually begins with an alteration in DNA. Within DNA are **oncogenes** and tumor **suppressor genes,** which normally work together to repair and replace cells. Defects in these genes—caused by external factors such as radiation, chemicals, and viruses, as well as internal factors such as immune conditions, hormones, and genetic mutations—ultimately allow the cell to grow into a tumor.

A healthy cell can duplicate as many as 100 times in its lifetime. Normally, the DNA molecule is duplicated perfectly during cell division. In the few cases when the DNA molecule is not replicated exactly, specialized enzymes make repairs quickly. Occasionally, however, cells with defective DNA keep dividing and ultimately form a small tumor. As more mutations occur, the altered cells continue to divide and can become malignant. A decade or more might pass between exposure to carcinogens or mutations and the time that cancer is diagnosed.

The process of abnormal cell division is related indirectly to chromosome segments called **telomeres** (see Figure 11.2). Each time a cell divides, chromosomes lose some telomeres. After many cell divisions, chromosomes eventually run out of telomeres and the cell then invariably dies.

Human tumors make an enzyme known as **telomerase.** In cancer cells, telomerase keeps the chromosome from running out of telomeres entirely. The shortened strand of telomeres (see Figure 11.3) now allows cells to reproduce indefinitely, creating a malignant tumor. Telomerase seems to have another function that is still under investigation: After many cell divisions, cancer cells grow old by nature, but telomerase is what apparently keeps them from dying. If scientists can confirm that telomerase plays such a crucial role in forming tumors, research will be directed to finding

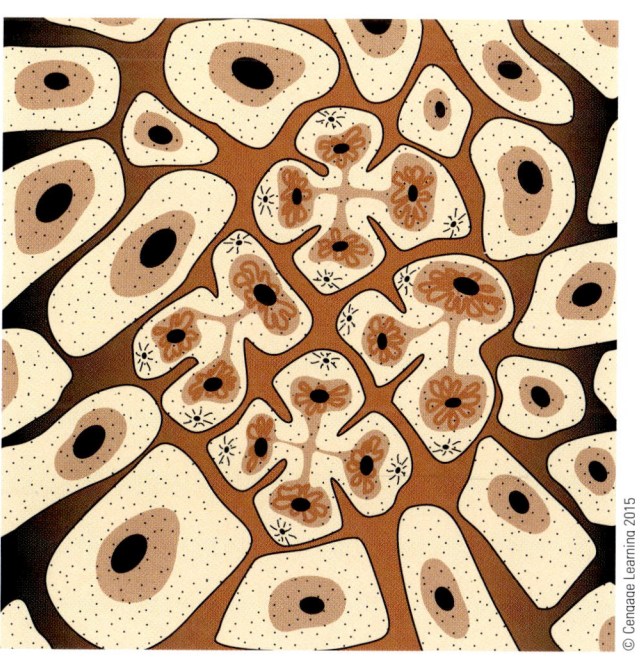

Figure 11.1 Mutant (cancer) cells.

Deoxyribonucleic acid (DNA) Genetic substance of which genes are made; molecule that contains cell's genetic code.

Ribonucleic acid (RNA) Genetic material that guides the formation of cell proteins.

Benign Noncancerous.

Malignant Cancerous.

Cancer Group of diseases characterized by uncontrolled growth and spread of abnormal cells.

Oncogenes Genes that initiate cell division.

Suppressor genes Genes that deactivate the process of cell division.

Telomeres A strand of molecules at both ends of a chromosome.

Telomerase An enzyme that allows cells to reproduce indefinitely.

Figure 11.2 Erosion of chromosome telomeres in normal cells.

Figure 11.3 Action of the enzyme telomerase.

a way to block the action of telomerase, thereby making cancerous cells die.

Cancer starts with the abnormal growth of one cell, which then can multiply into billions of cancerous cells. A critical turning point in the development of cancer is when a tumor reaches about a million cells. At this stage, it is referred to as **carcinoma in situ.** The undetected tumor may go for months or years without any significant growth. While it remains encapsulated, it does not pose a serious threat to human health. To grow, however, the tumor requires more oxygen and nutrients.

In time, a few of the cancer cells start producing chemicals that enhance **angiogenesis,** or capillary (blood vessel) formation into the tumor. Angiogenesis is the precursor of **metastasis.** Through the new blood vessels formed by angiogenesis, cancerous cells now can break away from a malignant tumor and migrate to other parts of the body, where they can cause new cancer (Figure 11.4).

Most adults have precancerous or cancerous cells in their bodies. By middle age, our bodies contain millions of precancerous cells. The immune system and blood turbulence destroy most cancer cells, but only one abnormal cell lodging elsewhere is enough to start a new cancer. These cells grow and multiply uncontrollably, invading and destroying normal tissue. The rate at which cancer cells grow varies from one type to another. Some types grow fast, and others take years.

Once cancer cells metastasize, treatment becomes more difficult. Although therapy can kill most cancer cells, a few cells might become resistant to treatment. These cells then can grow into a new tumor that will not respond to the same treatment.

11.1 Incidence of Cancer

According to the most recent mortality statistics from the National Center for Health Statistics, cancer causes about 23 percent of all deaths in the United States. It is the second lead-

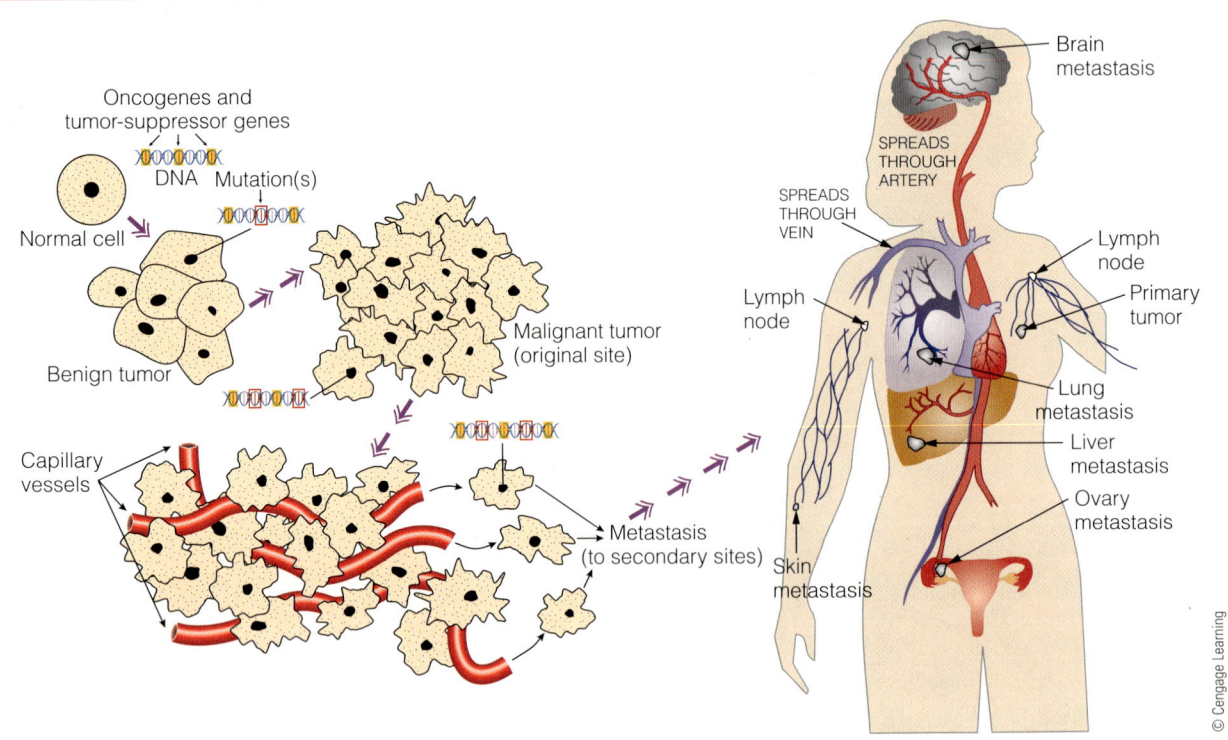

Figure 11.4 How cancer starts and spreads.

ing cause of death in the country and the leading cause in children between ages 1 and 14. The major contributor to the increase in incidence of cancer during the last five decades is lung cancer. Tobacco use alone is responsible for 30 percent of all deaths from cancer. Another third of all deaths from cancer are related to unhealthy nutrition, physical inactivity, and excessive body weight (fat).

Worldwide, experts predict that cancer will be the number one cause of death in the near future. This rise in cancer deaths is due primarily to the large increase in tobacco use in developing countries, particularly in India and China, home to 40 percent of the world's smokers.

Cancer is predicted to develop in approximately 1 of every 2 men and 1 of 3 women in the United States, affecting approximately 3 of every 4 families. The incidence is also higher in African Americans than in any other racial or ethnic group. Close to 600,000 people die from cancer in the United States every year and more than 1.6 million new cases are diagnosed per year.[1] The U.S. death rates for the major cancer sites are given in Figure 11.5.

Critical Thinking

Have you ever had, or do you now have, any family members with cancer? • Can you identify lifestyle or environmental factors as possible contributors to the disease? • If not, are you concerned about your genetic predisposition, and, if so, are you making lifestyle changes to decrease your risk?

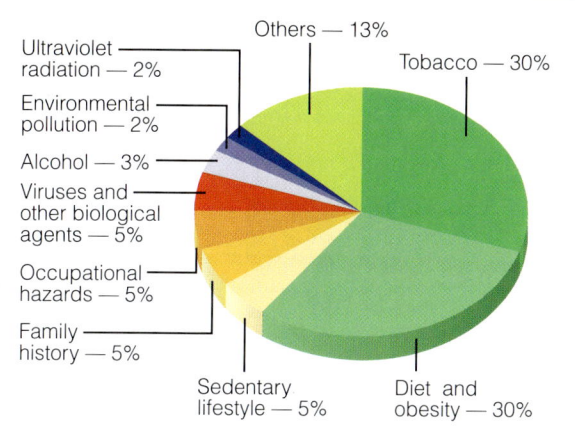

Figure 11.6 Your estimates of the relative role of the major cancer-causing factors.

- Ultraviolet radiation — 2%
- Environmental pollution — 2%
- Alcohol — 3%
- Viruses and other biological agents — 5%
- Occupational hazards — 5%
- Family history — 5%
- Sedentary lifestyle — 5%
- Diet and obesity — 30%
- Tobacco — 30%
- Others — 13%

SOURCE: Harvard Center for Cancer Prevention, "Causes of Human Cancer," *Harvard Report on Cancer Prevention* 1 (1996).

Like coronary heart disease, cancer is largely preventable. As much as 80 percent of all human cancer is related to lifestyle or environmental factors. The American Cancer Society released updated guidelines on nutrition and physical activity for cancer prevention.[2] These guidelines recommend that people:

1. Maintain healthy body weight throughout life
2. Adopt a physically active lifestyle
3. Adopt a healthy diet
4. Limit alcohol consumption if they drink alcoholic beverages

Additional existing general guidelines for cancer prevention for several decades now indicate that people should not use tobacco in any form (and limit exposure to secondhand smoke) and avoid exposure to occupational hazards (see Figure 11.6). Most cancers could be prevented by following the previously listed positive lifestyle habits and reducing environmental contaminants that may cause cancer (see box on page 376).

Research sponsored by the American Cancer Society and the National Cancer Institute showed that individuals who have a healthy lifestyle have some of the lowest cancer mortality rates ever reported in scientific studies. In a landmark study, a group of about 10,000 members of the Church of Jesus Christ of Latter-day Saints (commonly referred to as the Mormon church) in California was reported to have only about one-third (men) to one-half (women) the rate of cancer mortality of the general white population[3] (see Figure 11.7). In this study, the investigators looked at three

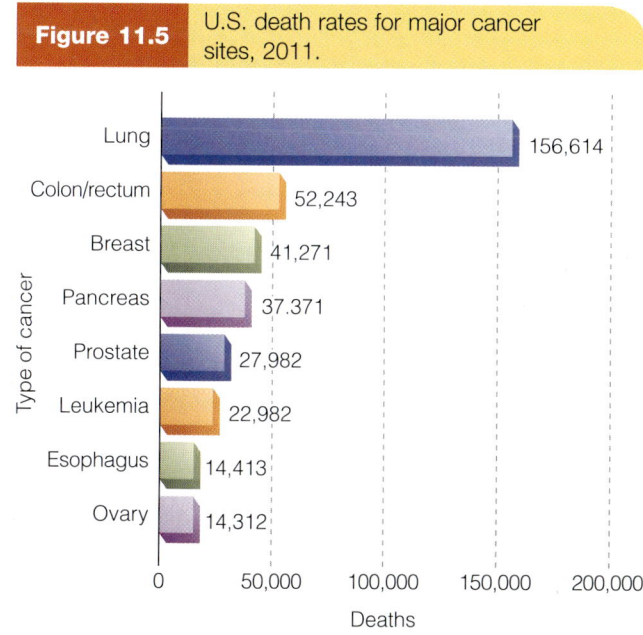

Figure 11.5 U.S. death rates for major cancer sites, 2011.

Type of cancer	Deaths
Lung	156,614
Colon/rectum	52,243
Breast	41,271
Pancreas	37,371
Prostate	27,982
Leukemia	22,982
Esophagus	14,413
Ovary	14,312

SOURCE: U.S. Department of Health and Human Services, Centers for Disease Control and Prevention, National Center for Health Statistics, *National Vital Statistics Reports, Deaths: Preliminary Data for 2011* 61, no. 6 (October 10, 2012).

Carcinoma in situ Encapsulated malignant tumor that has not spread.

Angiogenesis Formation of blood vessels (capillaries).

Metastasis The movement of cells from one part of the body to another.

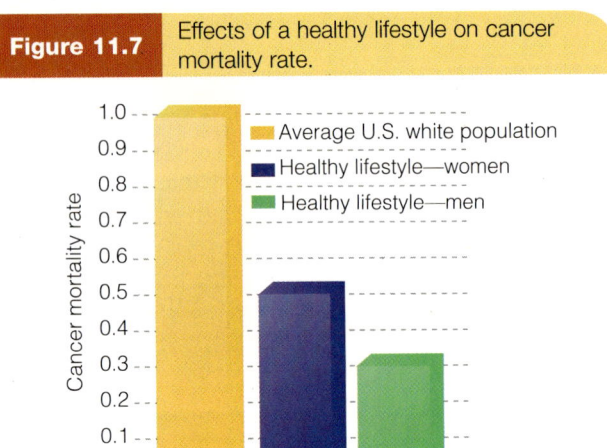

Figure 11.7 Effects of a healthy lifestyle on cancer mortality rate.

Healthy lifestyle factors include proper nutrition, abstinence from cigarette smoking, regular sleep (7–8 hours per night), and regular physical activity.

SOURCE: J.E. Enstrom, "Health Practices and Cancer Mortality Among Active California Mormons," *Journal of the National Cancer Institute* 81 (1989): 1807–1814.

general health habits in the participants: lifetime abstinence from smoking, regular physical activity, and sufficient sleep. Healthy lifestyle guidelines (encouraged by the church since 1833) include abstaining from all forms of tobacco, alcohol, and drugs, and adhering to a well-balanced diet based on grains, fruits, and vegetables, and moderate amounts of poultry and red meat.

Additional 2009 data from more than 23,000 German participants indicated that people who never smoked, had a BMI less than 30, exercised at least 3.5 hours per week, and consumed a diet rich in fruits and vegetables and low in meat, had a 36 percent lower risk of cancer.[4] The conclusion of the latter two studies is that lifestyle is definitely an important factor in the risk for cancer.

Equally important is that approximately 14 million Americans with a history of cancer were alive in 2012. Currently, six in ten people diagnosed with cancer are expected to be alive five years after their initial diagnosis.[5]

Behavior Modification Planning

Reducing Environmental Contaminants That May Cause Cancer

Since its creation in 1971, the U.S. President's Cancer Panel monitors exposure by the public to potential environmental cancer risks in daily life. The public remains by and large unaware of most of these widespread and underestimated risks, factors that are critical in any cancer prevention efforts. Exposure to environmental contaminants poses a threat to health because they may alter or interfere with a variety of biologic processes. Among the recommendations released in 2010 by the presidential panel are:

1. Filter tap water or well water and whenever possible use filtered water instead of commercially bottled water.
2. Properly dispose of pharmaceuticals, household chemicals, paints, and other products to minimize drinking water and soil contamination.
3. Eliminate exposure to secondhand smoke (and tobacco use in general).
4. Use stainless steel, glass, or BPA-free plastic water bottles.
5. Microwave in ceramic or glass instead of plastic containers.
6. Remove shoes before entering a home to avoid bringing in toxic chemicals, including pesticides.
7. Limit the consumption of food that is grown with pesticides and meats from animals raised with antibiotics and growth hormones.
8. Limit the consumption of processed, charred, or well-done meats that are high in heterocyclic amines and polyaromatic hydrocarbons.
9. Practice safe-sun exposure and avoid overexposure to ultraviolet light when the sunlight is most intense.
10. Reduce radiation exposure (x-rays) from medical sources.
11. Avoid exposure to three highly carcinogenic chemicals: formaldehyde, benzene, and radon.*
12. Use headsets and text, instead of talking on cell phones, and keep cell-phone calls brief to reduce exposure to electromagnetic energy. Although not scientifically proven, there is concern that frequent exposure to electromagnetic energy from cell phone use increases cancer risk.
13. Contaminant exposure in children is of significant concern because per pound of body weight they take in more food, water, air, and other substances than adults do. Toxic chemicals remain active longer in their developing brain and organs, placing them at far greater risk through chemical exposure.

*Formaldehyde is used in particle board, plywood, carpet, draperies, foam insulation, furniture, toiletries, and permanent press fabrics. Exposure is highest when newly installed. Benzene exposure is widespread and found primarily in vehicle exhaust. Radon exposure, which forms naturally and collects in homes, should be checked on a regular basis.

Behavior Modification Planning

Tips for a Healthy Cancer-Fighting Diet

I PLAN TO / I DID IT

I. Increase intake of phytonutrients, fiber, cruciferous vegetables, and antioxidants by

- ❏ ❏ Eating a predominantly vegetarian diet
- ❏ ❏ Eating more fruits and vegetables every day (six to eight servings per day maximize anticancer benefits)
- ❏ ❏ Increasing the consumption of broccoli, cauliflower, kale, turnips, cabbage, kohlrabi, Brussels sprouts, hot chili peppers, red and green peppers, carrots, sweet potatoes, winter squash, spinach, garlic, onions, strawberries, tomatoes, pineapple, and citrus fruits in your regular diet
- ❏ ❏ Eating vegetables raw or quickly cooked by steaming or stir-frying
- ❏ ❏ Substituting tea and fruit and vegetable juices for coffee and soda
- ❏ ❏ Eating whole-grain breads
- ❏ ❏ Including calcium in the diet (or from a supplement)
- ❏ ❏ Including soy products in the diet
- ❏ ❏ Using whole-wheat flour instead of refined white flour in baking
- ❏ ❏ Using brown (unpolished) rice instead of white (polished) rice

II. Limit saturated and trans fats by

- ❏ ❏ Using primarily unsaturated fats (olive oil, canola oil, nuts, seeds, avocado, fish, flaxseeds, and flaxseed oil)

III. Balancing caloric input

- ❏ ❏ Balancing caloric input with caloric output to maintain recommended body weight

Try It

Make a copy of these "Cancer-Fighting Diet" tips and each week incorporate into your lifestyle two additional dietary behaviors from the list.

11.2 Guidelines for Preventing Cancer

The biggest factor in fighting cancer today is health education. People need to be informed about the risk factors for cancer and the guidelines for early detection. The most effective way to protect against cancer is to change negative lifestyle habits and behaviors. Following are some guidelines for preventing cancer. For most Americans who do not use tobacco, increased physical activity and dietary choices are the most important modifiable risk factors.

Dietary Changes The American Cancer Society estimates that one-third of all cancer in the United States is related to nutrition and lack of physical activity. A healthy diet, therefore, is crucial to decrease the risk for cancer. The diet should be predominately vegetarian. **Cruciferous vegetables,** tea, vitamin D, soy products, calcium, and omega-3 fats are encouraged. If alcohol is used, it should be used in moderation. Obesity should be avoided.

Green and dark yellow vegetables, cruciferous vegetables (cauliflower, broccoli, cabbage, Brussels sprouts, and kohlrabi), and beans (legumes) seem to protect against cancer. Folate—found naturally in dark green leafy vegetables, dried beans, and orange juice—may reduce the risk for colon and cervical cancers. Brightly colored fruits and vegetables also contain **carotenoids**

Cruciferous vegetables are recommended in a cancer-prevention diet.

> **Cruciferous vegetables** Plants that produce cross-shaped leaves (cauliflower, broccoli, cabbage, Brussels sprouts, kohlrabi), which seem to have a protective effect against cancer.
>
> **Carotenoids** Pigment substances in plants that are often precursors to vitamin A. More than 600 carotenoids are found in nature, about 50 of which are precursors to vitamin A, the most potent one being beta-carotene.

and vitamin C. Lycopene, one of the many carotenoids (a phytonutrient—see the following discussion), has been linked to lower risk for cancers of the prostate, colon, and cervix. Lycopene is especially abundant in cooked tomato products.

The evidence for vitamin D in protecting against cancer continues to mount each day. Vitamin D is the most powerful regulator of cell growth and keeps cells from becoming malignant. The protective effect of vitamin D appears to be strongest against breast, colon, and prostate cancers, and possibly lung and digestive cancers. You should strive for "safe sun" exposure, that is, 10 to 20 minutes of unprotected sun exposure, on most days of the week between the hours of 10:00 a.m. and 4:00 p.m. For people living in the northern United States and Canada with limited sun exposure during the winter months, a vitamin D3 supplement of up to 2,000 IUs per day is strongly recommended. The cancer-protective benefits of this vitamin have already been discussed in detail in Chapter 3 (see "Vitamin D," page 107).

Some researchers believe that the antioxidant effect of vitamins and the mineral selenium helps to protect the body. During normal metabolism, most of the oxygen in the human body is converted into stable forms of carbon dioxide and water. A small amount, however, ends up in an unstable form known as oxygen-free radicals, which are thought to attack and damage the cell membrane and DNA, leading to the formation of cancers. Antioxidants are thought to absorb free radicals before they can cause damage and also interrupt the sequence of reactions once damage has begun. Research is still required in this area because a clear link has not been established.

Phytonutrients

Phytonutrients are compounds found in abundance in fruits, vegetables, beans, nuts, and seeds. These nutrients may prevent cancer by blocking the formation of cancerous tumors and perhaps even disrupting the process once it has started. Each plant contains hundreds of phytonutrients. Examples of these nutrients and their effects are found in Table 11.1. To obtain the best possible protection, a minimum of five servings of a variety of fruits and vegetables should be consumed each day. Fruits and vegetables should be consumed several times a day (instead of in one meal) to maintain phytonutrients at effective levels throughout the day. Phytonutrient blood levels drop within 3 hours of consuming foods containing these nutrients.

Fiber

Initial studies linked low intake of fiber to increased risk for colorectal cancer. Recent data, however, have been inconclusive.[6] While high fiber intake may not decrease the risk of colorectal cancer, a high-fiber diet is still encouraged because it decreases the risk for other chronic conditions such as cardiovascular disease and diabetes. Daily consumption of 25 (women) to 38 (men) grams of fiber is recommended. Whole grains are high in fiber and contain vitamins and minerals (folate, selenium, and calcium). Selenium protects against prostate cancer and, possibly, lung cancer. Calcium may protect against colon cancer by preventing the rapid growth of cells in the colon, especially in people with colon polyps.

Table 11.1 Selected Phytonutrients: Their Effects and Sources

Phytonutrient	Effect	Good Sources
Sulforaphane	Removes carcinogens from cells	Broccoli
PEITC	Keeps carcinogens from binding to DNA	Broccoli
Genistein	Prevents small tumors from accessing capillaries to get oxygen and nutrients	Soybeans
Flavonoids	Helps keep cancer-causing hormones from locking onto cells	Most fruits and vegetables
p-coumaric and chlorogenic acids	Disrupts the chemical combination of cell molecules that can produce carcinogens	Strawberries, green peppers, tomatoes, and pineapple
Capsaicin	Keeps carcinogens from binding to DNA	Hot chili peppers

© Cengage Learning

Tea

Polyphenols (a group of phytonutrients) are potent cancer-fighting antioxidants found in fresh fruits and vegetables and many grains. A prime source is tea. Green, black, and red tea all seem to provide protection. Evidence also points to certain components in tea that can block the spread of cancers to other parts of the body. Polyphenols are known to block the formation of **nitrosamines** and quell the activation of **carcinogens.** Polyphenols also are thought to fight cancer by shutting off the formation of cancer cells, turning up the body's natural detoxification defenses, and thereby suppressing progression of the disease. Different types of tea contain different mixtures of polyphenols. White tea appears to have the highest amount, followed by green and black tea. Herbal teas do not provide the same benefits as regular tea.

Observational data on tea-drinking habits in China showed that people who regularly drank green tea had about half the risk for chronic gastritis and stomach cancer, and the risk decreased further as the number of years of drinking green tea increased.[7] In Japan, where people drink green tea regularly but smoke twice as much as people in the United States, the incidence of lung cancer is half that of the United States.

The antioxidant effect of one of the polyphenols in green tea, epigallocatechin gallate, or EGCG, is at least 25 times more effective than vitamin E and 100 times more effective than vitamin C at protecting cells and DNA from damage believed to cause cancer, heart disease, and other diseases associated with free radicals.[8] Other research suggests that green tea inhibits the growth of cancer cells. EGCG also is twice as strong as the red wine antioxidant resveratrol in helping to prevent heart disease.

Many of the benefits of regular tea consumption warrant further investigation. Optimistic results in animal studies are still unclear in humans. Drinking two or more cups of tea daily, preferably white or green, in place of popular high-sugar/nutrient-deficient sodas is encouraged.

Although still in the early stages, research is uncovering cancer-fighting phytonutrients in many traditional spices. These phytonutrients may alter damaging carcinogenic pathways, provide antioxidant effects, promote cancer-fighting enzymes, decrease inflammation, stimulate the immune system, and suppress the development of tumors.[9] Ginger, oregano, curry, pepper, cloves, fennel, rosemary, and turmeric are all encouraged for use in cooking and at the table.

Sugar

New evidence indicates that frequent consumption of sugar and high-sugar foods may be associated with greater risk for pancreatic cancer, one of the most deadly forms of cancer.[10] Sugar is rapidly absorbed into the blood, quickly raising glucose and insulin levels. Researchers theorize that excessive glucose poisons and kills pancreatic cells, increasing cancer risk. Excessive insulin results in insulin-like growth factor, believed to increase cell proliferation and cancer.

The data showed that people who consumed the most sugar, including creamed fruit, syrup-based drinks, soft drinks, and foods such as coffee, tea, and cereal to which sugar is added had almost a 70 percent higher risk of developing pancreatic cancer compared with those with the lowest sugar consumption. Individuals who drank more than two soft drinks a day almost doubled the risk for pancreatic cancer.

Dietary Fat

Although previously viewed as a risk factor, minimal evidence exists that total fat intake affects cancer risk. There is far greater evidence that being overweight or obese increases cancer risk. Excessive caloric intake leads to weight gain and high fat foods are typically calorie dense. Thus, indirectly, a high-fat diet can increase cancer risk through excessive body weight.

In any healthy diet, fat intake should be primarily monounsaturated and omega-3 polyunsaturated fats (found in flaxseed and several types of cold-water fish). These types of fat seem to offer protection against colorectal, pancreatic, breast, oral, esophageal, and stomach cancers. Omega-3 fats also block the synthesis of prostaglandins, bodily compounds that promote growth of tumors.

Processed Meat and Protein

Salt-cured, smoked, and nitrite-cured foods have been associated with cancers of the esophagus, stomach, colon, and rectum. Processed meats (hot dogs, ham, bacon, sausage, and lunch meats) should be consumed sparingly and always with vitamin C–rich foods such as orange juice, as vitamin C seems to discourage the formation of nitrosamines. These potentially cancer-causing compounds are formed when nitrites and nitrates, which are used to prevent the growth of harmful bacteria in processed meats, combine with other chemicals in the stomach. According to the American Institute for Cancer Research, a daily intake of 3.5 ounces of processed meat increases colorectal cancer risk by 42 percent.

Cooking protein at higher temperature to "medium well" or "well done" should be done only occasionally as such leads to the formation of carcinogenic substances on the surface of meats.

The combination of the heme protein with iron, both found abundantly in red meat (but not poultry and fish), also contributes to the formation of nitrosamines in the large intestine, increasing the risk for colorectal cancer.

Further, nutritional guidelines discourage the excessive intake of protein. Too much animal protein appears to decrease blood enzymes that prevent precancerous cells from developing into tumors. According to the National Cancer Institute, eating substantial amounts of red meat may increase the risk for colorectal, pancreatic, breast, prostate, and renal cancer.

Cooking protein at a high temperature should be avoided or done so only occasionally. The data suggest that grilling, broiling, or frying meat, poultry, or fish at high temperatures to "medium well" or "well done" leads to the formation of carcinogenic substances known as heterocyclic amines (HCAs) and polycyclic aromatic hydrocarbons (PAHs). Individuals who prefer their meat medium well or well done have a much higher risk for colorectal and stomach cancers.

When proteins are cooked at high temperatures, amino acids are changed into HCAs that collect on the surface of meats. Charring meat increases

---

Phytonutrients Compounds found in fruits and vegetables that block formation of cancerous tumors and disrupt the progress of cancer.

Nitrosamines Potentially cancer-causing compounds formed when nitrites and nitrates, which prevent the growth of harmful bacteria in processed meats, combine with other chemicals in the stomach.

Carcinogens Substances that contribute to the formation of cancers.

their formation to an even greater extent. PAHs are formed when fat drips onto the rocks or coals of the grill. The subsequent fire flare-up releases smoke that coats the food with PAHs.

An electric contact grill such as a George Foreman grill is preferable when cooking meats because cooking temperatures are easily controlled. When cooking on an outdoor grill, line the grill with foil to minimize flare-up damage. Microwaving the meat for a couple of minutes before barbecuing also decreases the risk, as long as the fluid released by the meat is discarded. Most of the potential carcinogens collect in this solution. Precooking in the microwave will also decrease grilling time.

For an occasional outdoor barbecue, what you grill and how you grill are the most important factors. Animal products (both red and white meat) are the culprits, whereas grilling fruit and vegetables does not produce HCAs or PAHs. When grilling meats, the following approach can decrease HCAs and PAHs up to 90 percent.

- Cook meats with natural antioxidants, which decrease or eliminate HCAs and PAHs. Always marinate meat for at least 4 hours using some combination of vinegar, oil (preferably olive oil), and herbs and condiments including rosemary, red and black pepper, paprika, allspice, garlic, mustard, turmeric, thyme, chives, oregano, basil, sage, or parsley, among others. The marinade is believed to act as a barrier against the heat.
- Keep the meat moist and trim off all excess fat to avoid flare-ups.
- Microwave meat, poultry, and fish for 90 seconds to 2 minutes prior to grilling as such eliminates most of the HCAs.
- Cook at lower heat, less than 350°F, to "medium" rather than "well" or "well done."
- Cook over aluminum foil with small holes cut in the foil so that drippings can pass through.
- Turn the meat over frequently, every three to four minutes.
- Remove all skin before serving.
- Add broccoli to your meal. Broccoli has been shown to break down HCAs.
- Eat less meat as such increases your risk for cancer.

Soy

Soy protein seems to decrease the formation of carcinogens during cooking of meats. Soy foods may help because soy contains chemicals that prevent cancer. Although further research is merited, isoflavones (phytonutrients) found in soy are structurally similar to estrogen and may prevent breast, prostate, lung, and colon cancers. Isoflavones, frequently referred to as "phytoestrogens" or "plant estrogens," also block angiogenesis. Presently, it is not known whether the health benefits of soy are derived from isoflavones by themselves or in combination with other nutrients found in soy.

One drawback of soy was found in studies in which animals with tumors were given large amounts of soy. The estrogen-like activity of soy isoflavones actually led to the growth of estrogen-dependent tumors. Experts, therefore, caution women with breast cancer or a history of this disease to limit their soy intake because it could stimulate cancer cells by closely imitating the actions of estrogen. No specific recommendations are presently available as to the recommended amount of daily soy protein intake to prevent cancer.

Based on the traditional diets of people (including children) in China and Japan who consume soy foods regularly, there doesn't seem to be an unsafe natural level of consumption. Soy protein powder supplementation, however, may elevate intake of soy protein to an unnatural (and perhaps unsafe) level.

Alcohol Consumption

The general recommendation has been that people should consume alcohol in moderation, because too much alcohol raises the risk for developing certain cancers, especially when it is combined with tobacco smoking or smokeless tobacco. In combination, these substances significantly increase the risk for cancers of the mouth, larynx, throat, esophagus, and liver. The combined action of heavy alcohol and tobacco use can increase the odds of developing cancer of the oral cavity fifteenfold.

A 2009 study of almost 1.3 million women between the ages of 45 and 75, however, indicated that as little as one drink of alcohol per day increases a women's risk of cancer by 13 percent, including cancers of the breast, esophagus, larynx, rectum, and liver.[11] The researchers concluded that even low-to-moderate alcohol consumption increases cancer risk in women and the risks outweigh any potential cardioprotective benefits. Based on these data, it is estimated that about 30,000 yearly female cancers in the United States are due to these low levels of alcohol consumption.

Nutrient Supplements

An expert panel of the World Cancer Research Fund and the American Institute of Cancer Research stated that unless recommended by your doctor, you should not use supplements to protect against cancer. There is strong evidence that high-dose supplements of certain nutrients increase the risk of certain cancers. The best source of nutrients is a healthy diet.

Excessive Body Weight

Maintaining recommended body weight is encouraged. Based on estimates, excess weight accounts for 14 to 20 percent of deaths from cancer.[12] Furthermore, obese men and women have a more than 50 percent increased risk for dying from any form of cancer.[13] Adult weight gain increases the risk for many cancers, including those of the breast, colon/rectum, endometrium, esophagus, and kidney. Obesity may also increase the risk for pancreatic, gallbladder, ovarian, thyroid, and cervical cancers. Investigators theorize that excess weight raises hormone levels in the body that stimulate tumor growth.

Heavy drinking and smoking greatly increase the risk of oral cancer.

Abstaining from Tobacco Cigarette smoking by itself is a major health hazard. The biggest carcinogenic exposure in the environment without question is tobacco use and exposure to secondhand smoke. If we include all related deaths, smoking is responsible for more than 443,000 unnecessary deaths and 160,000 lung cancer deaths in the United States each year. The World Health Organization estimates that smoking causes 5 million deaths worldwide annually. The average life expectancy for a chronic smoker is about 13 to 14 years shorter than for a nonsmoker.[14]

Of all cancers, at least 30 percent are tied to smoking, and 87 percent of lung cancers are linked to smoking. Cigarette smoking contributes to at least 15 additional types of cancer, including oral, lip, nasal, pharyngeal, laryngeal, esophageal, uterine, stomach, and pancreatic. Use of smokeless tobacco can also lead to nicotine addiction and dependence, as well as increased risk for cancers of the mouth, larynx, throat, and esophagus. If you smoke or use any other tobacco products, STOP NOW! If you do not smoke, DON'T EVER START. If you are ever around people who are smoking, claim your right to clean air, or distance yourself from them as much as you possibly can.

Avoiding Excessive Exposure to Sun Near-daily "safe sun" exposure, that is, 10 to 20 minutes of unprotected exposure during peak hours of the day is beneficial to health; but too much exposure to ultraviolet radiation is a major contributor to skin cancer. The most common sites of skin cancer are the areas exposed to the sun most often (face, neck, and back of the hands). Ultraviolet rays are strongest when the sun is high in the sky. Therefore, you should avoid prolonged sun exposure between 10:00 a.m. and 4:00 p.m. Take the shadow test: If your shadow is shorter than you, the ultraviolet (UV) rays are at their strongest.

The three types of skin cancer are:

1. Basal cell carcinoma
2. Squamous cell carcinoma
3. Malignant melanoma

Nearly 90 percent of the almost 1 million cases of basal cell or squamous cell skin cancers reported yearly in the United States could have been prevented by protecting the skin from excessive sun exposure. **Melanoma,** the most deadly type, caused approximately 12,650 deaths in 2013. About 20 percent of Americans will develop skin cancer in their lifetime. Treatment for nonmelanoma skin cancer increased by more than 75 percent between 1992 and 2006. Melanoma, the most life-threatening form of skin cancer, increased 800 and 400 percent in young women and young men respectively between 1970 and 2009.

One to two blistering sunburns can double the lifetime risk for melanoma, even more so if the sunburn takes place prior to age 18, when cells divide at a much faster rate than later in life. Furthermore, nothing is healthy about a "healthy tan." Tanning of the skin is the body's natural reaction to permanent and irreversible damage from too much exposure to the sun. Even small doses of sunlight add up to a greater risk for skin cancer and premature aging. The tan fades at the end of the summer season, but the underlying skin damage does not disappear.

The stinging sunburn comes from **ultraviolet B (UVB) rays,** which are also thought to be the main cause of premature wrinkling and skin aging, roughened/leathery/sagging skin, and skin cancer. Unfortunately, the damage may not become evident until up to 20 years later. By comparison, skin that has not been overexposed to the sun remains smooth and unblemished and, over time, shows less evidence of aging.

Sun lamps and tanning parlors provide mainly **ultraviolet A (UVA) rays.** Once thought to be safe, they too are now known to be damaging and have been linked to melanoma. As little as 15 to 30 minutes of exposure to UVA rays can be as dangerous as a day spent in the sun. Similar to regular exposure to sun, short-term exposure to recreational tanning at a salon causes DNA alterations that can lead to skin cancer.[15]

Sunscreen lotion should be applied about 30 minutes before lengthy exposure to the sun because the skin takes that long to absorb the protective ingredients. Select sunscreens labeled "broad spectrum," as these products block both UVA and UVB rays. A **sun protection factor (SPF)** of at least 15 is recommended. SPF 15 means that the skin takes 15 times longer to burn than it would with no lotion. If you ordinarily get a mild sunburn after 20 minutes of noonday sun, an SPF 15 allows you to remain in the sun about 300

> **Melanoma** The most virulent, rapidly spreading form of skin cancer.
>
> **Ultraviolet B (UVB) rays** Ultraviolet rays that cause sunburn and lead to skin cancers.
>
> **Ultraviolet A (UVA) rays** Ultraviolet rays that pass deeper into the skin and are believed to cause skin damage and skin cancers.
>
> **Sun protection factor (SPF)** Degree of protection offered by ingredients in sunscreen lotion; at least SPF 15 is recommended.

Tanned skin is the body's natural reaction to permanent and irreversible damage—a precursor to severe or fatal skin cancer.

minutes before burning. Sunscreens with stronger SPF factors are not necessarily better. They should be applied just as often and they block only an additional 3 to 4 percent of ultraviolet rays. SPF 15 is adequate for most people.

Medical experts are also concerned about hormone-mimicking active ingredients in some sunscreens that are absorbed into the skin and possibly the bloodstream. Although the jury is still out on any potential harmful health effects of these ingredients, preferably choose a sunscreen that contains zinc oxide, titanium dioxide, or both. These are finely crushed minerals in sunscreens that shield the skin from the sun's ultraviolet rays.

When swimming or sweating, you should reapply sunscreens more often, because all sunscreens lose strength when they are diluted. Look for "water resistant" or "very water resistant" sunscreens, as such will adhere to the skin for 40 to 80 minutes, respectively. "Waterproof," "sweat-proof," and "continuous protection" sunscreens are not as effective.

If you plan on being out in the sun for a lengthy period of time, even better than sunscreen, is wearing protective clothing, including long-sleeved shirts, long pants, and a hat with a two to three-inch brim all the way around. This sun-protection strategy is even more critical for fair-skinned individuals who burn readily or turn red after only a few minutes of unprotected sun exposure, have a large number of moles, or have a personal or family history of skin cancer risk. Sun-protective fabrics, such as those manufactured by Coolibar® or Sun Precautions®, offer additional protection. You can also use RIT Sun Guard, a laundry additive that when used in washing penetrates the fibers and subsequently absorbs ultraviolet rays during sun exposure. The additive blocks up to 96 percent of UVA and UVB rays.

Monitoring Estrogen, Radiation Exposure, and Potential Occupational Hazards Estrogen use has been linked to endometrial cancer in some studies. Although the exposure to radiation from x-rays increases the risk for cancer, the benefits of x-rays may outweigh the risk involved, and most medical facilities use the lowest dose possible to keep the risk to a minimum. Occupational hazards—such as exposure to asbestos fibers, nickel and uranium dusts, chromium compounds, vinyl chloride, and bischlormethyl ether—increase the risk for cancer. Cigarette smoking magnifies the risk from occupational hazards.

Physical Activity An active lifestyle has been shown to have a protective effect against cancer. Although the mechanism is not clear, physical fitness and cancer mortality in men and women may have a graded and consistent inverse relationship (see Figure 11.8). A daily 30-minute, moderate-intensity exercise program lowers the risk for colon, breast, and uterine cancers between 20 and 50 percent; and vigorous physical activity may lower the risk of more aggressive and fatal types of prostate cancer.[16]

Research among 38,410 men followed for an average period of 17.2 years indicated a strong inverse relationships between cardiorespiratory fitness and cancer mortality; that is, the less-fit men had greater cancer deaths rates than the more-fit men.[17] A 2009 study on more than 2,200 men 49 years of age and older that were followed up for more than 35 years found that at least 30 minutes a day of moderate to high-intensity physical activity is inversely associated with the risk of premature death from cancer in men.[18] The researchers concluded that the activity needed to be at least moderate intensity to achieve the benefit of reducing overall cancer mortality. After 10 years, men who switched from low- or medium- to high-intensity physical activity (greater than 5.2 METs) were found to have half the risk of dying from cancer. There were no changes in mortality rate when switching from low to medium level physical activity. Other data suggest that in men 65 or older, exercising vigorously at least three times per week decreases the risk for advanced or fatal prostate cancer by 70 percent.[19]

Data on more than 6,300 women indicate that regular exercise lowers the risk for breast cancer by up to 40 percent, regardless of race or ethnicity.[20] Other studies have found similar results. Women who are active throughout life also cut their risk for endometrial cancer by about 40 percent. Those who started exercise in adulthood cut their risk by about 25 percent.[21] Among women diagnosed with breast cancer, those who walk 2 to 3 miles per hour one to three times per week are 20 percent less likely to die of the disease. Those who walk three to five times per week cut their risk in

Figure 11.8 Association between physical fitness and cancer mortality.

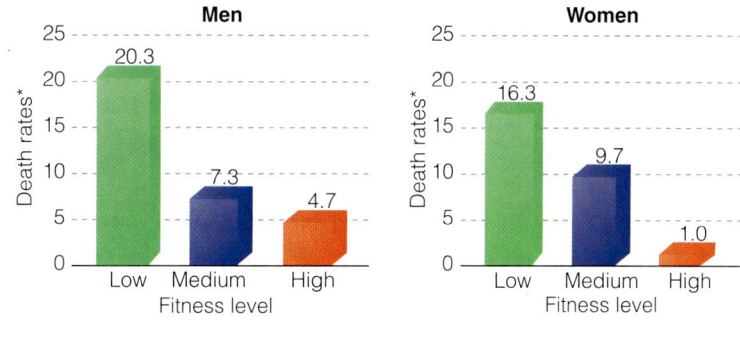

*Age adjusted per 10,000 person-years at follow-up.

Source: S. N. Blair et al., "Physical Fitness and All-Cause Mortality: A New Prospective Study of Healthy Men and Women," *Journal of the American Medical Association* 262 (1989): 2394-2401.

half.[22] Researchers believe that the decreased levels of circulating ovarian hormones through physical activity decrease breast cancer risk. Physical activity also decreases inflammation and body fat, both risk factors for cancer.

Regular strength-training also contributes to lower cancer mortality. A total of 8,677 men between the ages of 20 and 82 were tracked for more than two decades. The data indicated that men who regularly worked out with weights and had the highest muscle strength were up to 40 percent less likely to die from cancer, even among men with a higher waist circumference and BMI.[23]

The risk for other forms of cancer may also decrease, but additional research is necessary before definitive statements can be made. Growing evidence suggests that the body's autoimmune system may play a role in preventing cancer and that moderate exercise improves the autoimmune system.

Early Detection Fortunately, many cancers can be controlled or cured through early detection. The real problem comes when cancerous cells spread, because they become more difficult to destroy. Therefore, effective prevention, or at least early detection, is crucial. Herein lies the importance of periodic screening. Once a month, women should practice breast self-examination (BSE); and men, testicular self-examination (TSE). Men should pick a regular day each month (e.g., the first day of each month) to practice TSE, and women should perform BSE two or three days after the menstrual period is over.

Other Factors The contributions of many of the other much-publicized factors are not as significant as those just pointed out. Intentional food additives, saccharin, processing agents, pesticides, and packaging materials currently used in the United States and other developed countries seem to have minimal consequences. High levels of tension and stress and poor coping may affect the autoimmune system negatively and render the body less effective in dealing with the various cancers. Chronic stress increases cortisol and inflammatory chemicals that sustain cancer growth.[24]

Behavior Modification Planning

Cancer Promoters
- Use or exposure to tobacco products
- Physical inactivity
- Being more than 10 pounds overweight
- Frequent consumption of red meat
- A diet high in fat
- Charred/burned foods
- Frequent consumption of nitrate/nitrite-cured, salt-cured, or smoked foods
- Alcohol consumption
- Excessive sun exposure
- Estrogens
- Methyleugenol (flavoring agent in packaged foods)
- Radon, formaldehyde, and benzene
- Wood dust (high levels)

Try It

In your Online Journal or class notebook, make a list of cancer promoters around you and note whether you take necessary actions to avoid them. If you do not, note what it would take for you to do so.

Genetics plays a role in susceptibility in about 10 percent of all cancers. Most of the effect is seen in the early childhood years. Some cancers are a combination of genetic and environmental liability; genetics may add to the environmental risk of certain types of cancers. "Environment" means more than pollution and smoke. It incorporates diet, lifestyle-related events, viruses, and physical agents such as x-rays and exposure to the sun.

11.3 Warning Signals of Cancer

Everyone should become familiar with the following seven warning signals for cancer and bring any that are present to a physician's attention:

1. Change in bowel or bladder habits
2. Sore that does not heal
3. Unusual bleeding or discharge
4. Thickening or lump in the breast or elsewhere
5. Indigestion or difficulty in swallowing
6. Obvious change in wart or mole
7. Nagging cough or hoarseness

In Activity 11.1, you will be able to determine how well you are doing in terms of a cancer-prevention program. Activity 11.2 provides a questionnaire to alert you to symptoms that may indicate a serious health problem. Although in most cases nothing serious will be found, any symptom calls for a physician's attention as soon as possible. Scientific evidence and testing procedures for the prevention and early detection of cancer do change. Studies continue to provide new information. The intent of cancer-prevention programs is to educate and guide people toward a lifestyle that will help prevent cancer and enable early detection of malignancy.

Treatment of cancer should always be left to specialized physicians and cancer clinics. Current treatment modalities include surgery, radiation, radioactive substances, chemotherapy, hormones, and immunotherapy.

11.4 Cancer: Assessing Your Risks

Figure 11.9 provides a self-testing questionnaire to help you assess your cancer risk. The factors listed in the questionnaire are the major risk factors for specific cancer sites and by no means represent the only ones that might be involved. Check your status against the factors contained in this questionnaire. Based on the number of risk factors that apply to you, rate yourself on a scale from 1 to 3 (1 for low risk, 2 for moderate risk, and 3 for high risk) for each cancer site. Explanations of the risk factors for each type of cancer follow. If you are at higher risk, you are advised to discuss the results with your physician. Record your risk level totals for each cancer site in Activity 11.3.

11.5 Common Sites of Cancer

Lung Cancer
Risk Factors

1. Smoking status. Tobacco smoke causes nearly 9 out of 10 cases of lung cancer (includes cigarette, cigar, and pipe smoking). Smoking low-tar or "light" cigarettes increases lung cancer risk as much as regular cigarettes. The rates for ex-smokers who have not smoked for 10 years is half that of nonsmokers.
2. Amount and length of time smoked. The risk increases with the number of cigarettes smoked per day and years the individual has smoked.
3. Secondhand smoke. Exposure to secondhand smoke increases lung cancer risk. For example, nonsmoking spouses who live with a smoker have a 20 percent greater risk of developing lung cancer than do spouses of nonsmokers. Some individuals have a greater susceptibility to lung cancer as a result of secondhand smoke exposure.
4. Radon gas exposure. Radon, a radioactive gas that tends to build up indoors, is a potential cancer risk. The risk is also much greater for smokers. Homes and buildings should be tested periodically for radon content. State and local EPA offices provide information on radon testing.
5. Type of industrial work. Exposure to certain mining materials, uranium and radioactive products, or asbestos has been demonstrated to be associated with lung cancer. Exposure to materials in other industries also carries a higher risk. Smokers who work in these industries have greatly increased risks. Exposure to arsenic, radiation from occupational/medical/environmental sources, and air pollution increase the risk for lung cancer.

Colon/Rectum Cancer
Risk Factors

1. Age. Colon cancer occurs more frequently after 50 years of age.
2. Family predisposition. Colon cancer is more common in families that have a previous history of this disease.
3. Personal history. Polyps and bowel diseases are associated with colon cancer.
4. Physical inactivity. Strong scientific evidence points to a higher risk for colorectal cancer in physically inactive individuals.
5. Race or ethnicity. African Americans and Jews of Eastern European descent have some of the highest colorectal cancer rates in the world.

In addition to the previously mentioned risk factors, smoking, alcohol consumption, a diet high in saturated fat and/or red meat, a diet low in fiber, inadequate consumption of fruits and vegetables, type 2 diabetes, and inflammatory bowel disease increase the risk for colon or rectal cancer.

Activity 11.1: Are You Taking Control of Your Lifestyle to Prevent Cancer?

Name _____ Date _____

Course _____ Section _____ Gender _____ Age _____

Scientists know that most cancers are related to lifestyle and environment—your nutrition, whether you use tobacco in any form, and where you work and play. Thus, you can reduce your cancer risk by taking control of how you live your daily life.

14 Steps to a Healthier Life and Reduced Cancer Risk

| | Yes | No |

1. **Are you eating more cruciferous vegetables?**
   They include broccoli, cauliflower, Brussels sprouts, all cabbages, kohlrabi, and kale. ☐ ☐

2. **Does your diet include high-fiber foods?** ☐ ☐

3. **Do you choose foods with vitamin A?**
   Fresh foods with beta-carotene, including carrots, peaches, apricots, squash, and broccoli are the best source—not vitamin pills. ☐ ☐

4. **Is vitamin C included in your diet?**
   You'll find it naturally in lots of fresh fruits and vegetables, including grapefruit, cantaloupe, oranges, strawberries, red and green peppers, broccoli, and tomatoes. ☐ ☐

5. **Do you eat sufficient selenium-bearing foods?**
   Selenium is found in fish, Brazil nuts (primarily unshelled), and whole grains. Strive to obtain at least 100 mcg of selenium per day—but no more than 400 mcg per day. ☐ ☐

6. **Are you physically active for at least 30 minutes, and do you avoid excessive sitting on most days of the week?**
   Total number of daily steps: ☐☐☐☐ Total minutes of daily physical activity: ☐☐☐☐ ☐ ☐

7. **Do you maintain healthy weight (a BMI between 18.5 and 25)?** ☐ ☐

8. **Do you limit barbecuing and cooking meats at high temperatures to the point that they are "medium well" or "well done"?** ☐ ☐

9. **Do you limit salt-cured, smoked, and nitrite-cured foods?**
   Choose bacon, ham, hot dogs, or salt-cured fish only occasionally if you like them a lot. ☐ ☐

10. **Do you smoke cigarettes or use tobacco in any other form?** ☐ ☐

11. **If you drink alcohol at all, is your intake moderate (no more than 2 drinks per day for men, 1 for women, or none at all for women with a family history of breast, esophagus, larynx, rectum, or liver cancers)?** ☐ ☐

12. **Do you get almost daily "safe sun" exposure, and yet respect the sun's rays?**
    "Safe sun" exposure means 10 to 20 minutes of unprotected sun exposure (without sunscreen) to the face, arms, and hands during peak daylight hours on most days of the week (10:00 a.m. to 4:00 p.m.), but yet you respect the sun's rays (your skin does not turn pink or red and you do not sunburn). If not, do you take a daily vitamin D_3 supplement? ☐ ☐

    Do you protect yourself with sunscreen (at least SPF 15) and wear long sleeves and a hat, especially during midday hours, if you are going to be exposed to the sun for a prolonged period of time. ☐ ☐

13. **Do you have a family history of any type of cancer? If so, have you brought this to the attention of your personal physician?** ☐ ☐

14. **Are you familiar with the seven warning signals for cancer?** ☐ ☐

If you answered "yes" to most of these questions, **congratulations**. You are taking control of simple lifestyle factors that will help you feel better and reduce your risk for cancer.

© Fitness & Wellness, Inc.

Activity 11.2: Early Signs of Illness

Name _____ Date _____

Course _____ Section _____ Gender _____ Age _____

Major illnesses often begin with minor symptoms that if recognized early, allow you to control or cure the condition. In many cases, nothing is seriously wrong. Should you experience any of the following symptoms, however, you are strongly encouraged to bring them to the attention of your physician as soon as possible. In the following statements, please check only the conditions that apply.

☐ 1. Persistent unusual fatigue.

☐ 2. Sudden change in sleeping habits or feeling sleepy most of the day.

☐ 3. Sudden unexplained weight gain or loss (about 6 to 10 lb. in 10 weeks).

☐ 4. Pain or discomfort anywhere in the body that is not easily explained.

☐ 5. Severe headaches with no apparent reason.

☐ 6. A sore anywhere in the body that does not heal within a month.

☐ 7. Changes in moles, warts, or a skin blemish that begin to bleed, itch, or change in color, shape, or size.

☐ 8. Difficulty in swallowing, sudden vomiting occurrences, vomiting blood, or blood in coughed-up phlegm.

☐ 9. Shortness of breath or pain in the chest that may radiate to the jaw, shoulders, arms, or between the shoulder blades.

☐ 10. Fainting spells without reason.

☐ 11. Blurred vision or changes in vision such as seeing haloes.

☐ 12. Hoarseness or loss of voice without apparent reason that lasts several days.

☐ 13. A nagging cough that is getting worse.

☐ 14. Excessive thirst.

☐ 15. Swelling in the limbs/ankles or abdomen.

☐ 16. Persistent indigestion or abdominal pain.

☐ 17. A significant change in bowel habits, interchanging attacks of diarrhea and constipation.

☐ 18. Bowel movements that look unusually dark or rectal bleeding.

☐ 19. In men, discomfort/difficulty urinating, cloudy or reddish-looking urine, or discharge from the tip of the penis.

☐ 20. In women, vaginal bleeding or spotting between regular menstrual periods or following menopause.

☐ 21. In women, a lump or unusual thickening in a breast, changes in the shape or size of the breast, dimpling of the skin, "depression" of the nipples, any alteration in the breast noticeable by a change in position of the body, or any clear or bloody discharge after gently squeezing each nipple between your thumb and index finger.

☐ 22. Excessive sweating.

© Fitness & Wellness, Inc.

Figure 11.9 Cancer questionnaire: assessing your risks.

Name:_____ Date:_____

Course:_____ Section:_____ Gender:_____ Age:_____

Assessing Your Risks for Cancer

Read each question concerning each site and its specific risk factors. Be honest in your responses. Your risk increases as you move beyond item 1 for each factor. For example, the risk for breast cancer increases progressively as you age. If none of the answers apply, skip to the next question. Based on the number of risk factors that apply to you, rate yourself on a scale from 1 to 3 (1 for low risk, 2 for moderate risk, and 3 for high risk) for each cancer site. Record your results in Activity 11.3.

Lung Cancer

- Smoking status
  1. Non-smoker
  2. Smoker

- Amount of cigarettes smoked per day
  1. NA
  2. Less than 1 pack
  3. 1–2 packs
  4. 2+ packs

- Years smoked
  1. None
  2. 1–15
  3. 15–25
  4. >25

- Radon gas exposure
  1. No
  2. Yes
  3. Yes and smoker

- Type of industrial work
  1. Mining
  2. Uranium and radioactive products
  3. Asbestos

Colon/Rectum Cancer

- Age
  1. ≤40
  2. 41–60
  3. >60

- Family predisposition
  1. No
  2. Yes

- Personal history
  1. No
  2. Polyps
  3. Bowel diseases

- Are you physically active?
  1. Yes
  2. No

- Are you African American or a Jew of Eastern European descent?
  1. No
  2. Yes

Skin Cancer

- Do you practice safe sun exposure?
  1. Yes
  2. No

- Complexion—fair and/or light skin
  1. No
  2. Yes

- Personal or family history
  1. No
  2. Yes

- Work in mines, around coal tar, radioactive materials, or arsenic?
  1. No
  2. Yes

- Radiation treatment
  1. No
  2. Yes

Breast Cancer

- Age
  1. ≤35
  2. 36–50
  3. ≥51

- Are you Caucasian?
  1. No
  2. Yes

- Family history
  1. No
  2. One family member
  3. Two or more family members

- Personal history of breast or ovarian cancer
  1. No
  2. Yes

- Maternity
  1. First pregnancy before age 30
  2. First child after age 30
  3. No children

- Hormone replacement therapy
  1. No
  2. Short-term use
  3. Long-term use

- Are you physically active?
  1. Yes
  2. No

- Alcohol
  1. No alcohol
  2. <1 drink per day
  3. 1 drink per day
  4. >1 drink per day

- Are you significantly overweight?
  1. No
  2. Yes and premenopausal
  3. Yes and postmenopausal

Cervical Cancer

- Human papilloma virus (HPV) infection
  1. Never been infected
  2. Previously or currently infected

- Smoking status
  1. Nonsmoker
  2. Ex-smoker
  3. Current smoker

- HIV and chlamydia infections
  1. Neither one
  2. HIV
  3. Chlamydia
  4. Both

- Fruits and vegetables
  1. ≥5 servings per day
  2. 3–4 servings per day
  3. 1–2 servings per day
  4. <1 serving per day

- Are you overweight?
  1. No
  2. Yes

- Are you using birth control pills?
  1. No
  2. Yes

- Pregnancy
  1. Two or fewer
  2. Prior to age 17
  3. Multiple pregnancies

- Family history
  1. No
  2. Yes

Endometrial Cancer

- Estrogen therapy
  1. No
  2. Yes

- Age
  1. ≤40
  2. 41–49
  3. ≥50

- Are you Caucasian?
  1. No
  2. Yes

- Pregnancy
  1. Yes
  2. No

- Body weight
  1. At recommended weight
  2. Overweight
  3. Obese

- Diabetes
  1. No
  2. Yes

- Total years of menstrual cycles
  1. "Normal"
  2. Greater than "normal" (early start and/or late cessation)

- Are you hypertensive?
  1. No
  2. Yes

- Are you physically active?
  1. Yes
  2. No

Prostate Cancer

- Age
  1. ≤64
  2. ≥65

- Family history
  1. No
  2. Yes

(continued)

Figure 11.9 Cancer questionnaire: assessing your risks. *(continued)*

- Are you African American?
  1. No
  2. Yes

- Diet
  1. Low in saturated fat
  2. High in saturated fat

- Are you physically active?
  1. Yes
  2. No

Testicular Cancer

- Did you have an undescended testicle?
  1. No
  2. Yes

- Did you have abnormal testicular development?
  1. No
  2. Yes

- Do you have a family history of testicular cancer?
  1. No
  2. Yes

- Are you Caucasian?
  1. No
  2. Yes

Pancreatic Cancer

- Age
  1. ≤55
  2. ≥56

- Tobacco use
  1. No
  2. Yes

- Sugar intake
  1. Low
  2. Moderate
  3. Excessive

- Are you obese?
  1. No
  2. Yes

- Do you now have or have you had chronic pancreatitis, cirrhosis, or diabetes?
  1. No
  2. Yes

- Are you physically active?
  1. Yes
  2. No

- Are you African American?
  1. No
  2. Yes

- Family history
  1. No
  2. Yes

Kidney and Bladder Cancer

- Smoking history
  1. Nonsmoker
  2. Ex-smoker
  3. Cigarette smoker

- Were you diagnosed with congenital (inborn) abnormalities of the kidneys or bladder?
  1. No
  2. Yes

- Have you been exposed to aniline dyes, naphthalenes, or benzidines?
  1. No
  2. Yes

- Do you have a history of schistosomiasis (a parasitic bladder infection)?
  1. No
  2. Yes

- Do you suffer from frequent urinary tract infections?
  1. No
  2. Yes

Oral Cancer

- Tobacco use
  1. Nonuser
  2. Ex-user
  3. Pipe, cigar, or smokeless tobacco
  4. Cigarettes

- Alcohol use
  1. Do not drink alcohol
  2. Less than 1 drink per day (women) or 2 drinks per day (men)
  3. More than 1 drink per day (women) or 2 drinks per day (men)

Esophageal and Stomach Cancer

- How many servings of fruits and vegetables do you consume daily?
  1. >8
  2. 5–8
  3. 3–5
  4. <3

- How often do you consume salt-cured, smoked, or nitrate-cured foods?
  1. Rarely
  2. Less than once per week
  3. 1–3 times per week
  4. >3 times per week

- Have you been told that you have an imbalance in stomach acid?
  1. No
  2. Yes

- Do you have a history of pernicious anemia?
  1. No
  2. Yes

- Have you been diagnosed with chronic gastritis or gastric polyps?
  1. No
  2. Yes

- Family history of esophageal or stomach cancer?
  1. No
  2. Yes

- Are you overweight?
  1. No
  2. Yes

- Do you use alcohol or tobacco in any form?
  1. No
  2. Yes

Ovarian Cancer

- Age
  1. <50
  2. 51–60
  3. 61–70
  4. >70

- Do you have a personal history of ovarian problems?
  1. No
  2. Yes

- Have you had estrogen postmenopausal hormone therapy?
  1. No
  2. Yes

- Do you have an extensive history of menstrual irregularities?
  1. No
  2. Yes

- Family history
  1. None
  2. Breast cancer
  3. Ovarian cancer

- Do you have a personal history of breast cancer?
  1. No
  2. Yes

- Have you had a child?
  1. Yes
  2. No

- Body weight
  1. Normal
  2. 10–50 pounds overweight
  3. >50 pounds overweight

- Do you have a family history of nonpolyposis colon cancer?
  1. No
  2. Yes

Thyroid Cancer

- Age
  1. <35
  2. 35–55
  3. 56–70
  4. >70

- Did you receive radiation therapy to the head and neck region in childhood or adolescence?
  1. No
  2. Yes

- Do you have a family history of thyroid cancer?
  1. No
  2. Yes

Liver Cancer

- Do you have a family history of cirrhosis of the liver?
  1. No
  2. Yes

- Do you have a personal history of hepatitis B or hepatitis C virus?
  1. No
  2. Yes

- Have you been exposed to vinyl chloride (industrial gas used in plastics manufacturing)?
  1. No
  2. Yes

- Have you been exposed to aflatoxin (natural food contaminant)
  1. No
  2. Yes

- Alcohol
  1. None
  2. ≤2 drinks per day
  3. ≥3 drinks per day

- Are you Asian American or Pacific Islander?
  1. No
  2. Yes

(continued)

Figure 11.9 Cancer questionnaire: assessing your risks. *(continued)*

Leukemia

- Family history
  1. No
  2. Yes

- Do you suffer from Down syndrome or other genetic abnormalities?
  1. No
  2. Yes

- Have you had excessive exposure to ionizing radiation?
  1. No
  2. Yes

- Are you exposed to environmental chemicals?
  1. No
  2. Yes

Lymphomas

- Are you physically active?
  1. Yes
  2. No

- Do you have a family history of lymphomas?
  1. No
  2. Yes

- Are you exposed to
  1. Herbicides
  2. Organic solvents

- Have you had an organ transplant?
  1. No
  2. Yes

- Have you been diagnosed with any of the following?
  1. Epstein-Barr virus
  2. HIV
  3. Human T-cell leukemia/lymphoma virus-I (HTLV-1) virus

© Cengage Learning

2. Complexion. Risk factors vary for different types of skin. Individuals with light complexions, natural blonde or red hair, and those who burn easily are at greater risk.
3. Personal and family history of melanoma and moles. Of particular note are large or unusual moles or a large number of moles.
4. Work environment. Work in mines, around coal tar, radioactive materials, or arsenic (used in some insecticides) can cause cancer of the skin.
5. Radiation. Individuals who have undergone radiation treatment run a much higher risk of skin cancer in the treated area.

Risks for skin cancer are difficult to state. For instance, a person with a dark complexion can work longer in the sun and be less likely to develop cancer than a light-skinned person. Furthermore, a person wearing a long-sleeved shirt and a wide-brimmed hat who spends hours working in the sun has less risk than a person wearing a swimsuit who sunbathes for only a short time. The risk increases greatly with age, and family history also plays a role.

> **Critical Thinking**
>
> What significance does a "healthy tan" have in your social life?
> - Are you a "sun worshiper," or are you concerned about skin damage, premature aging, and potential skin cancer in your future?

If any of the previous risk factors apply to you, you need to protect your skin from the sun or any other toxic material. Changes in moles, warts, or skin sores are important and should be evaluated by your doctor (see Figure 11.10).

Skin Cancer

Risk Factors

1. UV light exposure. Excessive UV light is a culprit in skin cancer. Always practice safe sun exposure, that is, only 10 to 20 minutes of daily unprotected sun exposure. For longer exposure, protect yourself with a sunscreen medication

Figure 11.10 Warning signs of melanoma: ABCDE rule.

A. *Asymmetry:* One-half of a mole or lesion doesn't look like the other half.

B. *Border:* A mole has an irregular, scalloped, or not clearly defined border.

C. *Color:* The color varies or is not uniform from one area of a mole or lesion to another, whether the color is tan, brown, black, white, red, or blue.

D. *Diameter:* The lesion is larger than 6 millimeters (1/4 inch) or larger than a pencil eraser.

E. *Elevation:* Does it raise off the skin?

Source: Adapted from FDA Consumer, May 1991.

Skin Self-Exam

One of the easiest and quickest self-exams is a brief survey to detect possible skin cancers (see Figure 11.11). A simple skin self-exam can reduce deaths from melanoma by as much as 63 percent, saving as many as 4,500 lives in the United States each year.

Figure 11.11 Skin self-examination.

The American Cancer Society recommends you stand in front of a mirror and

Examine your face (especially the nose, mouth, and lips), front and back of the ears, neck, chest, abdomen, and upper back. Women should also lift their breasts to examine the skin underneath.

Check both sides of your arms, underarms, both sides of the hands, between the fingers, and under the fingernails.

With the aid of a handheld mirror, scan your lower back, buttocks, and genital area.

Using a comb, a hair blow dryer, and if possible, the assistance of a friend or family member, thoroughly examine the entire scalp.

Sit down on a chair or bench and

Inspect the front of your thighs, lower legs, the top and soles of your feet, between the toes, and under the toenails. Using a handheld mirror, inspect the back of your thighs and the lower legs.

Excessive sun exposure, cigarette smoking, and excessive body weight are major risk factors for cancer.

- Make a drawing of yourself. Include a full frontal view, a full back view, and close-up views of your head (both sides), the soles of your feet, the tops of your feet, and the backs of your hands.
- After you get out of the bath or shower, examine yourself closely in a full-length mirror. On your sketch, make note of any moles, warts, or other skin marks you find anywhere on your body. Pay particular attention to areas that are exposed to the sun constantly, such as your face, the tops of your ears, and your hands.
- Briefly describe each mark on your sketch—its size, color, texture, and so on.
- Repeat the exam about once a month. Watch for changes in the size, texture, or color of moles, warts, or other skin marks. If you notice any difference, contact your physician. You also should contact a doctor if you have a sore that does not heal.

Breast Cancer

Risk Factors

1. **Age.** The risk for breast cancer increases significantly after 50 years of age.
2. **Race.** Breast cancer occurs slightly more frequently in white women than African American women. The latter, however, are more likely to die from the disease.
3. **Family history.** The risk for breast cancer is higher in women with a family history of breast and ovarian cancers. The risk is even higher if more than one family member has developed these cancers and is further enhanced by the closeness of the relationship (e.g., a mother or sister with breast cancer indicates a higher risk than a cousin with breast cancer).
4. **Genes.** Inherited mutations in genes (breast cancer gene 1, or BRCA1, and breast cancer gene 2, or BRCA2) are found in families with high rates of breast cancer. Women who carry this genetic mutation have a greater than 80 percent chance of developing breast cancer and 50 percent higher chance of ovarian cancer. Prophylac-

Activity 11.3: Cancer Risk Profile

Name _____ Date _____

Course _____ Section _____ Gender _____ Age _____

I. Risk Assessment

Instructions—Read the section "Cancer: Assessing Your Risks" (beginning on page 384) and complete the Cancer Questionnaire: Assessing Your Risks in Figure 11.9 (pages 387–389). Rate yourself on a scale from 1 to 3 (1 = low risk, 2 = moderate risk, 3 = high risk) according to the risk factors provided for each site and write the scores and risk categories in the blanks provided.

Cancer Site	Total Points — Men	Total Points — Women	Risk Category
Lung	☐	☐	☐
Colon-Rectum	☐	☐	☐
Skin	☐	☐	☐
Breast		☐	☐
Cervical		☐	☐
Endometrial		☐	☐
Prostate	☐		
Testicular	☐		
Pancreatic	☐	☐	☐
Kidney and Bladder	☐	☐	☐
Oral	☐	☐	☐
Esophageal and Stomach	☐	☐	☐
Ovarian		☐	
Thyroid	☐	☐	☐
Liver	☐	☐	☐
Leukemia	☐	☐	☐
Lymphomas	☐	☐	☐

II. Stage of Change for Cancer Prevention
Using Figure 2.5 (page 63) and Table 2.3 (page 62), identify your current stage of change for participation in a cancer-prevention program:

III. Personal Interpretation
In the space provided, discuss your results for the various cancer sites. State your feelings about cancer and comment on any experiences that you may have had with cancer patients.

IV. Cancer Prevention: Behavior Modification
Discuss lifestyle habits that you should eliminate and habits that you need to adopt to reduce your own risk of cancer. Also indicate how you can best implement and adhere to these changes.

tic removal of the breasts and/or ovaries significantly decreases the risk of breast cancer. Not all women who opt to have the surgery necessarily would develop breast cancer. As an extremely emotional and personal decision, women who are contemplating preventive surgery should seek professional counseling prior to undertaking this option.

5. Personal history. A previous history of breast or ovarian cancer indicates a higher risk.
6. Maternity. The risk is higher in women who have never had children and in women who bear children after 30 years of age. Women are encouraged to breast feed their babies at least up to six months as such also reduces the risk for breast cancer.
7. Physical inactivity. Physically inactive women are at higher risk. Regular aerobic exercise has consistently been associated with a lower risk of breast cancer. Some research even indicates that the risk of dying from breast cancer decreases by more than 40 percent in women with high aerobic fitness as compared to less fit women. Vigorous aerobic activity at least three times per week seems most effective. Adding strength training twice a week is also helpful.
8. Hormone replacement therapy (HRT). Long-term use of a combination of progesterone and estrogen increases the risk. The risk seems to apply to current and recent users.
9. Alcohol. Even one alcoholic drink per day slightly enhances breast cancer risk in women. Two or more drinks per day clearly enhance the risk.
10. Obesity. Adipose tissue increases estrogen levels. Higher estrogen levels, particularly following menopause, increase the risk.

About 5 to 10 percent of breast cancers may be related to gene mutations; the most common are BRCA1 and BRCA2. These are tumor suppressor genes located on chromosomes 17 and 13. Women with such mutations have up to 80 percent greater risk of developing breast cancer.

Women with low to moderate risk should practice monthly BSE (see Figure 11.12) and have their breasts examined by a doctor as a part of a cancer-related checkup. Periodic mammograms should be included as recommended. Women at high risk should practice monthly BSE and have their breasts examined regularly by a doctor. See your doctor for the recommended examinations (including mammograms and physical exam of breasts).

Clinical breast exams by a physician are recommended every 3 years for women between ages 20 and 40 and every year for women older than age 40. The American Cancer Society also recommends an annual **mammogram** for women older than age 40. The 2009 guidelines by the U.S. Preventive Service Task Force, although heatedly debated by many health care practitioners, recommended that women get a mammogram every 2 years starting at age 50. According to Dr. Otis Brawley, Chief Medical Officer of the American Cancer Society, "This is one screening test I recommend unequivocally, and would recommend to any woman 40 and over." Frequency of mammograms is currently an area of debate among health care practitioners, and personal risk factors should be considered to determine when to start and how often they should be done.

Other possible risk factors for breast cancer that are not listed in the questionnaire are high breast-tissue density (a mammographic measure of the amount of glandular breast tissue relative to fatty breast tissue), a long menstrual history (onset of menstruation prior to age 13 and ending later in life), postmenopausal hormone therapy, recent use of oral contraceptives or postmenopausal estrogens, high saturated fat intake, high refined carbohydrate intake, chronic cystic disease, and ionizing radiation. To decrease the risk, increase fiber, folic acid, monounsaturated fat, and vegetable consumption, and increase daily physical activity.

Men should not feel immune to breast cancer. Although not common in men, approximately 2,000 men in the United States are diagnosed with breast cancer and 400 die from it each year.

Cervical Cancer (Women)
Risk Factors

1. Human papilloma virus (HPV). The most significant risk factor is infection with the HPV, a group of more than 100 related viruses, some of which can cause cervical cancer. The virus is frequently transmitted through vaginal, anal, or oral sex; or simply by skin-to-skin contact with a body area infected with HPV. Most infected women do not develop cervical cancer but other factors (see the following) can contribute to its development.
2. Smoking. The risk doubles in women who smoke. Tobacco by-products are found in cervical mucus of women who smoke.
3. Infections. Both human immunodeficiency virus (HIV) and chlamydia (bacterial infection—see Chapter 14) infections increase the risk of cervical cancer.
4. Diet. Low consumption of fruits and vegetables has been linked to higher cervical cancer risk.
5. Overweight. Women who are overweight are at higher risk.
6. Birth control pills. Long-term use of birth control pills increases the risk. The risk decreases once their use is stopped.
7. Pregnancies. Multiple pregnancies (three or more) increase the risk. Pregnancy prior to age 17 also increases the risk.
8. Family history. Cervical cancer may run in families because women in these families are less able to fight off the HPV.

Early detection through regular screening is critical for cancer prevention. A Pap

Mammogram Low-dose x-rays of the breasts used as a screening technique for the early detection of breast tumors.

Figure 11.12 Breast self-examination.

Looking

Stand in front of a mirror with your upper body unclothed. Look for changes in the shape and size of the breast, and for dimpling of the skin or "pulling in" of the nipples. Any changes in the breast may be made more noticeable by a change in position of the body or arms. Also look for changes in shape from one breast to the other.

1. Stand with your arms down.

2. Raise your arms overhead.

3. Place your hands on your hips and tighten your chest and arm muscles by pressing firmly.

Feeling

1. Lie flat on your back. Place a pillow or towel under one shoulder, and raise that arm over your head. With the opposite hand, you'll feel with the pads, not the fingertips, of the three middle fingers, for lumps or any change in the texture of the breast or skin.

2. The area you'll examine is from your collarbone to your bra line and from your breastbone to the center of your armpit. Imagine the area divided into vertical strips. Using small circular motions (the size of a dime), move your fingers up and down the strips. Apply light, medium, and deep pressure to examine each spot. Repeat this same process for your other breast.

3. Gently squeeze the nipple of each breast between your thumb and index finger. Any discharge, clear or bloody, should be reported to your doctor immediately.

Source: From D. Hales, *An Invitation to Health,* 11th ed. © 2005. Cengage Learning.

---

test, which screens for precancerous cells, should be done at age 21 and then repeated every three years up to age 65. Starting at age 30, if you choose to do so, an HPV test that looks for the virus that causes cellular changes may be used with the Pap test. When both tests are performed, it is referred to as co-testing. If your test results are normal, your chance of getting cervical cancer in the next few years is very low. Your physician may then inform you that you can wait five years prior to your next screening.

HPV vaccines are available to prevent cervical cancer and other diseases caused by HPV (see page 394). Both vaccines protect against HPV types 16 and 18, which cause most cervical cancers. The vaccines are recommended for women between the ages of 11 and 26. To get the full benefits of the vaccine, women should get vaccinated before they become sexually active.

Endometrial Cancer (Women)
Risk Factors

1. Estrogen use. Cancer of the endometrium is associated with high cumulative exposure to estrogen. Obesity and hormone replacement therapy increase estrogen exposure. You should consult your physician before starting or stopping any estrogen therapy.
2. Age. Endometrial cancer is seen in older age groups.
3. Race. White women have a higher occurrence but African American women have a higher incidence of death.
4. Pregnancy. The fewer children the woman has delivered, the greater is the risk for endometrial cancer.
5. Excessive weight. Women who are significantly overweight or obese are at greater risk.

6. Diabetes. Cancer of the endometrium is associated with diabetes.
7. Total number of menstrual cycles (periods). The greater the number of lifetime menstrual cycles (periods), the greater the risk.
8. Hypertension. Cancer of the endometrium is associated with high blood pressure.
9. Physical inactivity. The risk for endometrial cancer is higher among physically inactive women.

Prostate Cancer (Men) The prostate gland is actually a cluster of smaller glands that encircle the top section of the urethra (urinary channel) at the point where it leaves the bladder. Although the function of the prostate is not entirely clear, the muscles of these small glands help squeeze prostatic secretions into the urethra.

Risk Factors

1. Age. The highest incidence of prostate cancer is found in men over age 65 (more than 70 percent of cases).
2. Family history.
3. Race. African American men have the highest rate in the world.
4. Diet. A diet high in red meat or high-fat dairy products may increase risk.
5. Physical inactivity. The risk may be greater in physically inactive men.

Prostate cancer is difficult to detect and control because the causes are not known. Death rates can be lowered through early detection and awareness of the warning signals. Detection is done by a digital rectal exam of the gland and a prostate-specific antigen (PSA) blood test once a year after the age of 50. Possible warning signals include difficulties in urination (especially at night), painful urination, blood in the urine, and constant pain in the lower back or hip area.

Factors that may decrease the risk include increasing the consumption of tomato-rich foods and fatty fish in the diet two or three times per week, avoiding a high-fat (especially animal fat) diet, increasing daily consumption of produce and grains, and maintaining recommended vitamin D intake (obtained through supplements, in multivitamins, in fortified milk, and manufactured by the body when exposed to sunlight).

Testicular Cancer (Men) Testicular cancer accounts for only 1 percent of all male cancers, but it is the most common type of cancer seen in men between ages 15 and 34. The incidence is higher in Caucasians than in African Americans. If diagnosed early, this type of cancer is highly curable.

Risk Factors

1. Undescended testicle.
2. Abnormal testicle development.
3. Family history of testicular cancer.
4. Race. White American men have the highest rate (five times greater than African Americans and three times greater than Asian American and Native American men).

The incidence of testicular cancer is quite high in males born with an undescended testicle. Therefore, this condition should be corrected before puberty. The risk, however, remains high and the individual should be vigilant about the condition.

Some of the warning signals associated with testicular cancer are a small lump on the testicle, slight enlargement (usually painless) and change in consistency of the testis, sudden buildup of blood or fluid in the scrotum, pain in the groin and lower abdomen or discomfort accompanied by a sensation of dragging and heaviness, breast enlargement or tenderness, and enlarged lymph glands.

Early diagnosis of testicular cancer is essential, because this type of cancer spreads rapidly to other parts of the body. Because in most cases no early symptoms or pain is associated with testicular cancer, most people do not see a physician for months after discovering a lump or a slightly enlarged testis. Unfortunately, this delay allows almost 90 percent of testicular cancer to metastasize (spread) before a diagnosis is made. TSE once a month following a warm bath or shower (when the scrotal skin is relaxed) is recommended. Guidelines for performing a TSE are given in Figure 11.13.

Figure 11.13 Testicular self-examination.

How to Examine the Testicles

You can increase your chances of early detection of testicular cancer by regularly performing a testicular self-examination (TSE). The following procedure is recommended:

- Perform the self-exam once a month. Select an easy day to remember such as the first day or first Sunday of the month.
- Learn how your testicle feels normally so that it will be easier to identify changes. A normal testicle should feel oval, smooth, and uniformly firm, like a hard-boiled egg.
- Perform TSE following a warm shower or bath, when the scrotum is relaxed.
- Gently roll each testicle between your thumb and the first three fingers until you have felt the entire surface. Pay particular attention to any lumps, change in size or texture, pain, or a dragging or heavy sensation since your last self-exam. Do not confuse the epididymis at the rear of the testicle for an abnormality.
- Bring any changes to the attention of your physician. A change does not necessarily indicate a malignancy, but only a physician is able to determine that.

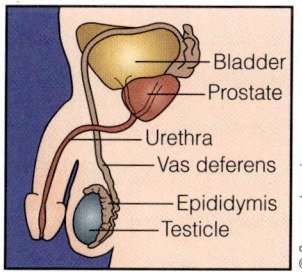

Pancreatic Cancer

The pancreas is a thin gland that lies behind the stomach. This gland releases insulin and pancreatic juice. Insulin regulates blood sugar, and pancreatic juice contains enzymes that aid in digesting food.

Possible Risk Factors

1. The risk increases with age. Almost 90 percent of cases are seen in people older than 55.
2. BRCA2 mutations.
3. Cigarette smoking, cigar smoking, and smokeless tobacco use significantly increase the risk.
4. Excessive sugar intake, which may increase the risk of developing pancreatic cancer by 70 percent.
5. Obesity.
6. Physical inactivity.
7. Chronic pancreatitis.
8. Cirrhosis.
9. Diabetes.
10. Family history.
11. African American race.

Detection of pancreatic cancer is difficult because no symptoms are apparent in the early stages and advanced disease symptoms are similar to those of other diseases. Only a biopsy can provide a definite diagnosis, but because pancreatic cancer is primarily a "silent" disease, the need for a biopsy is apparent only when the disease is already in an advanced stage.

Warning signals that may be related to pancreatic cancer include pain in the abdomen or lower back; jaundice; loss of weight and appetite; nausea; weakness, weariness, and loss of energy; agitated depression; dizziness; chills; muscle spasms; double vision; and coma.

Kidney and Bladder Cancer

The kidneys are the organs that filter the urine, and the bladder stores and empties the urine. Most of these two types of cancer are caused by environmental factors. Bladder cancer occurs most frequently between the ages of 50 and 70. Of all bladder cancers, 80 percent are seen in men, and the incidence among Caucasian males is twice that among African American males.

Possible Risk Factors

1. Heavy cigarette smoking, responsible for almost half of all deaths from bladder cancer in men and one-third of deaths from bladder cancer in women.
2. Congenital abnormalities of either organ, detectable by a physician.
3. Exposure to certain chemical compounds, such as aniline dyes, naphthalenes, or benzidines, cadmium, some herbicides, and asbestos.
4. History of schistosomiasis, a parasitic bladder infection.
5. Frequent urinary tract infections, particularly after age 50.
6. The rate is higher in men.

Avoiding cigarette smoking and occupational exposure to cancer-causing chemicals is important to decrease the risk. Bloody urine, especially in repeated occurrences, is always a warning sign and requires immediate evaluation. Bladder cancer is diagnosed through urine analysis and examination of the bladder with a cystoscope (a small tube that is inserted into the tract through the urethra).

Oral Cancer

Oral cancer affects the mouth, lips, tongue, salivary glands, pharynx, larynx, and floor of the mouth. Most of these cancers seem to be related to cigarette smoking and excessive consumption of alcohol.

Risk Factors

1. Heavy use of tobacco (cigarette, cigar, pipe, or smokeless).
2. Excessive alcohol consumption.

Regular examinations and good dental hygiene help in prevention and early detection of oral cancer. Warning signals include a sore that doesn't heal or a white patch in the mouth, a lump, problems with chewing and swallowing, or a constant feeling of having "something" in the throat. A person with any of these conditions should be evaluated by a physician or a dentist. A tissue biopsy normally is conducted to diagnose the presence of cancer.

Esophageal and Stomach Cancer

The incidence of gastric cancer in the United States has dropped significantly the last few decades. Cancer experts attribute this drastic decrease to changes in dietary habits and refrigeration. This type of cancer is more common in men, and the incidence is higher in African American males than in Caucasian males.

Risk Factors

1. A diet low in fresh fruits and vegetables.
2. High consumption of salt-cured, smoked, and nitrate-cured foods.
3. Imbalance in stomach acid, heartburn, or gastroesophageal reflex disease (GERD).
4. History of pernicious anemia.
5. Chronic gastritis or gastric polyps.
6. Excessive body weight.
7. Tobacco and alcohol use.
8. Family history of these types of cancer.

Prevention is accomplished primarily by increasing dietary intake of complex carbohydrates and fiber and decreasing the intake of salt-cured, smoked, and nitrate cured foods. In addition, regular guaiac testing for occult blood (hemoccult test) is recommended. Warning signals for this type of cancer include indigestion for 2 weeks or longer, blood in the stools, vomiting, and rapid weight loss.

Ovarian Cancer (Women) The ovaries are part of the female reproductive system that produces and releases the egg and the hormone estrogen. Ovarian cancer develops more frequently after menopause.

Risk Factors

1. Higher risk with age.
2. History of ovarian problems.
3. Inherited BRCA1 or BRCA2 mutations.
4. Estrogen postmenopausal hormone therapy.
5. Extensive history of menstrual irregularities.
6. Family history of breast or ovarian cancer.
7. Personal history of breast cancer.
8. Nulliparity (no pregnancies).
9. Excessive body weight.
10. Hereditary nonpolyposis colon cancer.

In most cases, ovarian cancer has no signs or symptoms. Therefore, regular pelvic examinations to detect signs of enlargement or other abnormalities are highly recommended. Some warning signals may be bloating, an enlarged abdomen, lower abdominal/pelvic pressure or pain, abnormal vaginal bleeding, unexplained digestive disturbances, trouble eating or feeling full quickly, "normal"-size (premenopause-size) ovaries after menopause, and frequent or urgent urination without infection. The previous symptoms may happen sporadically, but if they are a change from "normal," occur more often, or worsen, consult your doctor. Mutations to the BRCA1 and BRCA2 genes are also a significant risk factor.

Thyroid Cancer The thyroid gland, located in the lower portion of the front of the neck, helps regulate growth and metabolism. Thyroid cancer occurs almost three times as often in women as in men. The incidence also is higher in Caucasians than African Americans.

Risk Factors

1. Age.
2. Radiation therapy of the head and neck region received in childhood or adolescence or exposure to high levels of radiation.
3. Family history of thyroid cancer.

Regular inspection for thyroid tumors is done by palpating the gland and surrounding areas during a physical examination. Thyroid cancer is slow-growing; therefore, it is highly treatable. Nevertheless, any unusual lumps in front of the neck should be reported promptly to a physician. Although thyroid cancer does not have many warning signals (besides a lump), these may include difficulty swallowing, choking, labored breathing, and persistent hoarseness.

Liver Cancer The incidence of liver cancer in the United States is low. Men are more prone than women, and the disease is more common after age 60.

Risk Factors

1. History of cirrhosis of the liver.
2. History of hepatitis B or hepatitis C virus.
3. Exposure to vinyl chloride (industrial gas used in plastics manufacturing) and aflatoxin (a natural food contaminant).
4. Excessive alcohol consumption.
5. Race/ethnicity. Asian Americans and Pacific Islanders have the highest rate.

Prevention consists primarily of avoiding the risk factors and being aware of warning signals. Possible signs and symptoms are a lump or pain in the upper right abdomen (which may radiate into the back and shoulder), fever, nausea, rapidly deteriorating health, jaundice, and tenderness of the liver.

Leukemia Leukemia is a type of cancer that interferes with blood forming tissues (bone marrow, lymph nodes, and spleen) by producing too many immature white blood cells. People who have leukemia cannot fight infection very well. The causes of leukemia are mostly unknown, although suspected risk factors have been identified.

Possible Risk Factors

1. Inherited susceptibility, but not transmitted directly from parent to child.
2. Greater incidence in individuals with Down syndrome and a few other genetic abnormalities.
3. Excessive exposure to ionizing radiation.
4. Environmental exposure to chemicals such as benzene, found in gasoline and cigarette smoke.

Detection is not easy because early symptoms can be associated with other serious ailments. When leukemia is suspected, the diagnosis is made through blood tests and a bone marrow biopsy.

Early warning signals include fatigue, pallor, weight loss, easy bruising, nosebleeds, loss of appetite, repeated infections, hemorrhages, night sweats, bone and joint pain, and fever. At a more advanced stage, fatigue increases, hemorrhages become more severe, pain and high fever continue, the gums swell, and various skin disorders occur.

Lymphoma Lymphomas are cancers of the lymphatic system. The lymphatic system consists of lymph nodes found throughout the body and a network of vessels that link these nodes. The lymphatic system participates in the body's immune reaction to foreign cells, substances, and infectious agents.

Possible Risk Factors

As with leukemia, the causes of lymphomas are unknown. Age is a strong risk factor. Because of the weakened immune system, the majority of cases are seen in people older than 60. Individuals who have received organ transplants are at higher risk. Some researchers suspect that a form of herpes virus (called Epstein-Barr virus) is active in the initial stages of lymphosarcomas. Risk of non-Hodgkin's lymphoma is higher in people who carry the human immunodeficiency virus (HIV) and human T-cell leukemia/lymphoma virus I (HTLV-I). A family history increases the risk as well.

Other researchers suggest that certain external factors may alter the immune system, making it more susceptible to the development and multiplication of cancer cells. Exposure to radiation, herbicides, organic solvents, and other chemicals may also increase risk, as may poor diet and insufficient physical inactivity.

Prevention of lymphoma is limited because little is known about its causes. Enlargement of a lymph node or a cluster of lymph nodes is the first sign of lymphoma. Other signs and symptoms are an enlarged spleen or liver, weakness, fever, back or abdominal pain, nausea/vomiting, unexplained weight loss, unexplained itching and sweating, and fever at night that lasts for a long time.

> **Critical Thinking**
>
> You have learned about many of the risk factors for major cancer sites. How will this information affect your health choices in the future? • Will it be valuable to you, or will you quickly forget all you have learned and remain in a contemplation stage at the end of this course?

11.6 What Can You Do?

If you are at high risk for any form of cancer, you are advised to discuss this with your physician. An ounce of prevention is worth a pound of cure. Although cardiovascular disease is the number one killer in the United States, cancer is the number one fear. Of all cancers, 60 to 80 percent are preventable, and about 50 percent are curable. Most cancers are lifestyle related, so being aware of the risk factors and following basic recommendations for preventing cancer will greatly decrease your risk for developing it.

Behavior Modification Planning

Lifestyle Factors That Decrease Cancer Risk

Factor	Function
Physical activity	Controls body weight, may influence hormone levels, strengthens the immune system.
Fiber	Contains anti-cancer substances, increases stool movement, blunts insulin secretion.
Fruits and vegetables	Contain phytonutrients and vitamins that thwart cancer.
Recommended weight	Helps control hormones that promote cancer.
Healthy grilling	Prevents formation of heterocyclic amines (HCAs) and polycyclic aromatic hydrocarbons (PAHs), both carcinogenic substances.
Tea	Contains polyphenols that neutralize free radicals, including epigallocatechin gallate (EGCG), which protects cells and the DNA from damage believed to cause cancer.
Spices	Provide phytonutrients and strengthen the immune system.
Vitamin D	Disrupts abnormal cell growth.
Monounsaturated fat	May contribute to cancer cell destruction.

Try It

In your Online Journal or class notebook, note ways you can incorporate all of these factors into your everyday lifestyle.

ASSESS YOUR BEHAVIOR

CENGAGEbrain.com To access course materials, including companion resources, please visit www.cengagebrain.com.

1. Are you physically active on most days of the week?
2. Does your diet include ample amounts of colorful fruits and vegetables and fiber, and is it low in red and processed meats?
3. Are you aware of your family history of cancer?
4. Do you practice monthly breast self-examination (women) or testicular self-examination (men)?
5. Do you respect the sun's rays? Do you use sunscreen lotion or wear protective clothing when you are in the sun for extended periods of time? Do you perform regular skin self-examinations?
6. Are you familiar with the seven warning signals of cancer?

ASSESS YOUR KNOWLEDGE

Evaluate how well you understand the concepts presented in this chapter using the chapter-specific quiz available in the online materials at www.cengagebrain.com.

1. Cancer can be defined as
   a. a process whereby some cells invade and destroy the immune system.
   b. uncontrolled growth and spread of abnormal cells.
   c. the spread of benign tumors throughout the body.
   d. interference of normal body functions through blood-flow disruption caused by angiogenesis.
   e. All are correct choices.

2. Cancer treatment becomes more difficult when
   a. cancer cells metastasize.
   b. angiogenesis is disrupted.
   c. a tumor is encapsulated.
   d. cells are deficient in telomerase.
   e. cell division has stopped.

3. The leading cause of deaths from cancer in women is
   a. lung cancer.
   b. breast cancer.
   c. ovarian cancer.
   d. skin cancer.
   e. endometrial cancer.

4. Cancer
   a. is primarily a preventable disease.
   b. is often related to tobacco use.
   c. has been linked to dietary habits.
   d. risk increases with obesity.
   e. All are correct choices.

5. About 60 percent of cancers are related to
   a. genetics.
   b. environmental pollutants.
   c. viruses and other biological agents.
   d. ultraviolet radiation.
   e. diet, obesity, and tobacco use.

6. A cancer-prevention diet should include
   a. ample amounts of fruits and vegetables.
   b. cruciferous vegetables.
   c. phytonutrients.
   d. soy products.
   e. all of the above.

7. The biggest carcinogenic exposure in the workplace is to
   a. asbestos fibers.
   b. cigarette smoke.
   c. biological agents.
   d. nitrosamines.
   e. pesticides.

8. Which of the following is not a warning signal for cancer?
   a. Change in bowel or bladder habits
   b. Nagging cough or hoarseness
   c. A sore that does not heal
   d. Indigestion or difficulty in swallowing
   e. All of the above are warning signals for cancer.

9. The risk for breast cancer is higher in
   a. women younger than age 50.
   b. women with more than one family member with a history of breast cancer.
   c. minority groups than white women.
   d. women who had children prior to age 30.
   e. all of the above groups.

10. The risk for prostate cancer can be decreased by
    a. consuming selenium-rich foods.
    b. adding fatty fish to the diet.
    c. avoiding a high-fat diet.
    d. including tomato-rich foods in the diet.
    e. all of the above.

Correct answers can be found at the back of the book.

Stress Assessment and Management Techniques

12

"If we all threw our problems in a pile and saw everyone else's, we'd grab ours back."
—Regina Brett

Objectives

- **Understand** the importance of the mind–body connection in the manifestation of emotions and disease.
- **Learn** the consequences of sleep deprivation on mental and physical health.
- **Define** stress, eustress, and distress.
- **Explain** the role of stress in maintaining health and optimal performance.
- **Identify** the major sources of stress in life.
- **Define** the two major types of behavior patterns.
- **Learn** to lower your vulnerability to stress.
- **Develop** time management skills.
- **Define** the role of physical exercise in reducing stress.
- **Describe** and learn to use various stress management techniques.
- **Learn** how you're affected by stress.
- **Find** out how vulnerable you are to stress.

CENGAGEbrain.com

Visit www.cengagebrain.com to access course materials and companion resources for this text, including quiz questions designed to check your understanding of the chapter contents. See the preface on page ix for more information.

FAQ

Is all stress detrimental to health and performance?

Living in today's world is nearly impossible without encountering stress. The good news is that stress can be self-controlled. Unfortunately, most people have accepted stress as a normal part of daily life, and even though everyone has to face it, few seem to understand it or know how to cope with it effectively. It is difficult to succeed and have fun in life without "runs, hits, and errors." In fact, stress should not be avoided entirely, because a certain amount is necessary for motivation, performance, and optimum health and well-being. When stress levels push you to the limit, however, stress becomes distress and you will no longer function effectively.

How can I most effectively deal with negative stress?

Feelings of stress are the result of the body's instinct to defend itself. If you start to experience mental, social, and physical symptoms such as exhaustion, headaches, sleeplessness, frustration, apathy, loneliness, and changes in appetite, you are most likely under excessive stress and need to take action to overcome the stress-causing event(s). Do not deal with these symptoms through alcohol, drugs, or other compulsive behaviors, as such will not get rid of the stressor that is causing the problem. Stress management is best accomplished by maintaining a sense of control when excessive demands are placed on you.

First, recognize when you are feeling stressed. Early warning signs include tension in your shoulders and neck and clenching of your fists or teeth. Now, determine if there is something that you can do to control, change, or remove yourself from the situation. Most importantly, change how you react to stress. Be positive, avoid extreme reactions (anger, hostility, hatred, depression), try to change the way you see things, work off stress through physical activity, and master one or more stress management techniques to help you in situations where it is necessary to cope effectively. Finally, take steps to reduce the demands placed on you by prioritizing your activities—"don't sweat the small stuff." Realize that it is not stress that makes you ill, but the manner in which you react to stress that leads to illness and disease.

Real Life Story | Sreevita's Experience

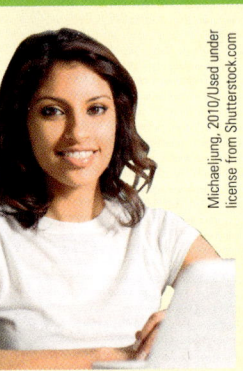

Throughout high school and college, the biggest source of stress for me has been my long habit of procrastination. Whenever I have a project I need to do, I automatically estimate the minimum amount of time it will take, and then wait until there is exactly that amount of time (or less!) before the project is due, and only then do I start. This means that everything is done in a mad rush, on a stress and adrenaline high, worrying that I might not make my deadline. I know this is a bad pattern. Not only does it cause me a lot of stress, but sometimes I underestimate how long something will take, and the amount of time left really isn't enough to finish the job or do it well. But the problem is that I am addicted to the pattern of having a flood of adrenaline carry me through the task, so I am not able to get motivated when the deadline is still far away. In fact, when I think of a task that I need to do, rather than feeling motivated to begin, I will often have thoughts that it will be horrible and hard and that I might fail. These thoughts are so unpleasant, that I will try to push the idea of the project out of mind entirely. But one of the strategies I have used recently to try to overcome my procrastination is baby steps. In fact, I will try to break a task down into the smallest pieces possible. For instance, if I have to start writing a report, my first step may be to just turn on the computer. Or to just open up the word-processing program. And then to just write one rough sentence (which doesn't even have to be good). By making each step as simple and unintimidating as possible, I can make a start. I celebrate the accomplishment of each baby step, even if it was just something as simple as turning on the computer. Once I start making progress, I usually find that the project is not as painful as I feared. I have also discovered something else surprising—exercising regularly and taking a yoga class have actually helped me procrastinate less! Since my procrastination is linked to feelings of anxiety about a task, and aerobic exercise and yoga give me a feeling of calm and well-being, when I exercise regularly, I procrastinate less.

> **PERSONAL PROFILE: Personal Stress Management Survey**
>
> I. Do you experience mostly eustress or distress in your daily life? Explain.
>
> II. Identify a recent life stressor and can you explain the general adaptation syndrome stage that you are currently experiencing?
>
> III. List three significant factors that cause stress in your life and indicate how you deal with those situations when they arise.
>
> IV. Explain personal time management techniques that you use given the many challenges and responsibilities you face in daily life.
>
> V. Have you ever used relaxation techniques to effectively manage stress? If so, explain the experience.

According to a growing body of evidence, virtually every illness known to modern humanity—from arthritis to migraine headaches, from the common cold to cancer—appears to be influenced for good or bad by our emotions. To a profound extent, emotions affect our susceptibility to disease and our **immunity**. The way we react to what comes along in life can determine in great measure how we will react to the disease-causing organisms that we face. The feelings we have and the way we express them can either boost our immune system or weaken it.

Emotional health is a key part of total wellness. Most emotionally healthy people take care of themselves physically—they eat well, exercise, and get enough rest. They work to develop supportive personal relationships. In contrast, many people who are emotionally unhealthy are self-destructive. For example, they may abuse alcohol and other drugs or may overwork and not have balance in their lives. Emotional health is so important that it affects what we do, who we meet, who we marry, how we look, how we feel, the course of our lives, and even how long we live.

12.1 The Mind–Body Connection

Emotions cause physiological responses that can influence health. Certain parts of the brain are associated with specific emotions and specific hormone patterns. The release of certain hormones is associated with various emotional responses, and those hormones affect health. These responses may contribute to development of disease. Emotions have to be expressed somewhere, somehow. If they are suppressed repeatedly, and/or if a person feels conflict about controlling them, they often reveal themselves through physical symptoms. These physiological responses may weaken the immune system over time.

The Brain The brain is the most important part of the nervous system. For the body to survive, the brain must be maintained. All other organs sacrifice to keep the brain alive and functioning when the entire body is under severe stress.

The brain directs nerve impulses that are carried throughout the body. It controls voluntary processes, such as the direction, strength, and coordination of muscle movements; the processes involved in smelling, touching, and seeing; and involuntary functions over which you have no conscious control. Among the latter are many automatic, vital functions in the body, such as breathing, heart rate, digestion, control of the bowels and bladder, blood pressure, and release of hormones.

The brain is the cognitive center of the body, the place where ideas are generated, memory is stored, and emotions are experienced. The brain has a powerful influence over the body via the link between the emotions and the immune system. That link is extremely complex.

The emotions that the brain produces are a mixture of feelings and physical responses. Every time the brain manufactures an emotion, physical reactions accompany it. The brain's natural chemicals form literal communication links among the brain, its thought processes, and the cells of the body, including those of the immune system.

The Immune System The immune system patrols and guards the body against attackers. This system consists of about a trillion cells called **lymphocytes** (the cells responsible for waging war against disease or infection) and many trillions of molecules called **antibodies**. The brain and the immune system are closely linked in a connection that allows the mind to influence both susceptibility and resistance to disease. A number of immune system cells—including those in the thymus gland, spleen, bone marrow, and lymph nodes—are laced with nerve cells.

Cells of the immune system are equipped to respond to chemical signals from the central nervous system. For example, the surface of the lymphocytes contains receptors for a variety of central nervous system chemical messengers, such as catecholamines, prostaglandins, serotonin, endorphins, sex hormones, the thyroid hormone, and the

> **Immunity** The function that guards the body from invaders, both internal and external.
>
> **Lymphocytes** Immune system cells responsible for waging war against disease or infection.
>
> **Antibodies** Substances produced by the white blood cells in response to an invading agent.

growth hormone. Certain white blood cells possess the ability to receive messages from the brain.

Because of these receptors on the lymphocytes, physical and psychological stress alters the immune system. Stress causes the body to release several powerful neurohormones that bind with the receptors on the lymphocytes and suppress immune function.

Sleep and Wellness Sleep is a natural state of rest that is vital for good health and wellness. It is an anabolic process that allows the body to restore and heal itself. During sleep, we replenish depleted energy levels and allow the brain, muscles, organs, and various body tissues to repair themselves.

Sleep deprivation weakens the immune system, impairs mental function, and has a negative impact on physical, social, academic, and job performance. Lack of sleep also impacts stress levels, mood, memory, behavioral patterns, and cognitive performance. Cumulative long-term consequences include an increase in the risk for cardiovascular disease, high blood pressure, obesity, diabetes, and psychological disorders. People who get less sleep have a threefold increased risk of getting a cold, are more likely to develop coronary heart disease earlier in life, increase body-wide inflammation, and have higher blood levels of the stress hormone cortisol. What most people notice is a chronic state of fatigue, exhaustion, and confusion.

Stress-wise, getting to bed too late often leads to oversleeping, napping, missing classes, poor grades, and distress. It further increases tension, irritability, intolerance, and confusion and may cause depression and life dissatisfaction. Not getting enough sleep can also lead to vehicle accidents with serious or fatal consequences as people fall asleep behind the wheel. More than 40,000 injuries and 1,500 deaths each year are attributed to sleepy drivers (sleepy drivers are just as dangerous as drunk drivers). Irregular sleep patterns, including sleeping in on weekends, also contribute to many of the aforementioned problems.

Although more than 100 sleep disorders have been identified, they can be classified into four major groups:

- Problems with falling and staying asleep
- Difficulties staying awake
- Difficulty adhering to a regular sleep schedule
- Sleep-disruptive behaviors (including sleep walking and sleep terror disorder)

College students are some of the most sleep-deprived people of all. On average, they sleep about 6 and a half hours per night and approximately 30 percent report chronic sleep difficulties. Only 8 percent report sleeping 8 or more hours per night. For many students, college is the first time they have complete control of their schedule, including when they go to sleep and how many hours they sleep.

Lack of sleep during school days and pulling all-nighters interferes with the ability to pay attention and to learn, process, and retain new information. You may be able to retain the information in short-term memory, but most likely it will not be there for a cumulative exam or when you need it for adequate job performance. Deep sleep that takes place early in the night, and a large portion of the REM (rapid eye movement) dream sleep that occurs near the end of the night, have both been linked to learning. The brain has been shown to consolidate new information for long-term memory while you sleep. Convincing sleep-deprived students to get adequate sleep is a real challenge because they often feel overwhelmed by school, work, and even family responsibilities. Students who go to sleep early and get about eight hours of sleep per night are more apt to succeed.

Compounding the problem is staying up late Friday and Saturday nights and crashing the next day. Doing so further disrupts the circadian rhythm, the biological clock that controls the daily sleep/wake schedule. Such disruption influences quantity and quality of sleep and keeps people from falling asleep and rising at the necessary times for school, work, or other required activities. In essence, the body wants to sleep and be awake at odd times of the 24-hour cycle.

A term used to describe the cumulative effect of needed sleep that you don't get is "sleep debt." Crashing on weekends, although it may help somewhat, does not solve the problem. You need to address the problem behavior by getting sufficient sleep each night so that you can be at your best the next day.

The exact amount of sleep that each person needs varies among individuals. Most people require around 8 hours. According to the National Sleep Foundation, currently most people get about 7 hours of sleep per night. Experts believe that the last 2 hours of sleep are the most vital for well-being. Thus, if you need 8 hours of sleep and you routinely get 6, you may be forfeiting the most critical sleep hours for health and wellness. Most students do not address sleep disorders until they start to cause mental and physical damage.

While there is no magic formula to determine how much sleep you need, if you don't need an alarm clock to get up every morning, you wake up at about the same time, and you are refreshed and feel alert throughout the day, you most likely have a healthy sleeping habit.

To improve your sleep pattern, you need to exercise discipline and avoid staying up late to watch a movie or leaving your homework or studying for an exam at the last minute. As busy as you are, your health and well-being is your most important asset. You only live once. Keeping your health and living life to its fullest potential includes a good night's rest. To enhance the quality of your sleep you should:

- Exercise and be physically active, but avoid vigorous exercise four hours prior to bedtime.
- Avoid eating a heavy meal or snacking 2 to 3 hours before going to bed (digestion increases your metabolism).
- Limit the amount of time that you spend (primarily in the evening) surfing and socializing on the Internet, texting, IMing (instant messaging), and watching television.

Figure 12.1 Relationship among stress and health and performance.

- Go to bed and rise at about the same time each day.
- Keep the bedroom cool, quiet, and dark.
- Develop a bedtime ritual (meditation, prayer, white noise).
- Use your bed for sleeping only (do not watch television, do homework, or use a laptop in bed).
- Relax and slow down 15 to 30 minutes before bedtime.
- Do not drink coffee or caffeine-containing beverages several hours before going to bed.
- Do not rely on alcohol to fall asleep (alcohol disrupts deep sleep stages).
- Avoid long naps (a 20- to 30-minute "power nap" is beneficial during an afternoon slump without interfering with night-time sleep).
- Have frank and honest conversations with roommates if they have different sleep schedules.
- Evaluate your mattress every 5 to 7 years for comfort and support. If you wake up with aches and pains or you sleep better when you are away from home, it is most likely time for a new mattress.

Stress Living in today's world is nearly impossible without encountering **stress**. In an unpredictable world that changes with every new day, most people find that working under pressure has become the rule rather than the exception. As a result, stress has become one of the most common problems we face and undermines our ability to stay well. Current estimates indicate that the annual cost of stress and stress-related diseases in the United States exceeds $100 billion, a direct result of health care costs, lost productivity, and absenteeism. Many medical and stress researchers believe that "stress should carry a health warning" as well.

Just what is stress? Dr. Hans Selye, one of the foremost authorities on stress, defined it as "the nonspecific response of the human organism to any demand that is placed upon it."[1] "Nonspecific" indicates that the body reacts in a similar fashion, regardless of the nature of the event that leads to the stress response. In simpler terms, stress is the body's mental, emotional, and physiological response to any situation that is new, threatening, frightening, or exciting.

The body's response to stress has been the same ever since humans were first put on Earth. Stress prepares the organism to react to the stress-causing event, also called the **stressor**. The problem arises in the way in which we react to stress. Many people thrive under stress; others under similar circumstances are unable to handle it. An individual's reaction to a stress-causing agent determines whether that stress is positive or negative.

Dr. Selye defined the ways in which we react to stress as either eustress or distress. In both cases, the nonspecific response is almost the same. In the case of **eustress**, health and performance continue to improve even as stress increases. On the other hand, **distress** refers to the unpleasant or harmful stress under which health and performance begin to deteriorate. The relationship between stress and performance is illustrated in Figure 12.1.

Stress is a fact of modern life, and every person does need an optimal level of stress that is most conducive to adequate health and performance. When stress levels reach mental, emotional, and physiological limits, however, stress becomes distress and the person no longer functions effectively.

Chronic distress raises the risk for many health disorders—among them, coronary heart disease, hypertension, eating disorders, ulcers, diabetes, asthma, depression, migraine headaches, sleep disorders, and chronic fatigue—and may even play a role in the development of certain types of cancers.[2] Recognizing this and overcoming the problem quickly and efficiently are crucial in maintaining emotional and physiological stability.

> **Stress** The mental, emotional, and physiological response of the body to any situation that is new, threatening, frightening, or exciting.
>
> **Stressor** Stress-causing event.
>
> **Eustress** Positive stress: Health and performance continue to improve, even as stress increases.
>
> **Distress** Negative stress: Unpleasant or harmful stress, which causes health and performance to begin to deteriorate.

Vandalism causes distress, or negative stress.

Marriage is an example of positive stress, also known as eustress.

Critical Thinking

Can you identify sources of eustress and distress in your personal life during this past year? Explain your emotional and physical response to each stressor and how the two differ.

12.2 Stress Adaptation

The body continually strives to maintain a constant internal environment. This state of physiological balance, known as **homeostasis**, allows the body to function as effectively as possible. When a stressor triggers a nonspecific response, homeostasis is disrupted. This reaction to stressors, best explained by Dr. Selye through the **general adaptation syndrome (GAS)**, is composed of three stages: alarm reaction, resistance, and exhaustion/recovery.

Alarm Reaction The alarm reaction is the immediate response to a stressor (whether positive or negative). During the alarm reaction, the body evokes an instant physiological reaction that mobilizes internal systems and processes to minimize the threat to homeostasis (see also "Coping with Stress" on page 417). If the stressor subsides, the body recovers and returns to homeostasis.

Resistance If the stressor persists, the body calls on its limited reserves to build up its resistance as it strives to maintain homeostasis. For a short while, the body copes effectively and meets the challenge of the stressor until it can be overcome (see Figure 12.2).

Exhaustion/Recovery If stress becomes chronic and intolerable, the body continues to resist, draining its limited reserves. The body then loses its ability to cope, and enters the exhaustion/recovery stage. During this stage, the body functions at a diminished capacity while it recovers from stress. In due time, following an "adequate" recovery period (which varies greatly), the body recuperates and is able to return to homeostasis. If chronic stress persists during the exhaustion stage, however, immune function is compromised, which can damage body systems and lead to disease.

An example of the stress response through the general adaptation syndrome can be illustrated in college test performance. As you prepare to take an exam, you experience an initial alarm reaction. If you understand the material, study for the exam, and do well (eustress), the body recovers and stress is dissipated. If, however, you are not adequately prepared and fail the exam, you trigger the resistance stage. You are now concerned about your grade, and you remain in the resistance stage until the next exam. If you prepare and do well, the body recovers. But, if you fail once again and can no longer bring up the grade, exhaustion sets in and physical and emotional breakdowns may occur. Exhaustion may be further aggravated if you are struggling in other courses as well.

Athletes and the most ardent fitness participants often manifest the exhaustion stage. Staleness is usually a manifestation of overtraining. Peak performance can be sustained for only about 2 to 3 weeks at a time. Any attempts to continue intense training after peaking leads to exhaustion, diminished fitness, and mental and physical problems associated with overtraining (see Chapter 9, page 327). Thus, athletes and some fitness participants also need an active recovery phase following the attainment of peak fitness.

12.3 Perceptions and Health

The habitual manner in which people explain the things that happen to them is their **explanatory style**. It is a way of thinking when all other factors are equal and when there are no clear-cut right and wrong answers. The contrasting explanatory styles are pessimism and optimism. People with a pessimistic explanatory style interpret events negatively; people with an optimistic explanatory style interpret events in a positive light—every cloud has a silver lining.

Figure 12.2 General adaptation syndrome: The body's response to stress can end in exhaustion, illness, or recovery.

Taking time out during stressful life events is critical for good health and wellness.

A pessimistic explanatory style can delay healing time and worsen the course of illness in several major diseases. For example, it can affect the circulatory system and general outlook for people with coronary heart disease. Blood flow actually changes as thoughts, feelings, and attitudes change. People with a pessimistic explanatory style have a higher risk of developing heart disease.

Studies of explanatory style verify that a negative explanatory style also compromises immunity. Blood samples taken from people with a negative explanatory style revealed suppressed immune function, a low ratio of helper/suppressor T-cells, and fewer lymphocytes.

In contrast, an optimistic style tends to increase the strength of the immune system. An optimistic explanatory style and the positive attitude it fosters can also enhance the ability to resist infections, allergies, autoimmunities, and even cancer. A change in explanatory style can lead to a remarkable change in the course of disease. An optimistic explanatory style and the positive emotions it embraces—such as love, acceptance, and forgiveness—stimulate the body's healing systems.

Self-Esteem Self-esteem is a way of viewing and assessing yourself. Positive self-esteem is a sense of feeling good about one's capabilities, goals, accomplishments, place in the world, and relationship to others. People with high self-esteem respect themselves. Self-esteem is a powerful determinant of health behavior and, therefore, of health status. Healthy self-esteem is one of the best things a person can develop for overall health, both mental and physical. A good, strong sense of self can boost the immune system, protect against disease, and aid in healing.

Whether people get sick—and how long they stay that way—may depend in part on the strength of their self-esteem. For example, low self-esteem worsens chronic pain. The higher the self-esteem, the more rapid the recovery. If we have strong self-esteem, the outlook is good. If our self-esteem is poor, however, our health can decline in direct proportion, as our attitude and negative perceptions worsen.

Belief in oneself is one of the

> **Homeostasis** A natural state of equilibrium; the body attempts to maintain this equilibrium by constantly reacting to external forces that attempt to disrupt this fine balance.
>
> **General adaptation syndrome (GAS)** A theoretical model that explains the body's adaptation to sustained stress that includes three stages: alarm reaction, resistance, and exhaustion/recovery.
>
> **Explanatory style** The way people perceive the events in their lives from an optimistic or a pessimistic perspective.
>
> **Self-esteem** A sense of positive self-regard and self-respect.

most powerful weapons people have to protect health and live longer, more satisfying lives. It has a dramatic and positive impact on wellness, and we can work to harness it to our advantage.

12.4 Fighting Spirit

A **fighting spirit** involves the healthy expression of emotions, whether they are negative or positive. At the other extreme is hopelessness, a surrender to despair. Fighting spirit can play a major role in recovery from disease. People with a fighting spirit accept their disease diagnosis, adopt an optimistic attitude filled with faith, seek information about how to help themselves, and are determined to fight the disease. A fighting spirit makes a person take charge.

A fighting spirit may be the underlying factor in what is called **spontaneous remission** from incurable illness. More and more physicians believe that the phenomenon is real and that the patient is the key in spontaneous remission. They believe the patient's attitude, especially the presence of a fighting spirit, is responsible for victory over disease. Fighters are not stronger or more capable than others—they simply do not give up as easily. They enjoy better health and live longer, even when physicians and laboratory tests say they should not. Fighters are intrinsically different from people who give up, and their health status reflects those differences.

12.5 Sources of Stress

Several instruments have been developed to assess sources of stress in life. A practical instrument to assess stressors is the **Stress Events Scale**, presented in Activity 12.1, which identifies life events within the past 12 months that may have an impact on your physical and psychological well-being.

The Stress Events Scale is divided into two sections. Section 1, to be completed by all respondents, contains a list of potential stress-causing life events with four additional blank spaces for other events experienced but not listed in the survey. Section 2 contains additional statements designed for students only (students should fill out both sections). Common stressors in the lives of college students are depicted in Figure 12.3.

The scale requires the testee to rate the extent to which his or her life events had a positive or negative impact on his or her life at the time these events occurred. The ratings are on a 7-point scale. A rating of −3 indicates an extremely undesirable impact (shocking). A zero (0) rating indicates neither a positive nor a negative impact (**neustress**). A rating of +3 indicates an extremely desirable impact (jubilation).

> ### Critical Thinking
> Technological advances provide many benefits to our lives.
> • What positive and negative effects do these advances have on your daily living activities, and what impact are they having on your stress level?

Figure 12.3 Stressors in the lives of college students.

Source: Adapted from W. W. K. Hoeger et al., *Wellness Guidelines for a Healthy Lifestyle*, (Belmont, CA: Wadsworth Cengage Learning, 2007).

After the person evaluates his or her life events, the negative and the positive points are totaled separately. Both scores are expressed as positive numbers (e.g., positive ratings of 2, 1, 3, and 3 = 9 points of positive score; negative ratings of −3, −2, −2, −1, and −2 = 10 points of negative score). A final "total life change" score can be obtained by adding the positive score and the negative score together as positive numbers (total stress events score: 9 + 10 = 19 points).

Because negative and positive changes alike can produce nonspecific responses, the total life change score is a good indicator of total life stress. Most research in this area, however, suggests that the negative change score is a better predictor of potential physical and psychological illness than the total change score. More research is necessary to establish the role of total change and the role of the ratio of positive to negative stress.

12.6 Behavior Patterns

Common life events are not the only source of stress in life. All too often, individuals bring on stress as a result of their behavior patterns. The two main types of behavior patterns, Type A and Type B, are based on several observable characteristics.

> **Fighting spirit** Determination; the open expression of emotions, whether negative or positive.
>
> **Spontaneous remission** Inexplicable recovery from incurable disease.
>
> **Stress Events Scale** A questionnaire used to assess sources of stress in life.
>
> **Neustress** Neutral stress; stress that is neither harmful nor helpful.

Activity 12.1: Stress Events Scale

Name _____ Date _____

Course _____ Section _____ Gender _____ Age _____

Introduction

The list of stress-causing life events below may have potential adverse effects on your physical and psychological well-being. Check only those events that occurred during the past 12 months and rate the event on a 7-point scale (−3, −2, −1, 0, +1, +2, +3) using the following guidelines:

Negative Effect	Indifferent	Positive Effect
−3 Shocked	0	+3 Jubilant
−2 Dismayed		+2 Delighted
−1 Dissatisfied		+1 Pleased

Section 1: General

	Life Event	Stress Rating			Life Event	Stress Rating
1. Death of a family member	☐	_____	10. Change/status of			
2. Death of a close friend or acquaintance	☐	_____		Self esteem	☐	_____
				Boyfriend/girlfriend	☐	_____
3. Substance abuse (addiction to drugs/alcohol)	☐	_____		Family relationships	☐	_____
4. Imprisonment	☐	_____		Personal health (illness/disease/injury)	☐	_____
5. Law violation (including traffic violations)	☐	_____		Family or friend(s) health status	☐	_____
6. Marriage	☐	_____		Fitness level	☐	_____
7. Sexual intimacy	☐	_____		Sleeping habits	☐	_____
8. Pregnancy	☐	_____		Nutrition habits	☐	_____
9. Divorce				Study habits	☐	_____
Your own	☐	_____		Friendship(s)	☐	_____
Your parents	☐	_____		Peer acceptance	☐	_____
Other close relative or friend	☐	_____		Social activities	☐	_____
				Recreational activities	☐	_____
				Mode of transportation	☐	_____

Section 1: General (continued)

	Life Event	Stress Rating
11. Ability to laugh and have fun	☐	_____
12. Financial status		
Sufficient for needs	☐	_____
Increase/decrease in income	☐	_____
Mortgage loan	☐	_____
Vehicle loan	☐	_____
Student loan(s)	☐	_____
Other (specify): _____	☐	
13. Work responsibilities		
New job	☐	_____
Loss of job	☐	_____
Change in work responsibilities	☐	_____
Change in work hours	☐	_____
Relationship with superior(s)	☐	_____
Relationship with coworkers	☐	_____
14. Time management	☐	_____
15. Exceptional personal accomplishment		
Specify: _____	☐	_____
16. Holidays		
Christmas	☐	_____
Thanksgiving	☐	_____
Other (specify): _____	☐	
17. Vacation	☐	_____
18. Ability to recoup from trials, tribulations, and challenges	☐	_____
19. Spirituality	☐	_____
20. Other(s), list: _____	☐	_____
21. _____	☐	_____
22. _____	☐	_____
23. _____	☐	

Section 2: Education

	Life Event	Stress Rating
24. Choice of school	☐	_____
25. Change in school	☐	_____
26. Starting or stopping school	☐	_____
27. Loneliness	☐	_____
28. Privacy	☐	_____
29. Military obligations	☐	_____
30. Selecting/changing a major or minor	☐	_____
31. School-related activities		
Missed classes	☐	_____
Grade(s)	☐	_____
Academic probation	☐	_____
Course(s)	☐	_____
Exam(s)	☐	_____
Assignment(s)	☐	_____
Academic workload	☐	_____
College instructor(s)	☐	_____
32. Joining a fraternity/sorority	☐	_____
33. Housing		
Satisfied	☐	_____
Relationship with roommates	☐	_____
Changing roommates	☐	_____
Dismissal from dorm or residence	☐	_____
Moving	☐	_____
34. Graduation	☐	_____
35. Career employment	☐	_____
36. Other(s), list: _____	☐	_____
37. _____	☐	
38. _____	☐	

How to Score

Upon completion of the questionnaire, add all the negative and positive scores separately (e.g., positive ratings: 2, 1, 3, and 3 = 9 points positive score; negative ratings: −3, −2, −2, −1, and −2 = 10 points negative score). A final "total stress score" can be obtained by adding the positive score and the negative score together as positive numbers (total stress score: 9 + 10 = 19 points). Stress ratings based on your score are given below. The negative score is the best indicator of stress (distress or negative stress) in your life.

Score Interpretation

Stress Category	Negative Score	Total Score
Poor	≥15	≥30
Fair	9–14	20–29
Average	6–8	15–19
Good	1–5	6–14
Excellent	0	1–5

Stress Events Scale Results

	Points	Stress Category
Negative score:	_____	_____
Positive score:	_____	NA
Total score:	_____	_____

Copyright © Fitness & Wellness, Inc., Boise, ID, 2010.

Several attempts have been made to develop an objective scale to identify Type A individuals properly, but these questionnaires are not as valid and reliable as researchers would like them to be. Consequently, the main assessment tool to determine behavioral type is still the **structured interview**, during which a person is asked to reply to several questions that describe Type A and Type B behavior patterns. The interviewer notes not only the responses to the questions but also the individual's mental, emotional, and physical behaviors as he or she replies to each question.

Based on the answers and the associated behaviors, the interviewer rates the person along a continuum, ranging from Type A to Type B. Along this continuum, behavioral patterns are classified into five categories: A-1, A-2, X (a mix of Type A and Type B), B-3, and B-4. The Type A-1 exhibits all of the Type A characteristics, and the B-4 shows a relative absence of Type A behaviors. The Type A-2 does not exhibit a complete Type A pattern, and the Type B-3 exhibits only a few Type A characteristics.

Type A behavior characterizes a primarily hard-driving, overambitious, aggressive, and at times hostile and overly competitive person. Type A individuals often set their own goals, are self-motivated, try to accomplish many tasks at the same time, are excessively achievement-oriented, and have a high degree of time urgency.

In contrast, **Type B** behavior is characteristic of calm, casual, relaxed, easygoing individuals. Type B people take one thing at a time, do not feel pressured or hurried, and seldom set their own deadlines.

Over the years, experts have indicated that individuals classified as Type A are under too much stress and have a significantly higher incidence of coronary heart disease. Based on these findings, Type A individuals have been counseled to lower their stress level by modifying many of their Type A behaviors.

Many of the Type A characteristics are learned behaviors. Consequently, if people can learn to identify the sources of stress and make changes in their behavioral responses, they can move along the continuum and respond more like Type Bs. The debate, however, has centered on which Type A behaviors should be changed, because not all of them are undesirable.

We also know that many individuals perform well under pressure. They typically are classified as Type A but do not demonstrate any of the detrimental effects of stress. Drs. Robert and Marilyn Kriegel came up with the term Type C to characterize people with these behaviors.[3]

Type C individuals are just as highly stressed as Type As but do not seem to be at higher risk for disease than Type Bs. The keys to successful Type C performance seem to be commitment, confidence, and control. Type C people are highly committed to what they are doing, have a great deal of confidence in their ability to do their work, and are in constant control of their actions. In addition, they enjoy their work and maintain themselves in top physical condition to be able to meet the mental and physical demands of their work.

Anger and hostility can increase the risk for disease.

Type A behavior by itself is no longer viewed as a major risk factor for coronary heart disease, but Type A individuals who commonly express anger and hostility are at higher risk. Therefore, many behavioral modification counselors now work on changing the latter behaviors to prevent disease.

Next time you feel like getting even with someone for what he/she has done to you, you may want to consider that your anger may be more likely to hurt you. Anger increases heart rate, blood pressure, and leads to constriction of blood vessels. Over time, these changes can cause damage to the arteries and eventually lead to a heart attack. Studies indicate that hostile people who get angry often, more intensely, and for longer periods of time, have up to a threefold increased risk for CHD and are seven times more likely to suffer a fatal heart attack by age 50.

Many experts also believe that emotional stress is far more likely than physical stress to trigger a heart attack. People who are impatient and readily annoyed when they have to wait for someone or something—an employee, a traffic light, a table in a restaurant—are especially vulnerable.

Research is also focusing on individuals who have anxiety, depression, and feelings of helplessness when they encounter setbacks and failures in life. People who lose control of their lives or who give up on their dreams in life,

> **Structured interview** Assessment tool used to determine behavioral patterns that define Type A and Type B personalities.
>
> **Type A** Behavior pattern characteristic of a hard-driving, overambitious, aggressive, at times hostile, and overly competitive person.
>
> **Type B** Behavior pattern characteristic of a calm, casual, relaxed, and easygoing individual.
>
> **Type C** Behavior pattern of individuals who are just as highly stressed as the Type A but do not seem to be at higher risk for disease than the Type B.

Behavior Modification Planning

Changing a Type A Personality

- Make a contract with yourself to slow down and take it easy. Put it in writing. Post it in a conspicuous spot, then stick to the terms you set up. Be specific. Abstracts ("I'm going to be less uptight") don't work.

- Work on only one or two things at a time. Wait until you change one habit before you tackle the next one.

- Eat more slowly and eat only when you are relaxed and sitting down.

- If you smoke, quit.

- Cut down on your caffeine intake, because it increases the tendency to become irritated and agitated.

- Take regular breaks throughout the day, even as brief as 5 or 10 minutes, when you totally change what you're doing. Get up, stretch, get a drink of cool water, walk around for a few minutes.

- Work on fighting your impatience. If you're standing in line at the grocery store, study the interesting things people have in their carts instead of getting upset.

- Work on controlling hostility. Keep a written log. When do you flare up? What causes it? How do you feel at the time? What preceded it? Look for patterns and figure out what sets you off. Then do something about it. Either avoid the situations that cause you hostility or practice reacting to them in different ways.

- Plan some activities just for the fun of it. Load a picnic basket in the car and drive to the country with a friend. After a stressful physics class, stop at a theater and see a good comedy.

- Choose a role model, someone you know and admire who does not have a Type A personality. Observe the person carefully, then try out some techniques the person demonstrates.

- Simplify your life so you can learn to relax a little bit. Figure out which activities or commitments you can eliminate right now, then get rid of them.

- If morning is a problem time for you and you get too hurried, set your alarm clock half an hour earlier.

- Take time out during even the most hectic day to do something truly relaxing. Because you won't be used to it, you may have to work at it at first. Begin by listing things you'd really enjoy that would calm you. Include some things that take only a few minutes: Watch a sunset, lie out on the lawn at night and look at the stars, call an old friend and catch up on news, take a nap, sauté a pan of mushrooms and savor them slowly.

- If you're under a deadline, take short breaks. Stop and talk to someone for 5 minutes, take a short walk, or lie down with a cool cloth over your eyes for 10 minutes.

- Pay attention to what your own body clock is saying. You've probably noticed that every 90 minutes or so, you lose the ability to concentrate, get a little sleepy, and have a tendency to daydream. Instead of fighting the urge, put down your work and let your mind wander for a few minutes. Use the time to imagine and let your creativity run wild.

- Learn to treasure unplanned surprises: a friend dropping by unannounced, a hummingbird outside your window, a child's tightly clutched bouquet of wildflowers.

- Savor your relationships. Think about the people in your life. Relax with them and give yourself to them. Give up trying to control others and resist the urge to end relationships that don't always go as you'd like them to.

From W. W. K. Hoeger, L. W. Turner, and B. Q. Hafen, *Wellness: Guidelines for a Healthy Lifestyle* (4th ed.) (Belmont, CA: Wadsworth, Cengage Learning, 2007).

Try It

If Type A describes your personality, pick three of these strategies and apply them in your life this week. At the end of each day determine how well you have done that day and evaluate how you can improve the next day.

---

knowing that they could and should be doing better, probably are more likely to have heart attacks than hard-driving people who enjoy their work.

12.7 Vulnerability to Stress

Researchers have identified a number of factors that can affect the way in which people handle stress. How people deal with these factors can actually increase or decrease vulnerability to stress. The questionnaire provided in Activity 12.2 lists these factors so that you can determine your vulnerability rating. Many of the items on this questionnaire are related to health, social support, self-worth, and nurturance (sense of being needed). All of these factors are crucial to a person's physical, social, mental, and emotional well-being and are essential to cope effectively with stressful life events. The more integrated people are in society, the less vulnerable they are to stress and illness.

Behavior Modification Planning

Tips to Manage Anger

- Commit to change and gain control over the behavior.
- Remind yourself that chronic anger leads to illness and disease and may eventually kill you.
- Recognize when feelings of anger are developing and ask yourself the following questions:
  - Is the matter really that important?
  - Is the anger justified?
  - Can I change the situation without getting angry?
  - Is it worth risking my health over it?
  - How will I feel about the situation in a few hours?
- Tell yourself, "Stop, my health is worth it" every time you start to feel anger.
- Prepare for a positive response: Ask for an explanation or clarification of the situation, walk away and evaluate the situation, exercise, or use appropriate stress management techniques (breathing, meditation, imagery) before you become angry and hostile.
- Manage anger at once; do not let it build up.
- Never attack anyone verbally or physically.
- Keep a journal and ponder the situations that cause you to be angry.
- Seek professional help if you are unable to overcome anger by yourself: You are worth it.

Try It

If you and others feel that anger is disrupting your health and relationships, these management strategies are critical to help restore a sense of well-being in your life. In your Online Journal or class notebook, list all of the strategies on a separate sheet of paper, study them each morning, and then evaluate yourself every night for the next week. If you gain control over the behavior, continue with the exercise until it becomes a healthy behavior. If you still struggle, professional help is recommended. "You are worth it."

Positive correlations have been found between social support and health outcomes. People can draw on social support to weather crises. Knowing that someone else cares, that people are there to lean on, that support is out there, is valuable for survival (or growth) in times of need.

The health benefits of physical fitness have already been discussed extensively. The questionnaire in Activity 12.2 will help you identify specific areas in which you can make improvements to help you cope more efficiently.

As you complete Activity 12.2, you will notice that many of the items describe situations and behaviors that are within your own control. To make yourself less vulnerable to stress, you will want to improve the behaviors that make you more vulnerable to stress. You should start by modifying the behaviors that are easiest to change before undertaking some of the most difficult ones. After completing the questionnaire, record the results in Activity 12.3 and in your fitness and wellness profile in Appendix A.

12.8 Time Management

According to Benjamin Franklin, "Time is the stuff life is made of." The present hurry-up style of American life is not conducive to wellness. The hassles involved in getting through a routine day often lead to stress-related illnesses. People who do not manage their time properly will quickly experience chronic stress, fatigue, despair, discouragement, and illness.

Surveys indicate that most Americans think time moves too fast for them, and more than half of those surveyed think they have to get *everything* done. The younger the respondents, the more they struggled with lack of time. Almost half wished they had more time for exercise and recreation, hobbies, and family. Healthy and successful people are good time managers, able to maintain a pace of life within their comfort zone, and attribute their success to smart work, not necessarily hard work.

Five Steps to Time Management Trying to achieve one or more goals in a limited time can create a tremendous amount of stress. Many people just don't seem to have enough hours in the day to accomplish their tasks. The greatest demands on our time, nonetheless, frequently are self-imposed—trying to do too much, too fast, too soon.

Some time killers, such as eating, sleeping, and recreation, are necessary for health and wellness, but, in excess, they'll lead to stress in life. You can follow five basic steps to make better use of your time (also see Activity 12.4):

1. Find the time killers. Many people do not know how they spend each part of the day. Keep a 4- to 7-day log and record at half-hour intervals the activities you do. Record the activities as you go through your typical day, so you will remember all of them. At the end of each day, decide when you wasted time. You may be shocked by the amount of time you spent on the phone, on the Internet, sleeping (more than 8 hours per night), or watching television.

Activity 12.2: Stress Vulnerability Questionnaire

Name _____ Date _____

Course _____ Section _____ Gender _____ Age _____

I. Stress Vulnerability Questionnaire

Item	Strongly Agree	Mildly Agree	Mildly Disagree	Strongly Disagree
1. I try to incorporate as much physical activity* as possible in my daily schedule.	1	2	3	4
2. I exercise aerobically for 20 minutes or more at least three times per week.	1	2	3	4
3. I regularly sleep 7 to 8 hours per night.	1	2	3	4
4. I take my time eating at least one hot, balanced meal a day.	1	2	3	4
5. I drink fewer than two cups of coffee (or equivalent) per day.	1	2	3	4
6. I am at recommended body weight.	1	2	3	4
7. I enjoy good health.	1	2	3	4
8. I do not use tobacco in any form.	1	2	3	4
9. I limit my alcohol intake to no more than one drink (women) or two (men) per day.	1	2	3	4
10. I do not use hard drugs.	1	2	3	4
11. There is someone I love, trust, and can rely on for help if I have a problem or need to make an essential decision.	1	2	3	4
12. There is love in my family.	1	2	3	4
13. I routinely give and receive affection.	1	2	3	4
14. I have close personal relationships with other people that provide me with a sense of emotional security.	1	2	3	4
15. There are people close by whom I can turn to for guidance in time of stress.	1	2	3	4
16. I can speak openly about feelings, emotions, and problems with people I trust.	1	2	3	4
17. Other people rely on me for help.	1	2	3	4
18. I am able to keep my feelings of anger and hostility under control.	1	2	3	4
19. I have a network of friends who enjoy the same social activities that I do.	1	2	3	4
20. I take time to do something fun at least once a week	1	2	3	4
21. My religious beliefs provide guidance and strength in my life.	1	2	3	4
22. I often provide service to others.	1	2	3	4
23. I enjoy my job (or major or school).	1	2	3	4
24. I am a competent worker.	1	2	3	4
25. I get along well with coworkers (or students).	1	2	3	4
26. My income is sufficient for my needs.	1	2	3	4
27. I manage time adequately.	1	2	3	4
28. I have learned to say "no" to additional commitments when I already am pressed for time.	1	2	3	4
29. I take daily quiet time for myself.	1	2	3	4
30. I practice stress management as needed.	1	2	3	4

Rating**
Excellent (great stress resistance)   0–30
Good (little vulnerability to stress)   31–40
Average (somewhat vulnerable to stress)   41–50
Fair (vulnerable to stress)   51–60
Poor (very vulnerable to stress)   ≥61

Total Points: _____

*Walk instead of driving, avoid escalators and elevators, or walk to neighboring offices, homes, and stores.

**Record total points and rating in Activity 12.3.

Activity 12.3: Stress Profile

Name _____ Date _____

Course _____ Section _____ Gender _____ Age _____

I. Assessments

Date:

Stress Events Scale

    Score (negative points only)

    Stress Rating

Stress Vulnerability Questionnaire

    Score

    Rating

Stress Management

Technique(s) to be used

II. In your own words, express how life stresses and your personality affect you in daily life.

_____
_____
_____
_____
_____
_____

III. In the space provided below, list, in order of priority, behaviors you would like to change to help you decrease your vulnerability to stress. Also, briefly outline how you intend to accomplish these changes.

Behavior(s)

1. _____

2. _____

How to accomplish the change(s)

_____
_____
_____

2. Set long-range and short-range goals. Setting goals requires some in-depth thinking and helps put your life and daily tasks in perspective. What do I want out of life? Where do I want to be 10 years from now? Next year? Next week? Tomorrow? You can use Activity 12.5 to list these goals.
3. Identify your immediate goals and prioritize them for today and this week (use Activity 12.6—make as many copies as necessary). Each day sit down and determine what you need to accomplish that day and that week. Rank your "today" and "this week" tasks in four categories: (a) top priority, (b) medium priority, (c) low priority, and (d) trash.

   Top-priority tasks are the most important ones. If you were to reap most of your productivity from 30 percent of your activities, which would they be? Medium-priority activities are those that must be done but can wait a day or two. Low-priority activities are those to be done only on completing all top- and middle-priority activities. Trash activities are not worth your time (e.g., cruising the hallways, channel surfing).
4. Use a daily planner to help you organize and simplify your day. In this way you can access your priority list, appointments, notes, references, names, places, phone numbers, and addresses conveniently from your coat pocket or purse. Many individuals think that planning daily and weekly activities is a waste of time. A few minutes to schedule your time each day, however, may pay off in hours saved.

   As you plan your day, be realistic and find your comfort zone. Determine the best way to organize your day. Which is the most productive time for work, study, and errands? Are you a morning person, or are you getting most of your work done when people are quitting for the day? Pick your best hours for top-priority activities. Be sure to schedule enough time for exercise and relaxation. Recreation is not necessarily wasted time. You need to take care of your physical and emotional well-being. Otherwise, your life will be seriously imbalanced.
5. Conduct nightly audits. Take 10 minutes each night to figure out how well you accomplished your goals that day. Successful time managers evaluate themselves daily. This simple task will help you see the entire picture. Cross off the goals you accomplished and carry over to the next day those you did not get done. You also may realize that some goals can be moved down to low priority or be trashed.

Time Management Skills In addition to the five major steps, the following can help you make better use of your time:

- Delegate. If possible, delegate activities that someone else can do for you. Having another person type your paper while you prepare for an exam might be well worth the expense and your time.
- Say "no." Learn to say no to activities that keep you from getting your top priorities done. You can do only so much in a single day. Nobody has enough time to do everything he or she would like to get done. Don't overload either. Many people are afraid to say no because they feel guilty if they do. Think ahead, and think of the

Behavior Modification Planning

Common Time Killers

Have you minimized the role of these time killers in your life?

I PLAN TO / I DID IT

- ☐ ☐ Watching television, listening to radio/music
- ☐ ☐ Excessive sleeping
- ☐ ☐ Surfing/socializing on the Internet
- ☐ ☐ Unnecessary texting, IMing, e-mailing
- ☐ ☐ Daydreaming
- ☐ ☐ Shopping
- ☐ ☐ Socializing/parties
- ☐ ☐ Excessive recreation
- ☐ ☐ Talking on the telephone
- ☐ ☐ Worrying
- ☐ ☐ Procrastinating
- ☐ ☐ Drop-in visitors
- ☐ ☐ Confusion (unclear goals)
- ☐ ☐ Indecision (what to do next)
- ☐ ☐ Interruptions
- ☐ ☐ Perfectionism (every detail must be done)

Try It

Using Activity 12.4, find the time killers in your life and make the necessary changes as required.

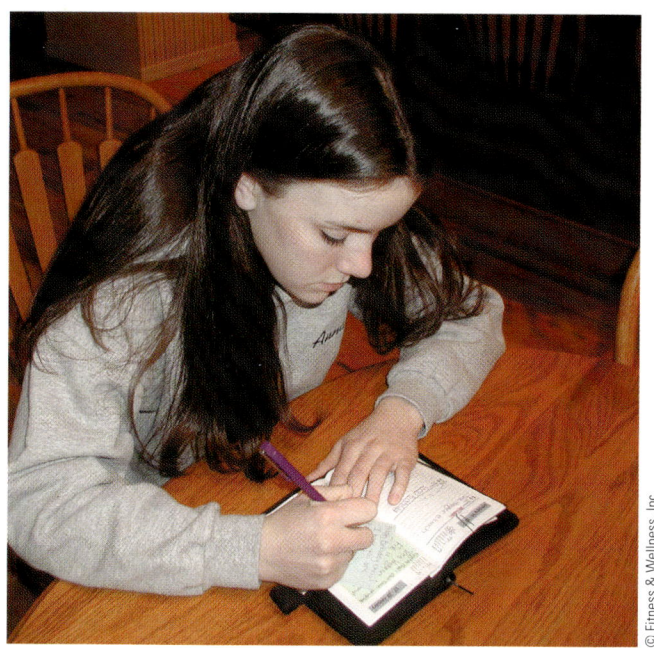
Planning and prioritizing activities will simplify your days.

- Plan time for you. Set aside special time for yourself daily. Life is not meant to be all work. Use your time to walk, read, or listen to your favorite music.
- Reward yourself. As with any other healthy behavior, positive change or a job well done deserves a reward. We often overlook the value of rewards, even if they are self-given. People practice behaviors that are rewarded and discontinue those that are not.

One more activity that you should perform weekly is to go through the list of strategies in Activity 12.7 to determine if you are becoming a good time manager. Provide a yes or no answer to each statement. If you are able to answer yes to most questions, congratulations. You are becoming a good time manager.

12.9 Coping with Stress

The ways in which people perceive and cope with stress seem to be more important in the development of disease than the amount and type of stress itself. If individuals perceive stress as a definite problem in their lives or if it interferes with their optimal level of health and performance, they can call on several excellent stress management techniques that can help them cope more effectively.

First, of course, the person must recognize the presence of a problem. Many people either do not want to believe that they are under too much stress or they fail to recognize some of the typical symptoms of distress. Noting some of the stress-related symptoms (see "Common Symptoms of Stress") will help a person respond more objectively and initiate an adequate coping response.

When people have stress-related symptoms, they should first try to identify and remove the stressor or stress-causing agent. This is not as simple as it may seem, because in some situations eliminating the stressor is not possible, or a person may not even know the exact causing agent. If the cause is unknown, keeping a log of the time and days when the symptoms occur, as well as the events preceding and following the onset of symptoms, may be helpful.

For instance, a couple noted that every afternoon around 6:00 p.m., the wife became nauseated and had abdominal pain. After seeking professional help, both were instructed to keep a log of daily events. It soon became clear that the symptoms did not occur on weekends but always started just before the husband came home from work during the week. Following some personal interviews with the couple, it was determined that the wife felt a lack of attention from her husband and responded subconsciously by becoming ill to the point at which she required personal care and affection from her husband. Once the stressor was identified, appropriate behavior changes were initiated to correct the situation.

In many instances, the stressor cannot be removed. Examples of such situations are the death of a close family member, the first year on the job, an intolerable boss, or a change in work responsibility. Nevertheless, stress can be managed through relaxation techniques.

consequences. Are you doing it to please others? What will it do to your well-being? Can you handle one more task? At some point you have to balance your activities and look at life and time realistically.
- Protect against boredom. Doing nothing can be a source of stress. People need to feel that they are contributing and that they are productive members of society. It is also good for self-esteem and self-worth. Set realistic goals and work toward them each day.
- Plan ahead for disruptions. Even a careful plan of action can be disrupted. An unexpected phone call or visitor can ruin your schedule. Planning your response ahead of time will help you deal with these saboteurs.
- Get it done. Select only one task at a time, concentrate on it, and see it through. Many people do a little here, do a little there, then do something else. In the end, nothing gets done. An exception to working on just one task at a time is when you are doing a difficult task. Rather than "killing yourself," interchange with another activity that is not as hard.
- Eliminate distractions. If you have trouble adhering to a set plan, remove distractions and trash activities from your eyesight. Television, radio, the Internet, magazines, open doors, or studying in a park might distract you and become time killers.
- Set aside "overtimes." Regularly schedule time that you did not think you would need as overtime to complete unfinished projects. Most people underschedule rather than overschedule time. The result is usually late-night burnout! If you schedule overtimes and get your tasks done, enjoy some leisure time, get ahead on another project, or work on some of your trash activities.

Activity 12.4: Finding Time Killers

Name _____ Date _____
Course _____ Section _____ Gender _____ Age _____

> Keep a 4- to 7-day log and record at half-hour intervals the activities you do (make additional copies of this form as needed). Record the activities as you go through your typical day, so you will remember them all. At the end of each day, decide when you wasted time. Using a highlighter, identify the time killers on this form and plan necessary changes for the next day.

Time	
6:00	
6:30	
7:00	
7:30	
8:00	
8:30	
9:00	
9:30	
10:00	
10:30	
11:00	
11:30	
12:00	
12:30	
1:00	
1:30	
2:00	
2:30	
3:00	
3:30	
4:00	
4:30	
5:00	
5:30	
6:00	
6:30	
7:00	
7:30	
8:00	
8:30	
9:00	
9:30	
10:00	
10:30	
11:00	
11:30	
12:00	

Activity 12.5: Planning Long- and Short-Range Goals

Name _____ Date _____

Course _____ Section _____ Gender _____ Age _____

Below, list your goals as indicated. You may want to keep this form and review it in years to come.

I. List three goals you wish to accomplish in life:

1. _____
2. _____
3. _____

II. List three goals you wish to see accomplished 10 years from now:

1. _____
2. _____
3. _____

III. List three goals you wish to accomplish this year:

1. _____
2. _____
3. _____

IV. List three goals you wish to accomplish this month:

1. _____
2. _____
3. _____

V. List three goals you wish to accomplish this week:

1. _____
2. _____
3. _____

Signature: _____ Date: _____

Activity 12.6: Daily and Weekly Goals and Priorities

Name _____ Date _____

Course _____ Section _____ Gender _____ Age _____

Take a few minutes each Sunday night to write down the goals or tasks you wish to accomplish that week. As with your daily goals, rank them as top, medium, low, or "trash" priorities. (Make as many copies of this form as needed.) At the end of the week, evaluate how well you accomplished your goals. Cross off the goals you accomplished and carry over to the next week those you did not get done.

Week: _____ / _____ to _____ / _____

Top-Priority Goals
1. _____
2. _____
3. _____
4. _____

Medium-Priority Goals
1. _____
2. _____
3. _____
4. _____

Low-Priority Goals
1. _____
2. _____
3. _____
4. _____

Trash (do only after all other goals have been accomplished)
1. _____
2. _____
3. _____
4. _____

Take 10 minutes each morning to write down the goals or tasks you wish to accomplish that day. Rank them as top, medium, low, or "trash" priorities. (Make as many copies of this form as needed.) At the end of the day, evaluate how well you accomplished your tasks for the day. Cross off the goals you accomplished and carry over to the next day those you did not get done.

Date: _____ / _____   Day of the Week: _____

Top-Priority Goals
1. _____
2. _____
3. _____
4. _____

Medium-Priority Goals
1. _____
2. _____
3. _____
4. _____

Low-Priority Goals
1. _____
2. _____
3. _____
4. _____

Trash (do only after all other goals have been accomplished)
1. _____
2. _____
3. _____
4. _____

Activity 12.7: Evaluating Time Management Skills

Name _____ Date _____

Course _____ Section _____ Gender _____ Age _____

> Weekly, go through the list of strategies below and write a "yes" or "no" response to each statement. If you are able to answer "yes" to most questions, congratulations, you are becoming a good time manager.

Strategy	Date:														
1. I evaluate my time killers periodically.															
2. I have written down my long-range goals.															
3. I have written down my short-term goals.															
4. I use a daily planner.															
5. I conduct nightly audits.															
6. I conduct weekly audits.															
7. I delegate activities that others can do.															
8. I have learned to say "no" to additional tasks when I'm already in overload.															
9. I plan activities to avoid boredom.															
10. I plan ahead for distractions.															
11. I work on one task at a time until it's done.															
12. I have removed distractions from my work.															
13. I set aside overtimes.															
14. I set aside special time for myself daily.															
15. I reward myself for a job well done.															

Behavior Modification Planning

Common Symptoms of Stress

Check those symptoms you experience regularly.

- Headaches
- Muscular aches (mainly in neck, shoulders, and back)
- Grinding teeth
- Nervous tic, finger tapping, toe tapping
- Increased sweating
- Increase in or loss of appetite
- Insomnia
- Nightmares
- Fatigue
- Dry mouth
- Stuttering
- High blood pressure
- Tightness or pain in the chest
- Impotence
- Hives
- Dizziness
- Depression
- Irritation
- Anger
- Hostility
- Fear, panic, anxiety
- Stomach pain, flutters
- Nausea
- Cold, clammy hands
- Poor concentration
- Pacing
- Restlessness
- Rapid heart rate
- Low-grade infection
- Loss of sex drive
- Rash or acne

Try It

If you regularly experience some of these symptoms, use your Online Journal or class notebook to keep a log of when these symptoms occur and under what circumstances. You may find out that a pattern emerges when experiencing distress in life.

The body responds to stress by activating the **fight-or-flight** mechanism, which prepares a person to take action by stimulating the vital defense systems. This stimulation originates in the hypothalamus and the pituitary gland in the brain. The hypothalamus activates the sympathetic nervous system, and the pituitary activates the release of catecholamines (hormones) from the adrenal glands.

These hormonal changes increase heart rate, blood pressure, blood flow to active muscles and the brain, glucose levels, oxygen consumption, and strength—all necessary for the body to fight or flee. For the body to relax, one of these actions must take place. However, if the person is unable to take action, the muscles tense up and tighten (see Figure 12.4). This increased tension and tightening can be dissipated effectively through some coping techniques.

Physical Activity The benefits of physical activity in reducing the physiological and psychological responses to stress are well established.[4] Exercise is one of the simplest tools to control stress. The value of exercise in reducing stress is related to several factors, the main one being a decrease in muscular tension. For example, a person can be distressed because he or she has had a miserable 8 hours of work with an intolerable boss. To make matters worse, it is late and, on the way home, the car in front is going much slower than the speed limit. The fight-or-flight mechanism—already activated during the stressful day—begins again: catecholamines rise, heart rate and blood pressure shoot up, breathing quickens and deepens, muscles tense up, and all systems say "go." No action can be initiated or stress dissipated, though, because the person cannot just hit the boss or the car in front.

A real remedy would be to take action by "hitting" the swimming pool, the tennis ball, the weights, or the jogging trail. Engaging in physical activity reduces the muscular tension and metabolizes the increased catecholamines (which were triggered by the fight-or-flight mechanism and brought about the physiological changes). Further, while you are concentrating on your tennis game, there isn't enough time to think about an irrational boss or other undesirable events. Although exercise does not solve problems at work or take care of slow drivers, it certainly helps the person cope with stress and prevents stress from becoming a chronic problem.

Stress management experts often recommend selecting activities like **yoga**, **tai chi**, and Pilates that combine physical

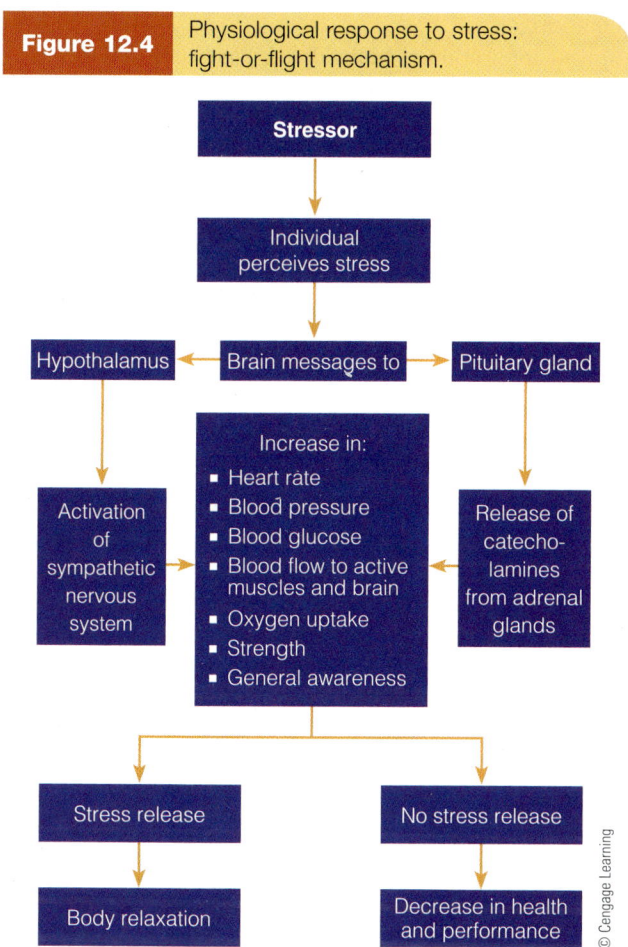

Figure 12.4 Physiological response to stress: fight-or-flight mechanism.

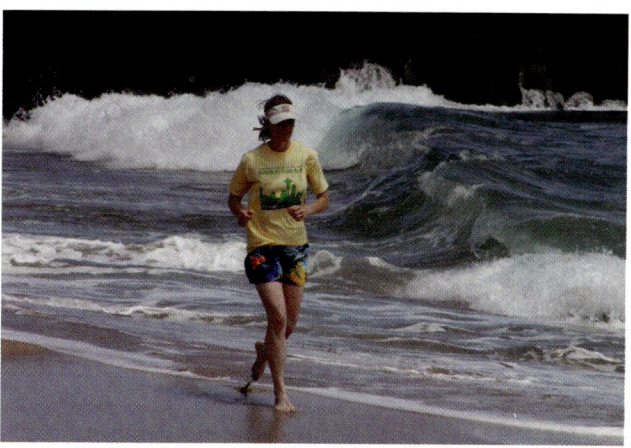

Physical activity: an excellent tool to control stress.

activity with additional stress reduction techniques. The latter activities regularly incorporate meditation, breathing, and/or muscle relaxation techniques—along with physical activity—to help people dissipate stress.

The early evening hours are a popular time to exercise for a lot of highly stressed executives. On the way home from work, they stop at the health club or the fitness center. Exercising at this time helps them to dissipate the stress accumulated during the day. Not only does evening exercise help to get rid of the stress, but it also provides an opportunity to enjoy the evening more. At home, the family will appreciate Dad or Mom coming home more relaxed, leaving work problems behind, and being able to dedicate all energy to family activities.

Many people can relate to exercise as a means of managing stress by remembering how good they felt the last time they concluded a strenuous exercise session after a long, difficult day at the office. A fatigued muscle is a relaxed muscle. For this reason, many people have said that the best part of exercise is the shower afterward.

Research also has shown that physical exercise requiring continuous and rhythmic muscular activity, such as aerobic exercise, stimulates alpha-wave activity in the brain. These are the same wave patterns seen commonly during meditation and relaxation.

Further, during vigorous aerobic exercise lasting 30 minutes or longer, morphine-like substances referred to as **endorphins** are thought to be released from the pituitary gland in the brain. These substances not only act as painkillers but also seem to induce the soothing, calming effect often associated with aerobic exercise. Research has also shown that moderate-intensity exercise has an immediate effect on a person's mood and the effects last up to 12 hours following activity. Thus exercise mitigates the daily stress the lead to mood alterations. Exercise is free and easily accessible to everyone. Pick an activity that you enjoy and use it to combat stress, blue moods, anxiety, and depression.

Another way by which exercise helps lower stress is to deliberately divert stress to various body systems. Dr. Hans Selye explains in his book *Stress without Distress* that, when one specific task becomes difficult, a change in activity can be as good or better than rest itself.[5] For example, if a person is having trouble with a task and does not seem to be getting anywhere, jogging or swimming for a while is better than sitting around and getting frustrated. In this way the mental strain is diverted to the working muscles, and one system helps the other to relax.

Other psychologists indicate that when muscular tension is removed from the emotional strain, the emotional strain disappears. In many cases, the

---

Fight-or-flight Physiological response of the body to stress that prepares the individual to take action by stimulating the body's vital defense systems.

Yoga A school of thought in the Hindu religion that seeks to help the individual attain a higher level of spirituality and peace of mind.

Tai chi A self-paced form of exercise often described as "meditation in motion" because it promotes serenity through gentle, balanced, low-impact movements that bring together the mind, body, and emotions.

Endorphins Morphine-like substances released from the pituitary gland in the brain during prolonged aerobic exercise, thought to induce feelings of euphoria and natural well-being.

change of activity suddenly clears the mind and helps put the pieces together.

Researchers have found that physical exercise gives people a psychological boost because exercise does all the following:

- Lessens feelings of anxiety, depression, frustration, aggression, anger, and hostility.
- Alleviates insomnia.
- Provides an opportunity to meet social needs and develop new friendships.
- Allows the person to share common interests and problems.
- Develops discipline.
- Provides the opportunity to do something enjoyable and constructive that will lead to better health and total well-being.

Beyond the short-term benefits of exercise in lessening stress, a regular aerobic exercise program actually strengthens the cardiovascular system itself. Because the cardiovascular system seems to be affected seriously by stress, a stronger system should be able to cope more effectively. For instance, good cardiorespiratory endurance has been shown to lower resting heart rate and blood pressure. Because both heart rate and blood pressure rise in stressful situations, initiating the stress response at a lower baseline will counteract some of the negative effects of stress. Cardiorespiratory-fit individuals can cope more effectively and are less affected by the stresses of daily living.

Relaxation Techniques Although benefits are reaped immediately after engaging in any of the several relaxation techniques, several months of regular practice may be necessary for total mastery. The relaxation exercises that follow should not be considered cure-alls. If these exercises do not prove to be effective, more specialized textbooks and professional help are called for. (Some symptoms may not be caused by stress but may be related to a medical disorder.)

Biofeedback

Clinical application of **biofeedback** has been used for many years to treat various medical disorders. Besides its successful application in managing stress, it is commonly used to treat medical disorders such as essential hypertension, asthma, heart rhythm and rate disturbances, cardiac neurosis, eczematous dermatitis, fecal incontinence, insomnia, and stuttering. Biofeedback as a treatment modality has been defined as a technique in which a person learns to influence physiological responses that are not typically under voluntary control or responses that normally are regulated but regulation has broken down as a result of injury, trauma, or illness.

In simpler terms, biofeedback is the interaction with the interior self. This interaction enables a person to learn the relationship between the mind and the biological response. The person actually can "feel" how thought processes influence biological responses (such as heart rate, blood pressure, body temperature, and muscle tension) and how biological responses influence the thought process.

As an illustration of this process, consider the association between a strange noise in the middle of a dark, quiet night and the heart rate response. At first the heart rate shoots up because of the stress the unknown noise induces. The individual may even feel the heart palpitating in the chest and, while still uncertain about the noise, attempts not to panic to prevent an even faster heart rate. On realizing that all is well, the person can take control and influence the heart rate to come down. The mind, now calm, is able to exert almost complete control over the biological response.

Complex electronic instruments are required to conduct biofeedback. The process itself entails a three-stage, closed-loop feedback system:

1. A biological response to a stressor is detected and amplified.
2. The response is processed.

Behavior Modification Planning

Thirty-Second Body Scan

This simple 30-second exercise helps you scan the body to raise stress awareness.

- ❏ Am I clenching my teeth?
- ❏ Am I furrowing my brow?
- ❏ Are my shoulders tense?
- ❏ Am I breathing rapidly?
- ❏ Am I tapping my fingers?
- ❏ Do I feel knots in my stomach?
- ❏ Are my arms, thighs, or calves tight?
- ❏ Am I nervously bouncing my leg or foot?
- ❏ Am I curling my toes?
- ❏ Do I feel uneasiness anywhere else in my body?

Try It

A body scan can be performed daily or several times a day to help you learn and recognize when you are distressed. People are often unaware of stress signals and activities that are causing excess stress. Increasing awareness allows you to initiate proper actions to more effectively manage stress. An example would be to breathe deeply for 1 to 3 minutes while doing the body scan and repeating positive affirmations (e.g., "I am at peace," or "I am calm and relaxed").

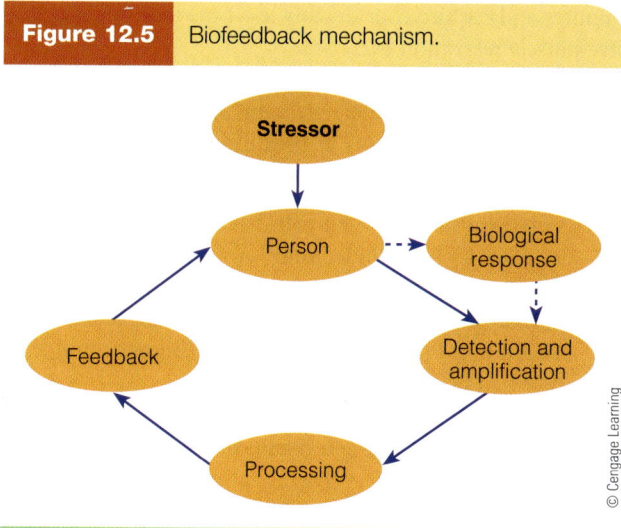

Figure 12.5 Biofeedback mechanism.

3. Results of the response are fed back to the individual immediately.

The person uses this new input and attempts to change the physiological response voluntarily—this attempt, in turn, is detected, amplified, and processed. The results then are fed back to the person. The process continues with the intent of teaching the person to reliably influence the physiological response for the better (see Figure 12.5). The most common methods used to measure physiological responses are monitoring the heart rate, finger temperature, and blood pressure; electromyograms; and electroencephalograms. The goal of biofeedback training is to transfer the experiences learned in the laboratory to everyday living.

Although biofeedback has significant applications in treating various medical disorders, including stress, it requires adequately trained personnel and, in many cases, costly equipment. Therefore, several alternative methods that yield similar results are frequently substituted for biofeedback. For example, research has shown that exercise and progressive muscle relaxation, used successfully in stress management, seem to be just as effective as biofeedback in treating essential hypertension.

Progressive Muscle Relaxation

Progressive muscle relaxation, developed by Dr. Edmund Jacobsen in the 1930s, enables individuals to relearn the sensation of deep relaxation. The technique involves progressively contracting and relaxing muscle groups throughout the body. Because chronic stress leads to high levels of muscular tension, acute awareness of how progressively tightening and relaxing the muscles feels can release the tension in the muscles and teach the body to relax at will.

Feeling the tension during the exercises also helps the person to be more alert to signs of distress, because this tension is similar to that experienced in stressful situations. In everyday life, these feelings then can cue the person to do relaxation exercises.

Relaxation exercises should be done in a quiet, warm, well-ventilated room. The recommended exercises and the duration of the routine vary from one person to the next. Most important is that the individual pay attention to the sensation he or she feels each time the muscles are tensed and relaxed.

The exercises should encompass all muscle groups of the body. Following is an example of a sequence of progressive muscle relaxation exercises. The instructions for these exercises can be read to the person, memorized, or tape-recorded. At least 20 minutes should be set aside to complete the entire sequence. Doing the exercises any faster will defeat their purpose. Ideally, the sequence should be done twice a day.

The individual performing the exercises stretches out comfortably on the floor, face up, with a pillow under the knees, and assumes a passive attitude, allowing the body to relax as much as possible. Each muscle group is to be contracted in sequence, taking care to avoid any strain. Muscles should be tightened to only about 70 percent of the total possible tension to avoid cramping or some type of injury to the muscle itself.

To produce the relaxation effects, the person must pay attention to the sensation of tensing up and relaxing. The person holds each contraction about 5 seconds and then allows the muscles to go totally limp. The person should take enough time to contract and relax each muscle group before going on to the next. An example of a complete progressive muscle relaxation sequence is as follows:

1. Point your feet, curling the toes downward. Study the tension in the arches and the top of the feet. Hold, continue to note the tension, and then relax. Repeat once.
2. Flex the feet upward toward the face and note the tension in your feet and calves. Hold and relax. Repeat once.
3. Push your heels down against the floor as if burying them in the sand. Hold and note the tension at the back of the thigh. Relax. Repeat once.
4. Contract the right thigh by straightening the leg, gently raising the leg off the floor. Hold and study the tension. Relax. Repeat with the left leg. Hold and relax. Repeat each leg.
5. Tense the buttocks by raising your hips ever so slightly off the floor. Hold and note the tension. Relax. Repeat once.
6. Contract the abdominal muscles. Hold them tight and note the tension. Relax. Repeat once.
7. Suck in your stomach. Try to make it reach your spine. Flatten your lower back to the

Biofeedback A stress management technique in which a person learns to influence physiological responses that are not typically under voluntary control or responses that typically are regulated but for which regulation has broken down as a result of injury, trauma, or illness.

Progressive muscle relaxation A stress management technique that involves sequential contraction and relaxation of muscle groups throughout the body.

Practicing progressive muscle relaxation on a regular basis helps reduce stress.

floor. Hold and feel the tension in the stomach and lower back. Relax. Repeat once.

8. Take a deep breath and hold it, then exhale. Repeat. Note your breathing becoming slower and more relaxed.
9. Place your arms at the sides of your body and clench both fists. Hold, study the tension, and relax. Repeat.
10. Flex the elbow by bringing both hands to the shoulders. Hold tight and study the tension in the biceps. Relax. Repeat.
11. Place your arms flat on the floor, palms up, and push the forearms hard against the floor. Note the tension on the triceps. Hold and relax. Repeat.
12. Shrug your shoulders, raising them as high as possible. Hold and note the tension. Relax. Repeat.
13. Gently push your head backward. Note the tension in the back of the neck. Hold and relax. Repeat.
14. Gently bring the head against the chest, push forward, hold, and note the tension in the neck. Relax. Repeat.
15. Press your tongue toward the roof of your mouth. Hold, study the tension, and relax. Repeat.
16. Press your teeth together. Hold, and study the tension. Relax. Repeat.
17. Close your eyes tightly. Hold them closed and note the tension. Relax, leaving your eyes closed. Do this one more time.
18. Wrinkle your forehead and note the tension. Hold and relax. Repeat.

When time is a factor during the daily routine and an individual is not able to go through the entire sequence, he or she may do only the exercises specific to the area that feels most tense. Performing a partial sequence is better than not doing the exercises at all. Completing the entire sequence, of course, yields the best results.

Breathing Techniques for Relaxation

Breathing exercises also can be an antidote to stress. These exercises have been used for centuries in the Orient and India to improve mental, physical, and emotional stamina. In breathing exercises, the person concentrates on "breathing away" the tension and inhaling a large amount of air with each breath. Breathing exercises can be learned in only a few minutes and require considerably less time than the progressive muscle relaxation exercises.

As with any other relaxation technique, these exercises should be done in a quiet, pleasant, well-ventilated room. Any of the three examples of breathing exercises presented here will help relieve tension induced by stress.

1. Deep breathing. Lie with your back flat against the floor and place a pillow under your knees. Feet are slightly separated, with toes pointing outward. (The exercise also may be done while sitting up in a chair or standing straight up.) Place one hand on your abdomen and the other hand on your chest.

   Slowly breathe in and out so that the hand on your abdomen rises when you inhale and falls as you exhale. The hand on the chest should not move much at all. Repeat the exercise about 10 times. Next, scan your body for tension and compare your present tension with the tension you felt at the beginning of the exercise. Repeat the entire process once or twice.

2. Sighing. Using the abdominal breathing technique, breathe in through your nose to a specific count (e.g., 4, 5, or 6). Now exhale through pursed lips to double the intake count (e.g., 8, 10, or 12). Repeat the exercise 8 to 10 times whenever you feel tense.

3. Complete natural breathing. Sit in an upright position or stand straight up. Breathing through your nose, gradually fill your lungs from the bottom up. Hold your breath for several seconds. Now exhale slowly by allowing your chest and abdomen to relax completely. Repeat the exercise 8 to 10 times.

Breathing exercises help dissipate stress.

Critical Thinking

List the three most common stressors that you face as a college student. • What techniques have you used to manage these situations, and in what way have they helped you cope?

Visual Imagery Visual or mental **imagery** has been used as a healing technique for centuries in various cultures around the world. In Western medicine, the practice of imagery is relatively new and not widely accepted among health care professionals.

Research is now being done to study the effects of imagery on the treatment of conditions such as cancer, hypertension, asthma, chronic pain, and obesity. Imagery induces a state of relaxation that rids the body of the stress that leads to illness. It improves circulation and increases the delivery of healing antibodies and white blood cells to the site of illness.[6] Imagery also helps with self-confidence, to regain control and power over the body, and to lower feelings of hopelessness, fear, and depression.

Visual imagery involves the creation of relaxing visual images and scenes in times of stress to elicit body and mind relaxation. Imagery works by offsetting the stressor with the visualization of relaxing scenes such as a sunny beach, a beautiful meadow, a quiet mountain top, lying in a hammock in a quiet backyard, soaking in a hot tub, or some other peaceful setting. If you are ill, you can also visualize your white blood cells attacking an infection or a tumor. Imagery is also used in conjunction with breathing exercises, meditation, and yoga.

As with other stress management techniques, imagery should be performed in a quiet and comfortable environment. You can either sit or lie down for the exercise. If you lie down, use a soft surface and place a pillow under your knees. Be sure that your clothes are loose and that you are as comfortable as you can be.

Visual imagery of beautiful and relaxing scenes helps attenuate the stress response.

To start the exercise, close your eyes and take a few breaths using one of the breathing techniques previously described. You then can proceed to visualize one of your favorite scenes in nature. Place yourself into the scene and visualize yourself moving about and experiencing nature to its fullest. Enjoy the people, the animals, the colors, the sounds, the smells, and even the temperature in your scene. After 10 to 20 minutes of visualization, open your eyes and compare the tension in your body and mind at this point with how you felt prior

> **Breathing exercises** A stress management technique wherein the individual concentrates on "breathing away" the tension and inhaling fresh air to the entire body.
>
> **Imagery** Mental visualization of relaxing images and scenes to induce body relaxation in times of stress or as an aid in the treatment of certain medical conditions such as cancer, hypertension, asthma, chronic pain, and obesity.

Behavior Modification Planning

Five-Minute De-Stress Technique

The following simple exercise can be used as an effective stress management technique, especially when coming home at the end of the day. De-stress by taking five minutes before getting into your evening routine by removing your shoes, lying on the carpet, and placing your feet up on a chair. Use a rolled up towel at the base of the skull for neck tension or along the middle of the spine for back tension. The lower back should be flat on the floor. Completely relax and practice deep breathing for five minutes.

Try It

This simple exercise will help you start your evening right and be kinder to those around you.

to the exercise. You can repeat this exercise as often as you deem necessary when you are feeling tension or stress.

You may not always be able to find a quiet/comfortable setting in which to sit or lie down for 10 to 20 minutes. If you think imagery works for you, however, you can perform this technique while standing or sitting in an active setting. If you are able, close your eyes and disregard your surroundings for a short moment and visualize one of your favorite scenes. Once you feel that you have regained some control over the stressor, open your eyes, and continue with your assigned tasks.

Autogenic Training Autogenic training is a form of self-suggestion in which people place themselves in an autohypnotic state by repeating and concentrating on feelings of heaviness and warmth in the extremities. This technique was developed by Johannes Schultz, a German psychiatrist who noted that hypnotized individuals developed sensations of warmth and heaviness in the limbs and torso. The sensation of warmth is caused by dilation of blood vessels, which increases blood flow to the limbs. Muscular relaxation produces the feeling of heaviness.

In this technique the person lies down or sits in a comfortable position, eyes closed, and concentrates progressively on six fundamental stages and says (or thinks) the following:

1. Heaviness
   My right (left) arm is heavy.
   Both arms are heavy.
   My right (left) leg is heavy.
   Both legs are heavy.
   My arms and legs are heavy.
2. Warmth
   My right (left) arm is warm.
   Both arms are warm.
   My right (left) leg is warm.
   Both legs are warm.
   My arms and legs are warm.
3. Heart
   My heartbeat is calm and regular. (Repeat four or five times.)
4. Respiration
   My body breathes itself. (Repeat four or five times.)
5. Abdomen
   My abdomen is warm. (Repeat four or five times.)
6. Forehead
   My forehead is cool. (Repeat four or five times.)

The autogenic training technique is more difficult to master than any of those mentioned previously. The person should not move too fast through the entire exercise, because this actually may interfere with learning and relaxation. Each stage must be mastered before proceeding to the next.

Meditation Meditation helps people draw attention inward and calm the mind. It is a mental exercise that brings about mental, spiritual, and physical benefits, including stress reduction and a feeling of well-being. It encompasses a combination of techniques such as thoughts, breathing, sounds, postures, visualization, and/or movement that help achieve a relaxed state of being. Regular meditation has been shown to decrease blood pressure, stress, anger, anxiety, fear, negative feelings, chronic pain, and increase activity in the brain's left

Behavior Modification Planning

Characteristics of Good Stress Managers

Good stress managers

- are physically active, eat a healthy diet, and get adequate rest every day.
- believe they have control over events in their life.
- understand their own feelings and accept their limitations.
- recognize, anticipate, monitor, and regulate stressors within their capabilities.
- control emotional and physical responses when distressed.
- use appropriate stress management techniques when confronted with stressors.
- recognize warning signs and symptoms of excessive stress.
- schedule daily time to unwind, relax, and evaluate the day's activities.
- control stress when called on to perform.
- enjoy life despite occasional disappointments and frustrations.
- look success and failure squarely in the face and keep moving along a predetermined course.
- move ahead with optimism and energy and do not spend time and talent worrying about failure.
- learn from previous mistakes and use them as building blocks to prevent similar setbacks in the future.
- give of themselves freely to others.
- have a deep meaning in life.

Try It

Change for many people is threatening, but often required. Pick three of these strategies and apply them in your life. After several days, determine the usefulness of these strategies to your physical, mental, social, and emotional well-being.

frontal region—an area associated with positive emotions.[7] The objective of meditation is to gain control over one's attention by clearing the mind and blocking out the stressor(s) responsible for the higher tension.

This technique can be learned rather quickly but first-time users often drop out before reaping benefits because they feel intimidated, confused, bored, or frustrated. In such cases, a group setting is best to get started. Many colleges, community programs, health clubs, and hospitals offer classes.

Initially the person who is learning to meditate should choose a room that is comfortable, quiet, and free of all disturbances (including telephones). After learning the technique, the person will be able to meditate just about anywhere. A time block of approximately 10 to 15 minutes is adequate to start, but as you become more comfortable with meditation you can lengthen the time to 30 minutes or longer. To use meditation effectively, meditate daily—as just once or twice per week may not provide noticeable benefits.

Meditation "101"

Of the several forms of meditation, the following routine is recommended to get started.

1. Sit in a chair in an upright position with the hands resting either in your lap or on the arms of the chair. Close your eyes and focus on your breathing. Allow your body to relax as much as possible. Do not try to consciously relax, because trying means work. Rather, assume a passive attitude and concentrate on your breathing.
2. Allow the body to breathe regularly, at its own rhythm, and repeat in your mind the word "one" every time you inhale, and the word "two" every time you exhale. Paying attention to these two words keeps distressing thoughts from entering into your mind.
3. Continue to breathe in this way about 15 minutes. Because the objective of meditation is to bring about a hypometabolic state leading to body relaxation, do not use an alarm clock to remind you that the 15 minutes have expired. The alarm will only trigger your stress response again, defeating the purpose of the exercise. Opening your eyes once in a while to keep track of the time is fine, but do not rush or anticipate the end of the session. This time has been set aside for meditation, and you need to relax, take your time, and enjoy the exercise.

Mindless Meditation

In addition to alleviating stress, mindless meditation is frequently used to help people relieve chronic pain and increase pain tolerance. Chronic pain increases stress hormones that lead a person to think that pain is much worse than it really is. Research indicates that chronic pain sufferers who use this technique not only have greater pain tolerance than nonpractitioners, but discomfort is eased by helping the brain stop anticipating the pain itself. As pain decreases, stress decreases, and the individual is able to sleep better, hurt less, and exercise more—all of which lead to greater comfort and relaxation.

Slightly different from Meditation 101, these steps can be followed to use this technique:

> ## Stress Coping Strategies
> - Balance personal, work, and family needs and obligations.
> - Have a sense of control and purpose in life.
> - Increase self-efficacy.
> - Be optimistic.
> - Express your emotions.
> - Get adequate sleep.
> - Eat well-balanced meals.
> - Be physically active every day.
> - Do not worry about things that you cannot control (the weather, for example).
> - Actively strive to resolve conflicts with other people.
> - Prepare for stressful events the best possible way (public speaking, job interviews, exams).
> - Limit or abstain from alcohol intake.
> - Do not use tobacco in any form.
> - View change as positive and not as a threat.
> - Obtain social support from family members and friends.
> - Use stress management programs and counselors available through work and school programs.
> - Seek help from church leaders.
> - Engage in nonstressful activities (reading, sports, hobbies, and social events).
> - Get involved in your community.
> - Practice stress management techniques.
> - Adopt a healthy lifestyle.

1. Close your eyes, breathe slowly and naturally, and focus on the feeling of each inhalation and exhalation.
2. Recognize your feelings, thoughts, and body sensations, but do not dwell on them.
3. Continue to focus on your breathing pattern and your feelings for about 15 minutes.
4. Open your eyes and notice your sur-

> **Autogenic training** A stress management technique using a form of self-suggestion, wherein an individual is able to place himself or herself in an autohypnotic state by repeating and concentrating on feelings of heaviness and warmth in the extremities.
>
> **Meditation** A stress management technique used to gain control over one's attention by clearing the mind and blocking out the stressor(s) responsible for the increased tension.

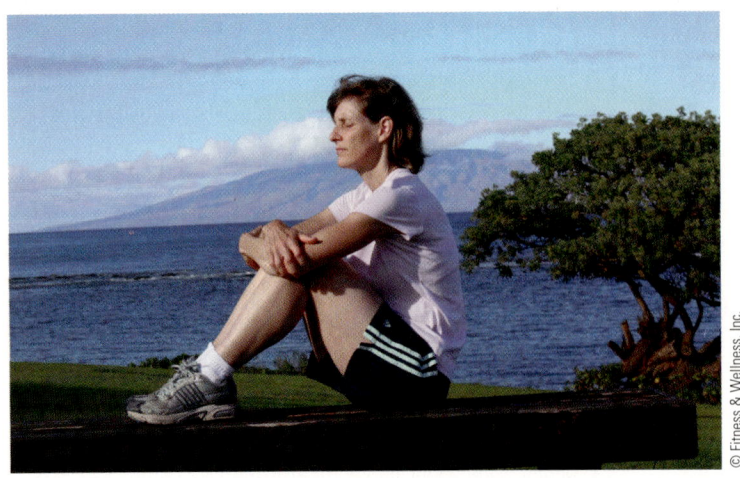

Meditation is an effective stress-reducing technique.

roundings while maintaining a calm and gentle breathing pattern.
5. You can now proceed to your daily activity schedule with this peaceful, calm, and serene feeling.

Mindfulness Meditation

Mindfulness can be defined as awareness of the present moment. In mindfulness meditation, you focus on becoming fully aware and accepting living in the present moment; paying particular attention to your feelings, thoughts, sensations, and emotions without passing judgment or dwelling in the past or projecting yourself into the future. Mindfulness has also been successfully used in helping people adhere to medical treatment and more effectively handle pain and manage anxiety and depression associated with illness.

Important during mindfulness meditation is not to worry about things that you have no control over. To live in the present, you must understand that the most significant event that you have control over is *your attitude*. While your confidence may be shaken because of life's challenges and stressors, you can control your attitude. Having a clear understanding that the "storm will pass" and that "there is light at the end of every tunnel," will allow you to navigate through life's stressors and ultimately overcome challenges and enjoy happiness while living in the present.

Let's look at an example. Your roommate agreed to clean up his three-day mess in the kitchen that evening. When you get home from the library that night, the kitchen looks worse and your roommate is sound asleep in the bedroom. You are extremely disappointed and upset. Your thoughts turn to the past and how much worse it may get in the future. The fight-or-flight mechanism kicks in and you are ready to wake your roommate up and let him have it. Your stress level rises with every thought of the past, present, and potential future. Should you act on your impulses, the situation may only get worse, not to mention your relationship with your roommate.

Now put yourself in the same situation, but stay in the present moment. Don't dwell in the past or worry about the future. Instead of allowing greater anger to build up, chose to stay with the uncomfortable feeling of disappointment for a moment. Recognize it, feel it, and acknowledge the disappointment. Maybe your roommate has a valid reason for not getting it done. Perhaps tomorrow you could tell your roommate about your disappointment, but after a night's rest you may choose not to do so. Now turn your attention to another task in the present moment. Eat a healthy meal and savor every bite, listen to your favorite music and enjoy the melody, go for a walk and appreciate the surroundings and beauty of the night, or take a moment to relish your good health. You can now pay attention to your breathing, notice the fresh air and your breathing pattern for a few minutes. Before retiring to bed, conduct your nightly audit and plan the next day's activities. At this point, notice that stress and the fight-or-flight mechanism have dissipated and the disappointment of the unclean kitchen, over which you had no control, would not have been worth the frustration and anger that you could have experienced. A few years from now, you can have a healthy laugh over the incident.

Yoga Yoga is an excellent stress-coping technique. It is a school of thought in the Hindu religion that seeks to help the individual attain a higher level of spirituality and peace of mind. Although its philosophical roots can be considered spiritual, yoga is based on principles of self-care.

Practitioners of yoga adhere to a specific code of ethics and a system of mental and physical exercises that promote control of the mind and the body. In Western countries, many people are familiar mainly with the exercise portion of yoga. This system of exercises (postures or asanas) can be used as a relaxation technique for stress management. The exercises include a combination of postures, diaphragmatic breathing, muscle relaxation, and meditation that help buffer the biological effects of stress. Although we are unable to avoid all life stressors, we can definitely change the emotional response through yoga postures, observing and controlling the breathing pattern, and reflecting on the moment, all of which are actions that help calm the mind and the body.

Western interest in yoga exercises developed gradually over the last century, particularly since the 1970s. The practice of yoga exercises helps align the musculoskeletal system and increases muscular flexibility, muscular strength and endurance, and balance.[8] People pursue yoga exercises to help dispel stress by raising self-esteem, clearing the mind, slowing respiration, promoting neuromuscular relaxation, and increasing body awareness. In addition, the exercises help relieve back pain and control involuntary body functions like heart rate, blood pressure, oxygen consumption, and metabolic rate. Yoga also is used in many hospital-based programs for cardiac patients to help manage stress and decrease blood pressure.

In addition, yoga exercises have been used to help treat chemical dependency, insomnia, and prevent injury. Research on patients with coronary heart disease who practiced yoga (among other lifestyle changes) has shown that it slows down or even reverses atherosclerosis. These patients were compared with others who did not use yoga as one of their lifestyle changes.[9]

Of the many different styles of yoga, more than 60 are presently taught in the United States. Classes vary according to their emphasis. Some styles of yoga are athletic, while others are passive in nature.

The most popular variety of yoga in the Western world is **hatha yoga**, which incorporates a series of static stretching postures performed in specific sequences (asanas) that help induce the relaxation response. The postures are held for several seconds while participants concentrate on breathing patterns, meditation, and body awareness.

Most yoga classes now are variations of hatha yoga and many of the typical stretches used in flexibility exercises today have been adapted from hatha yoga. Examples include:

1. *Integral yoga* and *viny yoga* that focus on gentle/static stretches
2. *Iyengar yoga*, promotes muscular strength and endurance
3. *Yogalates*, incorporates Pilates exercises to increase muscular strength
4. *Power yoga* or *yogarobics*, a high-energy form that links many postures together in a dance-like routine to promote cardiorespiratory fitness.

As with flexibility exercises, the stretches in hatha yoga should not be performed to the point of discomfort. Instructors should not push participants beyond their physical limitations. Similar to other stress management techniques, yoga exercises are best performed in a quiet place for 15 to 60 minutes per session. Many yoga participants like to perform the exercises daily.

To appreciate yoga exercises, a person has to experience them. The discussion here serves only as an introduction. Although yoga exercises can be practiced with the instruction of a book or video, most participants take classes. Many of the postures are difficult and complex, and few individuals can master the entire sequence in the first few weeks.

Individuals who are interested in yoga exercises should initially pursue them under qualified instruction. Many universities offer yoga courses, and you also can check the phone book for a listing of yoga instructors or classes. Yoga courses are offered at many health clubs and recreation centers. Because instructors and yoga styles vary, you may want to sit in on a class before enrolling. The most important thing is to look for an instructor whose views on wellness parallel your own. Instructors are not subject to any national certification standards. If you are new to yoga, you are encouraged to compare a couple of instructors before you select a class.

Tai Chi Tai chi chuan (full name) originated in China centuries ago and is practiced today for defense training and physical and mental health benefits. The martial side, however, is no longer the focus of its practice, so young and old, and even the very old, can perform the activity. Many fitness practitioners use it in conjunction with aerobic and strength training.

Tai chi is often described as "meditation in motion" because it is performed with flowing/rhythmic movements that focus heavily on breathing and the slow execution of its movements. The main objective is to promote tranquility and reflection through postures that combine meditation and dance. The postures are performed in sequences known as "sets" that require concentration, coordination, controlled breathing, muscle relaxation, strength, flexibility, gait, and body balance.

Research has attributed many health benefits to tai chi, including diabetes management, arthritis relief, lower blood pressure, faster recovery from heart disease and injury, improved strength and flexibility, better sleep, and improved physical work capacity. Among older adults, improved gait and the capability to perform activities of daily living are frequently reported.

Tai chi is frequently used for stress management to relieve tension, stress, and anxiety. The mental aspect of having to concentrate on leading the movement and paying attention to detail through gentle actions dissipates stress. The activity leaves no room to think or worry about other problems, thus calming and relaxing the mind and body.

To master tai chi, you need initial professional guidance. You are encouraged to join a group or a class available at many college campuses or community health clubs. The class should emphasize fitness and health benefits rather than combat techniques. Once you have mastered many of the sets available, you can practice the activity on your own.

12.10 Which Technique Is Best?

Each person reacts to stress differently. Therefore, the best coping strategy depends mostly on the individual. Which technique is used does not really matter, as long as it works. An individual may want to experiment with several or all of them to find out which works best. A combination of two or more is best for many people.

All of the coping strategies discussed here help to block out stressors and promote mental and physical relaxation by diverting the attention to a different, nonthreatening action. Some of the techniques are easier to learn and may take less time per session. As a part of your class experience, you may participate in a stress management session (see Activity 12.8). Regardless of which technique you select, the time spent doing stress management exercises (several times a day, as needed) is well worth the effort when stress becomes a significant problem in life. After completing your stress management experience, use Activity 12.9 to conduct a self-assessment of the impact of stress in your life and ways by which you can personally counteract or avoid stress-inducing events.

Keep in mind that most individuals need to learn to relax and take time for themselves. Stress is not what makes people ill; it's the way they react to the stress-causing agent. Individuals who learn to be diligent and start taking control of themselves find that they can enjoy a better, happier, and healthier life.

> **Hatha yoga** A form of yoga that incorporates specific sequences of static stretching postures to help induce the relaxation response.

Activity 12.8: Stress Management Experience

Name _____ Date _____
Course _____ Section _____ Gender _____ Age _____

I. Stage of Change for Stress Management
Using Figure 2.5 (page 63) and Table 2.3 (page 62), identify your current stage of change for a stress management program:

[   ]

II. Stress Management
Instructions: The class should be divided into groups of about five students per group. Each group should select and go through a minimum of two of the following stress management techniques outlined in this chapter:

1. Progressive Muscle Relaxation
2. Breathing Techniques for Relaxation
3. Visual Imagery
4. Autogenic Training
5. Meditation

A group leader is chosen who will lead the exercise according to the instructions provided for each relaxation technique in this chapter. Be sure this experience is conducted in a comfortable room that is as free of noise as possible. If trained personnel or a tape-recording for progressive muscle relaxation exercises is available, the entire class may participate in this experience at once. Institutions that have biofeedback equipment may use it in this activity as well.

After completing this activity, answer the four questions given below.

1. Indicate the two relaxation techniques used in your class:

   A. [   ]   B. [   ]

2. In your own words, relate your feelings as you were going through exercises A and B above:

   Exercise A: _____
   _____

   Exercise B: _____
   _____

3. Indicate how you felt mentally, emotionally, and physically after participating in this experience:

   _____
   _____

4. Are there situations in your daily life in which you think you would benefit from practicing the selected stress management exercises?

   _____
   _____

5. Number of daily steps: [   ]   Activity category (see Table 1.2, page 12): [   ]

Activity 12.9: Self-Assessment Stress Evaluation

Name _____ Date _____

Course _____ Section _____ Gender _____ Age _____

1. Do you currently perceive stress to be a problem in your life? ☐ Yes ☐ No

2. Do you experience any of the typical stress symptoms listed in the box on page 422? If so, which ones?

3. Indicate any specific events in your life that trigger a stress response.

   _____
   _____
   _____
   _____

4. Write specific objectives to either avoid or help you manage the various stress-inducing events listed above, including one or more stress management techniques.

   _____
   _____
   _____
   _____

5. Do you have any behavior patterns you would like to modify? List those you would like to change.

   _____
   _____
   _____
   _____

6. List specific techniques of change you will use to change undesirable behaviors (see Table 2.2, page 62).

   _____
   _____
   _____
   _____

ASSESS YOUR BEHAVIOR

CENGAGEbrain.com To access course materials, including companion resources, please visit www.cengagebrain.com.

1. Are you able to channel your emotions and feelings to exert a positive effect on your mind, health, and wellness?
2. Do you use time management strategies on a regular basis?
3. Do you use stress management techniques and do they allow you to be in control over the daily stresses of life?

ASSESS YOUR KNOWLEDGE

Evaluate how well you understand the concepts presented in this chapter using the chapter-specific quiz available in the online materials at www.cengagebrain.com.

1. Positive stress is also referred to as
   a. eustress.
   b. posstress.
   c. functional stress.
   d. distress.
   e. physiostress.

2. Which of the following is *not* a stage of the general adaptation syndrome?
   a. alarm reaction
   b. resistance
   c. compliance
   d. exhaustion/recovery
   e. All are stages of the general adaptation syndrome.

3. The behavior pattern of highly stressed individuals who do not seem to be at higher risk for disease is known as Type
   a. A.
   b. B.
   c. C.
   d. E.
   e. X.

4. Effective time managers
   a. delegate.
   b. learn to say "no."
   c. protect from boredom.
   d. set aside "overtimes."
   e. do all of the above.

5. Hormonal changes that occur during a stress response
   a. decrease heart rate.
   b. sap the body's strength.
   c. diminish blood flow to the muscles.
   d. induce relaxation.
   e. increase blood pressure.

6. Physical activity decreases stress levels by
   a. deliberately diverting stress to various body systems.
   b. metabolizing excess catecholamines.
   c. diminishing muscular tension.
   d. stimulating alpha-wave activity in the brain.
   e. doing all of the above.

7. Biofeedback is
   a. the interaction with the interior self.
   b. the biological response to stress.
   c. the nonspecific response to a stress-causing agent.
   d. used to identify biological factors that cause stress.
   e. most readily achieved while in a state of self-hypnosis.

8. The technique where a person breathes in through the nose to a specific count and then exhales through pursed lips to double the intake count is known as
   a. sighing.
   b. deep breathing.
   c. meditation.
   d. autonomic ventilation.
   e. release management.

9. During autogenic training, a person
   a. contracts each muscle to about 70 percent of capacity.
   b. concentrates on feelings of warmth and heaviness.
   c. visualizes relaxing scenes to induce body relaxation.
   d. learns to reliably influence physiological responses.
   e. notes the positive and negative impact of frequent stressors on various body systems.

10. Yoga exercises have been successfully used to
    a. stimulate ventilation.
    b. increase metabolism during stress.
    c. slow down atherosclerosis.
    d. decrease body awareness.
    e. accomplish all of the above.

Correct answers can be found at the back of the book.

Addictive Behavior 13

Addictive behaviors are lifetime nightmares that focus on immediate self-gratification without thought or concern for one's well-being or that of others—ultimately, taking away the control the person has over life itself.

Objectives

- **Address** the detrimental effects of addictive substances, including marijuana, cocaine, methamphetamine, MDMA (Ecstasy), heroin, Spice, inhalants, and alcohol.
- **List** the detrimental health effects of tobacco use in general.
- **Recognize** cigarette smoking as the largest preventable cause of premature illness and death in the United States.
- **Enumerate** the reasons people smoke.
- **Explain** the benefits and the significance of a smoking-cessation program.
- **Learn** how to implement a smoking-cessation program to help yourself (if you smoke) or someone else go through the quitting process.
- **Find** out if you're prone to addictive behavior.
- **Plan** for a drug-free future (including freedom from tobacco use).

CENGAGE brain.com
Visit **www.cengagebrain.com** to access course materials and companion resources for this text, including quiz questions designed to check your understanding of the chapter contents. See the preface on page ix for more information.

FAQ

What is drug addiction and how quickly can someone become addicted to drugs?

Drug addiction (addictive behavior, substance abuse, or chemical dependency) is a complex brain disease characterized by compulsive and uncontrollable drug cravings even at the peril of serious negative consequences. How quickly addictive behavior develops cannot be predicted. There are vast individual differences among people in sensitivity to different drugs.

Psychological and physiological factors, as well as the type of drug used, influence a person's response to the drug and subsequent addiction to it. Whereas one individual may use a certain drug several times without harmful effects, someone else may seriously overdose the first time that this same drug is used. All drugs have potentially damaging effects, and some have life-threatening consequences. One single moment of weakness, or caving in to peer pressure, can easily result in a lifetime nightmare, not just for users, but for everyone around them as well.

How can I tell if someone is addicted to drugs?

People with addictive behavior compulsively seek and use drugs despite potential serious repercussions, such as physical and family problems, loss of a job, or problems with the law. Some individuals realize that they need to cut down on their drinking/drug use, or they are told to do so by others. At times they crave alcohol or drugs when they first get up in the morning and they feel bad or guilty about their addictive behavior. If you see any of these signs in someone you know, that person is most likely addicted to drugs.

How is drug addiction treated?

In the early stages of substance abuse, most people believe that they can stop using the drug(s) on their own. Most of these attempts, however, fail to achieve long-term abstinence. Long-term drug use results in altered brain functions that linger on long after the person stops using drugs. Effective treatment of drug addiction is rarely accomplished without professional help. Treatment modalities are behavioral-based therapies, oftentimes combined with medication to help the body detoxify and effectively manage symptoms of withdrawal. Responses to these therapies vary among individuals, and several courses of rehab may be necessary to overcome the problem. For some individuals, it becomes a lifetime battle, and relapses are possible even after prolonged periods of abstinence.

Real Life Story | Steve's Experience

In high school I used to get teased and bullied a lot. It was so bad that I hated being the person I was, and I wanted to become somebody else. The way I tried to do that was through drugs. I started out drinking and doing marijuana. When I was drunk or high, I felt calm, confident, and popular. My self-doubts and self-hatred would go away for a while. The problem was, the bad feelings always came back. Eventually, some friends offered me meth, so I tried it. For me, the effects of meth were very intense. When I was using it, I felt like the king of the world. As soon as it wore off, I felt so horrible, I would do pretty much anything just to feel better again. That began a period of a couple years where meth crowded out everything else in my life. I stopped caring about school, and about any goals I had had for the future. I didn't care if I disappointed my parents or my friends. I didn't even care anymore about my younger brother, and he has always been my best friend and one of the people I love most in the world. Meth just completely took over my life. I dropped out of school and left home for several months. I camped out with several other addicts where we set up our own meth lab. We lived in really filthy conditions. Eventually I got disgusted with the way I was living, and I became terrified by the fact that I needed bigger and bigger doses of meth for a high that lasted only a fraction of the amount of time it used to. No matter how much I used, I was miserable much more often than I felt good. I finally moved back home and reached out for help to overcome my addiction. At first, I attended 12-step meetings almost constantly, and I finally managed to get clean. Now, the fact that I was able to go back and get my high school diploma, and now am in college, is a miracle to me. I have a second chance to make something of my life. That chance could easily have been lost forever due to drugs.

© Renars Jurkovskis/Shutterstock.com

> **PERSONAL PROFILE: Addictive Behavior Survey**
>
> I. Have you ever suffered from addiction to any legal or illicit drug?
>
> II. Do you regularly—on a weekly or nearly weekly basis—exceed the recommended one to two alcoholic beverages per day?
>
> III. Have you absolutely/positively decided to forgo instant gratification and peer pressure by saying *NO* to substance abuse (legal or illicit) that may or will harm your health and long-term life satisfaction? What led to this decision and how long ago did you make this choice?
>
> IV. What are your feelings about tobacco use in general and exposure to secondhand smoke?
>
> V. If you smoked cigarettes, have you quit? If you never smoked, have you helped someone else successfully quit smoking? If so, what approach did you use and why were you successful in accomplishing this goal?

Substance abuse remains one of the most serious health problems afflicting society. Chemical dependency is extremely destructive, having ruined and ended millions of lives. When addictive behaviors are at issue, education is vital—more, perhaps, than with any other unhealthy behavior. Education concerning these subjects may assist in the search for answers, treatment, and a more productive and better life. The information in this chapter will help you make informed decisions. The time to make healthy choices is *now*.

13.1 Addiction

When most people think of **addiction,** they probably think of dark and dirty alleys, an addict shooting drugs into a vein, or a wino passed out next to a garbage can after having spent an evening drinking alcohol. Psychotherapists have described addiction as a problem of imbalance or unease within the body and mind.

Almost anything can be addicting. Of the many types of addiction, some addictive behaviors are more detrimental than others. The most serious form is chemical dependency on drugs such as tobacco, alcohol, cocaine, methamphetamine, MDMA (Ecstasy), heroin, marijuana, or prescription drugs. Less serious are addictions to work, coffee, shopping, and even exercise.

People who are addicted to food eat to release stress or boredom or to reward themselves for every small personal achievement. Many people are addicted to television and the Internet. Others become so addicted to their jobs that all they think about is work. It may start out as enjoyable, but when it totally consumes a person's life, work can become an unhealthy behavior. If you find that you are readily irritated, moody, grouchy, constantly tired, not as alert as you used to be, or making more mistakes than usual, you may be becoming a workaholic and need to slow down or take time off work.

Even though exercise has enhanced the health and quality of life of millions of people, a relatively small number become obsessed with exercise, which has the potential for overuse and addiction. Compulsive exercisers feel guilty and uncomfortable when they miss a day's workout. Often, they continue to exercise even when they have injuries and sicknesses that require proper rest for adequate recovery. People who exceed the recommended guidelines to develop and maintain fitness (see Chapters 6, 7, 8, and 9) are exercising for reasons other than health—including addictive behavior.

Addiction to caffeine can have undesirable side effects. In some individuals, caffeine doses in excess of 200 to 500 mg can produce an abnormally rapid heart rate, abnormal heart rhythms, higher blood pressure, and increased secretion of gastric acids, leading to stomach problems and possible birth defects in offspring. It also may induce symptoms of anxiety, depression, nervousness, and dizziness.

The caffeine content of drinks varies according to the product. In 6 ounces of coffee, for example, the content varies from 65 mg in instant coffee to as high as 180 mg in drip coffee. Soft drinks, mainly colas, range in caffeine content from about 30 to 70 mg per 12-ounce can. The Food and Drug Administration (FDA) states that 100 mg to 200 mg of caffeine per day is safe as a stimulant for most adults.

Emergency department (ED) visits involving high-caffeine consumption increased 10-fold between 2005 and 2009. Fifty-six percent of the more than 13,000 ED visits were attributed directly to energy drinks. The trend continues to escalate. In 2011, there were some 20,000 ED visits, a 36 percent increase over 2010. Reported symptoms in the ED include lightheadedness, headaches, dizziness, and heart palpitations. An even greater concern is when energy drinks are mixed with alcohol. Young people reported that they thought they would be able to consume more alcohol because the energy drinks would keep them awake longer. Data also indicate that men are more likely to mix energy drinks with alcohol and illicit drugs, whereas women mix alcohol with pharmaceuticals.

Energy drinks on the market, such as Red Bull, Full Throttle, Monster, and Rock Star, usually have even higher caffeine content—somewhere in the range of 70 to 200 mg in an 8- to 12-ounce drink. Also quite popular at this time are 2-ounce 5-hour energy drinks or shots with a caffeine content equivalent to one cup of coffee, but the actual caffeine content is not made available. For energy drinks, the FDA requires that caffeine be listed on the label, but it does not mandate that the amount be specified.

Caffeine is now advertised as an energy booster

> **Addiction** Compulsive and uncontrollable behavior(s) or use of substance(s).

and is added to a variety of other food items such as energy bars, candy, gum, waffles, syrup, and even oatmeal. This trend is quite alarming to the FDA. Individuals who are caffeine sensitive should read all food labels for potential caffeine in those items.

Although previous examples may be the first addictions you think of, they are by no means the only forms. Other addictions can be to gambling, pornography, sex, people, places, and on and on.

According to the 2011 National Survey on Drug Use and Health (NSDUH) by the U.S. Department of Health and Human Services,[1] more than 22.5 million Americans use illicit drugs, including marijuana, prescription-type psychotherapeutics used nonmedically, cocaine, hallucinogens, and heroin (Figure 13.1). Approximately two-thirds of the world's production of illegal drugs is consumed in the United States. Each year, Americans spend more than $60 billion on illegal drugs.

Risk Factors for Addiction Although addictive behaviors cover a wide spectrum, they have factors in common that predispose people to addiction. Among these factors are the following[2]:

- The behavior is reinforced.
- The addiction is an attempt to meet basic human needs, such as physical needs, the need to feel safe, the need to belong, the need to feel important, or the need to reach one's potential.
- The addiction seems to relieve stress temporarily.
- The addiction results from peer pressure.
- The addiction can be present within the person's value system (a person whose values wouldn't let him or her shoot heroin may be able to rationalize compulsive eating or obsessive playing of computer games, for example).
- A serious physical illness is present, and the addiction may provide escape from pain or the fear of disfigurement.
- The addict feels pressured to perform or succeed.
- The addict has self-hate.
- A genetic link is present. Heredity might dictate susceptibility to some addictions.
- Society allows addiction. Advertising even encourages it (you can sleep better with a pill; snacking helps you enjoy life more fully; parties and sports are more fun with alcohol; shop 'til you drop; and so on).

The same general traits and behaviors are involved in all kinds of addictions, whether they involve food, sex, gambling, shopping, or drugs.

Most people with addictions deny their problem. Even when the addiction is clear to people around them, addicts continue to deny that they are addicted. Instead, they tend to get angry when someone tries to talk about the behavior and are likely to make excuses for their actions. Many addicts also blame others for their problem. In some cases, an addict admits the problem but fails to take any steps to change.

Recognizing that all forms of addiction are unhealthy, this chapter focuses on some of today's most self-destructive addictive substances: psychotherapeutics, marijuana, cocaine, methamphetamine, MDMA, heroin, Spice, inhalants, alcohol, and tobacco. About half a million Americans die each year from tobacco, alcohol, and illegal drug use.

13.2 Drugs and Dependence

A drug is any substance that alters the user's ability to function. Drugs encompass over-the-counter drugs, prescription medications, and illegal substances. Many drugs lead to physical and psychological dependence.

Any drug can be misused and abused. "Drug misuse" implies the intentional and inappropriate use of over-the-counter or prescribed medications.[3] Examples include taking more medication than prescribed, mixing drugs, not following prescription instructions, or discontinuing a drug prior to a physician's approval. "Drug abuse" is the intentional and inappropriate use of a drug resulting in physical, emotional, financial, intellectual, social, spiritual, or occupational consequences of the abuse.[4] Many substances, if used in the wrong manner, can be abused.

When drugs are used regularly, they integrate into the body's chemistry, increasing the user's tolerance to the drug and forcing the user to increase the dosage constantly to obtain similar results. Drug abuse leads to serious health problems, and more than half of all adolescent suicides are drug related. Often, drug abuse opens the gate to other illegal activities. According to the National Center on Addiction and Substance Abuse (CASA), the majority of convicted criminals—about 85 percent of federal and state inmates—have abused drugs.

According to the U.S. Department of Education, today's drugs are stronger and more addictive, and they pose a

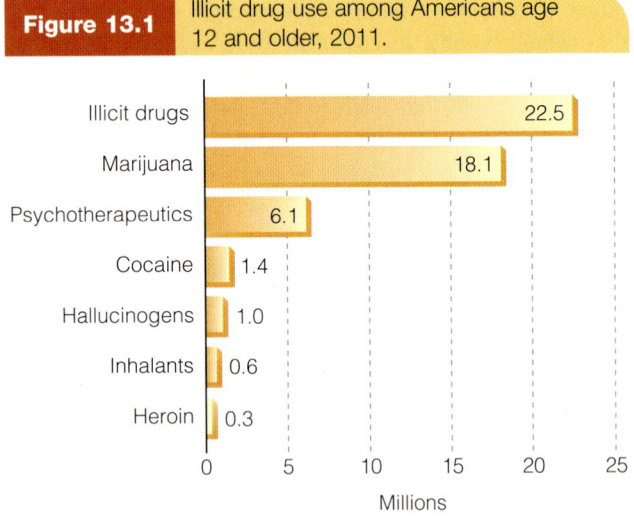

Figure 13.1 Illicit drug use among Americans age 12 and older, 2011.

SOURCE: http://www.samhsa.gov/data/NSDUH/2k11Results/NSDUHresults2011.htm#Fig2-1, downloaded June 24, 2013.

greater risk than ever before. Alcohol, tobacco, and illegal drug use lead to many negative health-related consequences—including cancers, cardiovascular diseases, stroke, bacterial endocarditis, fatal and nonfatal overdose, hepatitis, human immunodeficiency virus (HIV) infection and acquired immune deficiency syndrome (AIDS), and other sexually transmitted infections. Substance abuse is also linked to increased risk of intentional and unintentional injuries, complications in pregnancy and delivery, and psychiatric disturbances, ranging from acute panic attacks to chronic mood disturbances. Furthermore, illegal drug use is associated with negative effects on employment, school achievement, socioeconomic status, and family stability; if only because illegal drug use, once detected, can lead to school suspension or expulsion and to arrest, conviction, and incarceration for drug-related crimes.[5]

If you are uncertain about addictive behavior(s) in your life, the Addictive Behavior Questionnaire in Activity 13.1 can help you identify a potential problem. Some of the most commonly abused drugs in our society are discussed next.

Nonmedical Use of Prescription Drugs

America's drug problem is shifting from illicit drugs to abuse of prescription drugs. As a result, the CDC has classified prescription drug abuse in the United States as an epidemic. Fifty-one million Americans aged 12 or older have reported nonmedical use of psychotherapeutic drugs at some point in their lifetime. Psychotherapeutic drugs include any prescription pain reliever, tranquilizer, stimulant, or sedative (but not over-the-counter drugs).

In 2011, about 14.6 million Americans abused prescription drugs leading to 15,000 deaths due to an overdose of these drugs. Currently, drug poisoning is the second leading cause of unintentional injury deaths in the United States. The most commonly abused prescription medications are:

- Opioids, commonly prescribed to treat pain. These include codeine, morphine, oxycodone (OxyContin®), and hydrocodone (Vicodin®).
- Central nervous system depressants, used to treat anxiety and sleep disorders. Examples include Mebaral®, Nembutal®, Valium®, Xanax®, Ambien®, and Lunesta®.
- Stimulants, prescribed to treat the sleep disorder narcolepsy, attention-deficit hyperactivity disorder (ADHD), and obesity. Examples include Dexedrine®, Adderall®, Ritalin®, and Concerta®.

Most individuals, in particular young people, obtain these drugs with or without consent from friends and family members. A major concern is that many abusers believe these substances are safer than illicit drugs because they are prescribed by a health care professional and dispensed by a pharmacist and cause no serious or life-threatening consequences. The risks associated with psychotherapy drug misuse or abuse varies depending on the drug. Some of the risks include respiratory depression or cessation, decreased or irregular heart rate, high body temperature, seizures, and cardiovascular failure. Abuse of prescription drugs, or using them in a manner other than exactly as prescribed, can lead to addictive behavior.

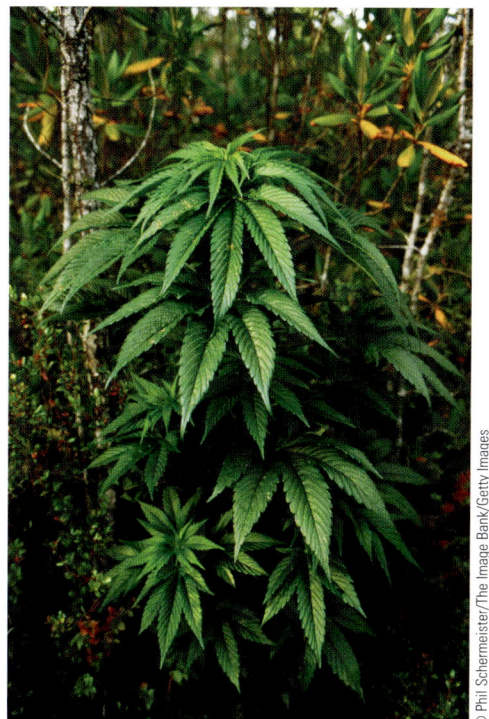

Cannabis sativa.

Marijuana

Marijuana (pot, grass, or weed as it is commonly called) is the most widely used illegal drug in the United States. Estimates by the Office of National Drug Control Policy indicate that 42 percent of Americans have smoked marijuana. Most users smoke loose marijuana that has been rolled into a joint or packed into a pipe. A few users bake it into foods such as brownies or use it to brew a tea. Marijuana cigarettes are often laced with other drugs such as crack cocaine.

In small doses, marijuana has a sedative effect. Larger doses produce physical and psychological changes. Studies in the 1960s indicated that the potential effects of marijuana were exaggerated and that the drug was relatively harmless. The drug as it is used today, however, is much stronger than when the initial studies were conducted.

The main, and most active, psychoactive and mind-altering ingredient in marijuana is thought to be delta-9-tetrahydrocannabinol (THC). In the 1960s, THC content in marijuana ranged from .02 to 2 percent. Users called the latter "real good grass." Today's THC content averages 11 percent, although it has been reported as high as 27 percent. The average potency has tripled over the last three decades.

THC reaches the brain within a few seconds after marijuana smoke is

> **Marijuana** A psychoactive drug prepared from a mixture of crushed leaves, flowers, small branches, stems, and seeds from the hemp plant *Cannabis sativa*.

inhaled, and the psychic and physical changes reach their peak in about 2 or 3 minutes. THC then is metabolized in the liver to waste metabolites, but 30 percent of it remains in the body a week after the marijuana was smoked. THC is not completely eliminated until 30 days or more after an initial dose of the drug. The drug always remains in the system of regular users.

Some of the short-term effects of marijuana are **tachycardia,** dryness of the mouth, reddened eyes, stronger appetite, decrease in coordination and tracking (the eyes' ability to follow a moving stimulus), difficulty in concentration, intermittent confusion, impairment of short-term memory and continuity of speech, interference with the physical and mental learning process during periods of intoxication, and increased risk for heart attack for a full day after smoking the drug. Another common effect is the **amotivational syndrome.** This syndrome persists after periods of intoxication but usually disappears a few weeks after the individual stops using the drug.

> **Critical Thinking**
>
> The legalization of marijuana is being heatedly debated across the United States. • Do you think this decision should rest with the government, medical personnel, or the individuals themselves?

Long-term harmful effects include atrophy of the brain (leading to irreversible brain damage), less resistance to infectious diseases, chronic bronchitis, lung cancer (marijuana smoke may contain as much as 50 to 70 percent more cancer-producing hydrocarbons than cigarette smoke), and possible sterility and impotence.

One of the most common myths about marijuana use is that it is not addictive. Lobbyists work to convince the federal government to legalize marijuana. Scientific evidence shows that regular users of marijuana do develop physical and psychological dependence. As with cigarette smokers, when regular users go without the drug, they crave the substance, go through mood changes, are irritable and nervous, and develop an obsession to get more.

The use of marijuana for medical purposes appears to be beneficial in selected conditions such as neuralgia, convulsive disorders, emaciation, and post-traumatic stress disorder (PTSD). A substantial amount of research is necessary, however, before we can fully understand its medicinal use.

Cocaine Similar to marijuana, **cocaine** was thought for many years to be relatively harmless. This misconception came to an abrupt halt when two well-known athletes in their 20s—Len Bias (basketball) and Don Rogers (football)—died suddenly following cocaine overdoses. Over the years, cocaine has been given several different names, including, among others, coke, C, snow, blow, nose candy, toot, flake, Peruvian lady, white girl, and happy dust. This drug can be sniffed or snorted, smoked, or injected.

When cocaine is snorted, it is absorbed quickly through the mucous membranes of the nose into the bloodstream. The drug is usually arranged in fine powder lines 1 to 2 inches long. Each line stimulates the autonomic nervous system for about 30 minutes. When cocaine is injected intravenously, larger amounts of cocaine can enter the body in a shorter time. The popularity of cocaine is based on the almost universal guarantee that users will find themselves in an immediate state of euphoria and well-being. It is an expensive drug—$400 to $1,800 per ounce for powdered cocaine. The addiction begins with a desire to get high, often at social gatherings, and usually with the assurance that "occasional use is harmless." Many of these first-time users will become addicted and for most it is the beginning of a lifetime nightmare.

Animal research with cocaine has shown that all laboratory animals can become compulsive cocaine users. Animals work more persistently at pressing a bar for cocaine than bars for other drugs, including opiates. In one instance, an addicted monkey pressed the bar almost 13,000 times until it finally got a dose of cocaine.

People respond in a similar way. Cocaine addicts prefer drug usage to any other activity and use the drug until the supply or the user is exhausted.

Cocaine users also exhibit unusual behaviors compared with their previous conduct, even to the point at which a user has been known to sell a child to obtain more cocaine. Educated people are not immune to cocaine addiction. Some, including lawyers, physicians, and athletes, have daily habits that cost them hundreds to thousands of dollars, with binges in the $20,000 to $50,000 range. Cocaine addiction can lead to loss of a job and profession, loss of family, bankruptcy, and death.

Increasingly more popular is crack cocaine, a smokable form of cocaine. It is many times more potent than powdered or injected cocaine and is highly addictive. Two-thirds of users in the United States who are addicted to cocaine use crack. Because it is so potent, crack doses are smaller and, therefore, less expensive, at $5 to $40 each, although users still spend hundreds of dollars a day to support their addiction. The crack high lasts about 12 minutes, which is shorter than the high from snorted or injected cocaine. Choosing to use cocaine in this form heightens the risk for emphysema and heart attack.

Powdered cocaine.

Cocaine seems to alleviate fatigue and raise energy levels, as well as lessen the need for food and sleep. Following the high comes a "crash," a state of physiological and psychological depression, often leaving the user with the desire to get more. This can produce a constant craving for the drug. Similar to alcoholics, cocaine users recover only by abstaining completely from the drug. A single "backslide" can result in renewed addiction.

Light to moderate cocaine use is typically associated with feelings of pleasure and well-being. Sustained cocaine snorting can lead to a constant runny nose, nasal congestion and inflammation, and perforation of the nasal septum. Long-term consequences of cocaine use include loss of appetite, digestive disorders, weight loss, malnutrition, insomnia, confusion, anxiety, and cocaine psychosis, characterized by paranoia and hallucinations. In one type of hallucination, referred to as formication, or "coke bugs," the chronic user perceives imaginary insects or snakes crawling on or underneath the skin.

High doses of cocaine can cause nervousness, dizziness, blurred vision, vomiting, tremors, seizures, strokes, angina, cardiac arrhythmias, and high blood pressure. As with smoking marijuana, there is an increased risk for heart attack following cocaine use. The user's risk may be 24 times higher than normal for up to 3 hours following cocaine use. Almost one-third of cocaine users who incurred a heart attack had no symptoms of heart disease prior to taking cocaine. In addition, users are at risk for hepatitis, HIV, and other infectious diseases because of the risky behaviors they engage in to obtain the drug.

Large overdoses of cocaine can precipitate sudden death from respiratory paralysis, cardiac arrhythmias, and severe convulsions. If individuals lack an enzyme used in metabolizing cocaine, as few as two to three lines of cocaine may be fatal.

Chronic users who constantly crave the drug often turn to crime, including murder, to sustain their habit. Some users view suicide as the only solution to this sad syndrome.

Methamphetamine Methamphetamine, or "meth," is a more potent form of amphetamine. **Amphetamines** in general are part of a large group of synthetic agents used to stimulate the central nervous system. A powerfully addictive drug, methamphetamine falls under the same category of psychostimulant drugs as amphetamines and cocaine. It is also known as a "club drug," a group of illegal substances used at dance clubs, rock concerts, and raves (all-night dance parties). Other club drugs include MDMA, LSD, GHB, Rohypnol, and ketamine.

Methamphetamine typically is a white, odorless, bitter-tasting powder that dissolves readily in water or alcohol. The drug is a potent central nervous system stimulant that produces a general feeling of well-being, decreases appetite, increases motor activity, and decreases fatigue and the need for sleep.

Unlike most other drugs, methamphetamine reaches rural and urban populations alike. Young people especially prefer methamphetamine because of its low cost and long-lasting effects—up to 12 hours following use.

Methamphetamine was easily manufactured in clandestine "meth labs" using over-the-counter pseudoephedrine, typically found in cold medications. Because of the ease of accessibility to methamphetamine ingredients, in March 2006 the federal *Combat Meth Act of 2005* was signed into law. This law requires retailers to keep cold medications behind the counter, and consumers are limited as to the amount they can purchase.

Methamphetamine labs are set up almost anywhere, including garages, basements, or hotel rooms. The abundance of potential meth lab sites makes it difficult for drug enforcement agencies to locate many of these facilities. The risk of injury in a meth lab, however, is high, because potentially explosive environmental contaminants are discarded during production of the drug.

U.S. production of methamphetamine is now limited and will likely remain at low levels in the near future. Mexico is the primary source of methamphetamine for the United States. Production in Canada, however, has increased significantly, primarily by Canadian-based Asian drug trafficking organizations. These organizations run large-capacity super labs.

Methamphetamine can be snorted, swallowed, smoked, or injected. It is commonly referred to as "speed" or "crystal" when snorted or taken orally, "ice" or "glass" when smoked, and "crank" when injected. Depending on how it is taken, methamphetamine affects the body differently. Smoked or injected methamphetamine provides an immediate intense, pleasurable rush that lasts only a few minutes. Negative effects, nonetheless, can continue for several hours. When the drug is snorted or taken orally, the user does not experience a rush but develops a feeling of euphoria that lasts up to 16 hours.

Users of methamphetamine experience increases in body temperature, blood pressure, heart rate, and breathing rate; a decrease in appetite; hyperactivity; tremors; and violent behavior. High doses produce irritability, paranoia, irreversible damage to blood vessels in the brain (causing strokes), and risk of sudden death from hypothermia and convulsions if not treated at once.

Chronic abusers experience insomnia, confusion, hallucinations, inflammation of the heart lining, schizophrenia like mental disorder, and brain cell damage similar to that caused by a stroke. Physical changes to the brain may last months or perhaps become permanent. Over time, methamphetamine use may reduce brain levels of **dopamine**, which can lead to symptoms similar to those of Parkinson's disease. In addition, users fre-

---

Tachycardia Faster than normal heart rate.

Amotivational syndrome A condition characterized by loss of motivation, dullness, apathy, and no interest in the future.

Cocaine 2-beta-carbomethoxy-3-betabenozoxytropane, the primary psychoactive ingredient derived from coca plant leaves.

Methamphetamine A potent form of amphetamine.

Amphetamines A class of powerful central nervous system stimulants.

Dopamine A neurotransmitter that affects emotional, mental, and motor functions.

"Ice," so named for its appearance, is a smokable form of methamphetamine.

quently are involved in violent crime, homicide, and suicide. Using methamphetamine during pregnancy may cause prenatal complications, premature delivery, and abnormal physical and emotional development of the child.

Similar to other stimulants, methamphetamine is often used in a binge cycle. Addiction takes hold quickly because the person develops tolerance to methamphetamine within minutes of using it. The "high" disappears long before blood levels of the drug drop significantly. The user then attempts to maintain the pleasurable feelings by taking in more of the drug, and a binge cycle ensues.

The binge cycle, which can last for a couple of weeks, consists of several stages. The initial rush lasts 5 to 30 minutes. During this stage, heart rate, blood pressure, and metabolism increase and the user receives a great sense of pleasure. The high follows, lasting up to 16 hours. During this stage, users become arrogant and more argumentative. The binge stage sets in next and lasts between 2 and 14 days. Addicts continue to use the drug in an attempt to maintain the high for as long as possible.

When addicts no longer can achieve a satisfying high, they enter the "tweaking stage," the most dangerous stage in the cycle. At this point, users may have gone without food for several days and without sleep anywhere from 3 to 15 days. They become paranoid, irritable, and violent. Tweakers crave more of the drug, but no amount of amphetamines will restore the pleasurable, euphoric feelings they achieved during the high. Thus, the addicts become increasingly frustrated, unpredictable, and dangerous to those around them (including police officers and medical personnel) and to themselves. Once they finally crash, they are no longer dangerous. The users now become lethargic and sleep for 1 to 3 days.

Following the crash, addicts fall into a 1- to 3-month period of withdrawal. During this stage, they can be paranoid, aggressive, fatigued, depressed, suicidal, and filled with an intense craving for another high. Reuse of the drug relieves these feelings. Therefore, the incidence of relapse in users who seek treatment is high.

MDMA (Ecstasy) MDMA, also known as Ecstasy, became popular among teenagers and young adults in the United States in the mid-1980s, when it evolved into the most common "club drug." Although its use already constituted a serious drug problem in Europe, MDMA was not illegal in the United States until 1985. Prior to 1985, few Americans abused this drug. In the 1970s, some therapists used MDMA as a tool to help patients open up and feel at ease. MDMA is named for its chemical structure: 3,4-methylenedioxymethamphetamine. Street names for the drug are X-TC, E, Adam, and love drug.

MDMA use, once popular primarily among Hispanic Americans and Caucasians, is now spread to a wide range of demographic subgroups. Typically, dealers push the drug as a way to increase energy, pleasure, and self-confidence. MDMA is now available in numerous settings, including high schools, private homes, malls, and other popular gathering places for teenagers and young adults.

The trafficking of MDMA is increasing at an alarming rate, and multiple agencies have reported large seizures of the drug. Most of the supply comes from Canada. All Canadian labs combined are believed to produce more than 2 million tablets per week.

Although MDMA usually is swallowed in the form of one or two pills in doses of up to 120 mg per pill, it can also be smoked, snorted, or, occasionally, injected. Because the drug often is prepared with other substances, users have no way of knowing the exact potency of the drug or additional substances found in each pill. Further, many users combine MDMA with alcohol, marijuana, or other drugs, which makes it even more dangerous to use.

MDMA shares characteristics with stimulants and hallucinogens. Its chemical structure closely parallels the hallucinogen **MDA** (methylenedioxyamphetamine) and methamphetamine, both man-made stimulants that damage the brain. The addictive properties of MDMA and stimulation of hyperactivity have been compared to stimulants such as amphetamines and cocaine. The chemical structure of MDMA and its appeal, however, are similar to hallucinogens, but with milder psychedelic effects.

Among young people, MDMA has a reputation for being fun and harmless as long as it is used sensibly. But it is not a harmless drug. Research is uncovering many negative side effects. The pleasurable effects peak about an hour after a pill is swallowed and last for two to six hours. Users claim to feel enlightened and introspective, accepting of themselves and trustful of others. Because they tend to act and feel closer to, or more intimate with, the people around them, some believe this drug to be an aphrodisiac, even though MDMA actually hampers sexual ability. MDMA also acts as a stimulant by increasing brain activity and making users feel more energetic.

Like most addictive drugs, the effects of MDMA are said to diminish with each use. MDMA users may experience rapid eye movement, faintness, blurred vision, chills, sweating, nausea, muscle tension, and teeth grinding. Users often bring infant pacifiers to raves to combat the latter side effect. Individuals with heart, liver, or kidney disease or high blood pressure are especially at risk because MDMA increases blood pressure, heart rate, and body temperature. Thus, its use may lead to seizures, kidney failure, a heart attack, or a stroke. The hot, crowded atmosphere at raves and dance clubs also heightens the risk to the user. Deaths are more likely when water is unavailable because the crowded atmosphere, combined with the stimulant effects of MDMA, causes dehydration (bottled water is often sold at inflated prices at raves). Other evidence suggests that a pregnant woman using MDMA may find long-term learning and memory difficulties in her child.

The damaging effects of the drug can be long-lasting and are possible after only a few uses. Long-term side effects, lasting for weeks after use, include confusion, depression, sleep disorders, anxiety, aggression, paranoia, and impulsive behavior. Questions still remain about other potential long-term effects. Verbal and visual memory may be significantly impaired for years after prolonged use. Researchers are focusing on these lasting side effects, which may be the result of depleted serotonin, a neurotransmitter that is released with each dose of MDMA. The short-term effect of serotonin release is increased brain activity. Serotonin helps to regulate sleep cycles, pain, emotion, and appetite. Because MDMA may damage the neurons that release serotonin, long-term effects could be dangerous.

Advocates of MDMA are attempting to get approval to study medical uses of the drug. For example, MDMA could relieve suffering in terminally ill cancer patients. It also could help people in therapy for marital problems by encouraging introspection and conversation. Because MDMA is heralded as an instant antidepressant, it may help people who are in mourning. Opponents, meanwhile, question the value of MDMA as an effective treatment modality because its effects diminish with continued use.

Heroin Heroin use has increased in recent years. Although the most common users are suburban, middle-class people and lower-income populations, its use is starting to appear in more affluent communities as well. Common nicknames for heroin include diesel, dope, dynamite, white death, nasty boy, china white, H. Harry, gumball, junk, brown sugar, smack, tootsie roll, black tar, and chasing the dragon. More recently, a heroin-based recreational drug referred to as "cheese" has become popular. The latter is a combination of heroin with crushed tablets of over-the-counter medications that contain acetaminophen and the antihistamine diphenhydramine. Most recently, an ultra-potent form of heroin, known as "black tar," has become available, and it is known to kill unsuspecting users before they even have a chance to remove the syringe or are done snorting the substance.

Heroin is classified as a narcotic drug. It is synthesized from morphine, a natural substance found in the seedpod of several types of poppy plants. In its purest form, heroin is a white powder, but on the streets it is typically available in yellow or brown powders. The latter colors are attained when pure heroin is combined with other drugs or substances such as sugar, cornstarch, chalk, brick dust, or laundry soap. Heroin also is sold in a hardened or solid form (black tar), which usually is dissolved with other liquids for use in injectable form. Many users combine heroin with cocaine, a risky process commonly called "speedballing."

Today's heroin is more pure, powerful, and affordable than ever before. Highly dangerous, heroin is a significant health threat to users in that they have no way of determining the strength of the drug purchased on the street, which places them at a constant risk for overdose and death.

Heroin can be injected intravenously or intramuscularly, sniffed/snorted, or smoked. Although injection is the predominant method of heroin use, users are turning away from intravenous injections because of the risk for HIV infection. The availability of relatively low-priced, high-purity heroin further contributes to the number of people who smoke or snort the drug. Some users have the misconception that heroin is less addictive when it is snorted or smoked. Whether injected, snorted, or smoked, heroin is an extremely addictive drug, and both physical and psychological dependence develop rapidly. Drug tolerance sets in quickly, and each time the drug is used, a higher dose is required to produce the same effects. Use of heroin induces a state of euphoria that comes within seconds of intravenous injection or within 5 to 15 minutes with other methods of administration. Because the drug is a sedative, during the initial rush the person has a sense of relaxation and does not feel any pain. In users who inhale the drug, however, the rush may be accompanied by nausea, vomiting, intense itching, and at times severe asthma attacks. As the rush wears off, users experience drowsiness, confusion, slowed cardiac function, and decreased breathing rate.

A heroin overdose can cause convulsions, coma, and death. During an overdose, heart rate, breathing, blood pressure, and body temperature drop dramatically. These physiological responses can induce vomiting and tight muscles and cause breathing to stop. Death is often the result of lack of oxygen or choking to death on vomit.

About four to five hours after taking the drug, withdrawal sets in. Heroin withdrawal is painful and usually lasts up to two weeks—but could go on for several months. Symptoms of short-term use include red/raw nostrils, bone and muscle pains, muscle spasms and cramps, sweating, hot and cold flashes, runny nose and eyes, drowsiness, sluggishness, slurred speech, loss of appetite, nausea, diarrhea, restlessness, and violent yawning. Heroin use can also kill a developing fetus or cause a spontaneous abortion.

Symptoms of long-term use of heroin include hallucinations, nightmares, constipation, sexual difficulties, impaired vision, reduced fertility, boils, collapsed veins, and a significantly elevated

> **MDMA** A synthetic hallucinogen drug with a chemical structure that closely resembles MDA and methamphetamine; also known as Ecstasy.
>
> **MDA** A hallucinogenic drug that is structurally similar to amphetamines.
>
> **Heroin** A potent drug that is a derivative of opium.

risk for lung, liver, and cardiovascular diseases, including bacterial infections in blood vessels and heart valves. The additives used in street heroin can clog vital blood vessels because these additives do not dissolve in the body, leading to infections and death of cells in vital organs. Sudden infant death syndrome (SIDS) also is seen more frequently in children born to addicted mothers.

Heroin addiction is treated with behavioral therapies and pharmaceutical agents. Medication suppresses withdrawal symptoms, which makes it easier for patients to stop using heroin. The combination of these two treatment modalities helps the individual learn to lead a more stable, productive, and drug-free lifestyle.

Spice Spice is a drug that provides a marijuana-like high, known as Spice, K2, Kind, Genie, Summit, potpourri, Yucatan Gold, Purple Passion, Train Wreck, or Ultra (among other names) and is popular among teenagers and young adults. Spice is a drug made of a mixture of herbs sprayed with synthetic cannabinoids, compounds similar to the chemical THC found in marijuana. According to the federal Drug Enforcement Agency (DEA) the adverse effects of Spice are far more dangerous than the side effects of marijuana, including seizures, high blood pressure, anxiety attacks, hallucinations, nausea, loss of consciousness, and chemical dependency. Some samples tested have been shown to be 100 times more potent than marijuana.

As of 2011, the chemical compounds used to manufacture Spice are illegally controlled substances in the United States. Manufacturers of this drug, however, try to evade the illegal restrictions by changing the mixture of chemicals in the drug with substances that are equally harmful. Users think it is a safe drug because the products used in manufacturing the drug are natural and thus harmless.

Inhalant Abuse A substance abuse trend increasingly popular among young people is inhaling the vapors or aerosol gases of a wide range of household and industrial chemical products. Also referred to as "huffing" or "sniffing glue," these drugs are taken by volatilization and not following burning and heating as is the case with tobacco, marijuana, or crack cocaine. Examples include whipped cream canisters, deodorants and hair sprays, glues, nail polish remover, spray paints, lighter and cleaning fluids.

Based on estimates, about 23 million Americans have used inhalants at least once in their lifetime. Approximately 13 percent of eighth graders have abused inhalants. Even occasional or single inhalant abuse can be extremely dangerous. The effects include alcohol-like intoxication, euphoria, hallucinations, drowsiness, disinhibition, lightheadedness, headaches, dizziness, slurred speech, agitation, loss of sensation, belligerence, depressed reflexes, impaired judgment, and unconsciousness. As with other drug abuse, users can be injured by the harmful effects of the vapors and detrimental intoxication behavior. More serious consequences include suffocation due to lack of oxygen supply, pneumonia, vomit aspiration, organ damage (including the brain, liver, and kidneys), abnormal heart rhythms, and sudden cardiac death. Inhalant abuse leads to a strong need to continue their use and these individuals are more likely to initiate other drug use and have a higher lifetime prevalence of substance abuse.

Alcohol Drinking **alcohol** has been a socially acceptable behavior for centuries. Alcohol is an accepted accompaniment at parties, ceremonies, dinners, sport contests, the establishment of kingdoms or governments, and the signing of treaties between nations. Alcohol also has been used for medical reasons as a mild sedative or as a painkiller for surgery.

For a short period of 14 years, from 1920 to 1933, by constitutional amendment, the sale and use of alcohol were declared illegal in the United States. This amendment was repealed because drinkers and nondrinkers alike questioned the right of government to pass judgment on individual moral standards. In addition, organized crime activities to smuggle and sell alcohol illegally expanded enormously during this period.

Alcohol is the most abused substance in the United States and the cause of one of the most significant health-related drug problems in the country today. According to *Dietary Guidelines for Americans 2010,* 79,000 yearly deaths in the United States are due to excessive drinking.

Based on the 2011 NSDUH, more than 133 million people 12 years and older (51.8 percent) used alcohol within a month of the survey, and 58.3 (22.6 percent) participated in binge drinking at least once in the 30 days prior to the survey. About 16 million (6.2 percent) were heavy drinkers; and 1 in 9 drove under the influence of alcohol at least once in the 12 months prior to the interview. The highest prevalence is among 21- to 25-year-olds, with 70 percent of this age group using alcohol within a month of the survey.

Alcohol drinkers are also more likely to misuse other drugs. More than half of lifetime drinkers have used 1 or more illicit drugs at some time in their lives, compared with less than 10 percent of lifetime nondrinkers.

Although modest health benefits are derived from moderate alcohol consumption, the media have extensively exaggerated these benefits. They like to discuss this topic because it seems to be "a vice that's good for you." Research supports the assertion that consuming no more than two alcoholic beverages a day for men and one for women provides modest benefits in decreasing the risk for cardiovascular disease.

What Constitutes a Standard Drink

In the United States a drink is considered to be 14 grams of pure alcohol (ethanol) or the equivalent of:

- 5 ounces of wine
- 12 ounces of beer
- 1.5 ounces of 80-proof liquor

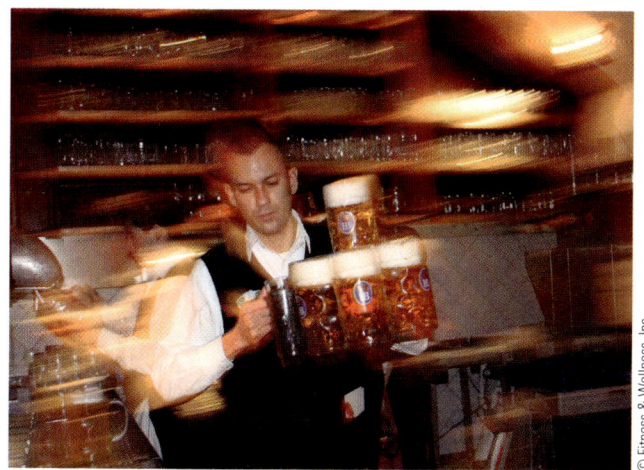

Approximately 18 million Americans will develop a drinking problem during their lifetime.

The benefits of modest alcohol use can be equated to those obtained through a small daily dose of aspirin (about 81 mg per day, or the equivalent of a baby aspirin) or eating a few nuts each day. Aspirin or a few nuts do not lead to impaired judgment or actions that you may later regret or have to live with for the rest of your life.

Consequences of Drinking Alcohol

Alcohol is not for everyone. **Alcoholism** seems to have both a genetic and an environmental component. The reasons some people can drink for years without becoming addicted, whereas others follow the downward spiral of alcoholism, are not understood. The addiction to alcohol develops slowly. Most people think they are in control of their drinking habits and do not realize they have a problem until they become alcoholics, when they find themselves physically and emotionally dependent on the drug. This addiction is characterized by excessive use of, and constant preoccupation with, drinking. Alcohol abuse, in turn, leads to mental, emotional, physical, and social problems.

The effects of alcohol intake include impaired peripheral vision, decreased visual and hearing acuity, slower reaction time, reduced concentration and motor performance (including increased swaying), and impaired judgment of distance and speed of moving objects. Further, alcohol alleviates fear, increases risk-taking, stimulates urination, and induces sleep. A single large dose of alcohol also may decrease sexual function. Two of the most serious consequences of alcohol abuse are increased risks of accidents and violent behavior. Excessive drinking has been linked to more than half of all deaths from car accidents. The risk for rape, domestic violence, child abuse, suicide, and murder also increases with alcohol abuse.

One of the most unpleasant, dangerous, and life-threatening effects of drinking is the **synergistic action** of alcohol when combined with other drugs, particularly central nervous system depressants. Each person reacts to a combination of alcohol and other drugs in a different way. The effects range from loss of consciousness to death.

Long-term effects of alcohol abuse are serious and often life-threatening (see Figure 13.2). Some of these detrimental effects are lower resistance to disease; **cirrhosis** of the liver; higher risk for breast, oral, esophageal, larynx, stomach, colon, and liver cancer; **cardiomyopathy;** irregular heartbeat; elevated blood pressure; greater risk for stroke; osteoporosis; inflammation of the esophagus, stomach, small intestine, and pancreas; stomach ulcers; sexual impotence; birth defects; malnutrition; damage to brain cells leading to loss of memory; depression; psychosis; and hallucinations.

Social Consequences of Alcohol Abuse

Alcohol abuse further leads to social problems that include loss of friends and jobs, separation of family members, child abuse, domestic violence, divorce, and problems with the law. Heavy drinking further contributes to decreased performance at work and school because drinkers are more likely to arrive late, make more mistakes, leave assignments incomplete, encounter problems with fellow workers or students, get lower grades and job evaluations, and flunk out of school or lose jobs.

Alcohol abuse also worsens financial concerns because drinkers have less money for needed items such as food and clothing, they fail to pay bills, and may have additional medical expenses, insurance premiums, and fines to pay.

Alcohol on Campus

Alcohol is the number one drug problem among college students. According to national surveys, about 61 percent of full-time college students reported using alcohol within the past month, and 39 percent had engaged in binge drinking (consumed 5 or more drinks in a row). Alcohol is a factor in about 25 percent of all college dropouts.

The statistics are sobering. For college students between the ages of 18 and 24,[6]

- 1,825 died from alcohol-related unintentional injuries.
- Almost 700,000 were assaulted by another student who had been drinking.
- 599,000 were unintentionally injured under the influence of alcohol.
- More than 150,000 developed alcohol-related health problems.
- About 97,000 were victims of alcohol-related sexual assault or date rape.

Alcohol (ethyl alcohol) A depressant drug that affects the brain and slows down central nervous system activity; has strong addictive properties.

Alcoholism Disease in which an individual loses control over drinking alcoholic beverages.

Synergistic action The effect of mixing two or more drugs, which can be much greater than the sum of two or more drugs acting by themselves.

Cirrhosis A disease characterized by scarring of the liver.

Cardiomyopathy A disease affecting the heart muscle.

Figure 13.2 Long-term risks associated with alcohol abuse.

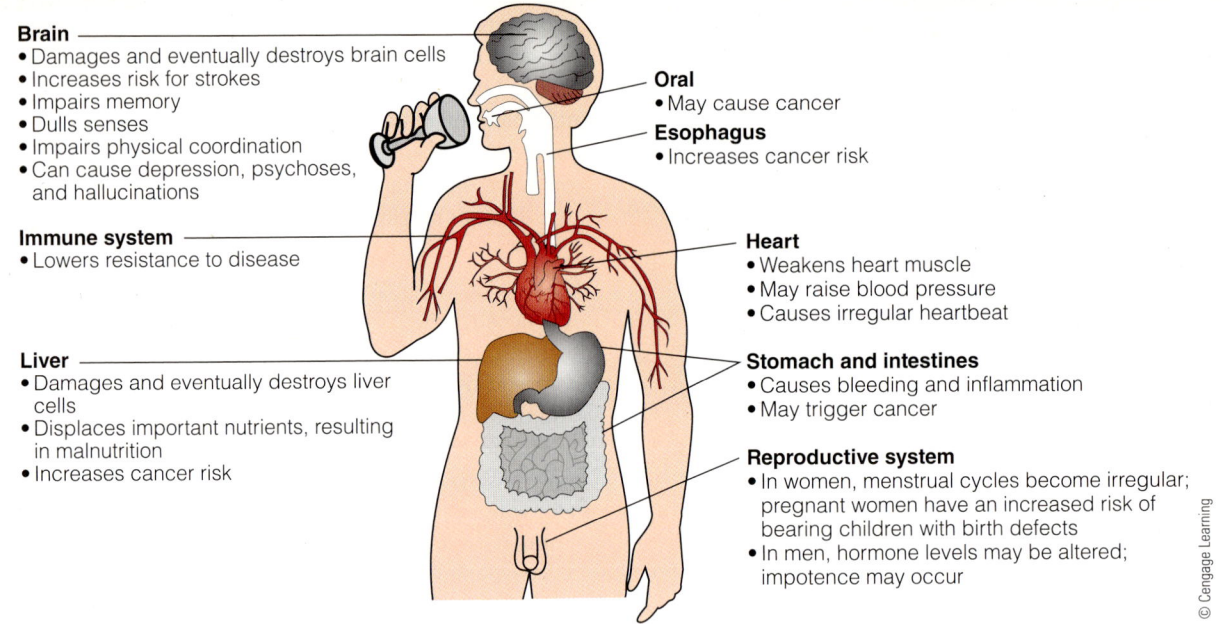

Brain
- Damages and eventually destroys brain cells
- Increases risk for strokes
- Impairs memory
- Dulls senses
- Impairs physical coordination
- Can cause depression, psychoses, and hallucinations

Immune system
- Lowers resistance to disease

Liver
- Damages and eventually destroys liver cells
- Displaces important nutrients, resulting in malnutrition
- Increases cancer risk

Oral
- May cause cancer

Esophagus
- Increases cancer risk

Heart
- Weakens heart muscle
- May raise blood pressure
- Causes irregular heartbeat

Stomach and intestines
- Causes bleeding and inflammation
- May trigger cancer

Reproductive system
- In women, menstrual cycles become irregular; pregnant women have an increased risk of bearing children with birth defects
- In men, hormone levels may be altered; impotence may occur

- 400,000 had unprotected sex.
- More than 100,000 were too intoxicated to know if they'd consented to having sex.
- Almost 3.4 million drove under the influence of alcohol in the past year.

In terms of academic work, a national survey involving about 94,000 college students from 197 colleges and universities conducted over 3 years showed that grade point average (GPA) was related to average number of drinks per week (see Figure 13.3).[7] Students with a "D" or "F" GPA reported a weekly consumption of almost 10 drinks. Students with "A" GPAs consumed about 4 drinks per week. Of significant concern, young adults ages 18 to 22 enrolled full-time in college are more likely than their peers (part-time students and those not enrolled in college) to use alcohol, binge drink, and drink heavily.

In another national survey of almost 55,000 undergraduate students from 131 colleges, close to 25 percent of students said that their academic problems resulted from alcohol abuse. Of greater concern, 20 percent of the surveyed students admitted driving while intoxicated. Of the more than 18 million college students in the United States, between 2 and 3 percent eventually will die from alcohol-related causes.

Another major concern is that more than half of college students participate in games that involve heavy drinking (consuming five or more drinks in one sitting). Often, students take part because of peer pressure and fear of rejection. Data show that one night of binge drinking results in an extra intake of around 2,000 calories from alcoholic beverages alone, plus another 800 calories from food and munchies consumed during the drinking episode. Some students even binge drink three days in a row on weekends.

Excessive drinking can also precipitate unplanned and unprotected sex (risking HIV infection), date rape, and alcohol poisoning. When some young people turn 21, they "celebrate" by having 21 drinks. Unaware of the risks of excessive alcohol intake in a relatively short period of time, drinking friends then try to let them "sleep it off," only to find out that they never wake up, but rather suffer death from alcohol poisoning.

How to Cut Down on Drinking

To find out if drinking is a problem in your life, refer to the questionnaire in Activity 13.2. A yes answer to any of these questions can be regarded as a warning sign to potential future problems. If you have answered three or more of them

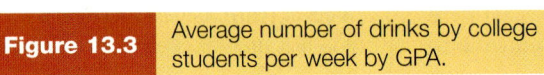

Figure 13.3 Average number of drinks by college students per week by GPA.

Number of alcoholic drinks per week:
- A: 4.12
- B: 6.03
- C: 7.76
- D or F: 9.97

Grade point average (GPA)

SOURCE. C. A. Presley, J. S. Leichliter, and P. W. Meilman, *Alcohol and Drugs on American College Campuses: Findings from 1995, 1996, and 1997 (A Report to College Presidents)* (Carbondale, IL: Southern Illinois University, 1999).

Activity 13.1: Addictive Behavior Questionnaire

Name _____ Date _____

Course _____ Section _____ Gender _____ Age _____

Could you be an addict?

I. Recognizing Addictive Behavior

The following questionnaire has been designed to identify possible addictive behavior (chemical dependency). This test is not designed to determine if you have an addictive disease, but rather to help recognize potential addictive behavior in yourself or the people around you. The term "drug" may imply illicit substances or drugs (such as marijuana, cocaine, heroin, Ecstasy, or methamphetamine), misuse of prescription drugs (painkillers, sleeping pills), or alcohol abuse.

1. Are you a compulsive person?
2. Are you a person of excesses?
3. Do you depend heavily on others or are you completely independent of others?
4. Do you spend a lot of time thinking about a drug(s)?
5. Do you use drugs other than for medical reasons?
6. Do you misuse prescription drugs?
7. Are you unable to stop using drugs or limit their use to required situations only?
8. Can you get through a week without misusing drugs?
9. Do friends or relatives sense or mention that you have a drug problem?
10. Has drug misuse ever created a problem between you and friends or relatives?
11. Have family members or friends ever sought help for problems associated with your misuse of drugs?
12. Have you ever sought help for drug misuse?
13. Do you deny or lie about the misuse of drugs?
14. Do you tend to associate with people who exhibit the same behaviors or take the same drugs you do?
15. Do you get angry at people who try to keep you from getting the drugs you desire?
16. Do you have a difficult time stopping the use of a drug when you start misusing it?
17. Do you experience withdrawal symptoms if you do not take the drugs you wish to have?
18. Has the misuse of drugs affected the way you function in life (school, work, recreation)?
19. Have you put yourself or others at risk by your actions while misusing drugs?
20. Have you unsuccessfully tried to cut back or stop the misuse of drugs?

Interpretation

If you answered "yes" to five or more of these questions, you may have an addictive behavior and should seek further evaluation by a physician, your institution's counseling center, or contact the local mental health clinic for a referral (see the Yellow Pages in your local phone book). You may also contact the National Center for Substance Abuse Treatment at 1-800-662-4357 for 24-hour substance abuse treatment centers in your area. Depending on the question (for example, 7, 8, 12, 15, 16, 17, 18, 20), note that even fewer than five "yes" answers may already be indicative of chemical dependency.

II. Stage of Change for Addictive Behavior

If chemical dependency is a problem in your life, use Figure 2.5 (page 63) and Table 2.3 (page 62) to identify your current stage of change for participation in a treatment program for addictive behavior.

III. Changing Addictive Behavior

On a separate sheet of paper indicate the steps that you are going to take to correct addictive behavior(s) and identify people or organizations that you will contact to help you get started.

Activity 13.2: Alcohol Use Questionnaire

Name _____ Date _____
Course _____ Section _____ Gender _____ Age _____

I. Alcohol Abuse

Use a separate sheet of paper to answer the following questions. This questionnaire can help you determine if your drinking (alcohol) patterns are a problem for you. If you do not consume alcohol, skip this questionnaire, as drinking does not interfere with your health and well-being.

Yes No

1. Do you consume more than one (women) or two (men) drinks per day? ☐ ☐
2. Does drinking interfere with your short- or long-term goals? ☐ ☐
3. Does drinking interfere with your school or work productivity? ☐ ☐
4. Have you missed school or work because of drinking? ☐ ☐
5. Do you skip workouts because of drinking? ☐ ☐
6. Do you drink to increase self-confidence? ☐ ☐
7. Do you drink to feel more at ease with others? ☐ ☐
8. Do you drink to be socially accepted by others? ☐ ☐
9. Are you annoyed by other people's comments about your drinking habits? ☐ ☐
10. Are you untruthful about the number of drinks you have had when questioned by others? ☐ ☐
11. To drink, do you associate with people who are not a good influence on you or that you normally don't relate to? ☐ ☐
12. Do you drink alone? ☐ ☐
13. At social gatherings, do you actively look for a refill before being offered one? ☐ ☐
14. Do you frequently serve yourself a more generous drink than the "going" amount for others? ☐ ☐
15. Do you drink to relieve stress, forget worries, or life's problems? ☐ ☐
16. Has drinking affected your reputation? ☐ ☐
17. Have you missed appointments due to drinking? ☐ ☐
18. Do you participate in binge drinking episodes? ☐ ☐
19. Do you have difficulty remembering what you have done because of drinking? ☐ ☐
20. Does drinking affect your family life or relationship with roommates? ☐ ☐
21. Are you ever abusive to others when drinking? ☐ ☐
22. Have you experienced financial difficulties as a result of drinking? ☐ ☐
23. Do you feel physically deprived if you cannot drink daily? ☐ ☐
24. Do you need a drink early in the day to get going? ☐ ☐
25. Do you need a drink at certain times of the day? ☐ ☐
26. Has drinking disrupted your sleeping pattern? ☐ ☐
27. Do you ever feel that you need to cut down on drinking? ☐ ☐
28. Do you ever feel bad or guilty about your drinking pattern? ☐ ☐
29. Have you been treated by a physician or health professional for drinking? ☐ ☐
30. Have you ever been treated in a hospital or other institution for drinking? ☐ ☐

A yes answer to any of these questions can be regarded as a warning sign to potential future problems. If you have answered three or more of them with a yes, your drinking habit can be harmful to your well-being and may indicate that you are alcohol dependent or an alcoholic. An evaluation by a healthcare professional is highly recommended.

> ## Behavior Modification Planning
>
> ### When Your Date Drinks . . .
>
> - **Don't** make excuses for his/her behavior, no matter how embarrassing.
> - **Don't** allow embarrassment to put you in a situation with which you are uncomfortable.
> - **Do** be sure that body language and tone of voice match verbal messages you send.
> - **Do** leave as quickly as you can, without your date. **Don't** stop to argue. Intoxicated people can't listen to reason.
> - **Do** call a cab, a friend, or your parents. **Don't** ride home with your date.
> - For women:
> - **Do** make your position clear. "No!" is much more effective than "Please stop!" or "Don't!"
> - **Do** make it clear that you will call the police if rape is attempted.
>
> ### Try It
>
> In your Online Journal or class notebook, write down strategies you can incorporate today to ensure your health and wellness.
>
> "Sexuality Under the Influence of Alcohol," *Human Sexuality Supplement to Current Health* 2 (October 1990): 3.

with a yes, your drinking habit can be harmful to your well-being and may indicate that you are alcohol dependent or an alcoholic. An evaluation by a health care professional is highly recommended.

If a person is determined to control the problem, it is not that difficult. The first and most important step is to want to cut down. If you want to do this but you cannot seem to do so, you had better accept the probability that alcohol is becoming a serious problem for you, and you should seek guidance from your physician or from an organization such as Alcoholics Anonymous. The next few suggestions also may help you cut down your alcohol intake.

- Set reasonable limits for yourself. Decide not to exceed a certain number of drinks on a given occasion, and stick to your decision. No more than two beers or two cocktails a day is a reasonable limit. If you set a target such as this and consistently do not exceed it, you have proven to yourself that you can control your drinking.
- Learn to say no. Many people have "just one more" drink because others in the group are doing this or because someone puts pressure on them, not because they really want a drink. When you reach the sensible limit you have set for yourself, politely but firmly refuse to exceed it. If you are being the generous host, pour yourself a glass of water or juice "on the rocks." Nobody will notice the difference.
- Drink slowly. Don't gulp down a drink. Choose your drinks for their flavor, not their "kick," and savor the taste of each sip.
- Dilute your drinks. If you prefer cocktails to beer, try tall drinks: Instead of downing gin or whiskey straight or nearly so, drink it diluted with a mixer such as tonic water or soda water in a tall glass. That way you can enjoy both the flavor and the act of drinking, but you will take longer to finish each drink. Also, you can make your two-drink limit last all evening or switch to the mixer by itself.
- Do not drink on your own. Confine your drinking to social gatherings. You may have a hard time resisting the urge to pour yourself a relaxing drink at the end of a hard day, but many formerly heavy drinkers have found that a soft drink satisfies the need as well as alcohol did. What may help you really unwind, even with no drink at all, is a comfortable chair, loosened clothing, and perhaps a soothing audio-tape, television program, good book to read, or even some low- to moderate-intensity physical activity.

13.3 Treatment of Addictions

Recovery from any addiction is more likely to be successful with professional guidance and support. The first step is to recognize the reality of the problem. The Addictive Behavior

The sooner treatment for addiction is started and the longer the user stays in treatment, the better are the chances for recovery and a more productive life.

Questionnaire in Activity 13.1 will help you recognize possible addictive behavior in yourself or someone you know. If the answer to five or more of these questions is positive, you may have a problem, in which case you should contact a physician, your institution's counseling center, or the local mental health clinic for a referral (see the Yellow Pages in your phone book).

You also may contact the Substance Abuse and Mental Health Services Administration (SAMHSA) at 1-800-662-HELP (1-800-662-4357) for referral to 24-hour substance abuse treatment centers in your local area. All information discussed during a phone call to this center is kept strictly confidential. Information also is available on the Internet at www.samhsa.gov. The national center provides printed information on drug abuse and addictive behavior.

About 2.3 million Americans received treatment for addictive behavior in 2011. An additional 19 million people were estimated to need treatment for illicit drug or alcohol abuse, but did not receive such treatment at any specialty facility.[8]

Among intervention and treatment programs for addiction are psychotherapy, medical care, and behavior modification. If addiction is a problem in your life, you need to act on it without delay. Addicts do not have to resign themselves to a lifetime of addiction. The sooner you start, and the longer you stay in treatment, the better are your chances to recover and lead a healthier and more productive life.

13.4 Tobacco Use

People throughout the world have used tobacco for hundreds of years. Before the 18th century, they smoked tobacco primarily in the form of pipes or cigars. Cigarette smoking per se did not become popular until the mid-1800s, and its use started to increase dramatically in the 20th century.

An estimated 68 million Americans aged 12 and older use tobacco products, including 57 million cigarette smokers, 13 million cigar smokers, 8.2 million using smokeless tobacco, and 2.1 million pipe smokers.[9] As depicted in Figure 13.4, tobacco use in general declines with education.

When tobacco leaves are burned, hot air and gases containing **tar** (chemical compounds) and **nicotine** are released in the smoke. More than 7,000 chemicals, hundreds of them toxic, have been found in tobacco smoke. About 70 are proven carcinogens. The harmful effects of cigarette smoking and tobacco use in general were not exactly known until the early 1960s, when research began to show a link between tobacco use and disease.

In 1964, the U.S. Surgeon General issued the first major report presenting scientific evidence that cigarettes were indeed a major health hazard in our society. More than 42 percent of the U.S. adult population smoked cigarettes at the time. In 2011, 22.1 percent of people 12 years and older smoked cigarettes. Young people who smoke are also more likely to abuse other illicit drugs. Smokers between the age of 12 and 17 are nine times more likely to use drugs than nonsmokers in this same age group.

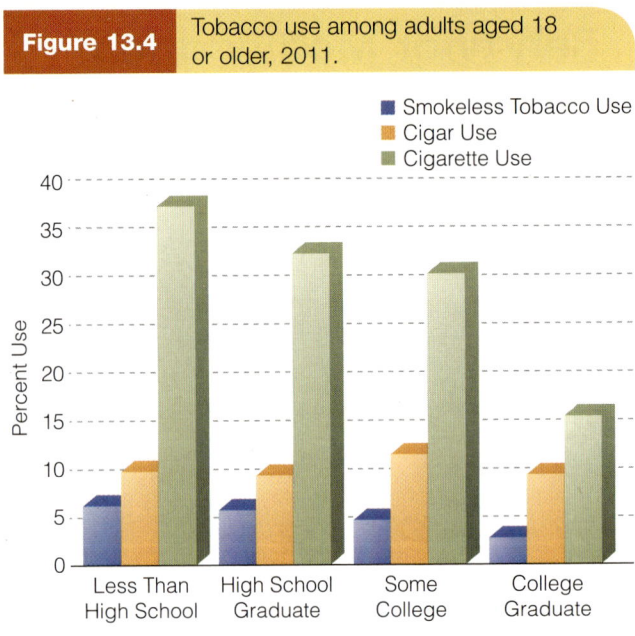

Figure 13.4 Tobacco use among adults aged 18 or older, 2011.

SOURCE: http://www.samhsa.gov/data/NSDUH/2011SummNatFindDetTables/Index.aspx. Downloaded June 24, 2013.

Morbidity and Mortality Tobacco use in all its forms is considered a significant threat to life. World Health Organization estimates indicate that 10 percent of the 7 billion people presently living will die as a result of smoking-related illnesses, which kill more than 5 million people each year. At the present rate of escalation, this figure is expected to climb to 8 million deaths annually by the year 2030. A total of 100 million tobacco-related deaths occurred in the 20th century, and based on estimates, that there will be 1 billion deaths in the 21st century.

To gain some perspective on the seriousness of the tobacco problem, CDC statistics indicate that drug overdoses and drug-related murders kill more than 40,000 people per year in the United States. By comparison, tobacco, a legal drug, kills about 11 times as many people as all illegal drugs combined.

> **Critical Thinking**
>
> Do you think the government should outlaw the use of tobacco in all forms? • Or does the individual have the right to engage in self-destructive behavior?

Cigarette smoking is the largest preventable cause of illness and premature death in the United States. Death rates from heart disease, cancer, stroke, aortic aneurysm, chronic bronchitis, emphysema, and peptic ulcers all increase with cigarette smoking.

In pregnant women, cigarette smoking has been linked to retarded fetal growth, higher risk for spontaneous abortion (miscarriage), and prenatal death. Smoking is also the most prevalent cause of injury and death from fire. The average life expectancy for a chronic smoker is 13 (men) to 14 (women) years shorter than for a nonsmoker, and the death rate among chronic smokers during their most productive years of life, between ages 25 and 65, is twice the national average. If we consider all related deaths, smoking is responsible for almost 443,000 unnecessary deaths each year—enough deaths to wipe out the entire population of Miami in a single year. For every tobacco-related death, there are 20 others, or 8.6 million people in the United States, who suffer from at least one serious illness associated with cigarette smoking. More deaths are caused each year by tobacco use than by all deaths from HIV, illegal drug use, motor vehicle injuries, alcohol use, suicides, and murders combined.

Based on a report by U.S. government physicians, each cigarette shortens life by 7 to 11 minutes. This figure represents 5.5 million years of potential life that Americans lose to smoking each year.

Effects on Cardiovascular System

Each year approximately 180,000 heart disease deaths are attributed to cigarette smoking. The CDC states that smoking increases the risk of coronary heart disease two- to fourfold. The mortality rate following heart attacks is higher for smokers because their attacks usually are more severe and their risk for deadly arrhythmias is much greater.

Cigarette smoking affects the cardiovascular system by increasing heart rate, blood pressure, and susceptibility to atherosclerosis, blood clots, coronary artery spasm, cardiac arrhythmia, and arteriosclerotic peripheral vascular disease. Evidence also indicates that smoking decreases high-density lipoprotein (HDL) cholesterol, the "good" cholesterol that lowers the risk for heart disease. Smoking further increases the amount of fatty acids, glucose, and various hormones in the blood. The carbon monoxide in smoke hinders the capacity of the blood to carry oxygen to body tissues. Both carbon monoxide and nicotine can damage the inner walls of the arteries and thereby encourage the buildup of fat on them. Smoking also causes increased adhesiveness and clustering of platelets in the blood, decreases platelet survival and clotting time, and increases blood thickness. Any of these effects can precipitate a heart attack.

Normal lung *(left)* is contrasted with diseased lung *(right)*. The white growth near the top of the diseased lung is cancer; the dark appearance on the bottom half is emphysema.

Smoking and Cancer

The American Cancer Society reports that 87 percent of lung cancer is attributable to smoking. Lung cancer is the leading cancer killer, accounting for approximately 160,000 deaths in the United States in the year 2013, or about 27 percent of all deaths from cancer.[10] Cigarette smoking also leads to chronic lower respiratory disease, the third leading cause of death in the United States (see also Chapter 1). Figure 13.5 illustrates normal and diseased **alveoli.**

The most common carcinogenic exposure in the work place is cigarette smoke. Both fatal and nonfatal cardiac events are increased greatly in people who are exposed to passive smoke. About 50,000 additional deaths result each year in the United States from secondhand smoke (also known as environmental tobacco smoke, or ETS), including 46,000 from cardiovascular diseases, 3,400 from lung cancer, and 430 from SIDS.[11] Furthermore, almost 22 million children between the ages of 3 and 11 are exposed to secondhand smoke, and approximately 30 percent of the indoor workforce is not protected by smoke-free work place policies. According to the U.S. Surgeon General, the evidence clearly shows that there is no risk-free level of exposure to ETS, prompting Dr. Richard Carmona, U.S. Surgeon General (2002–2006), to state: "Based on the science, I wouldn't allow anyone in my family to stand in a room with someone smoking."

Figure 13.5 Normal and diseased alveoli in lungs.

Tar Chemical compound that forms during the burning of tobacco leaves.

Nicotine Addictive compound found in tobacco leaves.

Alveoli Air sacs in the lungs where gas exchange (oxygen and carbon dioxide) takes place.

Adverse Effects of Secondhand Smoke

- A 30-percent increase in coronary heart disease risk. (Some adverse effects begin within minutes to hours of exposure.)
- Increases blood clotting, enhancing the risk of heart attacks and strokes.
- Lowers HDL (good) cholesterol.
- Increases oxidation of LDL cholesterol, enhancing atherosclerosis.
- Increases oxygen free radicals.
- Decreases levels of antioxidants.
- Increases chronic inflammation.
- Increases insulin resistance, leading to higher blood sugar levels and risk for diabetes.
- Increases lung and overall cancer risk.
- Increases risk for pulmonary diseases.
- Increases risk for adverse effects during pregnancy.
- Increases sudden infant death syndrome (SIDS) risk.

Two large-scale reviews of research studies on American, Canadian, and European communities that have passed laws to curb secondhand smoke by banning it in public places, including bars and restaurants, have shown an average drop of 17 percent in heart attacks in the first year as compared to communities without such a ban. There is a further 26 percent decline in heart attacks for at least 3 years each year thereafter. Within 20 minutes of secondhand smoke inhalation, chemical changes can be detected in the body's blood clotting mechanism, increasing the risk for heart attack or stroke. Nonsmokers exposed to secondhand smoke at home or at the office have up to a 30 percent greater risk of suffering a heart attack.

Although the 5-year survival rate for all cancers in the United States, Canada, and Europe is now at 67 percent (up from 49 percent in 1977), the five-year survival rate for lung cancer is about 16 percent. In addition to lung cancer, cigarette smoking increases the risk for cancers of the oral cavity, lip, nasopharynx, nasal cavity and paranasal sinus, pharynx, larynx, esophagus, stomach, colorectum, pancreas, uterine cervix, ovary, kidney, and bladder and acute myeloid leukemia cancers (also see Figure 13.6).

> **Critical Thinking**
>
> You are in a designated nonsmoking area and the person next to you lights up a cigarette. • What can you say to this person to protect your right to clean air?

Other Forms of Tobacco Many tobacco users are aware of the health consequences of cigarette smoking but may fail to realize the risk of pipe smoking, cigar smoking, and tobacco chewing. As a group, pipe and cigar smokers have lower risks for heart disease and lung cancer than ciga-

Figure 13.6 The health effects of smoking.

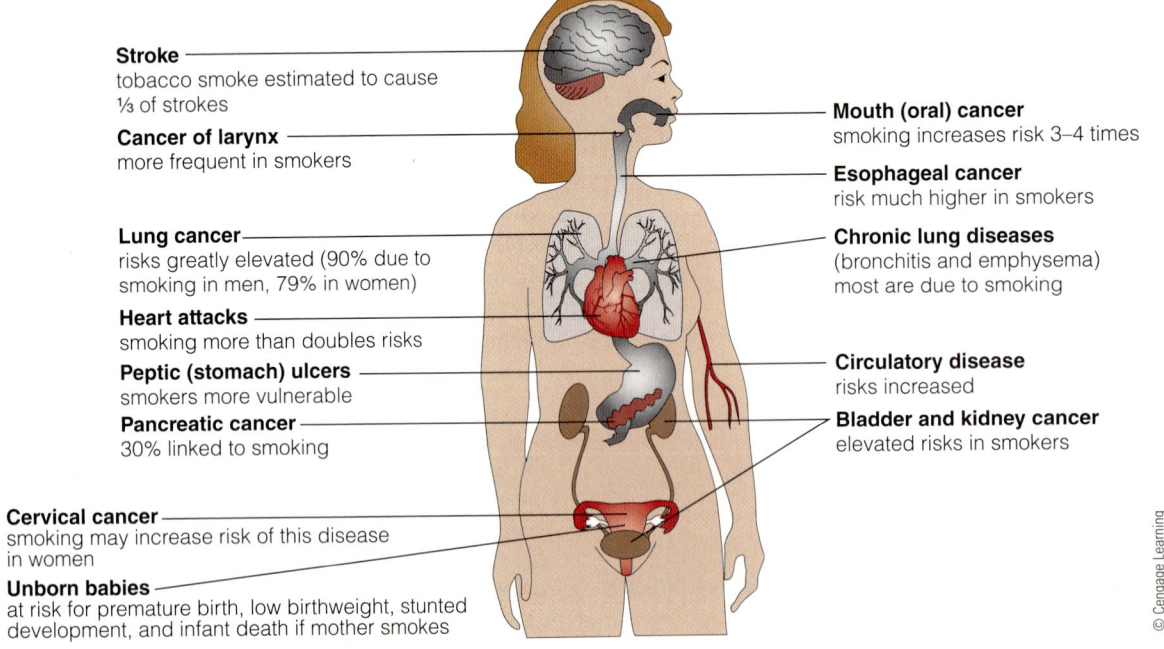

rette smokers. Nevertheless, blood nicotine levels in pipe and cigar smokers have been shown to approach those of cigarette smokers, because nicotine is still absorbed through the membranes of the mouth. Therefore, these tobacco users still have a higher risk for heart disease than nonsmokers do.

Cigarette smokers who substitute pipe or cigar smoking for cigarettes usually continue to inhale the smoke, which actually results in more nicotine and tar being brought into their lungs. Consequently, the risk for disease is even higher if pipe or cigar smoke is inhaled. The risk and mortality rates for lip, mouth, and larynx cancer for pipe smoking, cigar smoking, and tobacco chewing are actually higher than for cigarette smoking.

Smokeless Tobacco

Smokeless tobacco has been promoted in the past as a safe alternative to cigarette smoking. The Advisory Committee to the U.S. Surgeon General has stated that smokeless tobacco represents a significant health risk and is just as addictive as cigarette smoking.

Approximately 8 million Americans use smokeless tobacco. The greatest concern is the increase in use of smokeless tobacco among young people. Surveys indicate that about 13 percent of high school males use smokeless tobacco. The average starting age for smokeless tobacco use is 10 years old.

Using smokeless tobacco can lead to gingivitis and periodontitis. It carries a fourfold increase in oral cancer, and in some cases even premature death. People who chew or dip also have a higher rate of cavities, sore gums, bad breath, and stained teeth. Their senses of smell and taste diminish; consequently, they tend to add more sugar and salt to food. These practices alone increase the risk for being overweight and having high blood pressure. Nicotine addiction and its related health risks also hold true for smokeless tobacco users. Nicotine blood levels approach those of cigarette smokers, increasing the risk for diseases of the cardiovascular system. Further, research has revealed changes in heart rate and blood pressure similar to those of cigarette smokers.

Using tobacco in any form can be addictive and poses a serious threat to health and well-being. Completely eliminating its use is the single most important lifestyle change a tobacco user can make to improve health, quality of life, and longevity.

Health Care Costs of Tobacco Use

Heavy smokers use the health care system, especially hospitals, twice as much as nonsmokers do. The yearly cost to a given company has been estimated to be up to $6,000 per smoking employee. These costs include employee health care, absenteeism, additional health insurance, morbidity/disability and early mortality, on-the-job time lost, property damage/maintenance and depreciation, worker compensation, and the impact of second hand smoke.

If every smoker were to give up cigarettes, in 1 year alone sick time would drop by approximately 90 million days, heart conditions would decrease by 280,000, chronic bronchitis and emphysema would number 1 million fewer cases, and total death rates from cardiovascular disease, cancer, and peptic ulcers would fall off drastically.

Every day, almost 1,200 Americans die from smoking-related illnesses. That is the equivalent of three fully loaded jumbo jets crashing every day with no survivors. Imagine what the coverage and concern would be if 443,000 people each year were to die in the United States alone because of airplane accidents! People would not even consider flying anymore. Most people would think of it as a form of suicide.

Smoking kills more Americans in a single year than died in battle during World War II and the Vietnam War combined. Think of the public outrage if 443,000 Americans were to die annually in a meaningless war. What if a single nonprescription drug were to cause more than 160,000 deaths from cancer and 180,000 deaths from heart disease? The U.S. public would not tolerate these situations. We would mount an intense fight to prevent the deaths.

Yet, are we not committing slow suicide by smoking cigarettes? Isn't tobacco a nonprescription drug available to almost anyone who wishes to smoke, killing more than 443,000 people each year? If cigarettes were invented today, the tobacco industry would be put on trial for mass murder.

Trends

The fight against all forms of tobacco use is stronger than ever. This was not always the case. It has been difficult to fight an industry that wields such enormous financial and political influence as does the tobacco industry in the United States. Tobacco is one of the top 10 cash crops in the United States. The tobacco industry has influenced elections cleverly by emphasizing the individual's right to smoke, avoiding the fact that so many people die because of it.

Philip Morris International, also known as Altria, one of the largest tobacco-producing companies in the world, receives nearly 70 percent of its profits from the sale of cigarettes. Philip Morris has donated millions of dollars to prominent organizations, so they no longer question the detrimental effects of tobacco use. Among the organizations that have received donations from Philip Morris are United Way, YMCA, Salvation Army, Pediatric AIDS Foundation, Red Cross, Cystic Fibrosis Foundation, March of Dimes, Easter

Smokeless tobacco can lead to gum and tooth damage as well as oral cancer (pictured).

Seals, Muscular Dystrophy Association, Multiple Sclerosis Society, Hemophilia Foundation, United Cerebral Palsy, American Civil Liberties Union, American Bar Association, Task Force for Battered Women, Boy Scouts, Boys and Girls Club, and Big Brothers and Big Sisters. We call drug runners unprincipled scum, yet we welcome Philip Morris with glee and we call it civic pride."[12]

Tobacco was socially accepted for many years. Cigarette smoking, however, is no longer acceptable in most social circles. Smoking is prohibited in most public places as a result of nonsmokers and ex-smokers alike fighting for their rights to clean air and health.

Many smokers are unaware of, or simply do not care to realize, how much cigarette smoke bothers nonsmokers. Smokers sometimes think that blowing the smoke off to the side is enough to get it out of the way. As a matter of fact, it is not enough. Smokers do not comprehend this until they quit and later find themselves in that situation. Suddenly they realize why cigarette smoke is so unpleasant and undesirable to most people.

The FDA Drug Abuse Advisory Committee has taken a strong stance against the use of all forms of tobacco products. Although the American Heart Association (AHA) commends the work initiated by the FDA, the AHA has further stated that the FDA and the federal government have an obligation to take regulatory action against the national problem of nicotine addiction and abuse of cigarettes and tobacco products in general. In a statement before the FDA Drug Abuse Advisory Committee, the AHA indicated that "it is a national health travesty that a product such as tobacco (which accounts for about 443,000 deaths in the U.S. each year), has escaped regulation under every major health and safety law enacted by Congress to protect the public health."[13] The U.S. Surgeon General has stated that health education combined with social, economic, and regulatory approaches is imperative to offset the tobacco industry's marketing and promotions and to promote nonsmoking environments.

13.5 Why People Smoke

People typically begin to smoke without realizing its detrimental effects on their health and life in general. Although people start to smoke for many different reasons, the three fundamental instigators are peer pressure, the desire to appear "grown up," and rebellion against authority. Smoking only three packs of cigarettes can lead to physiological addiction, turning smoking into a nasty habit that has become the most widespread example of drug dependency in the United States.

Smoking Addiction and Dependency
The drug nicotine has strong addictive properties. Within seconds of inhalation, nicotine affects the central nervous system and can act simultaneously as a tranquilizer and a stimulant. The stimulating effect produces strong physiological and psychological dependency. The physical addiction to nicotine is six to eight times more powerful than the addiction to alcohol, and most likely greater than that of some of the hard drugs currently used.

Psychological dependency develops over a longer time. People smoke to help themselves relax, and they also gain a certain amount of pleasure from the ritual of smoking. Smokers automatically associate many activities of daily life with cigarettes—coffee drinking, alcohol drinking, being part of a social gathering, relaxing after a meal, talking on the telephone, driving, reading, and watching television. In many cases, the social rituals of smoking are the most difficult to eliminate. The dependency is so strong that years after people have stopped smoking, they may still crave cigarettes when they engage in certain social activities.

Most of the remaining information in this chapter is written directly to smokers. Nonsmokers, however, will gain a better understanding of smokers by reading it. The following material also provides valuable information so that you can help others implement a smoking-cessation program.

"Why Do You Smoke?" Test
Most people smoke for a variety of reasons. To find out why people smoke, the National Clearinghouse for Smoking and Health developed the simple "Why Do You Smoke?" Test. This test, contained in Activity 13.3, lists some statements by smokers describing what they get out of smoking cigarettes. Smokers are asked to indicate how often they have the feelings described in each statement when they are smoking.

The scores obtained on this test assess smokers for each of six factors that describe individuals' feelings when they smoke. The first three highlight the positive feelings that people derive from smoking. The fourth factor relates to reducing tension and relaxing. The fifth reveals the extent of dependence on cigarettes. The sixth factor differentiates habit smoking and purely automatic smoking. Each of the remaining factors fits one of the six reasons for smoking discussed next. A score of 11 or greater on any factor indicates that smoking is an important source of satisfaction for you. The higher you score (15 is the highest), the more important a given factor is in your smoking, and the more useful a discussion of that factor can be in your attempt to quit.

If you do not score high on any of the six factors, chances are that you do not smoke much or have not been smoking for long. If so, giving up smoking, and staying off, should be fairly easy.

1. Stimulation. If you score high or fairly high on the stimulation factor, you are one of those smokers who is stimulated by the cigarette. You think it helps wake you up, organize your energies, and keep you going. If you try to give up smoking, you may want a safe substitute—a brisk walk or moderate exercise, for example—whenever you feel the urge to smoke.

2. Handling. Handling things can be satisfying, but you can keep your hands busy in many ways without lighting up or playing with a cigarette. Why not toy with a pen or pencil? Try doodling. Play with a coin, a piece of jewelry, or some other harmless object.

3. Pleasure/Pleasurable Relaxation. Finding out whether you use the cigarette to feel good—you get real, honest pleasure from smoking—or to keep from feeling bad (Factor 4) is not always easy. About two-thirds of smokers score high or fairly high on accentuation of pleasure, and about half of those also score as high or higher on reduction of negative feelings. Those who do get real pleasure from smoking often find that honest consideration of the harmful effects of their habit is enough to help them quit. They substitute social and physical activities and find that they do not seriously miss cigarettes.

4. Crutch: Tension Reduction. Many smokers use cigarettes as a crutch during moments of stress or discomfort. Ironically, the heavy smoker—the person who tries to handle severe personal problems by smoking many times a day—is apt to discover that cigarettes do not help deal with problems effectively. This kind of smoker may stop smoking readily when everything is going well but may be tempted to start again in a time of crisis. Again, physical exertion or social activity may be a useful substitute for cigarettes, especially in times of tension.

5. Craving: Psychological Addiction. Quitting smoking is difficult for people who score high on this factor. The craving for a cigarette begins to build the moment the previous cigarette is put out, so tapering off is not likely to work. This smoker must go **cold turkey**. If you are dependent on cigarettes, you might try smoking more than usual for a day or two to spoil your taste for cigarettes, then isolating yourself completely from cigarettes until the craving is gone.

6. Habit. If you are smoking from habit, you no longer get much satisfaction from cigarettes. You light them frequently without even realizing you are doing it. You may have an easy time quitting and staying off if you can break the habitual patterns you have built up. Cutting down gradually may be effective if you change the way you smoke cigarettes and the conditions under which you smoke them. The key to success is to become aware of each cigarette you smoke. You can do this by asking yourself, "Do I really want this cigarette?" You might be surprised at how many you do not want.

Smoking Cessation If you are contemplating a smoking-cessation program or are preparing to stop cigarette smoking, you need to know that quitting smoking is not easy. Annually, only about 20 percent of smokers who try to quit the first time succeed. The addictive properties of nicotine and smoke make quitting difficult.

The American Psychiatric Association and the National Institute on Drug Abuse have indicated that nicotine is perhaps the most addictive drug known to humans. The U.S. Surgeon General has concluded that[14]:

- Cigarettes and other forms of tobacco are addicting.
- Nicotine is the drug responsible for the addictive behavior.
- Pharmacological and behavioral traits that determine addiction to tobacco are similar to those that determine addiction to drugs such as heroin and cocaine.

Smokers develop a tolerance to nicotine and tobacco smoke. They become dependent on both and get physical and psychological withdrawal symptoms when they stop smoking. Even though giving up smoking can be extremely difficult, it is by no means impossible, as attested by the many people who have quit. During the last four decades, cigarette smoking in the United States declined gradually among smokers of all ages.

Surveys have shown that approximately 70 percent of all smokers would like to quit. In 1964 (when the U.S. Surgeon General first reported the link between smoking and increased risk for disease and mortality), 40 percent of the adult population—53 percent of men and 32 percent of women—smoked. In 2011, only 21.6 percent of adult men and 16.5 percent of adult women smoked. Almost 50 million Americans have given up cigarettes.

Further, more than 91 percent of successful ex-smokers have been able to do it on their own, either by quitting cold turkey or by using self-help kits available from organizations such as the American Cancer Society, the American Heart Association, and the American Lung Association. Smokers' information and treatment centers can be readily found online.

"Do You Want to Quit?" Test

The most important factor in quitting cigarette

Cigarette smoking is the single largest preventable cause of illness and premature death in the United States.

> **Cold turkey** Eliminating a negative behavior all at once.

smoking is the person's sincere desire to do so. Although a few smokers can simply quit, this usually is not the case.

Those who can quit easily are primarily light or casual smokers. They realize that the pleasure of an occasional cigarette is not worth the added risk for disease and premature death. For heavy smokers, quitting most likely will be a difficult battle. Even though many do not succeed the first time around, the odds of quitting are much better for those who repeatedly try to stop.

If you are a smoker and want to find your readiness to quit, the "Do You Want to Quit?" Test, developed by the National Clearinghouse for Smoking and Health contained in Activity 13.4, will measure your attitude toward the four primary reasons you want to quit smoking. The results indicate whether you are ready to start the program. On this test, the higher you score in any category, say, the Health category, the more important that reason is to you. A score of 9 or greater in one of these categories indicates that this is one of the most important reasons you may want to quit.

1. Health. Knowing the harmful consequences of cigarettes, many people have stopped smoking and many others are considering doing so. If your score on the Health factor is 9 or greater, the health hazards of smoking may be enough to make you want to quit now. If your score on this factor is low (6 or less), consider the hazards of smoking. You may be lacking important information or may even have incorrect information. If so, health considerations are not playing the role they should in your decision to keep smoking or to quit.
2. Example. Some people stop smoking because they want to set a good example for others. Parents quit to make it easier for their children to resist starting to smoke. Doctors quit so that they can be role models for their patients. Teachers quit to discourage their students from smoking. Sports stars want to set an example for their young fans. Husbands quit to influence their wives to quit, and vice versa. Examples have a significant influence on our behavior. Surveys show that almost twice as many high school students smoke if both parents are smokers, compared with those whose parents are nonsmokers or former smokers. If your score is low (6 or less), you might not be interested in giving up smoking to set an example for others. Perhaps you do not realize how important your example could be.
3. Aesthetics. People who score high (9 or greater) in this category recognize and are disturbed by some of the unpleasant aspects of smoking. The smell of stale smoke on their clothing, bad breath, and stains on their fingers and teeth might be reason enough to consider quitting.
4. Mastery. If you score 9 or greater on this factor, you are bothered by knowing that you cannot control your desire to smoke. You are not your own master. Awareness of this challenge to your self-control may make you want to quit.

Breaking the Habit The following seven-step plan has been developed as a guide to help you quit smoking. You should complete the total program in 4 weeks or less. Steps One through Four combined should take no longer than 2 weeks. A maximum of 2 additional weeks is allowed for the rest of the program.

Step One
Decide positively that you want to quit. Avoid negative thoughts of how difficult this can be. Think positive. You can do it.

Now prepare a list of the reasons why you smoke and why you want to quit (Activity 13.5). Make several copies of the list and keep them in places where you commonly smoke. Frequently review the reasons for quitting, because this will motivate and prepare you psychologically to quit.

When the reasons for quitting outweigh the reasons for smoking, you will have an easier time quitting. Read as much information as possible on the detrimental effects of tobacco and the benefits of quitting.

Step Two
Initiate a personal diet and exercise program. About one-third of the people who quit smoking gain weight. This could be caused by one or a combination of the following reasons:

1. Food becomes a substitute for cigarettes.
2. Appetite increases.
3. Basal metabolism may slow down.

If you start an exercise and weight-control program prior to quitting smoking, weight gain should not be a problem. If anything, exercise and lower body weight create more awareness of healthy living and strengthen the motivation for giving up cigarettes.

Even if you gain some weight, the harmful effects of cigarette smoking are much more detrimental to human health than a few extra pounds of body weight. Experts have indicated that as far as the extra load on the heart is concerned, giving up one pack of cigarettes a day is the equivalent of losing between 50 and 75 pounds of excess body fat!

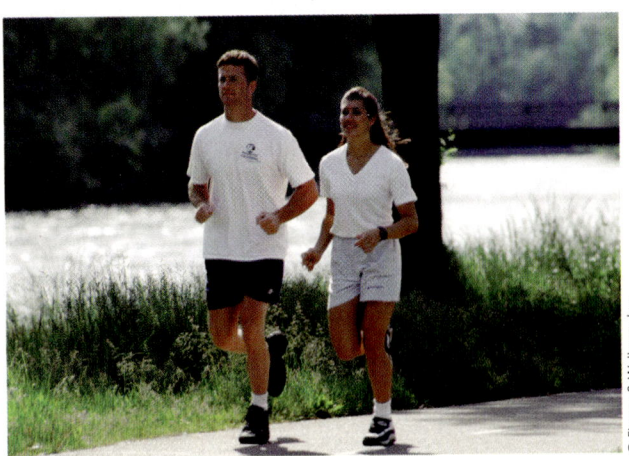

Starting an exercise program prior to giving up cigarettes encourages cessation and helps with weight control during the process.

Activity 13.3: "Why Do You Smoke?" Test

Name _____ Date _____

Course _____ Section _____ Gender _____ Age _____

	Always	Frequently	Occasionally	Seldom	Never
A. I smoke cigarettes to keep myself from slowing down.	5	4	3	2	1
B. Handling a cigarette is part of the enjoyment of smoking it.	5	4	3	2	1
C. Smoking cigarettes is pleasant and relaxing.	5	4	3	2	1
D. I light up a cigarette when I feel angry about something.	5	4	3	2	1
E. When I have run out of cigarettes, I find it almost unbearable until I can get them.	5	4	3	2	1
F. I smoke cigarettes automatically without even being aware of it.	5	4	3	2	1
G. I smoke cigarettes for stimulation, to perk myself up.	5	4	3	2	1
H. Part of the enjoyment of smoking a cigarette comes from the steps I take to light up.	5	4	3	2	1
I. I find cigarettes pleasurable.	5	4	3	2	1
J. When I feel uncomfortable or upset about something, I light up a cigarette.	5	4	3	2	1
K. I am very much aware of the fact when I am not smoking a cigarette.	5	4	3	2	1
L. I light up a cigarette without realizing I still have one burning in the ashtray.	5	4	3	2	1
M. I smoke cigarettes to give me a "lift."	5	4	3	2	1
N. When I smoke a cigarette, part of the enjoyment is watching the smoke as I exhale it.	5	4	3	2	1
O. I want a cigarette most when I am comfortable and relaxed.	5	4	3	2	1
P. When I feel "blue" or want to take my mind off cares and worries, I smoke cigarettes.	5	4	3	2	1
Q. I get a real gnawing hunger for a cigarette when I haven't smoked for a while.	5	4	3	2	1
R. I've found a cigarette in my mouth and didn't remember putting it there.	5	4	3	2	1

Scoring Your Test:

Enter the numbers you have checked on the test questions in the spaces provided below, putting the number you have circled to question A on line A, to question B on line B, and so on. Add the three scores on each line to get a total for each factor. For example, the sum of your scores over lines A, G, and M gives you your score on "Stimulation"; lines B, H, and N give the score on "Handling." Scores can vary from 3 to 15. Any score 11 and above is high; any score 7 and below is low.

A _____ + G _____ + M _____ = _____ Stimulation
B _____ + H _____ + N _____ = _____ Handling
C _____ + I _____ + O _____ = _____ Pleasure/Relaxation
D _____ + J _____ + P _____ = _____ Crutch: Tension Reduction
E _____ + K _____ + Q _____ = _____ Craving: Psychological Addiction
F _____ + L _____ + R _____ = _____ Habit

From *A Self-Test for Smokers*, U.S. Department of Health and Human Services, 1983.

Activity 13.4: "Do You Want to Quit?" Test

Name _____ Date _____

Course _____ Section _____ Gender _____ Age _____

	Strongly Agree	Mildly Agree	Mildly Disagree	Strongly Disagree
A. Cigarette smoking might give me a serious illness.	4	3	2	1
B. My cigarette smoking sets a bad example for others.	4	3	2	1
C. I find cigarette smoking to be a messy kind of habit.	4	3	2	1
D. Controlling my cigarette smoking is a challenge to me.	4	3	2	1
E. Smoking causes shortness of breath.	4	3	2	1
F. If I quit smoking cigarettes, it might influence others to stop.	4	3	2	1
G. Cigarettes cause damage to clothing and other personal property.	4	3	2	1
H. Quitting smoking would show that I have willpower.	4	3	2	1
I. My cigarette smoking will have a harmful effect on my health.	4	3	2	1
J. My cigarette smoking influences others close to me to take up or continue smoking.	4	3	2	1
K. If I quit smoking, my sense of taste or smell will improve.	4	3	2	1
L. I do not like the idea of feeling dependent on smoking.	4	3	2	1

How to Score: (See page 455, "Do You Want to Quit?" Test, to interpret your results.)

Write the number you have checked after each statement on the test in the corresponding space to the right. Add the scores on each line to get your totals. For example, the sum of your scores A, E, and I gives you your score for the Health factor. Scores can vary from 3 to 12. Any score of 9 or over is high; any score 6 or under is low.

A [____] + E [____] + I [____] = [____] Health
B [____] + F [____] + J [____] = [____] Example
C [____] + G [____] + K [____] = [____] Aesthetics
D [____] + H [____] + L [____] = [____] Mastery

From *A Self-Test for Smokers*, U.S. Department of Health and Human Services, 1983.

Step Three

Decide on the approach you will use to stop smoking. You may quit cold turkey or gradually cut down the number of cigarettes you smoke daily. Base your decision on your scores obtained on the "Why Do You Smoke?" Test. If you score 11 points or higher in either the "Crutch: Tension Reduction" or the "Craving: Psychological Addiction" categories, your best chance for success is quitting cold turkey. If your highest scores occur in any of the other four categories, you may choose either approach.

People still argue about which approach is more effective. Quitting cold turkey may cause fewer withdrawal symptoms than tapering off gradually. When you are cutting down slowly, the fewer cigarettes you smoke, the more important each one becomes. Therefore, you have a greater chance for relapse and returning to the original number of cigarettes you smoked. But when the cutting-down approach is accompanied by a definite target date for quitting, the technique has been shown to be quite effective. Smokers who taper off without a target date for quitting are the most likely to relapse.

The simple pleasures of life, such as taste and smell, improve with smoking cessation.

Step Four

Keep a daily log of your smoking habit for a few days. This will help you understand the situations in which you smoke. To assist you in doing this, make copies of Activity 13.6, or develop your own form. Keep this form with you, and every time you smoke, record the required information. Keep track of the number of cigarettes you smoke, times of day you smoke them, events associated with smoking, amount of each cigarette smoked, and a rating of how badly you needed that cigarette. Rate each cigarette from 1 to 3:

- 1 = desperately needed
- 2 = moderately needed
- 3 = no real need

This daily log will assist you in three ways:

1. You will get to know your habit.
2. It will help you eliminate cigarettes you do not crave.
3. It will help you find positive substitutes for situations that trigger your desire to smoke.

Step Five

Set the target date for quitting. If you are going to taper off gradually, read the instructions under the "Cutting Down Gradually" discussion before you proceed to Step Six. When you set the target date, choose a special date to add a little extra incentive. An upcoming birthday, anniversary, vacation, graduation, family reunion—all are examples of good dates to free yourself from smoking. Dates when you are going to be away from events and environments that trigger your desire to smoke may be especially helpful. Once you have set the date, do not change it. Do not let anyone or anything interfere with this date.

Let your friends and relatives know of your intentions and ask for their support. Consider asking someone else to quit with you. That way, you can support each other in your efforts to stop. Avoid anyone who will not support you in your effort to quit. When you are attempting to quit, other people can be a prime obstacle. Many smokers are intolerable when they first stop smoking, so some friends and relatives prefer that the person continue to smoke.

Step Six

Stock up on low-calorie foods—carrots, broccoli, cauliflower, celery, popcorn (butter-and salt-free), fruits, sunflower seeds (in the shell), sugarless gum—and drink plenty of water. Keep the food handy on the day you stop and the first few days following cessation. Substitute this food for a cigarette when you want one.

Step Seven

On your quit day and the first few days thereafter, do not keep cigarettes handy. Stay away from friends and events that trigger your desire to smoke, and drink a lot of water and fruit juices. To replace the old behavior with new behavior, replace smoking time with new, positive substitutes that will make smoking difficult or impossible.

When you want a cigarette, take a few deep breaths and then occupy yourself by doing any of a number of things, such as talking to someone else, washing your hands, brushing your teeth, eating a healthy snack, chewing on a straw, doing dishes, playing sports, going for a walk or a bike ride, going swimming, and so on. Engage in activities that require the use of your hands. Try gardening, sewing, writing letters, drawing, doing household chores, or washing the car. Visit nonsmoking places such as libraries, museums, stores, and theaters. Plan an outing or a trip away from home. Any of these activities can keep your mind off cigarettes. Record your choice of activity or substitute under the Remarks/Substitutes column in Activity 13.6.

Quitting Cold Turkey

Many people have found that quitting all at once is the easiest way to do it. Most smokers have tried this approach at least once. Even though it might not work the first time, they don't allow themselves to get discouraged, and they eventually succeed. Many times, after several attempts, all of a sudden they are able to overcome smoking without too much difficulty.

On the average, as few as three smokeless days are sufficient to break the physiological addiction to nicotine. The psychological addiction may linger for years but will get weaker as time goes by.

Cutting Down Gradually

Tapering off cigarettes can be done in several ways:

1. Eliminate cigarettes you do not strongly crave (those ranked numbers 3 and 2 on your daily log).
2. Switch to a brand lower in nicotine/tar every few days.
3. Smoke less of each cigarette.
4. Smoke fewer cigarettes each day.

Most people prefer a combination of these four suggestions.

Before you start cutting down, set a target date for quitting. Once the date is set, don't change it. The total time until your quit date should be no longer than 2 weeks. Reduce the total number of cigarettes you smoke each day by 10 to 25 percent. As you smoke less, be careful not to take more puffs or inhale more deeply as you smoke, because this would offset the principle of cutting down.

As an aid in tapering off, make several copies of Activity 13.6. By now you should have already completed the first daily log of your smoking habit—see Step Four under "Breaking the Habit" on page 456. Start a new daily log and every night review your data and set goals for the following day.

Decide and record which cigarettes will be easiest to give up, what brand you will smoke, the total number of cigarettes to be smoked, and how much of each you will smoke. Log any comments or situations you want to avoid, as well as any substitutes you could use to help you in the program. For example, if you always smoke while drinking coffee, substitute juice for coffee. If you smoke while driving, arrange for a ride or take a bus to work. If you smoke with a certain friend at lunch, avoid having lunch with that friend for a week or so. Continue using this log until you have stopped smoking completely.

Nicotine-Substitution Products

Nicotine-substitution drug products such as nicotine transdermal patches and nicotine gum were developed to help people kick the tobacco habit. These products are most effective when they are used in a physician-supervised cessation program. As with tapering off, these products gradually decrease the amount of nicotine used until the person no longer craves the drug.

Nicotine patches supply a steady dose of nicotine through the skin. According to a nicotine-replacement patch website, the program consists of a 10-week plan with three levels of nicotine patches. The person is asked to stop smoking before beginning the program; otherwise, the individual ends up with a very high blood nicotine level. A 21-mg patch is used during the first 6 weeks of the program, followed by a 14-mg patch for 2 weeks, and a final 7-mg patch for the last 2 weeks. The intent is to simulate a gradual weaning from the nicotine with fewer side effects. The instructions are specific, and the individual must carefully follow the instructions for the program to be effective. The site is clear that the program only works if the person is committed to quit the habit, because the patch does not override the mind.

At present, evidence shows that patches are not more effective for quitting smoking than doing so without patches. However, one study showed that patches are more effective when used in conjunction with exercise.[15] About 8 out of 10 smokers who exercised along with the use of nicotine-replacement therapy successfully quit smoking.

Nicotine-replacement patches are available in various dosages, delivering anywhere from about 5 to 21 mg of nicotine in a 24-hour period. The retail cost for a 10-week program ranges from $100 to $200, significantly cheaper than smoking a pack a day for 10 weeks. Public safety concerns regarding the use of nicotine patches, including indications, precautions, warnings, contraindications, potential abuse, and marketing and labeling issues are monitored and regulated by the FDA. People contemplating their use should pay careful attention to contraindications and potential side effects. Pregnant and lactating women and people with heart disease or high blood pressure or who have had a recent heart attack should check with their physician prior to using nicotine-substitution products. Skin redness, swelling, or rashes are sometimes associated with the use of nicotine patches. Other undesirable side effects are listed on the label and should be monitored closely.

Electronic Cigarettes

Electronic cigarettes, more commonly known as e-cigarettes, personal vaporizers, or simply VP, were introduced to the U.S. market in 2007 as alternative devices to simulate the act of tobacco smoking. The electronic inhaler heats up a liquid nicotine solution into an aerosol mist that smokers inhale. Health risks are unknown at this time because limited research is available on these products. Although e-cigarettes are marketed as safer alternatives because they have far fewer of the toxic chemical compounds found in cigarette smoke, the FDA warns of potential addiction and abuse of these products.

E-cigarettes are now being used as an alternative to nicotine patches. In 2011, about 21 percent of traditional-cigarette adult smokers had tried e-cigarettes. The real concern is that if smokers use both traditional and e-cigarettes, rather than using e-cigarettes to quit cigarettes completely, the health consequences could be exponentially greater.

> **Critical Thinking**
>
> If you ever smoked or now smoke cigarettes, discuss your perceptions of how others accepted your behavior. • If you smoked and have quit, how did you accomplish the task, and has it changed the way others view you? • If you never smoked, how do you perceive smokers?

Life after Cigarettes

When you first quit smoking, you can expect a series of withdrawal symptoms for a few days; among them are lower heart rate and blood pressure, headaches, gastrointestinal discom-

Activity 13.5: Reasons for Smoking Versus Quitting

Name _____ Date _____
Course _____ Section _____ Gender _____ Age _____

> Make several copies of this list and keep them in places where you commonly smoke. Frequently review the reasons for quitting to help motivate and prepare you psychologically to quit.

Reasons for Smoking Cigarettes

1. _____
2. _____
3. _____
4. _____
5. _____
6. _____
7. _____
8. _____
9. _____
10. _____

Reasons for Quitting Cigarette Smoking

1. _____
2. _____
3. _____
4. _____
5. _____
6. _____
7. _____
8. _____
9. _____
10. _____

Activity 13.6: Daily Cigarette Smoking Log

Name _____ Date _____

Course _____ Section _____ Gender _____ Age _____

Make copies of this form. Keep one copy with you every day and, every time you smoke, record the required information. This log will help you get to know your habit, eliminate cigarettes you really do not crave, and find positive substitutes for situations that trigger your desire to smoke.

Today's Date: _____ Quit Date: _____ Decision Date: _____

Cigarettes to be smoked today: _____ Brand: _____

No.	Time	Activity	Amount Smoked[a]	Rating[b]	Remarks/Substitutes
1.					
2.					
3.					
4.					
5.					
6.					
7.					
8.					
9.					
10.					
11.					
12.					
13.					
14.					
15.					
16.					
17.					
18.					
19.					
20.					

[a]Amount smoked: entire cigarette, two thirds, half, etc.
[b]Rating: 1 = desperately needed, 2 = moderately needed, 3 = no real need

Additional comments, list of friends and/or activities to avoid.

_____
_____
_____
_____
_____

fort, mood changes, irritability, aggressiveness, and difficulty sleeping.

The physiological addiction to nicotine is broken only 3 days following your last cigarette. Thereafter, you should not crave cigarettes as much. For the habitual smoker, the psychological dependency could be the most difficult to break. The first few days probably will not be as difficult as the first few months. Any of the activities of daily life that you have associated with smoking—either stress or relaxation, joy or unhappiness—may trigger a relapse even months, or at times years, after quitting.

Ex-smokers should realize that even though some harm may have been done already, it is never too late to quit. The greatest early benefit is a lower risk for sudden death. Furthermore, the risk for illness starts to decrease the moment you stop smoking. You will have fewer sore throats and sores in the mouth, less hoarseness, no more cigarette cough, and lower risk for peptic ulcers.

Circulation to the hands and feet will improve, as will gastrointestinal and kidney and bladder functions. Everything will taste and smell better. You will have more energy, and you will gain a sense of freedom, pride, and well-being. You no longer will have to worry whether you have enough cigarettes to last through a day, a party, a meeting, a weekend, or a trip.

When you first quit and you think how tough it is and how miserable you feel because you cannot have a cigarette, try the opposite: Think of the benefits and how great it is not to smoke! The ex-smoker's risk for heart disease approaches that of a lifetime nonsmoker 15 years following cessation. Stroke risk approaches that of a nonsmoker in less than five years. In terms of cancer, the time frame varies. The risk for certain cancer sites is cut in half as early as five years following cessation.

If you have been successful and stopped smoking, a lot of events can still trigger your urge to smoke. When confronted with these events, some people rationalize and think, "One cigarette won't hurt. I've been off for months (years in some cases)" or "I can handle it. I'll smoke just today." It won't work! Before you know it, you will be back to the regular nasty habit. Be prepared to take action in those situations by finding substitutes such as those provided in the "Tips to Help Stop Smoking" box.

Start thinking of yourself as a nonsmoker—no "butts" about it. Remind yourself how difficult it has been and how long it has taken you to get to this point. If you have come this far, you certainly can resist brief moments of temptation. It will get easier rather than harder as time goes on.

Behavior Modification Planning

Tips to Help Stop Smoking

Check the suggestions that may work for you and incorporate them into your own retraining program.

I PLAN TO / I DID IT

Preparing to Quit

- ❏ ❏ Create a personal list of reasons to quit. Keep the list handy, review it frequently, and add to it as needed.
- ❏ ❏ Know what to expect. Information is available from government sources, health organizations, doctors, hospitals, or on the Web. Talk with people who have quit or contact a local group or a hotline.
- ❏ ❏ Review any past attempts to quit. Determine what worked and what didn't work for you.
- ❏ ❏ Get a physical examination and discuss your desire to quit smoking with your doctor. Ask whether medication may help you quit.
- ❏ ❏ Create a stop-smoking plan customized to your personality, preferences, and schedule. If you are tapering off, set intermediate goals. Make sure to plan for times of intense desire for a cigarette. Be prepared and determine what you can use as a substitute for that cigarette. Is there anyone you can call for assistance or to help you distract your mind? Do not forget to include rewards for your success. Sign a contract and ask a friend to sign it as a witness.
- ❏ ❏ Determine your quit day. Choose a special day, such as a birthday, an anniversary, or a holiday. Select a day on which you will not feel a strong temptation to smoke—for instance, a stressful work day. Once you pick a date, do not alter this date.
- ❏ ❏ Enlist the support of friends, loved ones, team members, coworkers—as many people as you can. Ask others not to smoke around you or leave cigarettes in view. If you can, find someone else who wants to quit with you.
- ❏ ❏ Inquire about counseling. Individual, group, and telephone counseling can improve your chances of success.
- ❏ ❏ Consider starting a weight loss and exercise program before you quit. Such positive action will increase your confidence in your ability to quit and can keep you from gaining weight when you stop smoking.
- ❏ ❏ Stage a farewell activity to cigarettes and smoking; perhaps by overindulging so that the idea of smoking is no longer appealing, or with a ceremony to destroy all cigarettes, lighters, and ashtrays.
- ❏ ❏ Change your environment. Clean your room or house, clothes, and car to remove the scent of tobacco smoke. Rearrange the furniture, paint the walls a different color, open windows to freshen the air, and buy plants or flowers.
- ❏ ❏ Plan changes in your routine. Reschedule regular activities, use different routes to get to places you normally go, go to bed earlier and get up earlier, avoid being rushed.
- ❏ ❏ Start a new hobby or other activity; for example, dancing, making videos, painting, acting, or learning to cook ethnic foods—something enjoyable that you've wanted to do for a long time.
- ❏ ❏ Stock up on healthy, low-calorie snacks.

While Tapering Off

- ❏ ❏ Keep cigarettes as hard to get as possible. Leave them with someone else, lock them up, wrap them up like gifts with lots of tape or ribbon.
- ❏ ❏ Don't store cigarettes—wait until one pack is finished before buying another.
- ❏ ❏ Never carry matches or a lighter.
- ❏ ❏ Each time you want to smoke, write down what you are doing and feeling and how important the cigarette is to you—before you light up.
- ❏ ❏ Smoke only in uninteresting or uncomfortable places.
- ❏ ❏ Put off the first cigarette of the day for as long as possible.
- ❏ ❏ Smoke just half a cigarette.

Behavior Modification Planning

After Quitting

- ❑ ❑ To help prevent relapse, rather than saying "I quit smoking," say "I don't want to smoke."
- ❑ ❑ Get plenty of sleep.
- ❑ ❑ Eat regular, healthy, appetizing meals; pay attention to the flavors and textures of the foods.
- ❑ ❑ Be mindful of negative thoughts and replace them with positive actions—from "I can't stand this" to "What else can I do right now to keep my mind off cigarettes?" for example.
- ❑ ❑ Spend time in places where smoking is not allowed—libraries, museums, churches, malls, movie theaters.
- ❑ ❑ Tune in to the sights and scents around you.
- ❑ ❑ Drink plenty of water and other low-calorie drinks (but avoid caffeine).
- ❑ ❑ Deal with one minute, one hour, and one day at a time.
- ❑ ❑ Plan something that will bring you pleasure every day.
- ❑ ❑ Be aware of life stressors and plan a variety of ways to relax without cigarettes.
- ❑ ❑ Avoid situations in which you used to smoke, including being with people who smoke.
- ❑ ❑ Be wary of alcohol: Drinking lowers your chances of success.
- ❑ ❑ Use your lungs more by increasing daily physical activity and sports participation. Try to notice how clean the air feels flowing in and out of your lungs.
- ❑ ❑ Celebrate and reward yourself for each success.
- ❑ ❑ Visit your dentist and have your teeth cleaned and whitened.
- ❑ ❑ Calculate how much money you are saving and use this money to reward yourself or someone else with a small luxury.
- ❑ ❑ Consult your doctor if you are concerned about your physical or emotional feelings.
- ❑ ❑ If you gain weight, don't attempt to lose the weight until after you get over the craving for cigarettes.

Instead of Smoking a Cigarette

- ❑ ❑ Take several deep breaths, focusing on your breathing and the fresh air that you are inhaling.
- ❑ ❑ Tell yourself to wait three minutes; redirect your thoughts by visualizing a serene landscape or planning a dream vacation or weekend away from home.
- ❑ ❑ Go for a walk. If you have a dog, take the dog for a walk.
- ❑ ❑ Chew gum or suck on hard, sugarless candy—always carry some with you.
- ❑ ❑ Talk to someone you can easily reach for support.
- ❑ ❑ Munch on carrots, celery sticks, or other healthy snacks.
- ❑ ❑ Use your hands: wash dishes, sweep the floor, brush your teeth, write in a journal, sketch a cartoon, play a musical instrument.
- ❑ ❑ Go swimming or take a shower.

If You Relapse

- ❑ ❑ Don't be discouraged—most people try several times before they are finally able to kick the habit.
- ❑ ❑ Instead of berating yourself, remember your successes and recommit to quitting.
- ❑ ❑ Reevaluate your smoking-cessation plan and modify it as necessary.
- ❑ ❑ Remember that relapse doesn't mean failure. Failure comes to those who give up. Instead, learn from your mistake and reach once more for your goal.

Excerpted from TIPS, American Cancer Society, High Plains Division.

Try It

Nicotine is believed to be the most addictive drug we know. Smokers who are trying to kick the habit need behavioral change strategies to enhance their rate of success. From these strategies, prepare a list of those that may work for you. On a daily basis, conduct nightly audits on how well you have done that day. Every third day, review all of the strategies and make changes to your list as necessary.

ASSESS YOUR BEHAVIOR

To access course materials, including companion resources, please visit www.cengagebrain.com.

1. Is your life free of addictive behavior? If not, will you commit right now to seek professional help at your institution's counseling center? Addictive behavior destroys health and lives—don't let it waste yours.

2. Are you prepared to walk away, even at the peril of losing close friendships and relationships, if you are put in a situation where you are pressured to drink, smoke, or engage in any other form of drug (legal or illegal) abuse?

ASSESS YOUR KNOWLEDGE

Evaluate how well you understand the concepts presented in this chapter using the chapter-specific quiz available in the online materials at www.cengagebrain.com.

1. The following substance is not an object of chemical dependency.
   a. Ecstasy
   b. Alcohol
   c. Cocaine
   d. Heroin
   e. All are objects of chemical dependency.

2. The most widely used illegal drug in the United States is
   a. marijuana.
   b. alcohol.
   c. cocaine.
   d. heroin.
   e. Ecstasy.

3. Cocaine use
   a. causes lung cancer.
   b. leads to atrophy of the brain.
   c. can lead to sudden death.
   d. causes amotivational syndrome.
   e. All these things are possible.

4. Methamphetamine
   a. is less potent than amphetamine.
   b. increases fatigue.
   c. helps a person relax.
   d. is a central nervous system stimulant.
   e. increases the need for sleep.

5. Ecstasy
   a. is popular among middle-aged people.
   b. is a relatively harmless drug.
   c. is used primarily by African American males.
   d. increases heart rate and blood pressure.
   e. All are correct choices.

6. Treatment of chemical dependency is
   a. accomplished primarily by the individual alone.
   b. most successful when there is peer pressure to stop.
   c. best achieved with the help of family members.
   d. seldom accomplished without professional guidance.
   e. usually done with the help of friends.

7. Cigarette smoking is responsible for approximately how many unnecessary deaths in the United States each year?
   a. 10,000
   b. 80,000
   c. 250,000
   d. 443,000
   e. 1,000,000

8. Cigarette smoking increases death rates from
   a. heart disease.
   b. cancer.
   c. stroke.
   d. aortic aneurysm.
   e. all of the above.

9. The percentage of lung cancer attributed to cigarette smoking is
   a. 25 percent.
   b. 43 percent.
   c. 58 percent.
   d. 64 percent.
   e. 87 percent.

10. Smoking cessation results in
    a. a decrease in sore throats.
    b. improved gastrointestinal function.
    c. a decrease in risk for sudden death.
    d. better tasting of foods.
    e. All of these changes occur.

Correct answers can be found at the back of the book.

Preventing Sexually Transmitted Infections

14

Anyone who has sexual contact can acquire a sexually transmitted infection. More than half of all Americans will be infected during their lifetime. Infections are most common among teens and young adults, with about half of all infections occurring in people younger than 25.

Objectives

- **Name** and describe the most common sexually transmitted infections (STIs).
- **Outline** the health consequences of STIs.
- **Define** the difference between human immunodeficiency virus (HIV) and acquired immune deficiency syndrome (AIDS).
- **Explain** the seriousness of the AIDS epidemic in the United States and worldwide.
- **Describe** ways to prevent acquiring STIs.
- **Evaluate** your risk of HIV/AIDS.

CENGAGEbrain.com

Visit **www.cengagebrain.com** to access course materials and companion resources for this text, including quiz questions designed to check your understanding of the chapter contents. See the preface on page ix for more information.

FAQ

What is the difference between a sexually transmitted infection (STI) and a sexually transmitted disease (STD)?

Health experts are beginning to replace the term "STD" with "STI." The concept of disease implies a clear medical condition that manifests itself through signs or symptoms that define a specific disease. In terms of STIs, once infected, a person may or may not develop signs or symptoms indicative of disease. The unfortunate reality is that in the early stages of infection, many individuals with STIs exhibit no signs or symptoms, or such that are so mild that they are often ignored.

What is "safe" sex?

Safe sex means taking precautions during sexual intercourse or other forms of sexual contact, designed to prevent the exchange of blood, semen, vaginal fluids, or breast milk that can keep you or your partner from getting an STI. These infections include chlamydia, gonorrhea, pelvic inflammatory disease, genital warts, genital herpes, syphilis, and human immunodeficiency virus (HIV), among others. When unsure about your partner, use a lubricated latex condom from start to finish for each sexual act. If you think your partner should use a condom but refuses to do so, say "no" to sex with that person. While a condom definitely reduces the risk for infection, you need to realize that even with condom use you may acquire an STI. Condoms may not totally cover surrounding infected areas, and sometimes they rupture.

How does HIV damage the immune system?

On HIV infection, the virus attacks and starts killing CD4 cells in the immune system. CD4 cells are a special type of white blood cell that fights off infections (viral, fungal, and parasitic). Initially, the body can make more CD4 cells to replace the cells damaged by HIV. Eventually, however, the body is unable to replace all damaged cells. As the number of CD4 cells decreases, the immune system weakens and the person is more susceptible to sickness, illness, and infections, including the development of acquired immune deficiency syndrome (AIDS).

Real Life Story | Annalisa's Experience

I started dating Seth my freshman year of college. He had had sex before; I was a virgin. When we started sleeping together, he didn't really want to wear a condom, and I decided it wasn't necessary. After all, I was in love with him. Seth had never been tested for STIs, but I remember thinking, "He's on the cross-country team. Nobody who manages to run that many miles a week could possibly be sick or have a disease." However, it turned out that I was wrong—he was actually infected with chlamydia, and he passed it on to me. I was infected for several years before I found out. It wasn't until my senior year, when I took a health class and we were advised to get tested for STIs, that I learned I had chlamydia. During the time it had gone untreated, the disease did permanent damage to my reproductive system. I'll probably never be able to have kids now, and that was something I really wanted to do someday. Seth and I broke up not long after the diagnosis. Part of me was very angry and wanted to blame him for the whole thing, but the fact is, I had heard my whole life that you have to have "safe sex" and use a condom. Yet I made justifications for why that didn't apply to me. I made the wrong choice, and now I have to live with the results. As traumatic as it was for me to have chlamydia, the truth is that I was lucky. Because I engaged in unprotected sex, I could have contracted HIV. Then while everyone else was planning for graduation and their new lives, I would be worrying about dying of AIDS.

PERSONAL PROFILE: Sexually Transmitted Infections (STIs) Survey

I. Are you aware that there are more than 25 STIs and some are incurable?

II. Do you understand that more than 50 percent of all Americans will acquire at least one STI in their lifetime and almost half of them are seen in people between the ages of 15 and 24?

III. Did you know that genital herpes is one of the most common STIs, it is caused by a virus, it is incurable, and that a "simple" cold sore (or fever blister) can lead to genital herpes?

IV. Can you explain the difference between HIV infection and AIDS?

V. Do you understand the concept of "safe" sex and guidelines to follow to prevent STIs?

VI. If you choose not to have sex, have you thought out an appropriate response in the event that you are asked or are pressured to have sex?

Based on estimates by the World Health Organization, about 1.3 million people worldwide are infected daily with **sexually transmitted infections,** not including human immunodeficiency virus (HIV). STIs have also reached epidemic proportions in the United States. Of the more than 25 known STIs, some are still incurable. According to the American Sexual Health Association, more than half of all Americans will acquire at least one STI in their lifetime.

Few people are willing to talk about STIs, but for the health of the nation, we cannot afford to avoid the dialogue any longer. Each year, about 20 million people in the United States are newly infected with STIs, almost half of which are seen in young people between the ages of 15 and 24.[1] The infection rate is about the same among young women and young men, but the health consequences of untreated STIs is more serious for women, including infertility. About 24,000 women in the United States become infertile each year because of an STI they may not even know they had, as most infections have no symptoms.

According to estimates, one in four college students has had or has an STI. Young people are most at risk because they are more likely to have multiple sex partners. To avoid embarrassment, stigma, or concerns about confidentiality, young people are reluctant to discuss their risky sexual behavior with a physician.

Center for Disease Control and Prevention's (CDC) STI Screening Recommendations:

The CDC has released general screening recommendations for all sexually active people. The CDC encourages you to talk to your health care provider about STI testing and which tests may be right for you.

Because STIs are preventable, significant reductions in new infections are not only possible, they are urgently needed. Prevention can minimize the negative, long-term consequences of STIs and also reduce health care costs. The high incidence and overall prevalence of STIs in the general population suggests that many Americans are at substantial risk of exposure to STIs, underscoring the need for STI prevention.

Abstaining from sex, reducing the number of sexual partners, and consistently and correctly using condoms are all effective STI prevention strategies. Safe, effective vaccines are also available to prevent hepatitis B virus (HBV) and some types of HPV that cause disease and cancer. And for all individuals who are sexually active—particularly young people—STI screening and prompt treatment (if infected) are critical to protect a person's health and prevent transmission to others. The following are the CDC guidelines:

- All adults and adolescents should be tested at least once for HIV.
- Annual chlamydia screening for all sexually active women age 25 and younger, as well as older women with risk factors such as new or multiple sex partners.
- Yearly gonorrhea screening for at-risk sexually active women (e.g., those with new or multiple sex partners, and women who live in communities with a high burden of disease).
- Syphilis, HIV, chlamydia, and hepatitis B screening for all pregnant women, and gonorrhea screening for at-risk pregnant women at the first prenatal visit, to protect the health of mothers and their infants.
- Trichomoniasis screening should be conducted at least annually for all HIV-infected women.
- Screening at least once a year for syphilis, chlamydia, gonorrhea, and HIV for all sexually active gay men, bisexual men, and other men who have sex with men (MSM). MSM who have multiple or anonymous partners should be screened more frequently for STIs (e.g., at 3- to 6-month intervals). In addition, MSM who have sex in conjunction with illicit drug use (particularly methamphetamine use) or whose sex partners participate in these activities should be screened more frequently.

Currently, the United States has the highest rate of sexually transmitted infections of any country in the industrialized world. Following are brief descriptions of the leading STIs, their symptoms, and their treatments (if any).

> **Sexually transmitted infections (STIs)** Communicable diseases spread through sexual contact.

14.1 Chlamydia

Chlamydia is a bacterial infection that spreads during vaginal, anal, or oral sex, or from the vagina to a newborn baby during childbirth. Chlamydia can seriously damage the reproductive system. This infection is considered to be a major factor in male and female infertility. Because symptoms are usually mild or absent, three of four people with the infection don't know they're ill until the infection has become quite serious. Infertility often occurs "silently" because the individual is unaware of the infection until it is too late to prevent the irreversible damage.

Chlamydia is the most commonly reported STI. In any given year there may be as many as 2.8 million cases of chlamydia in the United States. Almost 55 percent of these cases are reported in women between the ages of 15 and 24. Only about 1.4 million cases are reported each year because most people are not aware of their infection.[2] Testing is also frequently skipped because patients are mistreated for symptoms that mimic other STIs. Women are frequently reinfected if their sex partners are not treated.

Symptoms of serious infection include abdominal pain, fever, nausea, vaginal bleeding, and arthritis. Although chlamydia can be treated successfully with oral antibiotics, its damage to the reproductive system is irreversible.

14.2 Gonorrhea

One of the oldest STIs, **gonorrhea** is caused by a bacterial infection. Gonorrhea is transmitted through contact with the vagina, penis, anus, or mouth of an infected person. According to the CDC approximately 820,000 individuals get new gonorrheal infections each year in the United States, less than half of the cases are reported, and about 570,000 are in the 15 to 24 age group.[3]

Typical symptoms in men include a pus-like secretion from the penis and painful urination. Infected women may have discharge and painful urination as well. Up to 80 percent of infected women, however, don't experience any symptoms until the infection has become fairly serious. At this stage, women develop fever, severe abdominal pain, and pelvic inflammatory disease (discussed next).

If untreated, gonorrhea can produce widespread bacterial infection, infertility, heart damage, and arthritis in men and women, and blindness in children born to infected women. At present gonorrhea is treated with penicillin and other antibiotics, but these will not repair any damage already done. There are signs from the CDC surveillance systems, however, that this disease may become resistant to the only available treatment option because drug-resistant strains are increasing and successful treatment is becoming more difficult.

14.3 Pelvic Inflammatory Disease

Estimates indicate that each year in the United States more than 750,000 women experience an acute episode of a condition known by the umbrella term **pelvic inflammatory disease (PID)**.[4] PID is not truly an STI but, rather, refers to complications resulting from STIs, especially chlamydia and gonorrhea. PID often develops when the STI spreads to the fallopian tubes, uterus, and ovaries. Sexually active women, especially those younger than age 25, are at higher risk for developing PID. These women are at higher risk because the cervix is not yet fully matured, increasing the risk for STIs that lead to PID. The more sex partners a woman has, the greater the risk for PID.

Complications associated with PID typically include scarring and obstruction of the fallopian tubes (which may lead to infertility), ectopic pregnancies, and chronic pelvic pain. If a woman with PID becomes pregnant, she could have an ectopic (tubal) pregnancy, which destroys the embryo and can kill the woman. Yearly, more than 100,000 women in the United States become infertile as a result of PID.

Typical symptoms of PID are fever, nausea, vomiting, chills, spotting between menstrual periods, heavy bleeding during periods, and pain in the lower abdomen during sexual intercourse, between menstrual periods, or during urination. Many times, however, women do not know they have PID because these symptoms are not always present.

PID is treated with antibiotics, bed rest, and sexual abstinence. Further, surgery may be required to remove infected or scarred tissue or to repair or remove the fallopian tubes or uterus.

More than 25 diseases are spread through sexual contact. More than half of all people will have an STI at some point in their lifetime.

14.4 Human Papillomavirus and Genital Warts

Human papillomavirus (HPV) is the most common sexually transmitted infection. There are more than 100 strains of HPV, and about 40 are sexually transmitted. "Low-risk" strains are wart-causing, whereas "high-risk" are cancer causing. Some strains of HPV infect the genital area, including the skin of the penis, the vulva, anus, lining of the vagina, cervix, and rectum, but they can also infect the mouth and throat as well. Others are known as "high risk" types and can lead to cancers of the cervix, vulva, vagina, anus, or penis.

Most HPVs have no signs or symptoms and the body's immune system clears them up within two years of infection without any form of treatment, while some forms persist. Presently, experts do not know why that is the case. When the body's immune system can't clear up a high-risk HPV infection, over time it turns normal cells into abnormal cells and subsequently cancer. Thirteen HPV types can cause cancer of the cervix; one of these types can cause cancers of the vulva, vagina, penis, anus, and certain head and neck cancers (specifically, the oropharynx, which includes the back of the throat, base of the tongue, and tonsils). HPV is responsible for nearly all cases of cervical cancer, 90 percent of anal, 65 percent of vaginal, 60 percent of oropharyngeal, 50 percent of vulvar, and 35 percent of penile cancers.

Approximately 14 million new cases of HPV are reported each year and at least 79 million Americans are infected.[5] Most sexually active people acquire HPV infection during their lifetime. At least 80 percent of women will acquire HPV infection by age 50. Most women are diagnosed with HPV through an abnormal Pap test. Infection is spread through genital or oral contact. Because most people have no signs or symptoms, they are unaware of the infection and can transmit the virus to a sex partner.

One of the potential health problems of HPV is **genital warts**, which show up between weeks or months after exposure. These warts may be flat or raised and usually are found on the penis or around the vulva and the vagina. They also can appear in the mouth, throat, rectum, on the cervix, or around the anus. Based on data from the CDC, as many as 1 million new cases of genital warts are diagnosed yearly in the United States. In some cities, nearly half of all sexually active teenagers have genital warts.

Critical Thinking

The high prevalence of STIs in our society makes the risk of acquiring a sexually transmitted infection extremely high. • To protect your health, wellness, and quality of life, are you willing to guard yourself in ALL CASES from getting an STI, and what is required of you to do so?

Health problems associated with genital warts include increased risk for cancers of the cervix, vulva, vagina, anus, penis, and enlargement and spread of the warts, leading to obstruction of the urethra, vagina, and anus. Because babies born to infected mothers commonly develop warts over their bodies, cesarean section is recommended for childbirth.

Treatment requires completely removing all warts. This can be done by freezing them with liquid nitrogen, dissolving them with chemicals, or removing them through electrosurgery or laser surgery. Infected patients may have to be treated more than once, because genital warts can recur.

Prevention of HPV infection is best accomplished through a mutually monogamous sexual relationship with an uninfected partner. It is difficult to know, however, if a person who has been sexually active in the past is currently infected.

Two HPV vaccines, Gardasil and Cervarix, are available to prevent cervical cancer and other diseases caused by HPV. Both vaccines protect against HPV types 16 and 18, which cause most cervical cancers. Additionally, Gardasil protects against HPV types 6 and 11 and most genital warts. To derive the benefits provided, HPV vaccines are routinely recommended for 11- and 12-year-old girls and boys and are highly recommended for all girls and women between the ages of 11 and 26. Gardasil has been approved for males between 11 and 21. To get the full benefits of the vaccine, people should get vaccinated before they become sexually active. The vaccines are most effective in women who have not been infected with any of the HPV types covered. Few women, however, are infected with all HPV types, thus vaccination still offers protection against those viruses that have not been acquired. The vaccine has not been widely tested in people older than 26. Licensing for this group may become available if the vaccine proves to be safe and effective for the older age group as well.

The HPV vaccines have surpassed all expectations in terms of disease prevention. Since the introduction of the vaccines in 2006, vaccine-type HPV prevalence decreased 56 percent among female teenagers 14–19 years of age. According to CDC Director Tom Frieden, "This report shows that HPV vaccine works well, and the report should be a wake-up call to our nation to protect the next generation by increasing HPV vaccination rates. Unfortunately only one-third of girls aged 13–17 have been fully vaccinated with HPV vaccine. Countries such as Rwanda have vaccinated more than 80 percent of their teen girls. Our low vaccination rates represent 50,000 preventable tragedies—50,000

Chlamydia A sexually transmitted infection, caused by a bacterial infection, that can cause significant damage to the reproductive system.

Gonorrhea A sexually transmitted infection caused by a bacterial infection.

Pelvic inflammatory disease (PID) An overall designation referring to the effects of other STIs, primarily chlamydia and gonorrhea.

Human papillomavirus (HPV) A group of viruses that can cause sexually transmitted infections.

Genital warts A sexually transmitted infection caused by a viral infection.

girls alive today will develop cervical cancer over their lifetime that would have been prevented if we reach 80 percent vaccination rates. For every year we delay in doing so, another 4,400 girls will develop cervical cancer in their lifetimes."

14.5 Genital Herpes

One of the most common STIs, **genital herpes** is caused by the herpes simplex virus (HSV). There are several types of HSV that produce different ailments, including genital herpes, oral herpes, shingles, and chicken pox. The two most common forms of HSV are types 1 and 2. In type 1—the HSV most often known to cause oral herpes—cold sores or fever blisters appear on the lips and mouth. HSV-2 is better known as the virus that causes genital herpes.

The fundamental difference between the two main types of HSV lies in their preferred "site of residence." The HSV-1 virus typically establishes latency in a collection of nerve cells near the ear known as trigeminal ganglion. HSV-2 usually establishes latency at the base of the spine in the sacral ganglion. The virus can remain dormant for a long time, but repeated outbreaks are common. The number of outbreaks tends to decrease over the years. Excessive fatigue, stress, cold, wind, wetness, heat, sun, sweating, rubbing, chafing, and friction, as well as lack of sleep, illness, and restrictive clothing, and diet can precipitate new outbreaks. Diet also plays a role as some foods such as popcorn, coffee, peanuts, chocolate, and alcohol may trigger outbreaks.

Unknown to most people, HSV-1 also causes genital herpes and an increasing number of genital herpes caused by HSV-1 has been found worldwide. Approximately 100 million Americans older than the age of 12 are infected with HSV-1. Most of these individuals acquired the virus as children. By age 50, more than 80 percent of the population has been exposed to HSV-1. Another 40 million are infected with HSV-2. One out of six people 14 to 49 years old are infected with the type 2 virus.[6] One in five women, one in nine men, and one in five adolescents are currently infected with genital herpes (HSV-2).

HSV is a highly contagious virus. Victims are most contagious during an outbreak, but the virus can also spread through virus-containing secretions. A few days following infection, a tingling sensation and lesions appear on the infected areas, most notably the mouth, genitals, and rectum, but can also surface on other parts of the body. Lesions can be somewhat painful.

Individuals infected with oral HSV-1 may shed the virus about 5 percent of the time, when they have no other symptoms of infection or visible lesions. In persons with asymptomatic HSV-2 infections, infected individuals can shed the virus up to 10 percent of days when they show no symptoms. At present, HSV-2 transmission most often occurs from an infected person who does not have a visible sore and may not even be aware of such an infection.

In conjunction with the lesions, victims usually have mild fever, swollen glands, and headaches. The symptoms disappear within a few weeks, causing some people to believe they are cured. Presently, though, herpes is incurable and its victims remain infected for life.

Society has typically labeled HSV-1 infection (cold sores) an "acceptable" viral infection, whereas infection with HSV-2 is viewed as a "bad" infection. The social stigma and emotional perspective of genital herpes make it difficult to objectively compare it with an oral infection, labeled as "just a cold sore" and acceptable to most people. HSV types 1 and 2, nonetheless, both cause oral and genital herpes. People who have an outbreak of oral herpes should not touch their own or someone else's genitals after touching the oral cold sores. Doing so can lead to a herpes infection of the genitals (genital HSV-1 infection). Oral sex can also result in transmission of HSV from the lips to the genitals. Thirty percent of *all new cases* of genital herpes result from HSV-1 infection. A 2011 study involving college students showed that HSV-1 accounts for 78 percent of female and 85 percent of male genital herpes infections.[7]

> **Critical Thinking**
>
> A "cold sore" or "fever blister," caused by an HSV-1 infection, is highly contagious and can lead to the development of genital herpes either by direct contact through oral sex or if the person with the outbreak touches the sore and then their own or their partner's genitals. • What can you do to protect yourself, loved ones, and others from a wider spread of the virus?

This startling finding is because of changing beliefs in what constitutes "safe" sex. The primary mode of HSV-1 transmission is by direct contact. College students assume that oral sex is safer and thus have vaginal intercourse and oral sex at about the same rate; giving HSV-1 a greater opportunity to spread.

The opposite is true as well: Oral sex with a genital HSV-2-infected person can cause oral HSV-2 infection (although there seems to be some degree of immunity against oral HSV-2 in people already infected with oral HSV-1). People with oral or genital sores should take care not to touch these sores. Following hand contact with cold or herpes sores, individuals should carefully wash themselves with soap. Avoid touching the eyes as such can cause vision damage as well.

During an outbreak, genital lesions may appear in areas that can be covered by a latex condom, but they can also appear in areas that cannot be covered. Use of a latex condom may protect against genital herpes only when the infected area is completely covered. Condoms, however, may not cover all infected areas. Thus genital herpes infections still occur. Individuals with HSV infection should abstain from sexual activity when lesions or other herpes symptoms are present. Sex partners of infected individuals should always be informed that they may become infected even if no lesions or symptoms are present. The best preventive approach is a mutually monogamous sexual relationship with an uninfected partner. Blood tests are available to determine HSV infection.

> **Critical Thinking**
>
> Many individuals who have sexually transmitted infections withhold this information from potential sexual partners. • Do you think it should be considered a criminal action if an individual knowingly transmits an STI to someone else?

14.6 Syphilis

Another common type of STI, also caused by bacterial infection, is **syphilis.** It is referred to as "the great imitator" because signs and symptoms are often indistinguishable from other diseases.

Once on the verge of elimination, syphilis began reappearing as a public health threat in 2001. More than 55,000 new cases are reported each year.[8] The incidence is highest in men between 20 and 29 years of age. A troubling statistic released in 2011 is that 72 percent of primary and secondary stage syphilis (see following discussion) cases occurred among men who have sex with men.

Syphilis is transmitted through direct contact with a syphilis sore during vaginal, anal, or oral sex. In the primary stage, between 10 and 90 days following infection (average 21 days) a painless sore appears where the bacteria entered the body (sometimes multiple sores appear). A sore also can appear on the lips or in the mouth. This sore disappears on its own in 3 to 6 weeks. If untreated, the infection progresses to the secondary stage.

During the secondary stage, as the initial sore is healing, or several weeks thereafter, skin rashes and mucous membrane lesions appear. A rough/reddish-brown rash can be seen on the palms of the hands and the bottom of the feet, although different types of rashes can appear on other parts of the body. Additional sores may also appear within six months of the initial outbreak. Signs and symptoms of the secondary stage will disappear with or without treatment. Untreated, the infection will progress into the latent stage.

A latent stage, during which the victim is not contagious, may last up to 30 years, lulling victims into thinking they are healed. During the last stage of the infection, some people develop paralysis, crippling, gradual blindness, heart disease, brain and organ damage, or dementia, or die as a direct result of the infection.

Syphilis is diagnosed by microscopic examination of material from a sore or through a simple blood test. One of the oldest known STIs, syphilis once killed its victims, but now penicillin and other antibiotics are used to treat it. A single injection of penicillin will cure individuals who have been infected for less than a year. Additional treatments are necessary for people infected longer than a year. Antibiotics are also available for individuals allergic to penicillin. People infected with syphilis must abstain from sexual activity until all syphilis sores have completely disappeared. Sexual partners must also be informed of potential infection so that they can seek treatment if necessary.

14.7 Trichomoniasis

Although not as well-known as other STIs, trichomoniasis or "trich" is a very common STI caused by infection with a protozoan parasite called *Trichomonas vaginalis*. Although symptoms of the disease vary, most women and men who have the parasite cannot tell they are infected. It is considered the most common curable STI. About 3.7 million people in the United States are infected, about 70 percent do not have any signs or symptoms of infection, and the incidence is more common in women than men. Presently it is unknown why some people with the infection get symptoms while others don't. Most likely it is related to the person's age and overall health. Asymptomatic infected individuals can still pass the infection on to others.

Men with trichomoniasis can experience itching or irritation inside the penis, a burning sensation after urination or ejaculation, or discharge from the penis. Women may also feel itching or burning, redness or soreness of the genitals, uncomfortable urination, or an unusual discharge that can be clear, white, yellowish, or greenish. Having trichomoniasis can make sex quite uncomfortable. Without treatment, the infection can last for months or even years.

Trichomoniasis increases the risk of getting or spreading other STIs. For example, trichomoniasis can cause genital inflammation that makes it easier to become HIV-infected or to pass the virus on to others.

Trichomoniasis can be cured with a single dose of prescription antibiotics, either metronidazole or tinidazole. Pregnant women can also be treated with these medications. Drinking alcohol within 24 hours of taking the medication can lead to uncomfortable side effects.

People who have been treated for trichomoniasis can get reinfected. About 20 percent of people get infected again within 3 months of antibiotic treatment. To avoid reinfection, be sure that all sex partners get treated as well, and do not engage in sexual activity until all of your symptoms have disappeared (about a week). See your physician if the symptoms return.

> **Genital herpes** A sexually transmitted infection caused by a viral infection of the herpes simplex virus types 1 and 2. The virus can attack different areas of the body but typically causes blisters on the genitals.
>
> **Syphilis** A sexually transmitted infection caused by a bacterial infection.

14.8 HIV and AIDS

Of all sexually transmitted infections, **HIV (human immunodeficiency virus)** infection is the most frightening because in most cases it is fatal if left untreated. AIDS—which stands for **acquired immunodeficiency syndrome**—is the end stage of infection by HIV. In Activity 14.1 you will have the opportunity to evaluate your basic understanding of HIV and AIDS.

HIV is a chronic infectious disease that is passed from one person to another through blood-to-blood and sexual contact. The virus spreads most commonly among individuals who engage in risky behavior such as having unprotected sex or sharing hypodermic needles. When a person becomes infected with HIV, the virus multiplies, then attacks and destroys white blood cells. These cells are part of the immune system, and their function is to fight off infections and diseases in the body.

As the number of white blood cells that are killed increases, the body's immune system gradually breaks down or may be destroyed completely. Without an immune system, a person becomes susceptible to various **opportunistic infections** and to cancers.

The only means to determine whether someone has HIV is through an HIV antibody test. Being HIV-positive does not mean that the person has AIDS. HIV is a progressive infection. At first, people who become infected with HIV might not know they are infected. An incubation period of weeks, months, or years may pass during which no symptoms appear. The virus may live in the body 10 years or longer before disease symptoms emerge. HIV infection can produce neurological abnormalities, leading to depression, memory loss, slower mental and physical response time, and sluggishness in limb movements that may progress to a severe disorder known as HIV dementia.

When the infection progresses to a point at which certain diseases develop, the person is said to have AIDS. HIV itself doesn't kill. Nor do people die from AIDS. "AIDS" is the term designating the final stage of HIV infection, and death is the result of a weakened immune system that is unable to fight off these opportunistic infections.

Earliest symptoms of AIDS include unexplained weight loss, constant fatigue, mild fever, swollen lymph glands, diarrhea, and sore throat. Advanced symptoms include loss of appetite, skin diseases, night sweats, and deterioration of mucous membranes.

Most of the illnesses that AIDS patients develop are harmless and rare in the general population but are fatal to AIDS victims. Two of the fatal conditions in AIDS patients, for example, are Pneumocystis jiroveci pneumonia (a parasitic infection of the lungs) and Kaposi's sarcoma (a type of skin cancer). HIV also attacks the nervous system, causing damage to the brain and spinal cord. An unsettling finding is that brain damage is seen even in patients who are on drug therapy. The brain appears to provide a haven for HIV where drugs cannot follow, leading to a selective destruction pattern of brain regions that control motor, language, and sensory functions. This finding may explain why individuals often display slower reflexes and disruption of balance and gait in the early stages of AIDS. Patients also frequently exhibit mild vocabulary loss, judgment problems, and difficulty planning.

On becoming infected, the immune system forms antibodies that bind to the virus. Most infected individuals will show these antibodies within 3 months of infection, the average being 25 days. In rare cases, they are not detectable until after 6 months or longer.

If HIV infection is suspected, seek medical attention *immediately*. Some evidence indicates that an immediate course of antiviral drugs reduces the chances that a person will be infected. This is referred to as post-exposure prophylaxis (PEP), frequently used to prevent transmission in health care workers injured by needle sticks. Less information is available about the effectiveness of PEP for people exposed to HIV through sexual activity or drug use injections, but it also appears to be effective. If you think you were exposed, discuss the possibility with a HIV specialist (local AIDS organizations provide the most recent information) as soon as possible. Sexual assault victims should consider the potential effects and benefits of PEP.

Following the initial consultation with a medical specialist, the individual may still need to wait three months to be tested. If the test is negative and the person still suspects infection, the test should be repeated three months later. During this time, and from then on, individuals should refrain from further endangering themselves and others through risky behaviors. Some people are tested to reassure themselves that their risky behaviors are acceptable. Even if the test turns up negative for HIV, this does not represent a "license" to continue risky behaviors.

No one has to become infected with HIV. At present,

Drug and alcohol use can make people more willing to have unplanned and unprotected sex, thereby risking HIV infection.

> **HIV (Human immunodeficiency virus)** Virus that leads to acquired immunodeficiency syndrome (AIDS).
>
> **AIDS (Acquired immunodeficiency syndrome)** Any of a number of diseases that arise when the body's immune system is compromised by HIV; the final stage of HIV infection.
>
> **Opportunistic infections** Infections that arise in the absence of a healthy immune system, which would fight them off in healthy people.

Activity 14.1: Self-Quiz on HIV and AIDS

Name _____ Date _____

Course _____ Section _____ Gender _____ Age _____

> Indicate whether the following statements are true or false, then turn the page to see how well you understand HIV and AIDS.

	True	False
1. AIDS—acquired immunodeficiency syndrome—is the end stage of infection caused by the human immunodeficiency virus, HIV.	☐	☐
2. HIV is a chronic infectious disease that spreads among individuals who choose to engage in risky behavior such as unprotected sex or the sharing of hypodermic needles.	☐	☐
3. AIDS is completely curable.	☐	☐
4. Abstaining from sex is the only 100 percent sure way to protect yourself from HIV infection through sexual activity.	☐	☐
5. A person infected with HIV can look and feel healthy.	☐	☐
6. Condoms are 100 percent effective in protecting you against HIV infection.	☐	☐
7. Using drugs and alcohol makes a person less likely to use a condom and use it correctly.	☐	☐
8. If you're sexually active, latex condoms provide the best protection against HIV infection.	☐	☐
9. Using drugs and alcohol can make you more likely to have unplanned and unprotected sex.	☐	☐
10. A pregnant woman who has HIV can transmit the virus to her baby during childbirth.	☐	☐
11. You can become HIV-infected by donating blood.	☐	☐
12. HIV can be transmitted by spending time with or through casual contact (shaking hands, hugging) with an infected person.	☐	☐
13. The only means to determine whether someone has HIV is through an HIV antibody test.	☐	☐
14. HIV can completely destroy the immune system.	☐	☐
15. The HIV virus may live in the body 10 years or longer before AIDS symptoms develop.	☐	☐
16. People infected with HIV have AIDS.	☐	☐
17. HIV infection is preventable.	☐	☐
18. Early treatment can reduce the symptoms of HIV-infected people.	☐	☐
19. Drugs are now available that can lengthen the life of an HIV-infected person.	☐	☐
20. Antiretroviral drugs delay the progress of HIV infection and can keep many people from developing AIDS.	☐	☐

(continued)

Selected items on this questionnaire are adapted from *Test Your Survival Smarts: Self-Quiz on Drugs and AIDS*, National Institute on Drug Abuse, U. S. Department of Health & Human Services.

Answers:

1. True. AIDS is the term used to define the manifestation of opportunistic diseases and cancers that occur as a result of HIV infection (also referred to as "HIV disease").
2. True. People do not get HIV because of who they are, but because of what they do. Almost all of the people who get HIV do so because they choose to engage in risky behaviors.
3. False. There is no cure for AIDS, although some medications are now available that delay the progress of HIV and keep some people from developing AIDS.
4. True. Abstinence will protect you from HIV infection. But you may still get the disease by sharing hypodermic needles.
5. True. The symptoms of HIV are often not noticeable until several years after a person has been infected. That's why—no matter who your partner is—it is important to always protect yourself against HIV and the risk of developing AIDS, either by abstaining from sex or by *always* practicing safe sex.
6. False. Only abstaining from sex gives you 100 percent protection, but condoms, if used correctly, are effective in protecting against HIV infection.
7. True. Teens who are drunk or high are less likely to use condoms because, under the influence, they forget or believe that nothing "bad" can happen.
8. True. Proper use is necessary to minimize the risk of infection, but condoms are not 100 percent foolproof as sometimes they break.
9. True. Otherwise-prudent people often act irrationally and engage in risky behaviors when they are under the influence of drugs and alcohol.
10. True. HIV transmission can occur between a pregnant woman and her baby during childbirth. A baby can also be infected through breast-feeding, although this occurs less frequently.
11. False. A myth regarding HIV is that it can be transmitted by donating blood. People cannot get HIV from giving blood. A brand-new needle is used by health professionals every time they draw blood. These needles are used only once and are destroyed and thrown away immediately after each individual has donated blood.
12. False. HIV is transmitted by the exchange of cellular body fluids, including blood and other body fluids containing blood, semen, vaginal secretions, and maternal milk. These fluids are most often exchanged during sexual intercourse, by using hypodermic needles previously used by infected individuals, or by contact with open wounds, cuts, or sores.
13. True. Not you, not a nurse, not even a doctor, can tell without an HIV antibody test. Upon HIV infection, the immune system's line of defense against the virus is the formation of antibodies that bind to the virus. On the average it takes 3 months for the body to manufacture enough antibodies to show positive in an HIV antibody test. Sometimes it takes 6 months or longer.
14. True. The virus multiplies, then attacks and destroys white blood cells. These cells are part of the immune system, and their function is to fight off infections and diseases in the body. As the number of white blood cells killed increases, the body's immune system gradually breaks down or may be completely destroyed.
15. True. Ten years or longer may go by before the person develops AIDS.
16. False. Being HIV-positive does not necessarily mean that the person has AIDS. It may be 10 years or longer following infection before the individual develops the symptoms that fit the case definition of AIDS. From that point on, the person may live another 2 to 3 years. In essence, from the point of infection, the individual may endure a chronic disease for about 12 or more years.
17. True. The best prevention technique is abstaining from sex until the time comes for a mutually monogamous sexual relationship (two people having a sexual relationship only with each other). That one behavior will almost completely remove you from any risk of HIV infection or developing any other sexually transmitted disease.
18. True. The sooner treatment is initiated, the better the prognosis is for a longer life.
19. True. Available antiretroviral drugs can delay the progress of infection.
20. True. Antiretroviral drugs allow HIV infected individuals to live healthier and longer lives and even keep some people from developing AIDS. However, these drugs do not cure HIV or AIDS.

once infected, with the exception of two rare cases, a person cannot become uninfected. There is no second chance. Everyone must protect himself or herself against this chronic infection. If people do not—and are so ignorant as to believe it cannot happen to them—they are putting themselves and their partners at risk.

New therapies are preventing AIDS from developing in a growing number of HIV-infected individuals. Professionals, however, disagree as to how many HIV carriers actually will develop AIDS. Even if individuals have not developed AIDS, they can pass on the virus to others, who then could easily develop AIDS.

Transmission of HIV HIV is transmitted by the exchange of cellular body fluids, including blood and other body fluids containing blood, semen, vaginal secretions, and maternal milk.

The most recent data available on HIV infection diagnoses among adults and adolescents in the United States by race/ethnicity are given in Figure 14.1. The percentage of adults and adolescents currently living with a diagnosis of HIV infection, by gender and transmission category, as of the end of 2010, are provided in Figure 14.2. Further, approximately 50,000 new infections are presently being reported each year. Of all new infections, about 63 percent are reported in men who had sex with men, 25 percent in men and women through heterosexual sex, 8 percent by injection drug use, 3 percent in male-to-male sexual contact and injection drug use combined, and less than 1 percent in other unidentified categories. Currently about 47 percent of the new infections occur in African Americans, followed by Caucasians (28 percent), Hispanics (21 percent), Asians (2 percent), and multiple races (2 percent). American Indians/Alaska Natives and Native Hawaiians/Pacific Islanders each account for 1 percent or less of diagnosis.

Today, the risk of being infected with HIV from a blood transfusion is slight. Prior to 1985, several cases of HIV infection came from blood transfusions because the blood had been donated by HIV-infected individuals. Now, all individuals who donate blood are first tested for HIV. To be absolutely safe, people who are planning to have surgery might consider storing their own blood in advance, so safe blood will be available if a transfusion becomes necessary.

A myth regarding HIV is that it can be transmitted by donating blood. People cannot get HIV from giving blood. Health professionals use a brand-new needle every time they withdraw blood from a person. They use these needles only once and destroy them immediately after each person has donated blood.

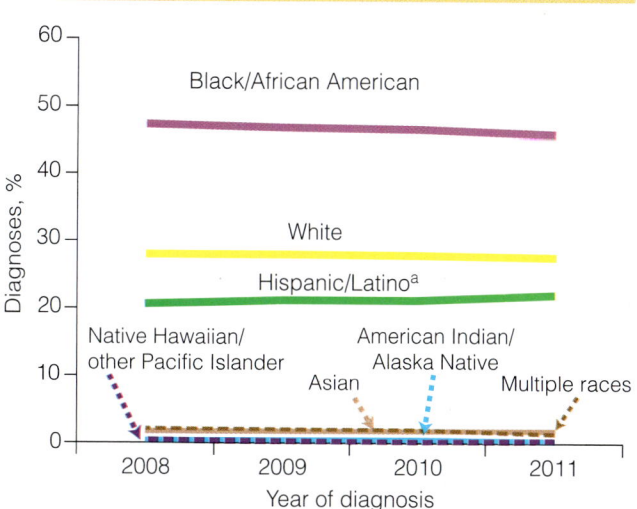

Figure 14.1 Diagnoses of HIV infection among adults and adolescents, by race/ethnicity, 2008–2011—United States and six U.S. dependent areas.

Note: Data include persons with a diagnosis of HIV infection regardless of stage of disease at diagnosis. All displayed data have been statistically adjusted to account for reporting delays, but not for incomplete reporting.
[a]Hispanics/Latinos can be of any race.

SOURCE: http://www.cdc.gov/hiv/pdf/statistics_surveillance_raceEthnicity.pdf, downloaded July 1, 2013.

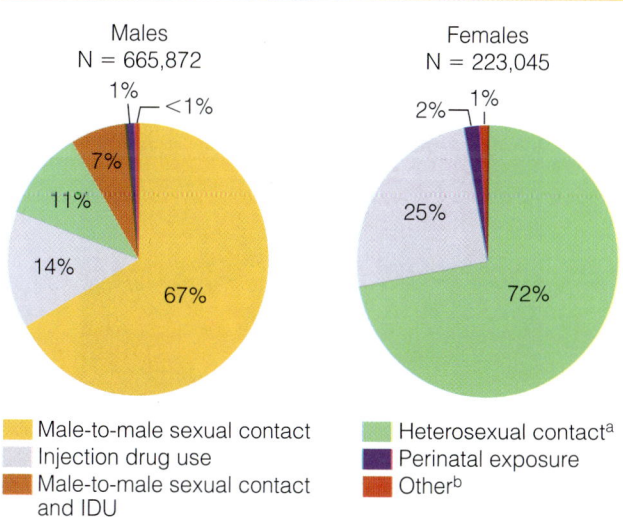

Figure 14.2 Adults and adolescents living with diagnosed HIV infection, by gender and transmission category, year-end 2010—United States and six U.S. dependent areas.

Note: Data include persons with a diagnosis of HIV infection regardless of stage of disease at diagnosis. All displayed data have been statistically adjusted to account for reporting delays and missing transmission category, but not for incomplete reporting.
[a]Heterosexual contact with a person known to have, or to be at high risk for, HIV infection.
[b]Includes hemophilia, blood transfusion, and risk factor not reported or not identified.

SOURCE: http://www.cdc.gov/hiv/pdf/statistics_surveillance_Epi-HIV-infection.pdf, downloaded July 1, 2013.

People do not get HIV because of who they are but, rather, because of what they do. HIV and AIDS can threaten anyone, anywhere: men, women, children, teenagers, young people, older adults, Caucasians, African Americans, Hispanic Americans, Asian Americans, Native Americans, Africans, Europeans, homosexuals, heterosexuals, bisexuals, drug users. Nobody is immune to HIV. HIV can be transmitted between males, between females, from male to female, or from female to male. Although HIV and AIDS are preventable, nearly all of the people who get HIV do so because they engage in risky behaviors.

Risky Behaviors You cannot tell if people are infected with HIV or have AIDS by simply looking at them or taking their word. Not you, not a nurse, not even a doctor can tell without an HIV antibody test. Therefore, every time you engage in risky behavior, you run the risk of contracting HIV. The two most basic risky behaviors are:

1. Having unprotected vaginal, anal, or oral sex with an HIV-infected person. Unprotected sex means having sex without using a condom properly. A person should select only latex (rubber or prophylactic) condoms that state "disease prevention" on the package. Although you might have unprotected sex with an infected person and not get the virus, you can get it by having unprotected sex only once with an infected individual.

    Rubbing during sexual intercourse often damages mucous membranes and causes unseen bleeding (even in the mouth). During vaginal, anal, or oral sexual contact, infected blood, semen, or vaginal fluids can penetrate the mucous membranes that line the vagina, the penis, the rectum, the mouth, or the throat. From the membrane, HIV then travels into the previously uninfected person's blood.

    Health experts believe that unprotected anal sex is the riskiest type of sex. Even though bleeding is not visible in most cases, anal sex almost always causes tiny tears and bleeding in the rectum. This happens because the rectum does not stretch easily, the mucous membrane is quite thin, and small blood vessels lie directly beneath the membrane. Condoms also are more likely to break during anal intercourse because more friction is produced in a smaller cavity. All of these factors greatly enhance the risk of transmitting HIV.

    Although latex condoms, if used correctly, provide for "safer" sex, they are not 100 percent foolproof. Abstaining from sex is the only 100 percent sure way to protect yourself from HIV infection and other STIs.

2. Sharing hypodermic needles or other drug paraphernalia with someone who is infected. Following an injection, a small amount of blood remains in the needle, and sometimes in the syringe itself. If the person who used the syringe is infected with HIV and someone else uses that same syringe to shoot up, regardless of the drug used (legal or illegal), that small amount of blood is sufficient to spread the virus. All used syringes should be destroyed and disposed of immediately.

In addition, a person must be cautious when getting acupuncture, getting a tattoo, or having the ears or other body parts pierced. If the needle had been used previously on an HIV-infected person and was not disinfected properly, the person risks getting HIV.

Otherwise-prudent people often act irrationally and engage in risky behaviors when they are under the influence of drugs. Getting high can make you willing to have sex when you really didn't plan to—thereby running the risk of contracting HIV.

Small concentrations of the virus have been found in saliva and teardrops. In principle, if both people have open cuts on the lips or in the mouth or gums, HIV could be transmitted through open-mouth kissing. Prolonged open-mouth kissing can damage the mouth or lips and allow HIV to be transmitted from an infected person to a partner through cuts or sores in the mouth. These cases, however, are rare.

Myths about HIV Transmission The HIV virus cannot be transmitted through perspiration. Sporting activities with no physical contact pose no risk to uninfected individuals unless they both have open wounds through which blood from an infected person can come in direct contact with the open wound of the uninfected person. The skin is an excellent line of defense against HIV. Blood from an infected person cannot penetrate the skin except through an opening in the skin. As an extra precaution, a person should use vinyl

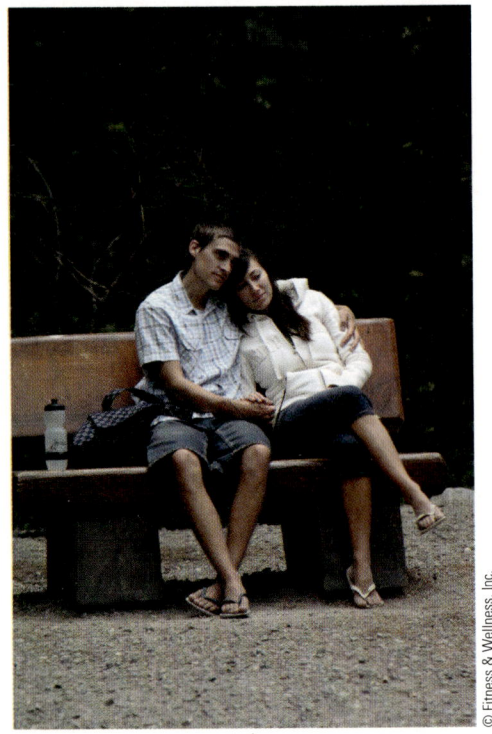

A monogamous sexual relationship almost completely removes people from risking HIV infection and the danger of developing other sexually transmitted infections.

or latex gloves when performing work that requires direct contact with someone else's blood or open wound.

HIV is not transmitted through casual contact. HIV cannot be caught by spending time with, shaking hands with, or hugging an infected person; from a toilet seat, dishes, or silverware used by an HIV patient; or sharing a drink, food, a towel, or clothes with a person who has HIV.

Some people fear getting HIV from health care professionals. The chances of getting infected during physical or medical procedures are rare. Health care workers take extra care to protect themselves and their patients from HIV.

Another myth regarding HIV transmission is that you can get it from insects or animals. The H in HIV stands for "human." You cannot catch HIV from insects or animals. Animals do not contract HIV.

Wise Dating With the advent of the Internet, people now search for sex partners online. Use of the Internet to find sexual partners may further increase the risk of contracting an STI. These people also are more likely to have characteristics that increase their chances of transmitting STIs.

Dating and getting to know other people are normal aspects of life. Dating, however, does not mean the same thing as having sex. Sexual intercourse as a part of dating can be risky, and one of the risks is HIV infection. You can't tell if someone you are dating or would like to date has been exposed to HIV. The good news is that as long as you avoid sexual activity and don't share drug needles, you are not at risk for contracting HIV.

Trends in HIV Infection and AIDS Based on 2010 estimates, about 34 million people worldwide are infected with HIV, and close to 2.7 million new worldwide infections were reported that year. More than 30 million have died from AIDS since the epidemic began in 1981. Women are becoming increasingly affected, with 16.8 million women now living with HIV.[9]

About 1.2 million people in the United States are infected with HIV and approximately 20 percent of them are unaware of the infection. One in every 260 Americans is infected, and about 24 percent of the newly reported cases are women.

Through the end of 2008, more than 1 million AIDS cases had been diagnosed in the United States and dependent areas (see Figure 14.3), and an estimated 600,000 people have died from the diseases caused by HIV. About 80 percent of the people who died are in the 25- to 49-year-old age group.

As with any other serious illness, HIV-infected people and AIDS patients deserve respect, understanding, and support. Rejection and discrimination are traits of immature, hateful, and ignorant people. Education, knowledge, and responsible behaviors are the best ways to minimize fear and discrimination.

HIV Testing A person can be tested for HIV in several ways. You may look up your local Public Health Department or AIDS Information Service (or related names) in the phone book. Testing results are kept confidential.

Many states also conduct anonymous testing. Your name is never recorded. You can call several toll-free hotlines or access the CDC Web site (www.cdc.gov/hiv) for more information on anonymous testing, treatment programs, support services, and information about HIV, AIDS, and STIs in general. All information discussed during a phone call to these hotlines is kept strictly confidential. The numbers to call are:

- National AIDS Hotline: 1-800-CDC-INFO (1-800-232-4636) in English and Spanish

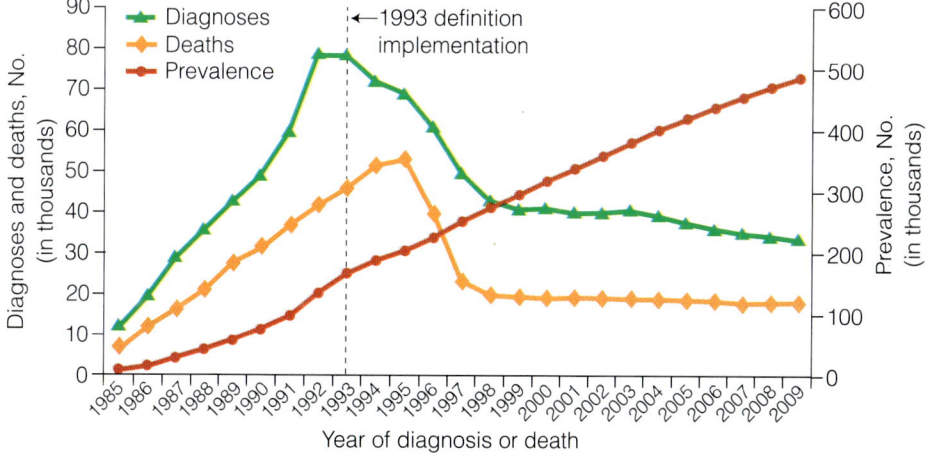

Figure 14.3 AIDS diagnoses, deaths, and persons living with AIDS, 1985–2009—United States and six U.S. dependent areas.

Note: All displayed data have been statistically adjusted to account for reporting delays, but not for incomplete reporting. Death may be due to any cause.

SOURCE: http://www.cdc.gov/hiv/pdf/statistics_surveillance_aidstrends.pdf, downloaded July 1, 2013.

- National AIDS Hotline for the hearing impaired (TTY): 1-888-232-6348
- STI Hotline: 1-800-227-8922

Information on local testing facilities is also available online at www.hivtest.org.

The CDC recommends HIV testing for all people between the ages of 13 to 64 and all pregnant women during the routine panel of prenatal screening tests. The recommendations further include annual screening for persons at high risk for infection. Consent for HIV testing is now included in the general consent form for medical care. Patients, however, can decline testing if they choose to do so.

HIV Treatment Even though several drugs are being tested to treat and slow the infection process, AIDS still has no known cure. To date, one leukemia patient, "the Berlin patient," is known to have been cured of HIV infection after undergoing a bone marrow transplant from a donor who had a rare genetic mutation that makes a person resistant to HIV infection. Other patients using a similar treatment, however, have not been as fortunate. At least 40 approaches to an AIDS vaccine are being explored. The best advice at this point is to take a preventive approach.

Antiretroviral drugs are available that delay the progress of HIV infection and even keep many people from developing AIDS. Antiretroviral drugs have turned HIV infection from an almost imminent predecessor of death to a lifelong chronic disease. Thanks to advances in the development of these drugs, many HIV-infected people can now look forward to decades of life. HIV-infected individuals, however, must take the drugs every day for the rest of their life. In most cases, failure to do so results in the virus coming back with full strength. The drugs don't eradicate HIV but rather suppress the virus and make it almost undetectable in the blood. The world, unfortunately, does not have the resources to make the drugs available to most HIV-infected people for decades to come.

About 30 drugs are available that suppress HIV. The drugs are usually used in combinations, commonly referred to as highly active antiretroviral therapy or "AIDS cocktails." Because the virus mutates rapidly and because some individuals don't tolerate some of the drugs, physicians often switch drug combinations to keep HIV under control.

A study sponsored by the National Institutes of Health was terminated early in May 2011 because of its significance in the prevention of HIV transmission. The study found that early treatment with antiretroviral drugs, at the time of HIV diagnosis, greatly decreased the risk of transmitting the virus to an uninfected partner. The research was conducted on 1,763 couples in nine countries throughout the world. Only one of the partners in each couple was infected with HIV. The results showed a 96 percent reduction in HIV infection risk only among patients who received the early drug treatment. (All couples in the study were urged to use condoms, which are still critical for protection.) Early treatment is thus critical to decrease transmission risk. HIV-infected individuals, nonetheless, cannot make the assumption that they will not pass on the virus simply because they are on antiretroviral medication.

At present, these drugs do not cure HIV infection or AIDS. They suppress the virus (decrease the viral load), even to undetectable levels, but they do not eliminate the virus. The sooner the treatment is initiated, the better the prognosis for a longer life.

For HIV-infected individuals, viral load tests are available to detect the amount of virus present in the blood. These tests measure HIV ribonucleic acid, the part of HIV that knows how to make more of the virus. Following drug therapy, an undetectable viral load does not mean the person is cured. It means that the amount of HIV in the blood is so low that it cannot be detected. Because there is no known cure,

---

Behavior Modification Planning

Protecting Yourself and Others from STIs

Are you sexually active? If you are not, read the following items to better educate yourself regarding intimacy. If you are sexually active, continue through all the following questions.

- Do you plan ahead before you get into a sexual situation?
- Do you know whether your partner now has or has ever had an STI? Are you comfortable asking your partner this question?
- Are you in a mutually monogamous sexual relationship and you know that your partner does not have an STI?
- Do you have multiple sexual partners? If so, do you *always* practice safe sex?
- Do you avoid alcohol and drugs in situations where you may end up having planned or unplanned sex?
- Do you abstain from sexual activity if you know or suspect that you have an STI and do you seek medical care and advice as to when you can safely resume sexual activity?

Try It

Taking chances during sexual contact is not worth the risk of an STI. Sex lasts a few minutes; the STI can last a lifetime, with potentially fatal consequences. Think ahead, know the facts, and don't place yourself in a situation where you may no longer be able to or have the desire to say no. Keep in mind that more than half of all Americans will acquire at least one STI in their lifetime. A few minutes of sexual pleasure can easily have consequences that you may regret for the rest of your life.

the person is still infected with HIV and can infect others. Although undetectable in the blood, the virus is still present in other body tissues and in the lymph system.

Development of a vaccine to prevent HIV infection or AIDS seems highly unlikely in the near future. People should not expect a medical breakthrough, although researchers are cautiously optimistic about finding a cure. Treatment modalities, however, continue to improve and allow HIV-infected individuals and AIDS patients to live longer and more productive lives.

Several AIDS clinical trials are available in the United States. These projects are cosponsored by the CDC, the FDA, the National Institute of Allergy and Infectious Diseases, the National Library of Medicine, and the National Institutes of Health. The purpose of AIDS clinical trials is to evaluate experimental drugs and various therapies for people at all stages of HIV infection. Interested individuals can call 1-800-TRIALS-A (1-800-874-2572). As with all HIV testing, calls are confidential. Eligibility to participate in an AIDS clinical trial varies, and all applicants are evaluated individually. By calling the telephone number, an interested person receives information on the purpose and location of the trials (studies) that are open, eligibility requirements and exclusion criteria, and names and telephone numbers of people to contact.

14.9 Guidelines for Preventing Sexually Transmitted Infections

The good news is that you can do things to prevent the spread of STIs and take precautions to keep yourself from becoming a victim. The facts are in: The best prevention technique is a mutually monogamous sexual relationship. This one behavior will remove you almost completely from any risk for developing an STI.

Unfortunately, in today's society, trust is elusive. You may be led to believe you are in a safe, monogamous relationship when your partner actually (a) may cheat on you and get infected, (b) has a one-night stand with someone who is infected, (c) got the virus several years ago before the current relationship and still doesn't know about the infection, (d) may choose not to tell you about the infection, or (e) shoots up drugs and becomes infected. In any of these cases, HIV can be passed on to you.

Because your future and your life are at stake, and because you may never know if your partner is infected, you should give serious and careful consideration to postponing sex until you believe you have found an uninfected person with whom you can have a lifetime monogamous relationship. In doing so, you will not have to live with the fear of catching HIV or other STIs or deal with an unplanned pregnancy.

As strange as this may seem to some, many people postpone sexual activity until they are married. This is the best guarantee against HIV. Young people should understand that

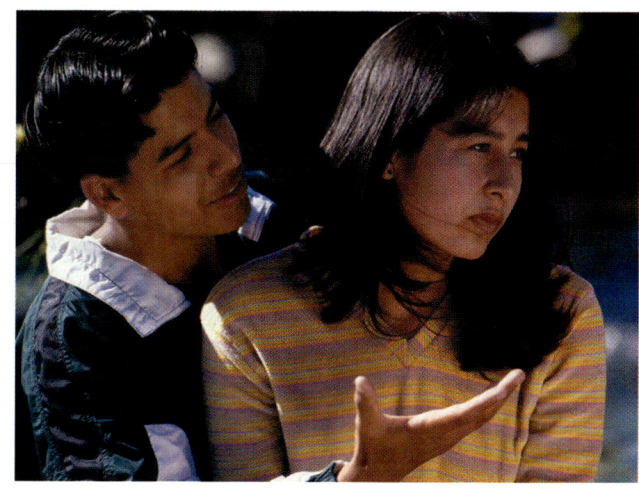

If someone does not respect your choice to wait, he or she certainly does not deserve your friendship or, for that matter, anything else.

married life will provide plenty of time for fulfilling and rewarding sex.

If you choose to delay sex, don't let peers pressure you into having sex. Some people would have you believe that you aren't a "real" man or woman if you don't have sex. Manhood and womanhood are not proven during sexual intercourse but, instead, through mature, responsible, and healthy choices.

Other people lead you to believe that love doesn't exist without sex. Sex in the early stages of a relationship is not the product of love. It is simply the fulfillment of a physical, and often selfish, drive. A loving relationship develops over a long time with mutual respect for each other.

Then there are those who enjoy bragging about their sexual conquests and mock people who choose to wait. Many of these conquests are only fantasies expounded in an attempt to gain popularity with peers.

Teenagers are especially susceptible to peer pressure leading to premature sexual intercourse. The result? About 330,000 teens gave birth in 2011. Presently, the U.S. teen pregnancy rate is one of the highest of the Western industrialized nations. Too many young people wish they had postponed sex and silently admire those who do. Sex lasts only a few minutes. The consequences of irresponsible sex may last a lifetime. And in some cases, they are fatal!

Sexual promiscuity never leads to a trusting, loving, and lasting relationship. Mature people respect others' choices. If someone doesn't respect your choice to wait, he or she certainly doesn't deserve your friendship or, for that matter, anything else.

There is no greater sex than that between two loving and responsible individuals who mutually trust, admire, and love each other. Contrary to many beliefs, these relationships are possible. They are built on unselfish attitudes and behaviors.

As you look around, you will find that many people hold these values. Seek them out and build your friendships and future around people who respect you for who you are and what you believe. You don't have to compromise your choices or values. In the end, you will reap the greater rewards of a lasting relationship free of HIV and other STIs.

Also, be prepared so that you will know your course of action before you get into an intimate situation. Look for common interests and work together toward them. Express your feelings openly: "I'm not ready for sex; I just want to have fun, and kissing is fine with me." If your friend doesn't accept your answer and isn't willing to stop the advances, be prepared with a strong response. Statements like, "Please stop" or "Don't!" are for the most part ineffective. Use a firm statement such as, "No, I'm not willing to have sex" or "I've already thought about this and I'm not going to have sex." If this still doesn't work, label the behavior as rape and say, "This is rape, and I'm going to call the police."

> ### Critical Thinking
> Discuss how the information presented in this chapter has affected your feelings and perceptions about sex. • What impact will this information have on your wellness lifestyle?

Reducing the Risk for STIs and HIV Infection

Based on recommendations from health experts, observing the following precautions can reduce your risk for STIs, including HIV infection and, subsequently, AIDS:

1. Postpone sex until you and your uninfected partner are prepared to enter into a lifetime monogamous relationship.
2. Unless you are in a monogamous relationship, and you know your partner isn't infected (which you may never know for sure), practice safe sex every time you have sex, and don't have sexual contact with anyone who doesn't practice safe sex. This means you should use a latex condom from start to finish for each sexual act. If your partner refuses to use a condom, say no to sex with that person.
3. Use "barrier" methods of contraception to help prevent the infection from spreading. Condoms, diaphragms, and spermicidal suppositories, foams, and jellies can all deter the spread of certain STIs. Spermicidal agents may act as a disinfectant as well. Young people are especially susceptible. Traditionally, teenagers have not used birth-control methods at all and therefore remain at high risk for STIs and unwanted pregnancies. At this time, take a few minutes and list at least three ways you might bring up the subject of condoms with your partner. Also, think of ways you might convince a person to use a condom. If your partner refuses to use a condom, your answer should be quite simple: "No condom, no sex."
4. Know your partner and limit your sexual relationships. The days are gone when safe sex resulted from anonymous encounters at a bathhouse or a singles bar. Having only one partner lowers your chances of becoming infected. Although you can still become infected by having unprotected sex with one person only, the more partners you have, the greater are your chances for infection.
5. Don't have sex with prostitutes.
6. Determine the conditions under which you will allow sex. Ask yourself: "Am I willing to have sex with this person?" If you decide to have sex, practice safe sex. There is no reason to accept anything else. You will feel better about yourself.
7. Plan before you get into a sexual situation. Discuss STIs with the person you are contemplating having sex with before you do so. Even though talking about STIs might be awkward, the short-lived embarrassment of addressing intimate questions can keep you from contracting or spreading infection. If you don't know the person well enough to address this issue or you are uncertain about the answers, don't have sex with this individual.
8. Negotiate safer sex. Focus on the problem and not the person. Describe your feelings about the problem, using "I" instead of "you." For example, you might say, "I'm feeling awkward and uncomfortable. The only way I can feel comfortable is by using a condom." You also can offer options and provide alternative solutions. You might indicate to your partner, "We can work this out together. Let's go for a drive and get a condom. We'll feel better about what we're doing."
9. If you are sexually promiscuous, have periodic physical checkups. You can easily get exposed to an STI from a person who does not have any symptoms and who is unaware of the infection. Sexually promiscuous men and women between ages 15 and 35 are a particularly high-risk group for developing STIs.
10. Avoid sexual contact with anyone who has had sex with one or more individuals at risk for getting HIV, even if they are now practicing safer sex.
11. If you do have sex with someone who might be infected with HIV or whose history is unknown to you, avoid exchanging body fluids.
12. Don't share toothbrushes, razors, or other implements that could become contaminated with blood with anyone who is, or who might be, infected with HIV.
13. If you suspect that your partner is infected with an STI, ask. He or she may not even be aware of the infection, so look for signs, such as sores, redness, inflammation, a rash, growths, warts, or a discharge. If you are unsure, abstain.
14. If you know you have an infection, be responsible enough to abstain from sexual activity. Go to a physician or a clinic for treatment and ask your doctor when you can safely resume sexual activity. Abstain until it is safe. Just as you want to be protected in a sexual relationship, you should want to protect your partner as well. If you are diagnosed with an STI and you believe you know the person who gave it to you, think of ways you might bring up the subject of STIs with this person. You need to take responsibility and discuss this matter with your partner. As a result of your conversation,

medical treatment can be initiated and other people can be protected from infection as well.

15. Wear loose-fitting clothes made from natural fibers. Tight-fitting clothing made from synthetic fibers (especially underwear and nylon pantyhose) can create conditions that encourage the growth of bacteria and can actually aggravate STIs.
16. Consider abstaining from sexual relations if you have any kind of an illness or disease, even a common cold. Any kind of illness makes you more susceptible to other illnesses, and lower immunity can make you more vulnerable to STIs. The same holds true for times when you are under extreme stress, when you are fatigued, and when you are overworked. Drugs and alcohol also can lower your resistance to infection.
17. Thoroughly wash immediately after sexual activity. Although washing with hot, soapy water will not guarantee safety against STIs, it can prevent you from spreading certain germs on your fingers and might wash away bacteria and viruses that have not entered the body yet.
18. Be cautious regarding procedures (such as acupuncture, tattooing, and ear piercing) in which needles or other nonsterile instruments may be used again and again to pierce the skin or mucous membranes. These procedures are safe if proper sterilization methods are followed or disposable needles are used. Before undergoing the procedure, ask what precautions are being taken.
19. If you are planning to undergo artificial insemination, insist that frozen sperm be obtained from a laboratory that tests all donors for infection with HIV. Donors should be tested twice before the lab accepts the sperm—once at the time of donation and again a few months later.
20. If you know you will be having surgery in the near future, and if you are able, consider donating blood for your own use. This will eliminate completely the already small risk of contracting HIV through a blood transfusion. It also will eliminate the more substantial risk for contracting other blood-borne diseases, such as hepatitis, from a transfusion.

Avoiding risky behaviors that destroy quality of life and life itself is crucial to a healthy lifestyle. Learning the facts and acting on your personal values so that you can make responsible choices can protect you and those around you from painful, embarrassing, startling, unexpected, or fatal conditions.

ASSESS YOUR BEHAVIOR

CENGAGEbrain.com   To access course materials, including companion resources, please visit www.cengagebrain.com.

1. Do you believe that a mutually monogamous sexual relationship is the best way to prevent STIs? If not, do you always take precautions to practice safer sex?
2. If you are not prepared to have a sexual relationship, are you prepared to say so? Have you prepared exactly what to say if you are asked to have sex?
3. Have you carefully considered the consequences of engaging in a sexual relationship, including the risk for STIs, HIV infection, your partner being untruthful about his/her sexual history and STIs, and the potential of an unplanned pregnancy?
4. Are you capable of discussing your and your partner's sexual history prior to engaging in a sexual relationship that could bring about detrimental consequences for the rest of your life?
5. If you have an STI or a history of STIs, are you sufficiently responsible to have an open and honest discussion with a potential partner about the risk for infection and consequences thereof?

ASSESS YOUR KNOWLEDGE

Evaluate how well you understand the concepts presented in this chapter using the chapter-specific quizzing available in the online materials at www.cengagebrain.com.

1. What percentage of Americans will develop at least one STI in their lifetime?
   a. 30 to 40 percent
   b. 20 to 30 percent
   c. More than 50 percent
   d. 15 to 20 percent
   e. 40 to 50 percent

2. Which of the following sexually transmitted infections is not caused by a bacterial infection?
   a. chlamydia
   b. genital warts
   c. syphilis
   d. gonorrhea
   e. All of the above are caused by bacterial infections.

3. Chlamydia
   a. can cause damage to the reproductive system that cannot be reversed by treatment, even if successful.
   b. can cause infertility.
   c. may occur without symptoms.
   d. may cause arthritis.
   e. All choices are correct.

4. Gonorrhea can cause
   a. widespread bacterial infection.
   b. infertility.
   c. heart damage.
   d. arthritis.
   e. all of the above.

5. Treatment of genital warts is done by
   a. dissolving the warts with chemicals.
   b. electrosurgery.
   c. freezing the warts with liquid nitrogen.
   d. All of the above choices apply.
   e. None of the above choices is correct.

6. Herpes
   a. is incurable.
   b. causes sores that are treated with electrosurgery.
   c. requires antibiotics for successful treatment and cure.
   d. is caused by a bacterial infection.
   e. is not a serious STI because the person becomes uninfected once the sores heal.

7. Cold sores or fever blisters
   a. can cause genital herpes.
   b. are not highly contagious.
   c. are treatable if caused by bacterial infection.
   d. All of the above choices are correct.
   e. None of the above choices is correct.

8. The only way to determine whether someone is infected with HIV is through
   a. an AIDS outbreak.
   b. a physical exam by a physician.
   c. a bacterial culture test.
   d. an HIV antibody test.
   e. All choices are correct.

9. HIV
   a. attacks and destroys white blood cells.
   b. readily multiplies in the human body.
   c. breaks down the immune system.
   d. increases the likelihood of developing opportunistic infections and cancers.
   e. All of the above are correct.

10. The best way to protect yourself against STIs is
    a. through the use of condoms for all sexual acts.
    b. by knowing about the people who have previously had sex with your partner.
    c. through a mutually monogamous sexual relationship.
    d. by having sex only with an individual who has no symptoms of STIs.
    e. All of the above choices provide equal protection against STIs.

Correct answers can be found at the back of the book.

15 Lifetime Fitness and Wellness

The human body is extremely resilient during young age—not so during middle and older age. Lifestyle choices you make today will affect your health, well-being, and quality of life tomorrow.

Objectives

- **Understand** the effects of a healthy lifestyle on longevity.
- **Learn** to differentiate between physiological and chronological age.
- **Estimate** your life expectancy and determine your real physiological age.
- **Learn** about complementary and alternative medicine practices.
- **Learn** guidelines for preventing consumer fraud.
- **Understand** factors to consider when selecting a health/fitness club.
- **Know** how to select appropriate exercise equipment.
- **Review** health/fitness accomplishments and chart a wellness program for the future.
- **Evaluate** how you have changed and plan for a healthy future.

CENGAGEbrain.com
Visit www.cengagebrain.com to access course materials and companion resources for this text, including quiz questions designed to check your understanding of the chapter contents. See the preface on page ix for more information.

How does regular physical activity affect chronological versus physiological age?

Chronological age is your actual age—that is, how old you are. Physiological age is used in reference to your functional capacity to perform physical work at any stage of your life. Data on individuals who have taken part in systematic physical activity throughout life indicate that these people maintain a higher level of functional capacity and do not experience the declines typical in later years. From a functional point of view, typical sedentary people in the United States are about 25 years older than their chronological age indicates. Thus, an active 60-year-old person can have a physical capacity similar to that of an inactive 35-year-old person. Similarly, a sedentary 20-year-old college student most likely has the physical capacity of a 45-year-old active individual.

What are the differences among conventional medicine, complementary and alternative medicine, and integrative medicine?

Conventional medicine implies the practice of traditional medicine by medical doctors, osteopaths, and allied health professionals such as registered nurses, physical therapists, and psychologists. Complementary and alternative medicine comprises a group of diverse medical and health care systems, practices, and products that are not presently considered to be part of conventional medicine. The safety and effectiveness of many of these practices have not been rigorously tested through well-designed scientific studies. Integrative medicine uses a combination of conventional medicine and complementary and alternative medicine treatments for which there is some scientific evidence of safety and effectiveness.

What is the greatest benefit of a lifetime wellness lifestyle?

There are many benefits derived from an active wellness lifestyle, including greater functional capacity, good health, less sickness, lower health care expenses and time under medical supervision, and a longer and more productive life. Without question, these benefits altogether translate into one great benefit: an optimum quality of life. That is, the freedom to live life to its fullest without functional and health limitations. Most people go through life wishing that they could live without these limitations. The power, nevertheless, is within each of us to do so. And it is accomplished only by taking action today and living a wellness way of life for the rest of our lives.

Real Life Story | Ken's Experience

Over the course of the fitness and wellness class I took last year, I made changes to my habits for the better. I started exercising regularly and eating better, and I even tried meditation. I can honestly say that by the end of the class, I was feeling as good and healthy as I ever have before. However, I have a history of going back and forth between being fit and being out of shape. When I was younger, I ran track, and when I was training and racing during the school year, I would be in excellent shape. Then when summer came, I would mostly stop running, eat whatever junk food I wanted, gain weight, and be a couch potato. When the new school year started, I would have to start from the very beginning to try to get back in shape. When I started college, I was no longer involved in track, so I followed the earlier pattern of letting myself go. It wasn't until my junior year, when I took the fitness class that I started exercising again. So as the class was ending, I was concerned that I would no longer have the motivation to work out and be healthy, once I didn't have my teacher and classmates there to reinforce the healthy habits. But I thought about it, and I realized that my reasons for being healthy shouldn't just be because of external factors, like doing well at track or getting a good grade in class and keeping up with my classmates. I wanted to be healthy for myself, so I can live a long, high quality life where I look and feel great. So when my class ended, rather than forgetting about fitness, I set new SMART goals for myself, and made a commitment to stick with it. Now, almost six months later, rather than turning back into a couch potato, I have become even more fit than I was when class ended. I intend to continue my healthy diet and exercise habits for a lifetime.

Chapter 15 Lifetime Fitness and Wellness

PERSONAL PROFILE: Lifetime Fitness and Wellness

I. Have you considered how long you would like to live and what type of health and well-being you desire to enjoy throughout life? If so, what lifestyle habits have you implemented that will contribute to this end? Can you elaborate?

II. Do you understand the difference between chronological and physiological age? What is your current physiological age?

III. Have you ever sought out complementary or alternative medical treatments? If you have done so and feel comfortable talking about it, what was it for and what results did you obtain?

IV. Have you ever been the victim of quackery and fraud? If such is the case, how were you entrapped? Can you discuss precautions that a person can take to prevent such occurrences?

V. Have you planned and written out short-term and long-range SMART goals to attain now that you are about to finish this course? What arrangements have you made to maintain your exercise program and other healthy lifestyle habits? What can you do to stay up-to-date on fitness and wellness concepts and future developments in the field? Explain.

Better health, higher quality of life, and longevity are the three most important benefits derived from a lifetime fitness and wellness program. You have learned that physical fitness in itself does not always lower the risk for chronic diseases and ensure better health. Thus, implementation of healthy behaviors is the only way to attain your highest potential for well-being. The real challenge will come now that you are about to finish this course: maintaining your own lifetime commitment to fitness and wellness. Adhering to a program in a structured setting is a lot easier, but from now on, you will be on your own.

In this chapter you will have an opportunity to evaluate how well you are adhering to health-promoting behaviors and how these behaviors will affect your **physiological age** and length of life. You will also learn how to chart a personal wellness program for the future.

Research data indicate that healthy (and unhealthy) lifestyle actions you take today will have an impact on health and quality of life in middle and advanced age. Whereas most young people don't seem to worry much about health and longevity, you may want to take a closer look at the quality of life of your parents or other middle-aged and older friends and relatives that you know. Though you may have a difficult time envisioning yourself at that age, their health status and **functional capacity** may help you determine how you would like to live when you reach your fourth, fifth, and subsequent decades of life.

Although previous research has documented declines in physiological function and motor capacity as a result of aging, no hard evidence at present proves that large declines in physical work capacity are related primarily to aging alone. Lack of physical activity—a common phenomenon in our society as people age—is accompanied by decreases in physical work capacity that are greater by far than the effects of aging itself.

Unhealthy behaviors precipitate premature aging. For sedentary people, any type of physical activity is seriously impaired by age 40 and productive life ends before age 60. Most of these people hope to live to be age 65 or 70 and often must cope with serious physical ailments. These people "stop living at age 60 but are buried at age 70" (see the theoretical model in Figure 15.1).

Good physical fitness provides freedom to enjoy many of life's recreational and leisure activities without limitations.

Scientists believe that a healthy lifestyle allows people to live a vibrant life—a physically, intellectually, emotionally, socially active, and functionally independent existence—to age 95. Such are the rewards of a wellness way of life. When death comes to active people, it usually is rather quick and not as a result of prolonged illness. In Figure 15.1, note the low, longer slope of the "sedentary/unhealthy lifestyle" before death.

15.1 Life Expectancy and Physiological Age

Aging is a natural process, but some people seem to age better than others. Most likely you know someone who looks much younger than his or her **chronological age** indicates—and vice versa, that is,

> **Physiological age** The biological and functional capacity of the body as it should be in relation to the person's maximal potential at any given age in the lifespan.
>
> **Functional capacity** The ability to perform the ordinary and unusual demands of daily living without limitations and excessive fatigue or injury.
>
> **Chronological age** Calendar age.

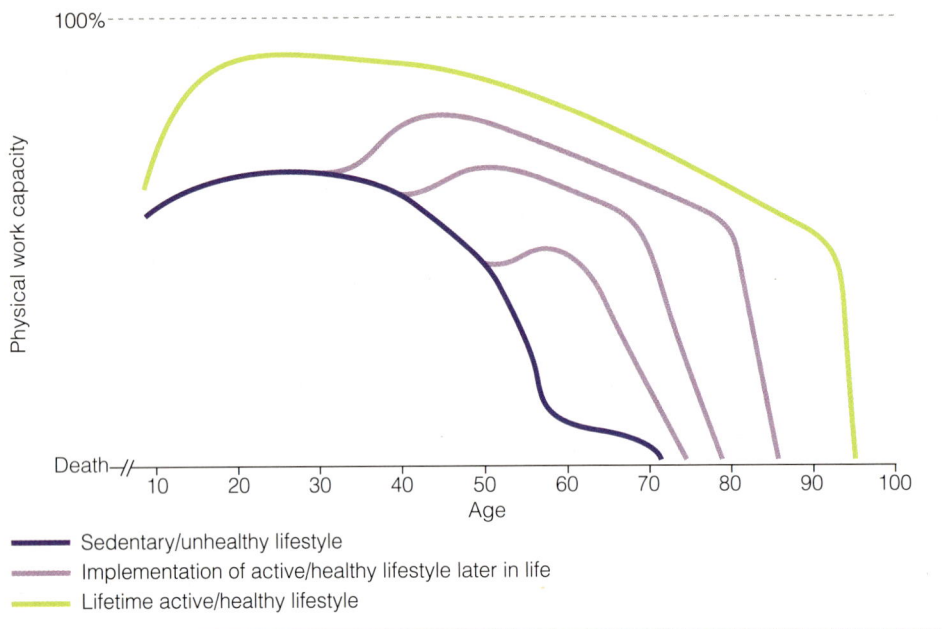

Figure 15.1 Relationships between physical work capacity, aging, and lifestyle habits.

— Sedentary/unhealthy lifestyle
— Implementation of active/healthy lifestyle later in life
— Lifetime active/healthy lifestyle

SOURCE: http://www.cdc.gov/hiv/pdf/statistics_surveillance_airtrends.pdf, downloaded July 1, 2013.

someone who appears much older than his or her chronological age indicates. For example, you may have an instructor who you would have guessed was about 40, but in reality is 52 years old. On the other hand, you may have a relative who looks 60 but is actually 50 years old. Why the differences?

During the aging process, natural biological changes occur within the body. Although no single measurement can predict how long you will live, the rate at which aging changes take place depends on a combination of genetic and lifestyle factors. Your lifestyle habits will determine to a great extent how your genes will affect your aging process. Hundreds of research studies now point to critical lifestyle behaviors that will determine your statistical chances of dying at a younger age or living a longer life. Research also shows that lifestyle behaviors have a far greater impact on health and longevity than your genes alone.

> **Critical Thinking**
>
> How long would you like to live, and are you concerned about how you will live the rest of your life?

Throughout this book, you have studied many of these factors. The question that you now need to ask yourself is: Are your lifestyle habits accelerating or decelerating the rate at which your body is aging? To help you determine how long and how well you may live the rest of your life, the **Life Expectancy** and Physiological Age Prediction questionnaire provided in Activity 15.1, can help answer this question. By looking at 48 critical genetic and lifestyle factors, you will be able to estimate your life expectancy and your real physiological age. Of greater importance, most of these factors are under your own control, and you can do something to make them work for you instead of against you.

As you fill out the questionnaire, you must be completely honest with yourself. Your life expectancy and physiological age prediction are based on your present lifestyle habits, should you continue those habits for life. Using the questionnaire, you will review factors you can modify or implement in daily living that may add years and health to your life. Please note that the questionnaire is not a precise scientific instrument, but rather an estimated life expectancy analysis according to the impact of lifestyle factors on health and longevity. Also, the questionnaire is not intended as a substitute for advice and tests conducted by medical and health care practitioners.

15.2 Conventional Western Medicine

Conventional Western medicine also known as allopathic medicine, has seen major advances in care and treatment modalities during the last few decades. Conventional medicine is based on scientifically proven methods, wherein medical treatments are tested through rigorous scientific trials. In addition to a **primary care physician** (medical doctor), people seek advice from other practitioners of conventional medicine, including **osteopaths, dentists, oral surgeons, orthodontists, ophthalmologists, optometrists, physician assistants**, and **nurses**.

Finding a physician: Invariably there are times when you will need medical attention. Finding the right physician isn't exactly the easiest task because there are no good resources available to do so. Preventive health care professionals caution that you should shop for a doctor the same way you do research to shop for other items and get the best quality care for your investment. Having a primary care physician is important to establish a relationship with your doctor while you are in good health and subsequently get the best possible care you deserve when truly needed. Attempting to get an appointment on short notice is often difficult for new patients and the choices can be limited.

Most people select a physician by word of mouth through family and friends, but your search requires more than that. You ought to be comfortable with your doctor, and a few questions and skepticism on your part may help. If you trust your doctor, you can be completely open about your health care concerns. If a follow-up consultation is needed, your physician can help direct you to the appropriate specialist to coordinate your care.

As you start your search, determine your medical needs. Now take a look at the list of doctors in your health care plan and cross-check the list with the top doctors in the area where you live. Location and hospital affiliations are important to consider as well. Having to travel a long distance discourages patients from seeking medical care when recommended or needed. Next, inquire about education, qualifications, skills, residency, and experience so that they meet your expectations. Additionally, because your association with your physician may become a lifetime relationship, you want to make sure that your personalities agree.

Other considerations include gender and age. Many women prefer female physicians for certain conditions, whereas men are more open to either gender. Older physicians are more experienced, while younger ones may be more in tune with recent advances and new medical procedures and technologies. You need to decide for yourself about your comfort zone and potential treatment options for your condition.

Finally, performing an Internet search provides valuable information about the physician's practice, friendliness, and availability to patients. Some sites provide information regarding board certification and possible disciplinary actions. Once you have narrowed your search, an introductory phone conversation is fully within your right. Most physicians are open to such a conversation. A choice not to do so gives you information about the doctor's personality, time constraints, or openness with patients.

Searching for a hospital: Another point to consider is the choice of hospital if a medical procedure is needed. An alarming statistic in the United States is that almost 100,000 hospital patients die each year from medical errors.[1] This figure represents more than double the number of people killed in automobile accidents each year. The data shows that about 5 percent of all hospital patients develop an infection while hospitalized. Selecting the appropriate facility is just as important as finding a good physician. Research has shown that patients get better medical care in some hospitals, experience fewer medical complications, and receive better attention for their needs. To decide on a hospital, follow these simple steps:

1. Does the hospital routinely handle your medical procedure? Check the hospital's record of treating patients with your condition in a safe and effective way. As with the physician of your choice, the more experienced the staff is with your procedure, the better the outcome for you.
2. Is the hospital accredited by The Joint Commission? The Joint Commission is an independent foundation that administers accreditation programs for hospitals and other healthcare organizations.
3. Does your doctor have privileges at the hospital (is he permitted to admit patients)?
4. Is the hospital covered by your health care plan?
5. What is the hospital readmission or bounce back rate? The bounce back rate is a medical term used to look at how many patients require rehospitalization within 30 days of the procedure. The higher the rate, the higher the risk for post-medical care complications. At present, one in five admissions results in

> **Life expectancy** How many years a person is expected to live.
>
> **Conventional Western medicine** Traditional medical practice based on methods that are tested through rigorous scientific trials; also called allopathic medicine.
>
> **Primary care physician** A medical practitioner who provides routine treatment for ailments; typically, the patient's first contact for health care.
>
> **Osteopath** A medical practitioner with specialized training in musculoskeletal problems who uses diagnostic and therapeutic methods of conventional medicine in addition to manipulative measures.
>
> **Dentist** Practitioner who specializes in diseases of the teeth, gums, and oral cavity.
>
> **Oral surgeon** A dentist who specializes in surgical procedures of the oral–facial complex.
>
> **Orthodontist** A dentist who specializes in the correction and prevention of teeth irregularities.
>
> **Ophthalmologist** Medical specialist concerned with diseases of the eye and prescription of corrective lenses.
>
> **Optometrist** Health care practitioner who specializes in the prescription and adaptation of lenses.
>
> **Physician assistant** Health care practitioner trained to treat most standard cases of care.
>
> **Nurse** Health care practitioner who assists in the diagnosis and treatment of health problems and provides many services to patients in a variety of settings.

readmission within 30 days. You can find out about the hospital bounce back rating at www.HospitalCompare.HHS.gov.

6. How well does the hospital check and improve its own safety record? Hospitals with effective staff communication, good team work, and regular patient care discussions have lower rates of infection than hospitals with a poor culture of safety. Although such data isn't readily available to the consumer, you can ask the hospital staff if they would trust their health care to their place of employment. Don't just accept a "yes" response, but evaluate the behavior, character, and choice of words in their response.

7. Have you discussed with former patients, family members, and friends their experience at the hospital? They can provide information on the treatment, response, friendliness, care, and helpfulness of the personnel, as well as privacy, comfort, and condition of the hospital.

8. Do you have a choice of procedures? If you do, always select a minimally invasive procedure. Discuss with your doctor all available options. If needed, opt for a second opinion. About one-third of second opinions differ from the initial diagnosis. Minimally invasive procedures have a lower risk of infection and involve shorter hospital stays and less pain.

9. What is the surgeon's experience? Death rates for any given surgical procedure are greatly reduced by the surgeon's experience with the procedure. Therein lies the importance of selecting a physician with ample experience in treating your condition.

10. Is the facility a teaching hospital with medical interns and residents? If so, inquire as to who will provide and oversee your care. If possible, avoid teaching hospitals during the month of July, when new interns and residents arrive and your medical care may not be as safe and efficient as the rest of the year.

11. Is the hospital a for-profit of not-for-profit hospital? For-profit hospitals may discharge you early or skip out on proper treatment because you are either uninsured or your health care plan only allows a certain amount of time in the hospital. If such is an issue, some consumer groups feel that you should think twice before going to a for-profit hospital.

12. Have you obtained a copy of your medical records? Request a copy of the physician's notes taken during your visit or procedure. Reviewing the notes can help clarify a diagnosis and the prescribed follow-up treatment. It will also allow you to correct any errors in information you provided your doctor. Under federal law, you have the right to obtain your records.

15.3 Complementary and Alternative Medicine

Notwithstanding modern technological and scientific advancements, many medical treatments either do not improve the patient's condition or create other ailments caused by the treatment itself. Only about 20 percent of conventional treatments have been proven to be clinically effective in scientific trials.[2] Thus, approximately 38 percent of adults (see Figure 15.2) and 12 percent of children in the United States are turning to **complementary and alternative medicine**, or CAM (also called "unconventional," or "nonallopathic," or "integrative" medicine) in search of answers to their health problems.[3] Unconventional medicine is referred to as complementary or alternative because patients use it to either augment their regular medical care or to replace conventional practices, respectively.

The reasons for seeking complementary and alternative treatments are diverse. Among the reasons commonly given by patients who seek unconventional treatments are lack of progress in curing illnesses and disease, frustration and dissatisfaction with physicians, lack of personal attention, testimonials about the effectiveness of alternative treatments, and rising health care costs. People who use CAM tend to be more educated and believe that body, mind, and spirit all contribute to good health.

The National Center for Complementary and Alternative Medicine (NCCAM) was established under the National Institutes of Health to examine methods of healing that have previously been unexplored by science. CAM includes treatments and health care practices not widely taught in medical schools, not generally used in hospitals, and not usually reim-

Complementary and alternative medicine (CAM) A group of diverse medical and health care systems, practices, and products that are not presently considered to be part of conventional medicine; also called unconventional, nonallopathic, or integrative medicine.

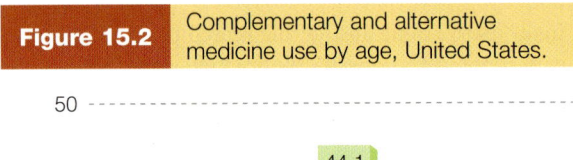

Figure 15.2 Complementary and alternative medicine use by age, United States.

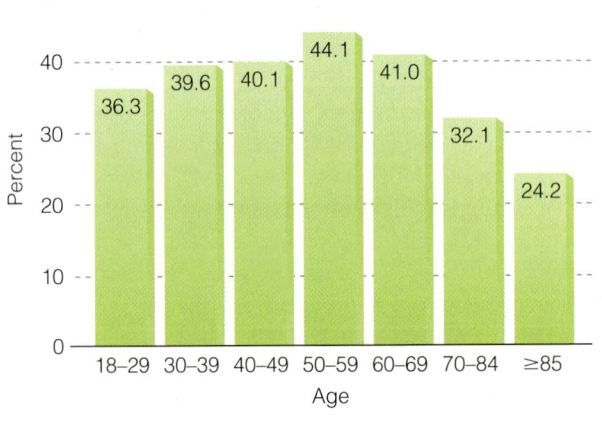

SOURCE: P. M. Barnes and B. Bloom. *Complementary and Alternative Medicine Use Among Adults and Children: United States 2007*. U.S. Department of Health and Human Service Centers for Disease Control and Prevention, National Health Statistics Reports, No. 12, December 10, 2008.

Chapter 15 Lifetime Fitness and Wellness   491

Activity 15.1: Life Expectancy and Physiological Age Prediction Questionnaire

Name _____ Date _____
Course _____ Section _____ Gender _____ Age _____

> **INSTRUCTIONS**
> Circle the points to the correct answer to each question. At the end of each page, obtain a net score for that page. Be completely honest with yourself. Your age prediction is based on your lifestyle habits, should you continue those habits for life. Using this questionnaire, you will learn about factors that you can modify or implement that can add years and health to your life. The scoring system is provided at the end of the questionnaire. Please note that the questionnaire is not a precise scientific instrument, but rather an estimated life expectancy analysis according to the impact of lifestyle factors on health and longevity. This questionnaire is not intended to substitute for advice and tests conducted by medical and healthcare practitioners.

Questionnaire

1. What is your current health status?
   - A. Excellent +2
   - B. Good +1
   - C. Average 0
   - D. Fair −1
   - E. Poor −2
   - F. Bad −3

2. How many days per week do you accumulate 30 minutes of moderate-intensity physical activity (at least 40 percent of heart rate reserve—see Chapter 6)?
   - A. More than 7 times per week +3
   - B. 6 or 7 +2
   - C. 3 to 5 0
   - D. 1 or 2 −1
   - E. Less than once per week −3

3. How often do you participate in a vigorous-intensity cardio-respiratory exercise (more than 60 percent of heart rate reserve) for at least 20 minutes?
   - A. 3 or more times per week +2
   - B. 2 times per week +1
   - C. Once a week −1
   - D. Less than once per week −2

4. How often do you perform strength-training exercises per week (a minimum of 8 exercises using 8 to 12 repetitions to near-fatigue on each exercise)?
   - A. 1–2 times +2
   - B. Less than once or less than 8 exercises with 8 to 12 reps per session 0
   - C. Do not strength train −1

5. How many times per week do you perform flexibility exercises (at least 15 minutes per stretching session)?
   - A. 3 or more +1
   - B. 1 to 3 times +.5
   - C. 1 time 0
   - D. Do not perform flexibility exercises −.5

6. How many servings of fruits and vegetables do you eat on a daily basis?
   - A. 9 or more +3
   - B. 6 to 8 +2
   - C. 5 +1
   - D. 3 or 4 0
   - E. 2 or less −2

7. How many grams of fiber do you consume on an average day?
   - A. 25 or over +1
   - B. Between 13 and 24 0
   - C. 10 to 12 or don't know −1
   - D. Less than 10 −2

8. As a percentage of total calories, what is your average fat intake daily?
   - A. 30% or less (mostly unsaturated) +1
   - B. 30% to 35% (mostly unsaturated) 0
   - C. More than 35% −2

9. As a percentage of total calories, what is your average saturated fat intake daily?
   - A. 5% or less +1
   - B. More than 5% but less than 7% 0
   - C. Don't know −1
   - D. More than 7% −2

10. How many servings of red meat (3 to 6 ounces) do you consume weekly?
    - A. 1 or none +1
    - B. 2 or 3 0
    - C. 4 to 7 −2
    - D. More than 7 −3

Page score: ☐

SOURCE: Fitness & Wellness, Inc., Boise, Idaho, ©2010. Reprinted with permission.

11. How many servings of omega-3-rich fish (3 to 6 ounces) do you consume weekly?
    A. 2 or more +2
    B. 1 0
    C. None −1

12. As a percentage of total calories, what is your average daily trans fatty acid intake?
    A. No trans fat intake +1
    B. Less than 1% 0
    C. 1% to 2% −1
    D. More than 2% −2

13. How many alcoholic drinks (a 12-ounce bottle of beer, a 4-ounce glass of wine, or a 1.5-ounce shot of 80-proof liquor) do you consume per day?
    A. Men 2 or less, women 1 or none +1
    B. None 0
    C. Men 3–4, women 2–4 −1
    D. 5 or more −3

14. How many milligrams of vitamin C do you get from food daily?
    A. Between 250 and 500 +1
    B. More than 90 but less than 250 +.5
    C. Less than 90 −1

15. How many micrograms of selenium do you get daily (preferably from food)?
    A. Between 100 and 200 +1
    B. Between 50 and 99 +.5
    C. Less than 50 −1

16. How many milligrams of calcium and how many international units of vitamin D do you get from food and supplements on an average day?
    A. Calcium = 1,200, vitamin D = 1,000 or more +1
    B. Calcium = 1,200, vitamin D = less than 1,000 +.5
    C. Calcium = 800 to 1,200, vitamin D = less than 1,000 0
    D. Calcium = less than 800, vitamin D = less than 1,000 −1

17. How many times per week do you eat breakfast?
    A. 7 +1
    B. 5 or 6 +.5
    C. 3 or 4 0
    D. Less than 3 −.5

18. How many cigarettes do you smoke each day?
    A. Never smoked cigarettes or more than 15 years since giving up cigarettes +2
    B. None for 5 to 14 years +1
    C. None for 1 to 4 years 0
    D. None for 0 to 1 year −1
    E. Smoker, less than 1 pack per day −3
    F. Smoker, 1 pack per day −5
    G. Smoker, up to 2 packs per day −7
    H. Smoker, more than 2 packs per day −10

19. Do you use tobacco products other than cigarettes?
    A. Never have 0
    B. Less than once per week −1
    C. Once per week −2
    D. 2 to 6 times per week −3
    E. More than 6 times per week −5

20. How often are you exposed to secondhand smoke or other environmental pollutants?
    A. Less than 1 hour per month 0
    B. Between 1 and 5 hours per month −1
    C. Between 5 and 29 hours per month −2
    D. Daily −3

21. Do you use addictive drugs, other than tobacco or alcohol?
    A. None 0
    B. 1 −3
    C. 2 or more −5

22. What is the age of your parents (or how long did they live)?
    A. Both older than 76 +3
    B. Only one older than 76 +1
    C. Both are still alive and younger than 76 0
    D. Only one younger than 76 −1
    E. Neither one lived past 76 −3

23. What is your body composition classification (see Table 4.11 on page 139)?
    A. Excellent +2
    B. Good +1
    C. Average 0
    D. Overweight −1
    E. Obese −2

24. What is your blood pressure?
    A. 120/80 or less (both numbers) +2
    B. 120–140 or 80–90 (either number) −1
    C. Greater than 140/90 (either number) −3

25. What is your HDL cholesterol?
    A. Men greater than 45, women greater than 55 +2
    B. Men 35 to 44, women 45 to 54 0
    C. Don't know −1
    D. Men less than 35, women less than 45 −2

26. What is your LDL cholesterol?
    A. Less than 100 +2
    B. 100 to 130 0
    C. 130 to 159 −1
    D. 160 or higher +2
    E. Don't know −2

27. Do you floss and brush your teeth regularly?
    A. Every day +.5
    B. 3 to 6 days per week 0
    C. Less than 3 days per week −.5

28. Are you a diabetic?
    A. No 0
    B. Yes, well-controlled −1
    C. Yes, poorly or not controlled −3

Page score: _____

29. How often do you get 10 to 20 minutes of unprotected ("safe") sun exposure between 10:00 a.m. and 4:00 p.m.?
   A. Almost daily +3
   B. 4 to 5 times per week +1
   C. 3 times per week 0
   D. 1 to 2 times per week −1
   E. Less than once per week −3

30. How often do you tan?
   A. Not at all +1
   B. Less than 3 times per year −1
   C. More than 3 times per year −2

31. How often do you wear a seat belt?
   A. All the time +1
   B. Most of the time −.5
   C. Less than half the time −1

32. How fast do you drive?
   A. Always at or less than the speed limit 0
   B. Up to 5 mph above the speed limit −.5
   C. Between 5 and 10 mph above the speed limit −1
   D. More than 10 mph above the speed limit −2

33. Do you drink and drive?
   A. Never 0
   B. Yes (even if only once) −5

34. Do you suffer from addictive behavior (misuse or abuse of alcohol, prescription and/or hard drugs)?
   A. No 0
   B. Yes −10

35. In terms of your sexual activity:
   A. I am not sexually active or I am in a monogamous sexual relationship +1
   B. I have more than one sexual partner but I always practice safe sex −1
   C. I have multiple sexual partners and I do not practice safe sex techniques −3

36. What is your marital status?
   A. Happily married +1
   B. Single and happy 0
   C. Single and unhappy −.5
   D. Divorced −1
   E. Widowed with a belief in life hereafter −1
   F. Widowed −2
   G. Married and unhappy −2

37. On the average, how many hours of sleep do you get each night?
   A. 8 +2
   B. 7 to 8 0
   C. 6 to 7 −1
   D. Less than 6 −2

38. Your stress rating according to the Stress Events Scale (see Activity 12.1, page 409) is:
   A. Excellent +1
   B. Good 0
   C. Average −.5
   D. Fair −1
   E. Poor −2

39. Your Type A behavior rating is:
   A. Low 0
   B. Medium −1
   C. High −2

40. When under stress (distress), how often do you practice stress management techniques?
   A. Always +1
   B. Most of the time +.5
   C. Not applicable (don't suffer from stress) 0
   D. Sometimes −1
   E. Never −2

41. Do you suffer from depression?
   A. Not at all 0
   B. Mild depression −1
   C. Severe depression −2

42. How often do you associate with people who have a positive attitude about life?
   A. Always +.5
   B. Most of the time 0
   C. About half of the time −.5
   D. Less than half the time −1

43. Do you have close family or personal relationships whom you can trust and rely on for help in times of need?
   A. Yes +1
   B. No −1

44. Do you feel loved and can you routinely give affection and love?
   A. Yes +1
   B. No −1

45. Do you have a good sense of humor?
   A. Yes +1
   B. No −1

46. How satisfied are you with your schoolwork?
   A. Satisfied +.5
   B. It's okay 0
   C. Not satisfied −.5

47. How do you rate your present job satisfaction?
   A. Love it +1
   B. Like it 0
   C. It's okay −.5
   D. Don't like it −1
   E. Hate it −2
   F. Not applicable 0

48. How do you rate yourself spiritually?
   A. Very spiritual +1
   B. Spiritual 0
   C. Somewhat spiritual −.5
   D. Not spiritual at all −1

Page score: ☐

Net score for all questions: ☐

How to Score

To estimate the total number of years that you will live, (a) determine a net score by totaling the results from all 48 questions, (b) obtain an age change score by multiplying the net score by the age correction factor given next, and (c) add or subtract this number from your base life expectancy age (76 for men and 81 for women—the current life expectancies in the United States). For example, if you are a 20-year-old male and the net score from the answers to all questions is −16, your estimated life expectancy would be 71.2 years (age change score = −16 × .3 = −4.8, life expectancy = 76 − 4.8 = 71.2).

You also can determine your real physiological age by subtracting a positive age-change score or adding a negative age-change score to your current chronological (calendar) age. For instance, in the previous example, the real physiological age would be 24.8 years (20 + 4.8). If the age change score had been +4.8, the real physiological age would have been 15.2 years (20 − 4.8). Thus, a healthy lifestyle will always make your physiological age younger than your chronological age. Your real physiological age will have much greater significance in middle and older age, when real-age reductions of 10 to 25 years occur in people who lead healthy lifestyles. Thus a 50-year-old person could easily have a real physiological age of 30.

Age Correction Factor (ACF)*

Age	ACF
≤30	.3
31–40	.4
41–50	.5
51–60	.6
61–70	.6
71–80	.5
81–90	.4
≥9	.3

*Adapted from M. F. Roizen, RealAge (New York: Cliff Street Books, 1999).

Age Change Score (ACS) = ☐ (net score) × ☐ (ACF) = ☐

Life Expectancy

Men = 76 ± ☐ (ACS) = ☐ years

Women = 81 ± ☐ (ACS) = ☐ years

Real Physiological Age**

Men = ☐ (your age) ± ☐ (ACS) = ☐ years

Women = ☐ (your age) ± ☐ (ACS) = ☐ years

**Subtract a positive ACS from, or add a negative ACS to, your current age.

Behavior Modification

State your feelings about the experience of taking this questionnaire, analyze your results, and list lifestyle factors that you can work on that will positively affect your health and longevity.

bursed by medical insurance companies. Many physicians now endorse complementary and alternative treatments, and an ever-increasing number of medical schools are offering courses in this area.

The NCCAM classifies CAM therapies into three broad categories[4]:

1. **Natural products**. Includes the use of a variety of herbal medicines (also known as botanicals), vitamins, minerals, and other "natural products." Many are sold over-the-counter as dietary supplements. (Some uses of dietary supplements—for example, taking a multivitamin to meet minimum daily nutritional requirements or taking calcium to promote bone health—are not considered CAM.) CAM "natural products," however, do include probiotics—live microorganisms (usually bacteria) that are similar to microorganisms normally found in the human digestive tract.

    Interest in and use of CAM natural products have grown considerably in recent decades. Approximately 17.7 percent of American adults use a nonvitamin/nonmineral natural product. The most commonly used product was fish oil/omega-3, reported by 37.4 percent of all adults who said they use natural products.

2. **Mind–body medicine**. This practice focuses on the interactions among the brain, mind, body, and behavior, with the intent to use the mind to affect physical functioning and promote health. Many CAM practices embody this concept in different ways. The most common are meditation, yoga, and acupuncture. Other examples of mind–body practices include deep-breathing exercises, guided imagery, progressive muscle relaxation, qi gong, and tai chi.

    Several mind–body approaches ranked among the top 10 CAM practices reported by adults. Data indicate that 12.7 percent of adults use deep-breathing exercises, 9.4 percent practice meditation, and 6.1 percent practice yoga. Progressive relaxation and guided imagery are also among the top 10 CAM therapies for adults.

3. **Manipulative and body-based practices**. This practice focuses primarily on the structures and systems of the body, including the bones and joints, soft tissues, and circulatory and lymphatic systems. Among the therapies within this category are spinal manipulation and massage therapy.

Spinal manipulation is performed by chiropractors and by other health care professionals such as physical therapists, osteopaths, and some conventional medical doctors. Practitioners use their hands or a device to apply a controlled force to a joint of the spine, moving it beyond its passive range of motion: The amount of force applied depends on the form of manipulation used. Spinal manipulation is among the treatment options used by people with low-back pain—a very common condition that can be difficult to treat. Massage therapy encompasses many different techniques. In general, therapists manipulate the muscles and other soft tissues of the body. People use massage for a variety of health-related purposes, including to relieve pain, rehabilitate sports injuries, reduce stress, increase relaxation, address anxiety and depression, and aid general well-being. About 8.6 percent of adults use chiropractic or osteopathic manipulation and 8.3 percent of adults use massage therapy.

Alternative medicine practices have not gone through the same standard scrutiny as conventional medicine. Nonallopathic treatments are often based on theories that have not been scientifically proven. This does not imply that unconventional medicine practices do not help people. Many people have found relief from ailments or been cured through unconventional treatments. In due time, however, these theories will need to be investigated using scientific trials similar to those in conventional medicine.

CAM includes a wide range of healing philosophies, approaches, and therapies. The practices most often associated with nonallopathic medicine are **acupuncture**, **chiropractics**, **herbal medicine**, **homeopathy**, **naturopathic medicine**, **ayurveda**, **magnetic therapy**, and **massage therapy**. Each of these practices offers a different approach to treatments based on its beliefs about the body, some of which are hundreds or thousands of years old.

Many of these practitioners believe that their treatment modality aids the body as it performs its own natural healing process. Because of their approach, alternative treatments usually take longer than conventional allopathic medical care. Nonallopathic treatments are usually less harsh on the patient, and practitioners tend to avoid surgery and extensive use of medications.

Unconventional therapies are frequently viewed as "holis-

> **Acupuncture** Chinese medical system that requires body piercing with fine needles during therapy to relieve pain and treat ailments and diseases.
>
> **Chiropractics** Health care system that proposes that many diseases and ailments are related to misalignments of the vertebrae and emphasizes the manipulation of the spinal column.
>
> **Herbal medicine** Unconventional system that uses herbs to treat ailments and disease.
>
> **Homeopathy** System of treatment based on the use of minute quantities of remedies that in large amounts produce effects similar to the disease being treated.
>
> **Naturopathic medicine** Unconventional system of medicine that relies exclusively on natural remedies to treat disease and ailments.
>
> **Ayurveda** Hindu system of medicine based on herbs, diet, massage, meditation, and yoga to help the body boost its own natural healing.
>
> **Magnetic therapy** Unconventional treatment that relies on magnetic energy to promote healing.
>
> **Massage therapy** The rubbing or kneading of body parts to treat ailments.

tic," implying that the practitioner looks at all the dimensions of wellness when evaluating a person's condition. Practitioners often persuade patients to adopt healthier lifestyle habits that not only help to improve current conditions but also prevent other ailments.

CAM also allows patients to better understand treatments, and patients are often allowed to administer self-treatment.

Costs for CAM practices are typically lower than conventional medicine costs. With the exception of acupuncture and chiropractic care, most nonallopathic treatments are not covered by health insurance. Typically, patients pay directly for these services. Estimates indicate that almost $34 billion out-of-pocket is spent a year on complementary and alternative medical treatments.[5] These costs exceeded the out-of-pocket expenses for all hospitalizations in the United States. If you are considering alternative medical therapies, consult with your health care insurance provider to determine which therapies are reimbursable.

CAM does have shortcomings, including the following:

1. Many of the practitioners do not have the years of education given to conventional medical personnel and often know less about physiological responses that occur in the body.
2. Some practices are completely devoid of science; hence, the practitioner can rarely explain the specific physiological benefits of the treatment used. Much of the knowledge is based on experiences with previous patients.
3. The practice of CAM is not regulated like that of conventional medicine. The training and certification of practitioners, malpractice liability, and evaluation of tests and methods used in treatments are not routinely standardized. Many states, however, license practitioners in the areas of chiropractic services, acupuncture, naturopathy, homeopathy, herbal therapy, and massage therapy. Other therapies, however, are unmonitored.
4. Unconventional medicine lacks regulation of natural and herbal products. The word "natural" does not imply that the product is safe. Many products, including some herbs, can be toxic in large doses.
5. About one-fifth of all prescription users combine high-dose vitamins and/or herbal supplements with prescription drugs.[6] Combinations such as these can yield undesirable side effects. Therefore, individuals should always let their health care practitioners know which medications and alternative (including vitamin and mineral) supplements are being taken in combination.

Herbal medicine has been around for centuries. Through trial and error, by design, or by accident, people have found that certain plant substances have medicinal properties. Today products that are safer and more effective and have fewer negative side effects have replaced many of these plant substances. Although science has found the mechanisms whereby some herbs work, much work remains to be done.

Many herbs or herbal remedies are not safe for human use and continue to meet resistance from the scientific community. One of the main concerns is that active ingredients in drug therapy must be administered in accurate dosages. With herbal medicine, the potency cannot always be adequately controlled.

Also, some herbs produce undesirable side effects. For example, ephedra (ma huang), a popular weight loss and energy supplement, can cause high blood pressure, rapid heart rate, tremor, seizures, headaches, insomnia, stroke, and even death. About 1,400 reports of adverse effects linked to herbal products containing ephedra, including 81 ephedra-related deaths, prompted its removal from the marketplace. St. John's wort, commonly taken as an antidepressant, can produce serious interactions with drugs used to treat heart disease. Ginkgo biloba impairs blood clotting, thus it can cause bleeding in people already on regular blood-thinning medication or aspirin therapy. Other herbs like yohimbe, chaparral, comfrey, and jin bu juan have been linked to adverse events.

Conventional health care providers are becoming more willing to refer you to someone who is familiar with alternative treatments, but you need to be an informed consumer. Ask your primary care physician to obtain valid information

A healthy lifestyle enhances functional capacity, quality of life, and longevity.

regarding the safety and effectiveness of a particular treatment. At times, nonetheless, the medical community resists and rejects unconventional therapies. If your physician is unable or unwilling to provide you with this information, medical, college, or public libraries and popular bookstores are good places to search for this information. You need to educate yourself about the advantages and disadvantages of alternative treatments, risks, side effects, expected results, and length of therapy.

Information on a wide range of medical conditions or specific diseases can also be obtained by calling the National Institutes of Health (NIH) at (301) 496-4000. Ask the operator to direct you to the appropriate NIH office. The NCCAM office also provides a Web site (http://nccam.nih.gov) with access to more than 180,000 bibliographic records of research published on CAM during the last 35 years.

When you select a primary care physician or a nonallopathic practitioner, consult local and state medical boards, other health regulatory boards and agencies, and consumer affairs departments for information about a given practitioner's education, accreditation, and license, and about complaints that may have been filed against this health care provider. Many of the unconventional medical fields also have a national organization that provides guidelines for practitioners and health consumers. These organizations can guide you to the appropriate regulatory agencies within your state where you can obtain information regarding a specific practitioner.

You may also talk to individuals who have undergone similar therapies and learn about the competence of the practitioner in question. Keep in mind, however, that patient testimonials do not adequately assess the safety and effectiveness of alternative treatments. Whenever possible, search for results of controlled scientific trials of the therapy in question and use this information in your decision process.

When undergoing any type of treatment or therapy, always disclose this information with all of your health care providers, whether conventional or unconventional. Adequate health care management requires that health care providers be informed of all concurrent therapies, so they will have a complete picture of the treatment plan. Lack of knowledge by one health care provider regarding treatments by another provider can interfere with the healing process or even worsen a given condition.

Millions of Americans have benefitted from CAM practices. You may also benefit from such services, but you need to make careful and educated decisions about the available options. By finding well-trained (and preferably licensed) practitioners, you increase your chances for recovery from ailments and disease.

> **Critical Thinking**
>
> Have you or someone you know ever used complementary or alternative medicine treatments? • What experiences did you have with these treatment modalities, and would you use them in the future?

Integrative Medicine Integrative medicine involves a combination of practices and methods of conventional Western medicine and alternative medicine. It takes into account the whole person and not just the disease. The approach encompasses all aspects of the individual's lifestyle. It is based on a partnership between the patient and the doctor, where the ultimate goal is to treat the body, mind, and spirit. It further involves principles of preventive medicine and therapies not accepted as "typical" medical practice, including prayer, meditation, social support, and recreation.

As a relatively new branch of medicine, departments are being instituted at some universities, and its practice is now available at several hospitals. The concept is not without its critics, as some physicians feel that the practice is driven by market forces and patients' need for hope. Patients are turning to integrative medicine because of their extreme dissatisfaction with physicians that rush them through appointments and seem to view them as simply another number going through the clinic.

15.4 Quackery and Fraud

The rapid growth of the fitness and wellness industry during the past four decades has spurred the promotion of fraudulent products that deceive consumers into "miraculous," quick, and easy ways to achieve total well-being. **Quackery** and **fraud** have been defined as the conscious promotion of unproven claims for profit.

Today's market is saturated with "special" foods, diets, supplements, pills, cures, equipment, books, and videos that promise quick, dramatic results. Advertisements for these products often are based on testimonials, unproven claims, secret research, half-truths, and quick-fix statements that the uneducated consumer wants to hear. In the meantime, the organization or enterprise making the claims stands to make a large profit from consumers' willingness to pay for astonishing and spectacular solutions to problems related to their unhealthy lifestyles.

Television, magazine, and newspaper advertisements are not necessarily reliable. For instance, one piece of equipment sold through television and newspaper advertisements promised to "bust the gut" through five minutes of daily exercise that appeared to target the abdominal muscle group. This piece of equipment consisted of a metal spring attached to the feet on one end and held in the hands on the other end. According to handling and shipping distributors, the equipment was "selling like hotcakes," and companies could barely keep up with consumer demand.

Three problems became apparent to the educated consumer: First, there is no such thing as spot reducing; therefore, the claims could not be true.

> **Integrative medicine** The combination of the practices and methods of alternative medicine with conventional Western medicine.
>
> **Quackery/fraud** The conscious promotion of unproven claims for profit.

Second, five minutes of daily exercise burn hardly any calories and therefore have no effect on weight loss. Third, the intended abdominal (gut) muscles were not really involved during the exercise. The exercise engaged mostly the gluteal and lower back muscles. This piece of equipment could then be found at garage sales for about a tenth of its original cost!

Although people in the United States tend to be firm believers in the benefits of physical activity and positive lifestyle habits as a means to promote better health, most do not reap these benefits because they simply do not know how to put into practice a sound fitness and wellness program that will give them the results they want. Unfortunately, many uneducated wellness consumers are targets of deception by organizations making fraudulent claims for their products.

Deception is not limited to advertisements. Deceit is all around us, in newspaper and magazine articles, trade books, radio, and television shows. To make a profit, popular magazines occasionally exaggerate health claims or leave out pertinent information to avoid offending advertisers. Some publishers print books on diets or self-treatment approaches that have no scientific foundation. Consumers should even be cautious about news reports of the latest medical breakthroughs. Reporters have been known to overlook important information or give certain findings greater credence than they deserve.

Precautions must also be taken when seeking health advice on the Internet. The Internet is full of both credible and dubious information. The following tips can help as you conduct a search on the Internet:

- Look for credentials of the person or organization sponsoring the site.
- Check when the site was last updated. Credible sites are updated often.
- Check the appearance of the information on the site. It should be presented in a professional manner. If every sentence ends with an exclamation point, you have a good cause for suspicion.
- Exercise caution if the site's sponsor is trying to sell a product. If so, be leery of opinions posted on the site. They could be biased, given that the company's main objective is to sell a product. Credible companies trying to sell a product on the Internet usually reference their sources of health information and provide additional links that support their product.

Behavior Modification Planning

Healthy Lifestyle Guidelines

1. Accumulate at least 30 minutes of moderate-intensity physical activity a minimum of 5 days per week.
2. Exercise aerobically in the proper cardiorespiratory training zone at least three times per week for a minimum of 20 minutes.
3. Accumulate at least 10,000 steps on a daily basis.
4. Strength-train at least once a week (preferably twice per week) using a minimum of eight exercises that involve all major muscle groups of the body.
5. Perform flexibility exercises that involve all major joints of the body at least two to three times per week.
6. Eat a healthy diet that is rich in whole-wheat grains, fruits, and vegetables and is low in saturated and trans fats.
7. Eat a healthy breakfast every day.
8. Do not use tobacco in any form, avoid secondhand smoke, and avoid all other forms of substance abuse.
9. Maintain healthy body weight (achieve a range between the high-physical fitness and health-fitness standards for percent body fat).
10. Get seven to eight hours of sleep per night.
11. Get 10 to 20 minutes of safe sun exposure on most days of the week.
12. Manage stress effectively.
13. Limit daily alcohol intake to two or less drinks per day if you are a man or one drink or less per day if you are a woman (or do not consume any alcohol at all).
14. Have at least one close friend or relative in whom you can confide and to whom you can express your feelings openly.
15. Be aware of your surroundings and take personal safety measures at all times.
16. Seek continued learning on a regular basis.
17. Subscribe to a reputable health/fitness/nutrition newsletter to stay up-to-date on healthy lifestyle guidelines.
18. Seek proper medical evaluations as necessary.

Try It

Now that you are about to complete this course, evaluate how many of the healthy lifestyle guidelines have become part of your personal wellness program. Prepare a list of those that you still need to work on and use Activity 15.4 to write SMART goals and specific objectives that will help you achieve the desired behaviors. Remember that each one of the guidelines will lead to a longer, healthier, and happier life.

© Cengage Learning

- Compare a site's content to other credible sources. The contents should be generally similar to that of other reputable sites or publications.
- Note the address and contact information for the company. A reliable company will list more than a P.O. box, an 800 number, and the company's e-mail address. When only the latter information is provided, consumers may never be able to locate the company for questions, concerns, or refunds.
- Be on the alert for companies that claim to be innovators while criticizing competitors or the government for being close-minded or trying to keep them from doing business.
- Watch for advertisers that use valid medical terminology in an irrelevant context or use vague pseudomedical jargon to sell their product.

Not all people who promote fraudulent products, however, know they are doing so. Some may be convinced that the product is effective. If you have questions or concerns about a health product, you may write to the National Council against Health Fraud (NCAHF), 119 Foster Street, Peabody, MA 01960. The purpose of this organization is to provide the consumer with responsible, reliable, evidence-driven health information. The organization also monitors deceitful advertising, investigates complaints, and offers public information regarding fraudulent health claims. You may also report any type of quackery to them on their website at www.ncahf.org/. The site contains an updated list of reliable and unreliable health websites for the consumer.

Other consumer protection organizations offer to follow up on complaints about quackery and fraud. The existence of these organizations, however, should not give the consumer a false sense of security. The overwhelming number of complaints made each year makes it impossible for these organizations to follow up on each case individually. The U.S. Food and Drug Administration's (FDA) Center for Drug Evaluation Research, for example, has developed a priority system to determine which health fraud product it should regulate first. Products are rated on how great a risk they pose to the consumer. With this in mind, you can use the following list of organizations to make an educated decision before you spend your money. You can also report consumer fraud to these organizations:

- Food and Drug Administration (FDA). The FDA regulates safety and the labeling of health products and cosmetics. You can search for the office closest to you in the federal government listings (blue pages) of the phone book.
- Better Business Bureau (BBB). The BBB can tell you whether other customers have lodged complaints about a product, a company, or a salesperson. You can find a listing for the local office in the business section of the phone book or you can check their Web site at www.bbb.com/.
- Consumer Product Safety Commission (CPS). This independent federal regulatory agency targets products that threaten the safety of American families. Unsafe products can be researched and reported on their website at www.cpsc.gov/.

Reliable Sources of Health, Fitness, Nutrition, and Wellness Information

Newsletter	Yearly Issues	Approx. Annual Cost
Bottom Line/Health www.BottomLinePublications.com 800-289-0409	12	$29.95
Consumer Reports on Health www.ConsumerReports.org/health 800-234-2188	12	$24
Environmental Nutrition www.environmentalnutrition.com 800-829-5384	12	$30
Tufts University Health & Nutrition Letter www.tuftshealthletter.com 800-274-7581	12	$28
University of California Berkeley Wellness Letter www.berkeleywellness.com 386-447-6328	12	$28

Another way to get informed before you make your purchase is to seek the advice of a reputable professional. Ask someone who understands the product but does not stand to profit from the transaction. As examples, a physical educator or an exercise physiologist can advise you regarding exercise equipment; a registered dietitian can provide information on nutrition and weight control programs; a physician can offer advice on nutritive supplements. Also, be alert to those who bill themselves as "experts." Look for qualifications, degrees, professional experience, certifications, and reputation.

Keep in mind that if it sounds too good to be true, it probably is. Fraudulent promotions often rely on testimonials or scare tactics and promise that their products will cure a long list of unrelated ailments; they use words like "quick fix," "time-tested," "newfound," "miraculous," "special," "secret," "all natural," "mail order only," and "money-back guarantee." Deceptive companies move often so that customers have no way of contacting the company to ask for reimbursement.

When claims are made, ask where the claims are published. Refereed scientific journals are the most reliable sources of information. When a researcher submits information for publication in a refereed journal, at least two qualified and reputable professionals in the field conduct blind reviews of the manuscript. A blind review means the author does not know who will review the manuscript, and the reviewers do not know who submitted the manuscript. Acceptance for publication is based on this input and relevant changes.

15.5 Looking at Your Fitness Future

Once you've decided to pursue a lifetime wellness program, you'll face several more decisions about exactly how to accomplish it. Following are a few issues you'll encounter.

Health/Fitness Club Memberships You may want to consider joining a health/fitness facility. Or, if you have mastered the contents of this book and your choice of fitness activity is one you can pursue on your own (walking, jogging, cycling), you may not need to join a health club. Barring injuries, you may continue your exercise program outside the walls of a health club for the rest of your life. You also can conduct strength training and stretching programs in your own home (see Chapters 7 and 8).

To stay up-to-date on fitness and wellness developments, you should buy a reputable and updated fitness/wellness book every four to five years. You may subscribe to a credible health, fitness, nutrition, or wellness newsletter to stay current. You can also surf the World Wide Web, but be sure that the sites you are searching are from credible and reliable organizations.

If you are contemplating membership in a fitness facility, do all of the following:

- Make sure that the facility complies with the standards established by the American College of Sports Medicine (ACSM) for health and fitness facilities. These standards are given in Figure 15.3.
- Examine all exercise options in your community: health clubs/spas, YMCAs, gyms, colleges, schools, community centers, senior centers, and the like.

Reliable Health Websites

- American Cancer Society
  www.cancer.org/
- American Heart Association
  www.heart.org
- American College of Sports Medicine
  www.acsm.org
- Clinical Trials Listing Service
  www.centerwatch.com
- Healthfinder—Your Guide to Reliable Health Information
  www.healthfinder.gov
- HospitalWeb
  http://neuro-www.mgh.harvard.edu/hospitalweb.shtml
- National Cancer Institute
  www.cancer.gov
- National Center for Complementary and Alternative Medicine
  http://nccam.nih.gov/
- The National Library of Medicine
  www.nlm.nih.gov/
- The National Institutes of Health
  www.nih.gov/
- The Centers for Disease Control and Prevention
  www.cdc.gov/
- The Medical Matrix (requires subscription)
  www.medmatrix.org/
- The National Council Against Health Fraud
  www.ncahf.org/
- The Food and Drug Administration
  www.fda.gov/
- WebMD
  http://webmd.com/
- World Health Organization
  www.who.int/en/

- Check to see if the facility's atmosphere is pleasant and nonthreatening to you. Will you feel comfortable with the instructors and other people who go there? Is it clean and well kept? If the answers are no, this may not be the right place for you.
- Analyze costs versus facilities, equipment, and programs. Take a look at your personal budget. Will you really use the facility? Will you exercise there regularly? Many people obtain memberships and permit dues to be withdrawn automatically from a credit card or local bank account, yet seldom attend the fitness center.

Figure 15.3 American College of Sports Medicine standards for health and fitness facilities.

1. A facility must have an appropriate emergency plan.
2. A facility must offer each adult member a preactivity screening that is relevant to the activities that will be performed by the member.
3. Each person who has supervisory responsibility must be professionally competent.
4. A facility must post appropriate signs in those areas of a facility that present potential increased risk.
5. A facility that offers services or programs to the youth must provide appropriate supervision.
6. A facility must conform to all relevant laws, regulations, and published standards.

SOURCE: *ACSM's Health/Fitness Facility Standards and Guidelines* (Champaign, IL: Human Kinetics, 2012).

- Find out what types of facilities are available: walking/running track, basketball/tennis/racquetball courts, aerobic exercise room, strength training room, pool, locker rooms, saunas, hot tubs, handicapped access, and so on.
- Check the aerobic, strength-training, and stretching equipment available. Does the facility have treadmills, bicycle ergometers, elliptical trainers, swimming pool, free weights, and strength-training machines? Make sure that the facilities and equipment meet your activity interests.
- Consider the location. Is the facility close, or do you have to travel several miles to get there? Distance often discourages participation.
- Check on times the facility is accessible. Is it open during your preferred exercise time (e.g., early morning or late evening)?
- Work out at the facility several times before becoming a member. Does it have ample space amidst all the equipment and people in the facility? Are people standing in line to use the equipment, or is it readily available during your exercise time?
- Evaluate the facility for cleanliness and hygiene. Is the equipment and facility regularly cleaned and disinfected? Sweat and body fluids are great environments for bacterial growth. The facility should also provide hand sanitizers, paper towels, facial tissue, and clean towels for members.
- Inquire about the instructors' knowledge and qualifications. Do the fitness instructors have college degrees or professional training certifications from organizations such as the ACSM, the American Council on Exercise (ACE), the National Strength and Conditioning Association (NSCA), or the National Academy of Sports Medicine (NASM)? These organizations have rigorous standards to ensure professional preparation and quality of instruction.
- Consider the approach to fitness (including all health-related components of fitness). Is it well rounded? Do the instructors spend time with members, or do members have to seek them out constantly for help and instruction?
- Ask about supplementary services. Does the facility provide or contract out for regular health and fitness assessments (cardiovascular endurance, body composition, blood pressure, blood chemistry analysis)? Are wellness seminars (nutrition, weight control, stress management) offered? Do these have hidden costs?

A personal trainer provides valuable guidance and helps motivate individuals to achieve fitness goals.

Personal Trainers The current way of life has opened an entire new job market for personal trainers who are presently in high demand by health and fitness participants. A **personal trainer** is a health/fitness professional who evaluates, motivates, educates, and trains clients to help them meet individualized healthy lifestyle goals. Rates typically range between $20 and $100 an hour. Some trainers offer reduced rates for extended packages or prepaid sessions. For most people, using the expertise of a personal trainer is an investment in fitness, health, and quality of life.

Exercise sessions are usually conducted at a health/fitness facility or at the client's own home. Experience and the ability to design safe and effective programs based on the client's current fitness level, health status, and fitness goals are important. Personal trainers also recognize their limitations and refer clients to other health care professionals as necessary.

Currently, anyone who prescribes exercise can make the claim to be a personal trainer without proof of education, experience, or certification. Although good trainers need to strive to maximize their own health and fitness, a good physique and previous athletic experience do not certify a person as a personal trainer.

Because of the high demand for personal trainers, more than 200 organizations now certify fitness specialists. This has led to great confusion by clients on how to evaluate the credentials of personal trainers. "Certification" and a "certificate" are different. Certification implies that the individual has met educational and professional standards of performance and competence. A certificate typically is awarded to individuals who attend a conference or workshop but are not required to meet any professional standards.

Presently, no licensing body is in place to oversee personal trainers. Thus, becoming a personal trainer is easy. At a minimum, personal trainers should have an undergraduate degree and certification from a reputable organization such as ACSM, ACE, NSCA, or NASM. Undergraduate

> **Personal trainer** A health/fitness professional who evaluates, motivates, educates, and trains clients to help them meet individualized, healthy, lifestyle goals.

(and graduate) degrees should be conferred in a fitness-related area such as exercise science, exercise physiology, kinesiology, sports medicine, or physical education. When looking for a personal trainer, always inquire about the trainer's education and certification credentials.

Before selecting a trainer, you must establish your program goals. Following are sample questions to ask yourself and consider when interviewing potential trainers prior to selecting one:

- Can the potential personal trainer provide you with a resume?
- What type of professional education and certification does the potential trainer possess?
- How long has the person been a personal trainer and are references available on request?
- Are you looking for a male or female trainer?
- What are the fees? Are multiple sessions cheaper than a single session? Can individuals be trained in groups? Are there cancellation fees if you are not able to attend a given session?
- How long will you need the services of the personal trainer: one session, multiple sessions, periodically, or indefinitely?
- What goals do you intend to achieve with the guidance of the personal trainer: weight loss, cardiorespiratory fitness, strength and/or flexibility fitness, improved health, or sport fitness conditioning?
- What type of personality are you looking for in the trainer—a motivator, a hard-challenging trainer, a gentle trainer, or professional counsel only?

When seeking fitness advice from a health/fitness trainer via the Internet, here's a final word of caution: Be aware that certain services cannot be provided over the Internet. An Internet trainer is not able to directly administer fitness tests, motivate, observe exercise limitations, or respond effectively in an emergency situation (spotting, or administering first aid or cardiopulmonary resuscitation [CPR]), and thus is not able to design the most safe and effective exercise program for you.

15.6 Purchasing Exercise Equipment

A final consideration is that of purchasing your own exercise equipment. The first question you need to ask yourself is: Do I really need this piece of equipment? Most people buy on impulse because of television advertisements or because a salesperson has convinced them it is a great piece of equipment that will do wonders for their health and fitness. Ignore claims that an exercise device or machine can provide "easy/no-sweat" results in a few minutes only. Keep in mind that the benefits of exercise are obtained only if you do exercise. With some creativity, you can implement an excellent and comprehensive exercise program with little, if any, equipment (see Chapters 6, 7, 8, and 9).

Many people buy expensive equipment only to find they really do not enjoy that mode of activity. They do not remain regular users. Stationary bicycles (lower body only) and rowing ergometers were among the most popular pieces of equipment a few years ago. Most of them now are seldom used and have become "fitness furniture" somewhere in the basement. Furthermore, be skeptical of testimonials and before-and-after pictures from "satisfied" customers. These results may not be typical, and it doesn't mean that you will like the equipment as well.

Exercise equipment does have its value for people who prefer to exercise indoors, especially during the winter months. It supports some people's motivation and adherence to exercise. The convenience of having equipment at home also allows for flexible scheduling. You can exercise before or after work or while you watch your favorite television show.

If you are going to purchase equipment, the best recommendation is to actually try it out several times before buying it. Ask yourself several questions: Did you enjoy the workout? Is the unit comfortable? Are you too short, tall, or heavy for it? Is it stable, sturdy, and strong? Do you have to assemble the machine? If so, how difficult is it to put together? How durable is it? Ask for references—people or clubs that have used the equipment extensively. Are they satisfied? Have they enjoyed using the equipment? Talk with professionals at colleges, sports medicine clinics, or health clubs.

Another consideration is to look at used units for signs of wear and tear. Quality is important. Cheaper brands may not be durable, so your investment would be wasted.

Finally, watch out for expensive gadgets. Monitors that provide exercise heart rate, work output, caloric expenditure, speed, grade, and distance may help motivate you, but they are expensive, need repairs, and do not enhance the actual fitness benefits of the workout. Look at maintenance costs and check for service personnel in your community.

> **Critical Thinking**
>
> Do you admire certain people around you and would like to emulate their wellness lifestyle? • What behaviors do these people exhibit that would help you adopt a healthier lifestyle?
> • What keeps you from emulating these behaviors, and how can you overcome these barriers?

15.7 Self-Evaluation and Behavioral Goals for the Future

The main objective of this book is to provide the information and experiences necessary to implement your personal fitness and wellness program. If you have implemented the programs in this book, including exercise, you should be convinced that a wellness lifestyle is the only way to attain a higher quality of life.

Activity 15.2: Fitness and Wellness Community Resources

Name _____ Date _____

Course _____ Section _____ Gender _____ Age _____

NECESSARY LAB EQUIPMENT
None required.

OBJECTIVE
To identify community resources available for you to continue your path toward lifetime fitness and wellness.

INSTRUCTION
Using a community directory, identify a minimum of three fitness, recreational, or wellness facilities that will allow you to maintain and further develop your personal fitness and wellness program. Initially, contact all three facilities by phone to obtain the pertinent information (see Item I). On completion of this task, make an appointment to personally visit at least one of the facilities during a time when you would work out, and evaluate the equipment, equipment availability, personnel, and programs that would be available to you. Keep in mind that one of the options available to you may be your own campus health/fitness/recreation center. College alumni, for a fee, often have the option to continue to use such a facility.

I. Initial Contact

	Facility I	Facility II	Facility III
Facility Name:			
Address:			
Distance from home:			
Mode of transportation to the facility:			
Travel time to the facility:			
Monthly fee:			
Hours of operation:			
Cardio equipment:			
Strength training:			
Flexibility equipment:			
Personal trainers, availability and costs:			
Personal trainers' certifications:			
Fitness tests, availability and costs:			
Exercise classes:			
Other services (nutrition, stress management, smoking cessation, cardiac profiles, etc.):			
Free trial of facility available?			

II. Facility Visit and Evaluation

1. Provide an overall impression of the facility:

   _____
   _____
   _____

2. Was the staff knowledgeable, accessible, and friendly?

   _____
   _____
   _____

3. Were you able to work out at the facility?   ___ Yes ___ No
   If so, was the equipment available and suitable to your preferences?

   _____
   _____
   _____

   Did you feel comfortable with other individuals using the facility (please indicate why or why not)?

   _____
   _____
   _____

4. Provide an overall evaluation of the locker facilities and other amenities available to you.

   _____
   _____
   _____

5. Overall letter grade for the facility: A   B   C   D   E   F

III. Ongoing Educational Program

1. Are there any other community resources available to you that would benefit your personal health, fitness, and wellness lifestyle program? Please list:

   _____
   _____
   _____

2. Contact at least one reliable health, fitness, nutrition, or wellness newsletter that you may subscribe to (see page 499) for a free copy and list the newsletter in the space provided. Also indicate if there are any other fitness/wellness materials that have provided valuable information to you.

   _____
   _____
   _____

3. List at least three reliable and helpful websites that you accessed this term and indicate why these sites were useful to you.

   _____
   _____
   _____

Most people who engage in a personal fitness and wellness program experience this new quality of life after only a few weeks of training and practicing healthy lifestyle patterns. In some instances, however—especially for individuals who have led a poor lifestyle for a long time—a few months may be required to establish positive habits and feelings of well-being. In the end, though, everyone who applies the principles of fitness and wellness will reap the desired benefits.

Prior to the completion of this course, you now need to identify community resources available to you that will support your path to lifetime fitness and wellness. Activity 15.2 will provide a road map to initiate your search for this support. You will find the process beneficial, one that will help you maintain your new wellness way of life.

Self-Evaluation Throughout this course you have had an opportunity to assess various fitness and wellness components and write goals to improve your quality of life. You now should take the time to evaluate how well you have achieved your own goals. Ideally, if time allows and facilities and technicians are available, reassess the health-related components of physical fitness. If you are unable to reassess these components, determine subjectively how well you accomplished your goals. You will find a self-evaluation form in Activity 15.3.

Behavioral Goals for the Future The real challenge will come now that you are about to finish this course: a lifetime commitment to fitness and wellness. Adhering to a program in a structured setting is a lot easier, but from now on you will be on your own. Realizing that you may not have achieved all of your goals during this course, or perhaps you need to reach beyond your current achievements, the Wellness Scale provided in Activity 15.3 will help you chart the future. This guide provides a list of various wellness components, each illustrating a scale from poor to excellent. Using the Wellness Scale, rate yourself for each component according to the following instructions:

1. Indicate with an "I" (I = Initial) the category from poor to excellent where you stood on each component at the beginning of the term. For example, if at the start of this course, you rated poor in cardiorespiratory endurance, place an "I" under the poor column for this component.
2. Mark with a "C" (C = Current) a second column (between poor and excellent) to indicate where you stand on each component at the current time. If your level of cardiorespiratory endurance improved to average by the end of the term, write a "C" under this column. If you were not able to work on a given component, simply make a "C" out of the "I."
3. Select one or two components you intend to work on in the next two months. Developing new behavioral patterns takes time, and trying to work on too many components at once most likely will lower your chances for success. Start with components in which you think you will have a high chance for success.

Next, place a "G" (G = Goal) under the intended goal column to accomplish by the end of this period. If your goal in the next 2 months is to achieve a "good" level of cardiorespiratory endurance, place a "G" under the good column for this component in the Wellness Scale.

Use Activity 15.4 to write the goals and actions for two components you intend to work on during the next two months. As you write and work on these goals and actions, review the goal-setting guidelines provided in Chapter 2, pages 61–68. Using these guidelines will help you design an effective plan of action to reach your goals. You are encouraged to keep this form (activity) in a place that you will remember so that you may review it in months and years to come.

One final assignment that you should complete is to summarize your feelings about your past and present lifestyle, what you have learned in this course, and changes that you were able to successfully implement. Activity 15.5 can be used for this experience.

15.8 The Fitness/Wellness Experience and a Challenge for the Future

Patty Neavill is a typical example of someone who often tried to change her life but was unable to do so because she did not know how to implement a sound exercise and weight control program. At age 24 and at 240 pounds, she was discouraged with her weight, level of fitness, self-image, and quality of life in general. She had struggled with her weight most of her life. Like thousands of other people, she had made many unsuccessful attempts to lose weight.

Patty put her fears aside and decided to enroll in a fitness course. As part of the course requirement, a battery of fitness tests was administered at the beginning of the semester. Patty's cardiovascular endurance and muscular (strength) fitness ratings were poor, her flexibility classification was average, and her percent body fat was 41.

Following the initial fitness assessment, Patty met with her course instructor, who prescribed an exercise and nutrition program like the one in this book. Patty fully committed to carry out the prescription. She walked/jogged five times a week. She enrolled in a weight-training course that met twice a week. Her daily caloric intake was set in the range of 1,500 to 1,700.

Determined to increase her level of activity further, Patty signed up for recreational volleyball and basketball courses. Besides being fun, these classes provided four additional hours of activity per week.

She took care to meet the minimum required servings from the basic food groups each day, which contributed about 1,200 calories to her diet. The remainder of the calories came primarily from complex carbohydrates.

At the end of the 16-week semester, Patty's cardiovascular endurance, muscular fitness, and flexibility ratings had all improved to the Good category, she had lost 50 pounds, and her percent body fat had decreased to 22.5!

Patty was tall. At 190 pounds, most people would have thought she was too heavy. Her percent body fat, however, was lower than the average for college female physical education major students (about 23 percent body fat).

A thank-you note from Patty to the course instructor at the end of the semester read:

Thank you for making me a new person. I truly appreciate the time you spent with me. Without your kindness and motivation, I would have never made it. It is great to be fit and trim. I've never had this feeling before, and I wish everyone could feel like this once in their life.

Thank you,
Your trim Patty!

Patty had never been taught the principles governing a sound weight loss program. In Patty's case, not only did she need this knowledge, but, like most Americans who never have experienced the process of becoming physically fit, she needed to be in a structured exercise setting to truly feel the joy of fitness.

Even more significant was that Patty maintained her aerobic and strength-training programs. A year after ending her calorie-restricted diet, her weight increased by 10 pounds, but her body fat decreased from 22.5 to 21.2 percent. As you may recall from Chapter 5, this weight increase is related mostly to changes in lean tissue that is lost during the weight-reduction phase.

In spite of only a slight drop in weight during the second year following the calorie-restricted diet, the 2-year follow-up revealed a further decrease in body fat, to 19.5 percent. Patty understood the new quality of life reaped through a sound fitness program, and at the same time, she finally learned how to apply the principles that regulate weight maintenance.

If you have read and successfully completed all of the assignments set out in this book, including a regular exercise program, you should be convinced of the value of exercise and healthy lifestyle habits in achieving a new quality of life.

Perhaps this new quality of life was explained best by the late Dr. George Sheehan, when he wrote[7]:

For every runner who tours the world running marathons, there are thousands who run to hear the leaves and listen to the rain, and look to the day when it is all suddenly as easy as a bird in flight. For them, sport is not a test but a therapy, not a trial but a reward, not a question but an answer.

Fitness and healthy lifestyle habits lead to improved health, quality of life, and wellness.

Activity 15.3: Self-Evaluation of Selected Wellness Components

Name _____ Date _____

Course _____ Section _____ Gender _____ Age _____

In the appropriate columns, enter I (for Initial), C (for Current), and G (for Goal) according to instructions on page 505.

Wellness Components	Wellness Rating				
	Poor	Fair	Average	Good	Excellent
Cardiorespiratory Endurance					
Muscular Fitness (Strength and Endurance)					
Muscular Flexibility					
Body Composition					
Nutrition					
Cardiovascular Disease Prevention					
Cancer Prevention					
Stress Control					
Tobacco Use					
Substance Abuse Control*					
Sexuality*					
Accident Prevention and Personal Safety					
Spirituality*					
Health Education					

Current Number of Daily Steps: ☐   Activity category (see Table 1.2, page 12): ☐

*These components are personal, and you are not required to reveal this information. If you think that counseling is necessary, you are encouraged to seek professional help.

Activity 15.4: Goal Setting: Behavioral Goals for the Future

Name _____ Date _____

Course _____ Section _____ Gender _____ Age _____

Select two wellness components that you will work on during the next couple of months. Specify your SMART goals and write specific actions that will lead to your accomplishing these goals (you may not need six objectives; write only as many as you need).

Goal: _____

Actions:

1. _____
2. _____
3. _____
4. _____
5. _____
6. _____

Goal: _____

Actions:

1. _____
2. _____
3. _____
4. _____
5. _____
6. _____

Number of Daily Steps Goal: [   ]   Activity category goal: [   ]

Activity 15.5: Wellness Lifestyle Self-Assessment

Name _____ Date _____
Course _____ Section _____ Gender _____ Age _____

I. Explain the exercise program that you implemented in this course. Express your feelings about the outcomes of this program, and evaluate how well you accomplished your fitness goals.

_____
_____
_____
_____
_____
_____
_____
_____
_____
_____
_____
_____
_____

II. List nutritional or dietary changes that you were able to implement this term and the effects of these changes on your body composition and personal wellness.

_____
_____
_____
_____
_____
_____
_____
_____
_____
_____
_____
_____
_____

III. List other lifestyle changes that you were able to make this term that may decrease your risk for disease. In a few sentences, explain how you feel about these changes and their impact on your overall well-being.

_____
_____
_____
_____
_____
_____
_____
_____
_____
_____

IV. Briefly evaluate this course and its impact on your quality of life. Indicate what you think you will need so that you are able to continue to adhere to an active and healthy lifestyle.

_____
_____
_____
_____
_____
_____
_____
_____
_____
_____

The real challenge will come now: a lifetime commitment to fitness and wellness. To make the commitment easier, enjoy yourself and have fun along the way. If you implement your program based on your interests and what you enjoy doing most, then adhering to your new lifestyle will not be difficult.

Your activities over the last few weeks or months may have helped you develop "positive addictions" that will carry on throughout life. If you truly experience the feelings Dr. Sheehan expressed, there will be no looking back. If you don't get there, you won't know what it's like. Fitness and wellness is a process, and you need to put forth a constant and deliberate effort to achieve and maintain a higher quality of life. Improving the quality of your life, and most likely your longevity, is in your hands. Only you can take control of your lifestyle and thereby reap the benefits of wellness.

ASSESS YOUR BEHAVIOR

CENGAGEbrain To access course materials, including companion resources, please visit www.cengagebrain.com.

1. Has your level of physical activity increased compared with the beginning of the term?
2. Do you participate in a regular exercise program that includes cardiorespiratory endurance, muscular strength, and muscular flexibility training?
3. Is your diet healthier now compared with a few weeks ago?
4. Are you able to take pride in the lifestyle changes that you have implemented over the last several weeks? Have you rewarded yourself for your accomplishments?

ASSESS YOUR KNOWLEDGE

Evaluate how well you understand the concepts presented in this chapter using the chapter-specific quizzing available in the online materials at www.cengagebrain.com.

1. From a functional point of view, typical sedentary people in the United States are about ___ years older than their chronological age indicates.
   a. 2
   b. 8
   c. 15
   d. 20
   e. 25

2. Which one of the following factors has the greatest impact on health and longevity?
   a. genetics
   b. the environment
   c. lifestyle behaviors
   d. chronic diseases
   e. gender

3. Your real physiological age is determined by
   a. your birthdate.
   b. lifestyle habits.
   c. amount of physical activity.
   d. your family's health history.
   e. your ability to obtain proper medical care.

4. Complementary and alternative medicine is
   a. also known as allopathic medicine.
   b. referred to as "Western" medicine.
   c. based on scientifically proven methods.
   d. a method of unconventional medicine.
   e. All are correct choices.

5. Complementary and alternative medicine health care practices and treatments are
   a. not widely taught in medical schools.
   b. endorsed by many physicians.
   c. not generally used in hospitals.
   d. not usually reimbursed by medical insurance companies.
   e. All of the above choices are correct.

6. In complementary and alternative medicine,
   a. practitioners believe that their treatment modality aids the body as it performs its own natural healing process.
   b. treatments are usually shorter than with typical medical practices.
   c. practitioners rely extensively on the use of medications.
   d. patients are often discouraged from administering self-treatment.
   e. All of the above choices are correct.

7. When the word "natural" is used with a product,
   a. it implies that the product is safe.
   b. it cannot be toxic, even when taken in large doses.
   c. it cannot yield undesirable side effects when combined with prescription drugs.
   d. there will be no negative side effects with its use.
   e. All choices are incorrect.

8. To protect yourself from consumer fraud when buying a new product,
   a. get as much information as you can from the salesperson.
   b. obtain details about the product from another salesperson.
   c. ask someone who understands the product but does not stand to profit from the transaction.
   d. obtain all the research information from the manufacturer.
   e. All choices are correct.

9. Which of the following should you consider when looking to join a health/fitness center?
   a. location
   b. instructor's certifications
   c. type and amount of equipment available
   d. verification that the facility complies with ACSM standards
   e. All choices are correct.

10. When you purchase exercise equipment, the most important factor is
    a. to try it out several times before buying it.
    b. a recommendation from an exercise specialist.
    c. cost effectiveness.
    d. that it provides accurate exercise information.
    e. to find out how others like this piece of equipment.

Correct answers can be found at the back of the book.

Physical Fitness and Wellness Profile

APPENDIX A

Figure A.1 Physical Fitness and Wellness Profile.

Fill out the following profile as you obtain the results for each fitness and wellness component. Attempt to determine the four fitness components (cardiorespiratory endurance, muscular strength/endurance, muscular flexibility, and body composition) during the first 2 or 3 weeks of the term so that you may proceed with your exercise program. After determining each component, discuss with your instructor the goals to be accomplished and the date of completion.

Name: _____ Course: _____ Section: _____ Gender: _____ Age: _____

Item	Pre-Assessment			Goal[a]	Post-Assessment		
	Date	Test Results	Category		Date	Test Results	Category
Cardiorespiratory Endurance							
VO_{2max}							
Daily min. of phys. activity							
Total daily steps							
Muscular Fitness (Strength)							
Muscular Flexibility							
Body Composition							
Body weight							
Percent body fat							
Lean body mass							
BMI							
Waist circumference							
Waist-to-Height Ratio							
Cardiovascular Risk							
Cancer Risk							
Lung							
Colorectal							
Skin							
Breast[b]							
Cervical[b]							
Endometrial[b]							
Prostate							
Testicular							
Pancreatic							
Kidney and Bladder							
Oral							
Esophageal and Stomach							
Ovarian							
Thyroid							
Liver							
Leukemia							
Lymphomas							
Stress							
Stress Events Scale							
Vulnerability Questionnaire							
Tobacco Use[c]							

INSTRUCTOR'S SIGNATURE: _____ STUDENT'S SIGNATURE: _____

[a]Indicate goal to complete by end of the term.
[b]Women only
[c]For test results, indicate type and amount smoked; for classification indicate smoker, ex-smoker, nonsmoker.

Nutritive Value of Selected Foods

APPENDIX B

Food Description	Qty	Measure	Wt (g)	Ener (cal)	Prot (g)	Carb (g)	Dietary Fiber (g)	Fat (g)	Fat Breakdown (g)				Chol (mg)	Calc (mg)	Iron (mg)	Sodi (mg)	Vit E (mg)	Folate (mcg)	Vit C (mg)	Selenium (mcg)
									Sat	Mono	Poly	Trans								
Almonds, dry roasted, no salt added	¼	cup(s)	35	206	8	7	4	18	1.40	11.61	4.36	—	0	92	1.56	<1	8.97	11	0	1
Apple juice, unsweetened, canned	½	cup(s)	124	58	<1	14	<1	<1	0.02	0.01	0.04	—	0	9	0.46	4	0.01	0	1	<1
Apples, raw medium, w/ peel	1	item(s)	138	72	<1	19	3	<1	0.04	0.01	0.07	—	0	8	0.17	1	—	4	6	0
Applesauce, sweetened, canned	½	cup(s)	128	97	<1	25	2	<1	0.04	0.01	0.07	—	0	5	0.45	4	0.27	1	2	<1
Apricot, fresh w/o pits	4	item(s)	140	67	2	16	3	1	0.04	0.24	0.11	—	0	18	0.55	1	1.25	13	14	<1
Apricot halves w/ skin, canned in heavy syrup	½	cup(s)	129	107	1	28	2	<1	0.01	0.04	0.02	—	0	12	0.39	5	0.77	3	4	<1
Asparagus, boiled, drained	½	cup(s)	90	20	2	4	2	0.19	0.06	0	0.12	—	0	20.7	0.81	12.6	1.35	134.1	6.92	5.48
Avocado, California, whole, w/o skin or pit	1	item(s)	170	284	3	15	12	26	3.59	16.61	3.42	—	0	22	1.00	14	3.35	105	15	1
Bacon, cured, broiled, pan fried, or roasted	2	slice(s)	13	68	5	<1	0	5	1.73	2.33	0.57	0	14	1	0.18	291	0.04	<1	1	8
Bagel chips, plain	3	item(s)	29	130	3	19	1	5	0.50	—	—	—	0	0	0.72	70	—	—	0	—
Bagel, plain, enriched, toasted	1	item(s)	66	195	7	38	2	1	0.16	0.09	0.49	—	0	53	2.52	379	0.08	64	0	23
Banana, fresh whole, w/o peel	1	item(s)	118	105	1	27	3	<1	0.13	0.04	0.09	—	0	6	0.31	1	0.12	24	10	1
Beans, black, boiled	½	cup(s)	86	114	8	20	7	<1	0.12	0.04	0.20	—	0	23	1.81	1	—	128	0	1
Beans, Fordhook lima, frozen, boiled, drained	½	cup(s)	85	88	5	16	5	<1	0.07	0.02	0.14	—	0	26	1.55	59	0.25	18	11	1
Beans, mung, sprouted, boiled, drained	½	cup(s)	62	13	1	3	<1	<1	0.02	0.00	0.02	—	0	7	0.40	6	0.04	18	7	<1
Beans, red kidney, canned	½	cup(s)	128	109	7	20	8	<1	0.06	0.03	0.24	—	0	31	1.61	436	0.77	65	1	2
Beans, refried, canned	½	cup(s)	127	119	7	20	7	2	0.60	0.71	0.19	—	10	44	2.10	378	0.00	14	8	2
Beans, yellow snap, string or wax, boiled, drained	½	cup(s)	62	22	1	5	2	<1	0.04	0.00	0.09	—	0	29	0.80	2	0.28	21	6	<1
Beef, chuck, arm pot roast, lean & fat, ¼" fat, braised	3	ounce(s)	85	282	23	0	0	20	7.97	8.68	0.77	—	84	9	2.64	51	0.19	8	0	21
Beef, corned, canned	3	ounce(s)	85	213	23	0	0	13	5.25	5.07	0.54	—	73	10	1.77	855	0.13	8	0	36
Beef, ground, lean, broiled, well	3	ounce(s)	85	238	24	0	0	15	5.89	6.56	0.56	—	86	10	2.08	76	—	9	0	22
Beef, ground, regular, broiled, medium	3	ounce(s)	85	246	20	0	0	18	6.91	7.70	0.65	—	77	9	2.07	71	—	8	0	16
Beef, liver, pan fried	3	ounce(s)	85	149	23	4	0	4	1.27	0.56	0.49	0.17	324	5	5.24	65	0.39	221	1	28
Beef, rib steak, small end, lean, ¼" fat,	3	ounce(s)	85	188	24	0	0	10	3.84	4.01	0.27	—	68	11	2.18	59	0.12	7	0	19
Beef, rib, whole, lean & fat, ¼" fat, roasted	3	ounce(s)	85	320	19	0	0	27	10.71	11.42	0.94	—	72	9	1.96	54	—	6	0	19
Beef, short loin, T-bone steak, lean, ¼" fat, broiled	3	ounce(s)	85	174	23	0	0	9	3.05	4.23	0.26	—	50	5	3.11	65	0.12	7	0	9
Beer	12	fluid ounce(s)	356	118	1	6	<1	<1	0.00	0.00	0.00	0	0	18	0.07	14	0.00	21	0	2
Beer, light	12	fluid ounce(s)	354	99	1	5	0	0	0.00	0.00	0.00	0	0	18	0.14	11	0.00	14	0	2
Beets, sliced, canned, drained	½	cup(s)	85	26	1	6	1	<1	0.02	0.02	0.04	0	0	13	1.55	165	0.03	26	3	<1
Biscuits	1	item(s)	41	121	3	16	1	5	1.40	1.41	1.82	—	<1	33	1.01	205	0.01	26	0	7
Blueberries, raw	1	cup(s)	72	41	1	10	2	<1	0.02	0.03	0.11	0	0	4	0.20	1	0.41	4	7	<1
Bologna, beef	1	slice(s)	28	90	3	1	0	8	3.50	4.26	0.31	—	20	0	0.36	310	—	4	0	—
Bologna, turkey	1	slice(s)	28	50	3	1	0	4	1.00	1.09	0.98	—	20	40	0.36	270	—	4	0	—
Brazil nuts, unblanched, dried	¼	cup(s)	35	230	5	4	3	23	5.30	8.59	7.20	—	0	56	0.85	1	2.01	8	<1	671
Bread, cracked wheat	1	slice(s)	25	65	2	12	1	1	0.23	0.48	0.17	—	0	11	0.70	135	—	15	0	6
Bread, French	1	slice(s)	25	69	2	13	1	1	0.16	0.30	0.17	—	0	19	0.63	152	0.08	37	0	8
Bread, mixed grain	1	slice(s)	26	65	3	12	2	1	0.21	0.40	0.24	—	0	24	0.90	127	0.09	31	<1	8
Bread, pita	1	item(s)	60	165	5	33	1	1	0.10	0.06	0.32	—	0	52	1.57	322	0.18	64	0	16
Bread, pumpernickel	1	slice(s)	32	80	3	15	2	1	0.14	0.30	0.40	—	0	22	0.92	215	0.13	30	0	8
Bread, rye	1	slice(s)	32	83	3	15	2	1	0.20	0.42	0.26	—	0	23	0.91	211	0.11	35	<1	10
Bread, white	1	slice(s)	25	67	2	13	1	1	0.18	0.17	0.34	—	0	38	0.94	170	0.05	28	0	4
Bread, whole wheat	1	slice(s)	46	128	4	24	3	2	0.37	0.53	1.35	—	0	15	1.43	159	0.35	30	0	18
Broccoli, chopped, boiled, drained	½	cup(s)	78	27	2	6	3	<1	0.06	0.03	0.13	—	0	31	0.52	32	1.13	84	51	1
Brownie, prepared from mix	1	item(s)	24	112	1	12	1	7	1.76	2.60	2.26	—	18	14	0.44	82	—	7	<1	3
Brussels sprouts, boiled, drained	½	cup(s)	78	28	2	6	2	<1	0.08	0.03	0.20	—	0	28	0.94	16	0.34	47	48	1
Bulgur, cooked	½	cup(s)	91	76	3	17	4	<1	0.04	0.03	0.09	—	0	9	0.87	5	0.01	16	0	1
Buns, hamburger, plain	1	item(s)	43	120	4	21	1	2	0.47	0.48	0.85	—	0	59	1.43	206	0.03	48	0	8
Butter	1	tablespoon(s)	15	108	<1	<1	0	12	6.13	5.00	0.43	—	32	4	0.00	86	0.35	<1	0	<1
Buttermilk, low fat	1	cup(s)	245	98	8	12	0	2	1.34	0.62	0.08	—	10	284	0.12	257	0.12	12	2	5
Cabbage, boiled, drained, no salt added	1	cup(s)	150	33	2	7	3	1	0.08	0.05	0.29	—	0	47	0.26	12	0.18	30	30	1
Cabbage, raw, shredded	1	cup(s)	70	17	1	4	2	<1	0.01	0.01	0.04	—	0	33	0.41	13	0.10	30	23	1
Cake, angel food, from mix	1	slice(s)	50	129	3	29	<1	<1	0.02	0.01	0.06	—	0	42	0.12	255	0.00	10	0	8
Cake, butter pound, ready to eat, commercially prepared	1	slice(s)	75	291	4	37	<1	15	8.67	4.43	0.80	—	166	26	1.04	299	—	0	<1	—

Food	Amt	Unit															
Cake, carrot, cream cheese frosting, from mix	1	slice(s)	111	5	52	1	29	5.43	7.24	15.10	—	60	28	1.39	273	—	13	1	—
Cake, chocolate, chocolate icing, commercially prepared	1	slice(s)	64	3	35	2	10	3.05	5.61	1.18	—	27	28	1.41	214	—	11	<1	2
Cake, devil's food cupcake, chocolate frosting	1	item(s)	35	2	20	1	4	1.80	1.60	0.60	—	19	21	0.70	92	—	2	0	2
Cake, white, coconut frosting, from mix	1	slice(s)	112	5	71	1	12	4.36	4.14	2.42	—	1	101	1.30	318	0.13	35	<1	12
Candy, Almond Joy bar	1	item(s)	49	2	29	2	13	9.00	3.63	0.74	0	3	20	0.36	70	—	—	0	0
Candy, Life Savers	1	item(s)	2	0	2	0	<1	0.00	—	—	0	0	<1	0.04	1	—	—	0	0
Candy, M & Ms peanut chocolate candy, small bag	1	item(s)	49	5	30	2	13	5.00	5.42	2.07	—	5	40	0.36	25	—	17	1	2
Candy, M & Ms plain chocolate candy, small bag	1	item(s)	48	2	34	1	10	6.00	3.30	0.30	—	5	40	0.36	30	—	3	1	1
Candy, milk chocolate bar	1	item(s)	91	8	53	2	28	16.69	7.20	0.63	—	22	228	0.83	92	0.04	11	2	—
Candy, Milky Way bar	2	item(s)	58	2	41	1	10	5.00	3.50	0.35	—	5	60	0.18	95	0.40	6	1	3
Candy, Reese's peanut butter cups	2	piece(s)	45	5	25	2	14	5.00	6.17	2.34	0	3	20	0.36	140	0.80	25	0	2
Candy, Special Dark chocolate bar	1	item(s)	41	2	24	3	13	8.00	4.59	0.41	0	3	0	0.72	0	0.32	1	0	0
Candy, Starburst fruit chews, original fruits	1	package	59	0	48	0	5	1.00	2.10	1.83	—	0	10	0.18	0	0.22	—	30	<1
Candy, York peppermint patty	1	item(s)	42	1	34	1	3	2.00	1.32	0.12	—	0	0	0.36	10	0.04	2	0	<1
Cantaloupe	1/2	cup(s)	80	1	7	1	<1	0.04	0.00	0.07	0	0	7	0.17	13	0.04	17	30	<1
Carrots, raw	1/2	cup(s)	61	2	25	2	<1	0.02	0.01	0.06	0	0	20	0.18	42	0.40	12	4	<1
Carrots, sliced, boiled, drained	1/2	cup(s)	78	2	6	2.33	0.14	0	0	0.08	—	0	23.39	0.26	45.24	0.80	10.92	2.8	0.54
Cashews, dry roasted	1/4	cup(s)	34	5	11	1	16	3.14	9.36	2.68	—	0	15	2.06	5	0.32	24	0	4
Catsup/ketchup	1	tablespoon(s)	15	<1	4	<1	<1	0.01	0.01	0.04	—	0	3	0.08	167	0.22	2	2	<1
Cauliflower, boiled, drained	1/2	cup(s)	62	1	3	2	<1	0.04	0.02	0.13	—	0	10	0.20	9	0.04	27	27	<1
Celery, stalk	2	item(s)	80	1	2	1	<1	0.03	0.03	0.06	0	0	32	0.16	64	0.22	29	2	<1
Cereal, All-Bran	1	cup(s)	62	8	46	20	2	0.00	0.00	1.00	—	0	300	9.00	160	—	800	12	6
Cereal, All-Bran Buds	1	cup(s)	91	6	73	42	3	—	—	—	0	0	0	13.64	606	—	1212	18	26
Cereal, Bran Flakes, Post	1	cup(s)	40	6	32	7	1	0.00	0.71	—	0	0	0	10.77	293	—	133	0	—
Cereal, Cap'n Crunch	1	cup(s)	36	2	30	1	2	0.53	0.39	0.27	0	0	5	6.00	269	—	133	0	2
Cereal, Cheerios	1	cup(s)	30	3	22	3	2	0.00	0.50	—	0	0	100	8.10	280	—	200	6	7
Cereal, Complete wheat bran flakes	1	cup(s)	39	4	31	7	1	0.00	0.00	0.00	—	0	0	23.94	279	—	532	80	11
Cereal, Corn Flakes	1	cup(s)	28	2	24	1	0	0.00	0.00	0.00	0	0	0	8.10	200	—	100	6	4
Cereal, Corn Pops	1	cup(s)	31	1	28	0	0	0.00	0.00	0.00	—	0	0	1.80	120	—	100	6	1
Cereal, Cracklin' Oat Bran	1/2	cup(s)	65	5	47	7	9	2.70	4.70	1.33	0	0	27	2.38	186	—	218	20	2
Cereal, Cream of Wheat, instant, prepared	1	cup(s)	121	2	13	2	<1	0.01	0.01	0.04	—	0	27	8.60	1	—	357	0	14
Cereal, Frosted Flakes	1	cup(s)	41	1	37	1	0	0.00	0.00	0.00	—	0	0	5.99	200	—	133	8	—
Cereal, Frosted Mini-Wheats	5	item(s)	51	2	41	5	1	0.00	0.00	0.50	—	0	0	15.30	5	0.12	100	0	2
Cereal, granola, prepared	1/2	cup(s)	61	9	32	5	15	2.76	4.7	6.53	—	0	48	2.59	13	3.59	51	1	16.95
Cereal, Kashi puffed	1	cup(s)	25	2	13	2	1	0.00	0.00	0.00	—	0	0	0.72	0	—	0	0	—
Cereal, Life	1	cup(s)	43	4	33	3	2	0.35	0.64	0.61	—	0	124	11.92	218	—	142	0	11
Cereal, Multi-Bran Chex	1	cup(s)	58	4	49	7	1	0.00	0.00	0.00	—	0	100	16.20	390	—	100	6	5
Cereal, Nutri-Grain golden wheat	1/2	cup(s)	40	4	31	5	1	0.00	0.00	0.67	—	0	0	1.46	279	—	133	20	9
Cereal, oatmeal, cooked w/water	1	cup(s)	117	6	13	4	2	0.19	0.37	0.44	—	0	9	0.80	1	—	5	0	9
Cereal, Product 19	1	cup(s)	30	2	25	1	0	0.00	0.00	0.00	—	0	0	18.00	210	—	400	60	4
Cereal, Raisin Bran	1	cup(s)	59	4	47	8	1	0.10	0.10	0.36	—	0	20	10.80	300	—	140	0	—
Cereal, Rice Chex	1	cup(s)	25	2	22	<1	0	0.00	0.00	0.00	—	0	80	7.20	232	—	160	5	1
Cereal, Rice Krispies	1	cup(s)	26	2	23	0	0	0.00	0.00	0.00	—	0	0	1.44	256	—	5	5	4
Cereal, Shredded Wheat	1	tablespoon(s)	5	3	20	3	1	0.04	0.01	0.10	—	0	10	1.08	2	—	3	0	—
Cereal, Smacks	1	cup(s)	36	3	32	1	0	0.00	0.00	0.00	—	0	0	0.48	67	—	12	0	1
Cereal, Special K	1	cup(s)	31	7	22	4	0	0.00	0.00	0.00	—	0	0	8.70	220	—	133	8	17
Cereal, Total whole grain	1	cup(s)	40	3	31	3	0	0.00	0.00	0.00	—	0	1330	23.94	253	31.24	400	15	7
Cereal, Wheaties	1	cup(s)	30	3	24	3	1	0.00	0.00	0.00	—	0	0	8.10	220	2.26	532	80	2
Cheese, American, processed	1	ounce(s)	28	6	<1	0	9	5.58	2.54	0.28	0	27	156	0.05	422	0.08	200	0	1
Cheese, blue, crumbled	1	ounce(s)	28	6	1	0	8	5.29	2.21	0.23	—	21	150	0.09	395	0.07	2	6	4
Cheese, cheddar, shredded	1/4	cup(s)	28	7	<1	0	9	5.96	2.65	0.27	—	30	204	0.19	175	0.08	10	0	4
Cheese, feta	1	ounce(s)	28	4	1	0	6	4.18	1.29	0.17	—	25	138	0.18	312	0.05	5	0	4
Cheese, Monterey jack	1	ounce(s)	28	7	<1	0	8	5.34	2.45	0.25	—	25	209	0.20	150	0.07	9	0	4
Cheese, mozzarella, part skim milk	1	ounce(s)	28	7	1	0	4	2.83	1.26	0.13	—	18	219	0.06	173	0.04	5	0	4
Cheese, Parmesan, grated	1	tablespoon(s)	5	2	<1	0	1	0.87	0.42	0.06	—	4	55	0.05	76	0.01	3	0	4
Cheese, ricotta, part skim milk	1/4	cup(s)	62	7	3	0	5	3.03	1.42	0.16	—	19	167	0.27	77	0.04	1	0	10
Cheese, Swiss	1	ounce(s)	28	8	2	0	8	4.98	2.04	0.27	—	26	221	0.06	54	0.11	8	0	5
Cherries, sweet, raw	1/2	cup(s)	73	1	12	2	<1	0.03	0.03	0.04	—	0	9	0.26	0	0.05	2	5	0
Chicken, broiler breast, meat & skin, flour coated, fried	3	ounce(s)	85	27	1	<1	8	2.08	2.98	1.67	—	76	14	1.01	65	—	3	0	20

Food Description	Qty	Measure	Wt (g)	Ener (cal)	Prot (g)	Carb (g)	Dietary Fiber (g)	Fat (g)	Fat Breakdown (g)				Chol (mg)	Calc (mg)	Iron (mg)	Sodi (mg)	Vit E (mg)	Folate (mcg)	Vit C (mg)	Selenium (mcg)
									Sat	Mono	Poly	Trans								
Chicken, broiler drumstick, meat & skin, flour coated, fried	3	ounce(s)	85	208	23	1	<.1	12	3.11	4.61	2.75	—	77	10	1.14	76	—	9	0	16
Chicken, light meat, roasted	3	ounce(s)	85	130	23	0	0	3	0.92	1.29	0.79	—	64	11	0.92	43	0.23	3	0	22
Chicken, roasted (meat only)	3	ounce(s)	85	142	21	0	0	6	1.54	2.13	1.28	—	64	10	1.03	64	—	4	0	21
Chickpeas or bengal gram, garbanzo beans, boiled	½	cup(s)	82	134	7	22	6	2	0.22	0.48	0.95	—	0	40	2.37	6	0.29	141	1	3
Chocolate milk, low fat	1	cup(s)	250	158	8	26	1	3	1.54	0.75	0.09	—	8	288	0.60	153	0.05	13	2	5
Cilantro	1	teaspoon(s)	2	<1	<.1	<.1	<.1	<.1	0.00	0.00	0.00	—	0	1	0.03	1	—	1	1	<.1
Cocoa, hot, prepared w/milk	1	cup(s)	250	193	9	27	3	6	3.58	1.69	0.09	0.18	20	263	1.20	110	0.08	13	1	7
Coconut, dried, not sweetened	¼	cup(s)	60	393	4	14	10	38	34.06	1.63	0.42	—	0	15	1.98	22	0.26	5	1	11
Cod, Atlantic cod or scrod, baked or broiled	3	ounce(s)	44	46	10	0	0	<1	0.07	0.05	0.13	—	24	6	0.22	35	—	5	<.1	17
Coffee, brewed	8	fluid ounce(s)	237	9	<1	0	0	0	0.00	0.00	0.00	—	0	2	0.02	2	0.02	5	0	0
Collard greens, boiled, drained	½	cup(s)	95	25	2	5	3	<1	0.04	0.02	0.16	—	0	133	1.10	15	0.84	88	17	<1
Cookies, animal crackers	12	piece(s)	30	134	2	22	<1	4	1.03	2.29	0.56	—	0	13	0.82	1118	0.04	50	0	4
Cookies, chocolate chip	1	item(s)	30	140	2	16	1	8	2.09	3.26	2.09	0.62	13	11	0.70	109	0.54	16	<.1	<1
Cookies, chocolate sandwich, extra crème filling	1	item(s)	13	65	<1	9	<1	3	0.50	1.39	1.22	1.10	0	3	0.37	64	0.25	6	0	<1
Cookies, Fig Newtons	1	item(s)	16	55	1	10	1	1	0.50	0.50	0.00	0.50	0	5	0.36	60	—	—	<1	17
Cookies, oatmeal	1	item(s)	69	234	6	45	3	4	0.70	1.28	1.85	0	<.1	26	1.94	311	0.23	30	<1	5
Cookies, peanut butter	1	item(s)	35	163	4	17	<1	9	1.65	4.72	2.43	0	13	28	0.67	157	0.74	21	<1	3
Cookies, sugar	1	item(s)	16	61	1	7	<1	3	0.63	1.27	0.87	—	18	5	0.32	50	0.28	8	<1	3
Corn, yellow sweet, frozen, boiled, drained	½	cup(s)	82	66	2	16	2	1	0.08	0.16	0.26	—	0	2	0.39	1	0.06	29	3	1
Cornbread	1	piece(s)	55	141	5	18	1	5	2.09	1.44	1.50	0	21	88	1.01	209	0.33	36	2	6
Cornmeal, yellow whole grain	½	cup(s)	61	221	5	47	4	2	0.31	0.58	1.00	—	0	4	2.10	21	0.26	15	0	9
Cottage cheese, low fat, 1% fat	½	cup(s)	113	81	14	3	0	1	0.73	0.33	0.04	—	5	69	0.16	459	0.01	14	0	10
Cottage cheese, low fat, 2% fat	½	cup(s)	113	102	16	4	0	2	1.38	0.62	0.07	—	9	78	0.18	459	0.02	15	0	12
Crab, blue, canned	2	ounce(s)	57	56	12	0	0	<1	0.14	0.12	0.25	—	50	57	0.48	189	1.04	24	2	18
Crackers, cheese (mini)	30	item(s)	30	151	3	17	1	8	2.81	3.63	0.74	—	4	45	1.43	299	0.66	46	0	3
Crackers, honey graham	4	item(s)	28	118	2	22	1	3	0.43	1.14	1.07	—	0	7	1.04	169	0.09	13	0	3
Crackers, matzo, plain	1	item(s)	28	112	3	24	1	<1	0.06	0.04	0.17	—	0	4	0.90	1	0.02	5	0	10
Crackers, Ritz	5	item(s)	16	80	1	10	<1	4	0.50	1.50	0.00	—	0	20	0.72	135	—	10	1	—
Crackers, rye crispbread	1	item(s)	10	37	1	8	2	<1	0.01	0.02	0.06	—	0	3	0.24	26	0.08	5	0	4
Crackers, saltine	5	item(s)	15	65	1	11	<1	2	0.44	0.96	0.25	0.54	0	18	0.81	195	0.15	19	0	2
Crackers, wheat	10	item(s)	30	142	3	19	1	6	1.55	3.43	0.84	—	0	15	1.32	239	0.15	35	0	2
Cranberry juice cocktail	½	cup(s)	127	72	0	18	0	<1	0.01	0.02	0.06	—	0	4	0.19	3	0.28	0	45	0
Cream cheese	2	tablespoon(s)	29	101	2	1	0	10	6.37	2.85	0.37	—	32	23	0.35	86	0.09	4	0	1
Cream, heavy whipping, liquid	1	tablespoon(s)	15	52	<1	<1	0	6	3.45	1.60	0.21	—	21	10	0.00	6	0.16	1	<.1	<.1
Cream, light whipping, liquid	1	tablespoon(s)	15	44	<1	<1	0	5	2.90	1.36	0.13	—	17	10	0.00	5	0.13	1	<.1	<.1
Croissant, butter	1	item(s)	57	231	5	26	2	12	6.59	3.15	0.62	—	38	21	1.16	424	—	35	<1	13
Cucumber	¼	cup(s)	75	11	<1	3	<1	<1	0.03	0.00	0.04	—	0	12	0.21	2	0.02	5	2	<1
Danish pastry, nut	1	item(s)	65	280	5	30	1	16	3.78	8.90	2.78	—	30	61	1.17	236	0.53	54	1	9
Dates, domestic, whole	¼	cup(s)	44.5	126	1	33	4	<1	0.01	0.01	0	—	0	17	0.45	<1	0.02	9	0	1
Distilled alcohol, 90 proof	1	fluid ounce(s)	28	73	0	0	0	0	0.00	0.01	0.00	0	0	0	0.01	<1	0.00	0	<.1	0
Doughnut, cake	1	item(s)	47	198	2	23	1	11	1.70	4.37	3.70	—	17	21	0.92	257	—	22	<.1	0
Doughnut, glazed	1	item(s)	60	242	4	27	1	14	3.49	7.72	1.74	—	4	26	0.36	205	—	13	<.1	5
Egg substitute, Egg Beaters	¼	cup(s)	61	30	6	1	0	0	0.00	0.00	0.00	—	0	20	1.08	115	0.02	60	0	—
Eggs, fried	1	item(s)	46	92	6	<1	0	7	1.98	2.92	1.22	—	210	27	0.91	94	0.56	23	0	16
Eggs, hard boiled	1	item(s)	50	78	6	<1	0	5	1.63	2.04	0.71	—	212	25	0.60	62	0.51	22	0	15
Eggs, poached	1	item(s)	50	74	6	<1	0	5	1.54	1.90	0.68	—	211	27	0.92	147	0.48	24	0	16
Eggs, raw, white	1	item(s)	33	17	4	<1	0	<.1	0.00	0.00	0.00	—	0	2	0.03	55	0.00	1	0	7
Eggs, raw, whole	1	item(s)	50	74	6	<1	0	5	1.55	1.91	0.68	—	212	27	0.92	70	0.49	24	0	16
Eggs, raw, yolk	1	item(s)	17	53	3	1	0	4	1.59	1.95	0.70	—	205	21	0.45	8	0.43	24	0	9
Eggs, scrambled, prepared w/ milk & butter	2	item(s)	122	203	14	3	0	15	4.49	5.82	2.62	—	429	87	1.46	342	1.04	37	<1	27
Figs, raw, medium	2	item(s)	101	74	1	19	3	<1	0.06	0.07	0.14	—	0	35	0.37	1	0.11	6	2	<1
Fish fillets, batter coated or breaded, fried	3	ounce(s)	85	197.19	12.46	14.42	0.42	10.44	2.39	2.19	5.32	—	28.89	15.3	1.79	452.2	—	17	0	7.73
Flounder, baked	3	ounce(s)	85	114	15	<1	<.1	6	1.15	2.17	1.44	0	44	19	0.35	281	0.41	7	3	34
Flour, all purpose, white, bleached, enriched	½	cup(s)	63	228	6	48	2	1	0.10	0.05	0.26	—	0	9	2.90	3	0.04	114	0	21
Flour, whole wheat	½	cup(s)	60	203	8	44	7	1	0.19	0.14	0.47	—	0	20	2.33	3	0.49	26	0	42

Food	Amt	Unit	Wt	Cal															
Frankfurter, beef & pork	1	item(s)	57	174	7	1	16	6.14	7.79	1.56	—	29	6	0.66	638	0.14	2	0	8
Frankfurter, beef	1	item(s)	45	149	5	2	13	5.26	6.44	0.53	—	24	6	0.68	513	0.09	2	0	4
Frankfurter, turkey	1	item(s)	45	102	6	1	8	2.65	2.51	2.25	—	48	48	0.83	642	0.28	4	0	7
Frozen yogurt, chocolate, soft serve	½	cup(s)	72	115	3	18	4	2.61	1.26	0.16	—	1	106	0.90	71	—	8	<1	2
Frozen yogurt, vanilla, soft serve	½	cup(s)	72	117	3	17	4	2.46	1.14	0.15	—	0	103	0.22	63	0.08	4	1	2
Fruit cocktail, canned in heavy syrup	½	cup(s)	124	91	<1	23	<1	0.01	0.02	0.04	0	0	7	0.36	7	0.50	4	2	1
Fruit cocktail, canned in juice	½	cup(s)	119	55	1	14	<1	0.01	0.00	0.00	0	0	9	0.25	5	0.47	4	3	1
Granola bar, plain, hard	1	item(s)	25	115	2	16	5	0.58	1.07	2.95	0	1	15	0.72	72	—	6	<1	4
Grape juice, sweetened, added vitamin C, from frozen concentrate	½	cup(s)	125	64	<1	16	<1	0.04	0.01	0.03	0	0	5	0.13	3	0.00	1	30	<1
Grapefruit juice, pink, sweetened, canned	½	cup(s)	125	58	1	14	<1	0.02	0.02	0.03	0	0	10	0.45	3	0.05	13	34	<1
Grapefruit juice, white	½	cup(s)	124	48	1	11	<1	0.02	0.02	0.03	0	0	11	0.25	1	0.27	12	47	<1
Grapefruit, raw, pink or red	½	cup(s)	115	48	1	12	<1	0.02	0.02	0.04	0	0	25	0.09	0	0.15	15	36	<1
Grapes, European, red or green, adherent skin	½	cup(s)	80	55	1	14	<1	0.04	0.01	0.04	0	0	8	0.29	2	0.15	2	9	<1
Haddock, baked or broiled	3	ounce(s)	44	50	11	0	<1	0.07	0.07	0.14	33	0	19	0.60	39	—	4	0	18
Halibut, Atlantic & Pacific, cooked, dry heat	3	ounce(s)	85	119	23	0	2	0.35	0.82	0.80	35	0	51	0.91	59	—	12	0	40
Ham, cured, boneless, 11% fat, roasted	3	ounce(s)	85	151	19	0	8	2.65	3.77	1.20	50	0	7	1.14	1275	0.01	3	0	17
Ham, deli sliced, cooked		slice(s)	28	30	5	0	1	0.50	0.39	0.11	15	0	1	0.00	240	—	—	—	—
Honey	1	tablespoon(s)	21	64	<1	17	0	0.00	0.00	0.00	0	0	1	0.09	1	—	<1	<1	1
Honeydew melon	½	cup(s)	89	32	<1	8	<1	0.03	0.00	0.05	0	0	5	0.15	16	0.02	17	16	1
Ice cream, chocolate	½	cup(s)	66	143	3	19	7	4.49	2.12	0.27	22	0	72	0.61	50	0.20	11	<1	2
Ice cream, chocolate, soft serve	½	cup(s)	87	177	3	24	8	5.17	2.43	0.31	22	0	103	0.33	44	0.22	5	1	—
Ice cream, light vanilla	½	cup(s)	66	109	4	18	3	1.71	0.57	0.10	17	0	77	0.05	49	0.08	3	1	—
Jams, jellies, preserves, all flavors	1	tablespoon(s)	20	56	<1	14	<1	0.00	0.01	0.00	0	0	4	0.10	6	0.00	2.20	1.76	—
Jams, jellies, preserves, all flavors, low sugar	1	tablespoon(s)	18	25	<1	6	<1	0.00	0.01	0.02	0	0	2	0.05	<1	0.01	—	4.93	—
Kale, frozen, chopped, boiled, drained	½	cup(s)	65	20	2	3	<1	0.04	0.02	0.15	0	61	90	0.61	10	0.60	9	16	36
Kiwifruit	1	item(s)	77	53	1	11	<1	0.02	0.03	0.19	0	5	30	0.38	2	—	<1	74	1
Lamb, chop, loin, domestic, lean & fat, ¼" fat, broiled	3	ounce(s)	85	269	21	0	20	8.36	8.25	1.43	85	0	17	1.54	65	0.11	15	0	23
Lamb, leg, domestic, lean & fat, ¼" fat, cooked	3	ounce(s)	85	250	21	0	18	7.51	7.50	1.28	82	0	14	1.60	61	0.12	15	0	22
Lemon juice	1	tablespoon(s)	15	4	<1	1	0	0.00	0.00	0.00	0	4	1	0.00	<1	0.02	2	7	<1
Lemonade, from frozen concentrate	8	fluid ounce(s)	248	131	<1	34	<1	0.02	0.02	0.04	0	5	10	0.52	7	0.02	2	13	<1
Lentils, boiled	½	cup(s)	99	115	9	20	8	0.05	0.06	0.17	0	179	19	3.30	2	0.11	179	1	3
Lentils, sprouted	1	cup(s)	77	82	7	17	<1	0.04	0.08	0.17	0	77	19	2.47	8	—	77	13	<1
Lettuce, butterhead, Boston, or bibb	1	cup(s)	55	7	1	1	<1	0.02	0.00	0.06	0	40	19	0.69	3	0.10	40	2	<1
Lettuce, romaine, shredded	1	cup(s)	56	10	1	2	<1	0.02	0.01	0.09	0	77	19	0.55	5	0.07	77	14	<1
Lobster, northern, cooked, moist heat	3	ounce(s)	85	83	17	1	<1	0.09	0.14	0.08	61	0	52	0.33	323	0.85	9	<1	36
Macadamias, dry roasted, no salt added	¼	cup(s)	34	241	3	4	25	4.00	19.86	0.50	0	1	23	0.89	1	0.19	3	<1	1
Mayonnaise w/ soybean oil	1	tablespoon(s)	14	99	<1	<1	11	1.64	2.70	5.89	5	0	2	0.07	78	0.72	1	0	<1
Mayonnaise, low calorie	1	tablespoon(s)	16	37	<1	3	3	0.53	0.72	1.70	4	0	<1	0.00	80	0.32	0	0	0
Milk, fat free, nonfat, or skim	1	cup(s)	245	83	8	12	<1	0.29	0.12	0.02	5	0	223	1.23	108	0.02	12	0	8
Milk, fat free, nonfat, or skim, w/ nonfat milk solids	1	cup(s)	245	91	9	12	1	0.40	0.16	0.02	5	0	316	0.12	130	0.00	12	2	5
Milk, low fat, 1%	1	cup(s)	244	102	8	12	2	1.54	0.97	0.09	12	0	264	0.85	122	0.02	12	2	8
Milk, low fat, 1% w/ nonfat milk solids	1	cup(s)	245	105	9	12	2	1.48	0.69	0.09	10	0	314	0.12	127	0.02	12	2	6
Milk, reduced fat, 2%	1	cup(s)	244	122	8	11	5	2.35	2.04	0.17	20	0	271	0.24	115	0.11	12	<1	6
Milk, reduced fat, 2%, w/ nonfat milk solids	1	cup(s)	245	125	9	12	5	2.93	1.36	0.17	20	0	314	0.12	127	0.07	12	2	6
Milk, whole, 3.3%	1	cup(s)	244	146	8	11	8	4.55	1.98	0.48	24	0	246	0.07	105	0.10	12	<1	6
Milk, whole, evaporated, canned	2	tablespoon(s)	32	42	2	3	2	1.45	0.74	0.08	9	0	82	0.06	33	0.07	3	1	9
Milkshakes, chocolate	1	cup(s)	227	270	7	48	6	3.81	1.77	0.23	25	0	299	0.70	252	0.85	11	0	4
Muffin, English, plain, enriched	1	item(s)	57	134	4	26	1	0.15	0.17	0.51	0	0	30	1.43	264	0.04	42	0	—
Muffin, English, wheat	1	item(s)	57	127	5	26	1	0.16	0.16	0.48	0	0	101	1.64	218	—	36	<1	17
Muffins, blueberry	1	item(s)	63	160	3	23	6	0.87	1.48	3.25	20	0	50	1.15	288	0.26	29	1	9
Mushrooms, raw	½	cup(s)	35	8	1	1	<1	0.02	0.00	0.05	0	0	1	0.18	1	0.76	6	1	3
Mustard greens, frozen, boiled, drained	½	cup(s)	75	14	2	2	<1	0.01	0.08	0.04	0	0	76	0.84	19	0.00	53	10	<1
Oil, canola	1	tablespoon(s)	14	120	0	0	14	0.97	8.01	4.03	0	0	0	0.00	0	1.01	0	0	0
Oil, corn	1	tablespoon(s)	14	120	0	0	14	1.73	3.29	7.98	0	0	0	0.00	0	2.33	0	0	0
Oil, olive	1	tablespoon(s)	14	119	0	0	14	1.82	9.98	1.35	0	0	0	0.09	<1	1.94	0	0	0
Oil, peanut	1	tablespoon(s)	14	120	0	0	14	2.28	6.24	4.32	0	0	<1	0.00	0	2.12	0	0	0
Oil, safflower	1	tablespoon(s)	14	120	0	0	14	0.84	10.15	1.95	0	0	0	0.00	0	4.64	0	0	0
Oil, soybean w/ cottonseed oil	1	tablespoon(s)	14	120	0	0	14	2.45	4.01	6.54	0	0	0	0.00	0	1.65	0	0	0

Food Description	Qty	Measure	Wt (g)	Ener (cal)	Prot (g)	Carb (g)	Dietary Fiber (g)	Fat (g)	Fat Breakdown (g)				Chol (mg)	Calc (mg)	Iron (mg)	Sodi (mg)	Vit E (mg)	Folate (mcg)	Vit C (mg)	Selenium (mcg)
									Sat	Mono	Poly	Trans								
Okra, sliced, boiled, drained	½	cup(s)	80	18	1	4	2	<1	0.04	0.02	0.04	—	0	62	0.22	5	0.22	37	13	<1
Onions, chopped, boiled, drained	½	cup(s)	106	47	1	11	1	<1	0.03	0.03	0.08	—	0	23	0.26	3	0.02	16	6	1
Orange juice, unsweetened, from frozen concentrate	½	cup(s)	125	56	1	13	<1	<.1	0.01	0.01	0.01	—	0	11	0.12	1	0.25	55	48	<1
Orange, raw	1	item(s)	131	62	1	15	3	<1	0.02	0.03	0.03	—	0	52	0.13	0	0.24	39	70	1
Oysters, eastern, farmed, raw	3	ounce(s)	85	50	4	5	0	1	0.38	0.13	0.50	—	21	37	4.91	151	—	15	4	54
Oysters, eastern, wild, cooked, moist heat	3	ounce(s)	85	116	12	7	0	4	1.31	0.53	1.65	—	89	77	10.19	359	—	12	5	61
Pancakes, blueberry, from recipe	3	item(s)	114	253	7	33	1	10	2.26	2.64	4.74	—	64	235	1.96	470	—	41	3	16
Pancakes, from mix w/egg & milk	3	item(s)	114	249	9	33	2	9	2.33	2.36	3.33	—	81	245	1.48	576	—	105	1	—
Papaya, raw	½	cup(s)	70	27	<1	7	1	<1	0.03	0.03	0.02	—	0	17	0.07	2	0.51	27	43	<1
Pasta, egg noodles, enriched, cooked	½	cup(s)	80	106	4	20	1	1	0.25	0.34	0.33	0.02	26	10	1.27	6	0.14	51	0	17
Pasta, macaroni, enriched, cooked	½	cup(s)	70	99	3	20	1	<1	0.07	0.06	0.19	—	0	5	0.98	1	0.04	54	0	15
Pasta, spaghetti, al dente, cooked	½	cup(s)	65	95	3	20	1	1	0.05	0.05	0.15	—	0	5	1.00	1	0.04	8	0	40
Pasta, spaghetti, whole wheat, cooked	½	cup(s)	70	87	4	19	3	<1	0.07	0.05	0.15	—	0	11	0.74	2	0.21	4	0	18
Pasta, tricolor vegetable macaroni, enriched, cooked	½	cup(s)	67	86	3	18	3	<.1	0.01	0.01	0.03	—	0	7	0.33	4	0.06	44	0	13
Peach, halves, canned in heavy syrup	½	cup(s)	131	97	1	26	2	<1	0.01	0.05	0.06	—	0	4	0.35	8	0.64	4	4	<1
Peach, halves, canned in water	½	cup(s)	122	29	1	7	2	<1	0.01	0.03	0.03	—	0	2	0.39	4	0.60	4	4	<1
Peach, raw, medium	1	item(s)	98	38	1	9	1	<1	0.02	0.07	0.08	—	0	6	0.25	0	0.72	4	6	<.1
Peanut butter, smooth	1	tablespoon(s)	16	96	4	3	1	8	1.60	3.96	2.38	—	0	8	0.30	80	1.44	12	0	1
Peanuts, oil roasted, salted	¼	cup(s)	36	216	10	5	3	19	3.12	9.33	5.49	—	0	22	0.54	115	2.50	43	<1	1
Pear, halves, canned in heavy syrup	½	cup(s)	133	98	<1	25	2	<1	0.01	0.04	0.04	—	0	7	0.29	7	0.11	1	1	0
Pear, raw	1	item(s)	166	96	1	26	5	<1	0.01	0.04	0.05	—	0	15	0.28	2	0.20	12	7	<1
Peas, green, canned, drained	½	cup(s)	85	59	4	11	3	<1	0.05	0.03	0.14	—	0	17	0.81	214	0.03	37	8	1
Peas, green, frozen, boiled, drained	½	cup(s)	80	62	4	11	4	<1	0.04	0.02	0.10	—	0	19	1.22	58	0.02	47	8	1
Pecans, dry roasted, no salt added	¼	cup(s)	57	403	5	8	5	42	3.56	24.92	11.66	—	0	41	1.59	1	0.74	9	<1	2
Pepperoni, beef & pork	1	slice(s)	11	55	2	<1	0	5	1.77	2.32	0.48	—	9	1	0.15	224	—	<1	0	0
Peppers, green bell or sweet, raw	1	tablespoon(s)	75	15	1	3	1	<1	0.04	0.01	0.05	—	0	7	0.25	2	0.28	8	60	0
Pickle relish, sweet	1	tablespoon(s)	15	20	<1	5	<1	<.1	0.01	0.03	0.02	—	0	<1	0.13	122	0.06	<1	<1	0
Pickle, dill	1	ounce(s)	28	5	<1	1	<1	<.1	0.01	0.00	0.02	—	0	3	0.15	363	0.03	<1	1	0
Pie crust, frozen, ready to bake, enriched, baked	1	slice(s)	16	82	1	8	<1	5	1.69	2.51	0.65	—	0	3	0.36	104	0.42	9	0	<1
Pie crust, prepared w/water, baked	1	slice(s)	20	100	1	10	<1	6	1.54	3.46	0.77	—	0	12	0.43	146	—	20	0	2
Pie, apple, from home recipe	1	slice(s)	155	411	4	58	2	19	4.73	8.36	5.17	—	0	11	1.74	327	—	37	3	12
Pie, pecan, from home recipe	1	slice(s)	122	503	6	64	0	27	4.87	13.64	6.97	—	106	39	1.81	320	—	32	<1	15
Pie, pumpkin, from home recipe	1	slice(s)	155	316	7	41	4	14	4.92	5.73	2.81	—	65	146	1.97	349	—	33	3	11
Pineapple, canned in extra heavy syrup	½	cup(s)	130	108	<1	28	1	<1	0.01	0.02	0.05	—	0	18	0.49	1	—	7	9	<1
Pineapple, canned in juice	½	cup(s)	125	75	1	20	1	<1	0.01	0.01	0.04	—	0	17	0.35	1	0.01	6	12	<1
Pineapple, raw, diced	½	cup(s)	78	37	<1	10	1	<1	0.01	0.01	0.03	—	0	10	0.22	1	0.02	12	28	<.1
Pinto beans, boiled, drained, no salt added	½	cup(s)	114	25	2	5	2	<1	0.04	0.03	0.21	—	0	17	0.75	58	—	146	7	1
Pomegranate	1	item(s)	154	105	1	26	1	<1	0.06	0.07	0.10	—	0	5	0.46	5	0.92	9	9	1
Popcorn, air popped	1	cup(s)	8	31	1	6	1	<1	0.05	0.09	0.15	—	0	1	0.22	<1	0.02	2	0	1
Popcorn, popped in oil	1	cup(s)	33	165	3	19	3	9	1.61	2.70	4.43	—	0	3	0.92	292	—	6	<.1	2
Pork, ribs, loin, country style, lean & fat, roasted	3	ounce(s)	85	279	20	0	0	22	7.83	9.36	1.71	—	78	21	0.90	44	—	4	<1	32
Potato chips, salted	20	item(s)	28	152	2	15	1	10	3.11	2.79	3.46	—	0	7	0.46	169	1.91	13	9	2
Potatoes, au gratin mix, prepared w/water, whole milk, & butter	½	cup(s)	114	106	3	15	1	5	2.94	1.34	0.15	—	17	94	0.36	499	—	8	4	3
Potatoes, baked, flesh & skin	1	item(s)	202	220	5	51	4	<1	0.05	0.00	0.09	—	0	20	2.75	16	—	22	26	2
Potatoes, baked, flesh only	½	cup(s)	61	57	1	13	1	<.1	0.02	0.00	0.03	—	0	3	0.21	3	0.02	5	8	<1
Potatoes, hashed brown	½	cup(s)	78	207	2	27	2	10	1.11	3.13	2.78	—	0	11	0.43	267	0.01	12	10	<1
Potatoes, mashed, from dehydrated granules w/milk, water, & margarine	½	cup(s)	105	122	2	17	1	5	1.27	2.05	1.41	—	2	34	0.22	181	0.54	8	7	6
Pretzels, plain, hard, twists	5	item(s)	30	114	3	24	1	1	0.23	0.41	0.37	—	0	11	1.30	515	—	51	0	2
Prune juice, canned	1	cup(s)	256	182	2	45	3	<.1	0.01	0.05	0.02	—	0	31	3.02	10	0.31	0	10	2

Food	Amount	Unit																		
Prunes, dried	2	item(s)	17	40	<1	11	1	<1	0.01	0.06	0.02	—	0	9	0.42	1	0.00	1	1	<1
Pudding, chocolate	½	cup(s)	144	154	5	23	1	5	2.78	1.94	0.23	—	35	138	1.04	135	0.00	7	<1	5
Pudding, tapioca, ready to eat	1	item(s)	142	169	3	28	1	5	0.85	2.24	1.93	0	1	119	0.33	226	0.43	4	1	2
Pudding, vanilla	½	cup(s)	136	116	<1	17	<1	3	1.31	1.21	0.16	—	35	133	0.25	134	0.00	6	<1	5
Quinoa, dry	½	cup(s)	85	318	11	59	5	5	0.50	1.30	1.99	0	0	51	7.86	18	—	42	0	<1
Raisins, seeded, packed	¼	cup(s)	41	122	1	32	3	<1	0.07	0.01	0.07	—	0	12	1.07	12	—	1	2	<1
Raspberries, raw	½	cup(s)	62	32	<1	7	4	<1	0.01	0.04	0.23	—	0	15	0.42	1	0.54	13	16	<1
Raspberries, red, sweetened, frozen	½	cup(s)	125	129	1	33	6	<1	0.01	0.02	0.11	—	0	19	0.81	1	0.90	33	21	10
Rice, brown, long grain, cooked	½	cup(s)	98	108	3	22	2	1	0.18	0.32	0.31	—	0	10	0.41	5	0.03	4	0	6
Rice, white, long grain, boiled	½	cup(s)	79	103	2	22	<1	<1	0.06	0.07	0.06	—	0	8	0.95	1	0.03	46	0	<1
Rice, wild brown, cooked	½	cup(s)	82	82.81	3.27	17.49	1.47	0.27	0.04	0.04	0.17	—	0	2.46	0.49	2.46	0.24	21.31	—	0.65
Roll, hard	1	item(s)	57	167	6	30	1	2	0.35	0.65	0.98	—	0	54	1.87	310	0.24	54	0	22
Salad dressing, blue cheese	2	tablespoon(s)	31	154	1	2	<1	16	3.03	3.76	8.51	5	10	25	0.06	335	1.84	9	1	<1
Salad dressing, French	2	tablespoon(s)	31	143	<1	5	<1	14	1.76	2.63	6.56	—	0	7	0.25	261	1.56	0	0	0
Salad dressing, French, low fat	2	tablespoon(s)	33	76	<1	10	<1	4	0.36	1.92	1.64	—	1	4	0.28	262	0.10	1	0	1
Salad dressing, Italian	2	tablespoon(s)	29	86	<1	3	<1	8	1.32	1.86	3.80	—	0	4	0.19	486	1.47	0	0	1
Salad dressing, Italian, diet	2	tablespoon(s)	30	23	<1	1	<1	2	0.14	0.66	0.51	—	2	3	0.20	410	0.06	0	0	2
Salad dressing, ranch	2	tablespoon(s)	30	146	<1	2	<1	16	2.32	3.85	8.92	—	4	4	0.03	354	1.85	<1	<1	—
Salad dressing, thousand island	2	tablespoon(s)	31	115	<1	5	<1	11	1.59	2.46	5.68	—	8	5	0.37	269	1.25	0	0	<1
Salad dressing, thousand island, low calorie	2	tablespoon(s)	31	62	<1	7	<1	4	0.23	1.98	0.82	—	<1	5	0.28	254	0.31	0	0	<1
Salami, pork, dry or hard	1	slice(s)	13	52	3	<1	0	4	1.52	2.05	0.48	—	10	2	0.17	289	—	<1	0	3
Salmon, broiled or baked w/butter	3	ounce(s)	85	155	23	0	0	6	1.16	2.29	2.33	—	40	15	1.02	99	1.15	4	2	41
Salmon, smoked chinook (lox)	3	ounce(s)	57	66	10	0	0	2	0.52	1.14	0.56	—	13	6	0.48	1134	—	1	0	22
Salsa	2	tablespoon(s)	16	4	<1	1	<1	<1	0.00	0.00	0.02	—	0	3	0.16	69	0.19	3	2	<1
Sardines, Atlantic, with bones, canned in oil	2	item(s)	24	50	6	0	0	3	0.36	0.92	1.23	—	34	108	0.70	121	0.49	3	<1	13
Sauerkraut, canned	1	cup(s)	114	22	1	5	3	<1	0.04	0.01	0.07	—	0	34	1.67	751	0.11	27	17	1
Sausage, Italian, pork, cooked	1	item(s)	68	220	14	1	0	17	6.14	8.13	2.23	—	53	16	1.02	627	—	3	1	15
Sausage, smoked, pork link	1	piece(s)	76	295	17	2	0	24	8.58	11.09	2.85	—	52	23	0.88	1137	—	4	0	16
Scallops, mixed species, breaded, fried	3	item(s)	47	100	8	5	0	5	1.24	2.09	1.32	—	28	20	0.38	216	—	23	0	13
Seaweed, spirulina, dried	2	tablespoon(s)	8	22	4	2	0	1	0.20	0.05	0.16	—	0	9	2.14	79	0.38	7	1	1
Shrimp, mixed species, breaded, fried	3	ounce(s)	85	205.69	18.18	9.74	<1	10.43	1.77	3.24	4.32	—	150.44	56.95	1.07	292.39	—	20.39	1.27	35.44
Shrimp, mixed species, cooked, moist heat	3	ounce(s)	85	84	18	0	0	1	0.25	0.17	0.37	—	166	33	2.63	190	1.17	3	2	34
Soda, Coca-Cola Classic cola	12	fluid ounce(s)	360	146	0	41	0	0	0.00	0.00	0.00	0	0	—	—	50	—	—	0	—
Soda, Coke diet cola	12	fluid ounce(s)	360	2	0	<1	0	0	0.00	0.00	0.00	0	0	—	—	42	—	—	0	—
Soda, cola	12	fluid ounce(s)	426	179	<1	46	0	0	0.00	0.00	0.00	0	0	13	0.09	17	0.00	0	0	<1
Soda, ginger ale	12	fluid ounce(s)	366	124	0	32	0	0	0.00	0.00	0.00	0	0	11	0.66	26	0.00	0	0	0
Soda, lemon lime	12	fluid ounce(s)	368	147	0	38	0	0	0.00	0.00	0.00	0	0	7	0.26	41	0.00	0	0	0
Soda, root beer	12	fluid ounce(s)	370	152	0	39	0	0	0.00	0.00	0.00	0	0	18	0.18	48	0.00	0	0	0
Sour cream	2	tablespoon(s)	24	51	1	1	0	5	3.13	1.45	0.19	—	11	28	0.01	13	0.14	3	<1	1
Sour cream, fat free	2	tablespoon(s)	32	24	1	5	0	0	0.00	0.00	0.00	—	3	40	0.00	45	0.00	4	0	<1
Soy sauce	½	cup(s)	18	10	1	2	<1	<1	0.00	0.00	0.01	—	0	3	0.36	1029	0.00	3	0	—
Spinach, canned, drained	½	cup(s)	108	25	3	4	3	1	0.09	0.02	0.23	—	0	138	2.49	29	2.10	106	16	2
Spinach, chopped, boiled, drained	½	cup(s)	90	21	3	3	2	<1	0.04	0.01	0.10	—	0	122	3.21	63	1.87	131	9	<1
Spinach, raw, chopped	1	cup(s)	30	7	1	1	1	<1	0.02	0.00	0.05	—	0	30	0.81	24	0.61	58	8	1
Squash, acorn, baked	½	cup(s)	103	57	1	15	5	<1	0.03	0.01	0.06	—	0	45	0.95	4	—	19	11	<1
Squash, summer, all varieties, sliced, boiled, drained	½	cup(s)	90	18	1	4	1	<1	0.06	0.02	0.12	—	0	24	0.32	1	0.13	18	5	<1
Squid, winter, all varieties, baked, mashed	½	cup(s)	103	38	1	9	3	<1	0.13	0.05	0.27	—	0	23	0.45	1	0.12	21	10	<1
Squid, mixed species, fried	3	ounce(s)	85	149	15	7	<1	6	1.60	2.34	1.82	—	221	33	0.86	260	—	12	4	44
Strawberries, raw	½	cup(s)	72	23	<1	6	1	<1	0.01	0.03	0.09	—	0	12	0.30	1	0.21	17	42	2
Strawberries, sweetened, frozen, thawed	½	cup(s)	128	99	1	27	2	<1	0.01	0.02	0.09	—	0	14	0.60	2	0.31	5	50	26
Sugar, brown, packed	1	teaspoon(s)	5	17	0	4	0	0	0.00	0.00	0.00	—	0	4	0.09	1	0.00	<1	0	1
Sugar, white, granulated	1	teaspoon(s)	4	15	0	4	0	0	0.00	0.00	0.00	—	0	<1	0.00	0	0.00	0	0	<1
Sweet potatoes, baked, peeled	½	cup(s)	100	90	2	21	3	<1	0.03	0.00	0.06	—	0	38	0.69	36	0.71	6	20	<1
Syrup, maple	¼	cup(s)	80	209	0	54	0	<1	0.03	0.05	0.08	—	0	54	0.96	7	—	0	<1	<1
Taco shell, hard	1	item(s)	13	62	1	8	1	3	0.43	1.19	1.13	—	0	21	0.33	49	0.22	17	0	2
Tangerine, raw	1	item(s)	84	37	1	9	2	<1	0.02	0.00	0.03	—	0	12	0.08	1	0.17	17	26	<1
Tea, decaffeinated, prepared	8	fluid ounce(s)	237	2	0	<1	0	0	0.00	0.00	0.00	0	0	5	0.05	7	0.00	12	0	<1
Tea, herbal, prepared	8	fluid ounce(s)	237	2	0	<1	0	0	0.00	0.00	0.00	0	0	5	0.19	2	0.00	2	0	<1
Tea, prepared	8	fluid ounce(s)	237	2	0	1	0	0	0.00	0.00	0.01	0	0	0	0.05	7	0.00	12	0	0
Teriyaki sauce	1	tablespoon(s)	18	15	1	3	<1	0	0.00	0.00	0.01	—	0	5	0.31	690	0.00	4	0	<1
Tofu, firm	3	ounce(s)	79	80	8	2	1	4	0.50	0.87	2.17	—	0	60	1.08	0	0.00	—	0	<1
Tomato juice, canned	½	cup(s)	122	21	1	5	1	<1	0.01	0.01	0.03	—	0	12	0.52	328	0.39	24	22	<1

Food Description	Qty	Measure	Wt (g)	Ener (cal)	Prot (g)	Carb (g)	Dietary Fiber (g)	Fat (g)	Fat Breakdown (g) Sat	Mono	Poly	Trans	Chol (mg)	Calc (mg)	Iron (mg)	Sodi (mg)	Vit E (mg)	Folate (mcg)	Vit C (mg)	Selenium (mcg)
Tomato sauce	½	cup(s)	112	46	2	8	2	1	0.18	0.29	0.72	0	0	21	1.08	199	0.39	15	15	1
Tomatoes, fresh, ripe, red	1	item(s)	123	22.13	1.08	4.82	1.47	0.24	0.05	0.06	0.16	—	0	12.3	0.33	6.15	0.66	18.45	15.62	0
Tomatoes, stewed, canned, red	½	cup(s)	128	33	1	8	2	<1	0.03	0.04	0.10	—	0	43	1.70	282	1.06	6	10	1
Tortilla chips, plain	6	item(s)	28	142	2	18	2	7	1.43	4.39	1.03	—	0	44	0.43	150	1	3	0	2
Tortillas, corn, soft	1	item(s)	26	58	1	12	1	1	0.09	0.17	0.29	—	0	46	0.36	42	0.07	26	0	5
Tortillas, flour	1	item(s)	32	104	3	18	1	2	0.56	1.21	0.34	—	0	40	1.06	153	0.06	33	0	7
Tuna, light, canned in oil, drained	2	ounce(s)	57	113	17	0	0	5	0.87	1.68	1.64	—	10	7	0.79	202	0.50	3	0	43
Tuna, light, canned in water, drained	2	ounce(s)	57	66	14	0	0	<1	0.13	0.09	0.19	—	17	6	0.87	192	0.19	2	0	46
Turkey, breast, processed, oven roasted, fat free	1	slice(s)	28	25	4	1	0	0	0.00	0.00	0.00	0	10	0	0.00	330	—	—	0	—
Turkey, breast, processed, traditional carved	2	slice(s)	45	40	9	0	0	1	0.00	0.07	0.14	—	20	0	0.72	540	—	—	0	—
Turkey, roasted, dark meat, meat only	3	ounce(s)	85	159	24	0	0	6	2.06	1.39	1.84	—	72	27	1.98	67	0.54	8	0	35
Turkey, roasted, light meat, meat only	3	ounce(s)	85	133	25	0	0	3	0.88	0.48	0.73	—	59	16	1.15	54	0.08	5	0	27
Turnip greens, chopped, boiled, drained	½	cup(s)	72	14	1	3	3	<1	0.04	0.01	0.07	—	0	99	0.58	21	1.35	85	20	<1
Turnips, cubed, boiled, drained	½	cup(s)	78	17	1	4	2	<1	0.01	0.01	0.03	—	0	26	0.14	12	0.02	7	9	<1
Vegetables, mixed, canned, drained	½	cup(s)	82	40	2	8	2	<1	0.04	0.01	0.10	—	0	22	0.86	121	0.28	20	4	1
Vinegar, balsamic	1	tablespoon(s)	15	10	0	2	0	0	0.00	0.00	0.00	0	0	0	0.00	0	—	0	0	—
Waffle, plain, frozen, toasted	2	item(s)	66	174	4	27	2	5	0.95	2.12	1.84	—	16	153	2.95	519	0.65	36	0	11
Walnuts, dried black, chopped	¼	cup(s)	31	193	8	3	2	18	1.05	4.69	10.96	—	0	19	0.98	1	0.56	10	1	5
Watermelon	½	cup(s)	77	23	<1	6	<1	<1	0.01	0.03	0.04	—	0	5	0.19	1	0.04	2	6	<1
Wheat germ, crude	2	tablespoon(s)	14	52	3	7	2	<1	0.24	0.20	0.86	—	0	6	0.90	2	—	40	0	11
Wine cooler	10	fluid ounce(s)	300	150	<1	18	<1	<1	0.01	0.00	0.02	—	0	17	0.81	25	0.02	5	<1	—
Wine, red, California	5	fluid ounce(s)	150	125	<1	4	0	<1	0.00	0.00	0.00	0	0	12	1.43	15	0.00	1	0	—
Wine, sparkling, domestic	5	fluid ounce(s)	150	105	<1	4	0	0	0.00	0.00	0.00	—	0	—	—	—	—	—	0	<1
Wine, white	5	fluid ounce(s)	148	100	<1	1	0	0	0.00	0.00	0.00	—	0	13	0.47	7	—	0	0	—
Yogurt, custard style, fruit flavors	6	ounce(s)	170	190	7	32	0	4	2.00	—	—	—	15	200	0.00	90	—	22	1	7
Yogurt, fruit, low fat	1	cup(s)	245	243	10	46	0	3	1.82	0.77	0.08	—	12	338	0.15	130	0.05	26	1	—
Yogurt, fruit, nonfat, sweetened w/low calorie sweetener	1	cup(s)	241	122	11	19	1	<1	0.21	0.10	0.04	—	3	370	0.62	139	0.17	27	2	8
Yogurt, plain, low fat	1	cup(s)	245	154	13	17	0	4	2.45	1.04	0.11	—	15	448	0.20	172	0.05			
VEGETARIAN FOODS																				
Prepared																				
Macaroni & cheese (lacto)	8	ounce(s)	226	181	8	17	<1	9	4.37	2.88	0.89	0	22	187	0.77	768	0.29	39	<1	16
Steamed rice & vegetables (vegan)	8	ounce(s)	228	265	5	40	3	10	1.84	3.91	4.07	—	0	41	1.43	1403	3.05	28	13	8
Vegan spinach enchiladas (vegan)	1	piece(s)	82	93	5	15	2	2	0.34	0.55	1.27	—	0	117	1.13	134	—	46	1	5
Vegetable chow mein (vegan)	8	ounce(s)	227	166	6	22	2	6	0.65	2.66	2.47	—	0	190	3.65	371	0.06	47	7	6
Vegetable lasagna (lacto)	8	ounce(s)	225	177	12	25	2	4	1.92	0.93	0.34	—	10	144	1.91	637	0.05	64	15	19
Vegetarian chili (vegan)	8	ounce(s)	227	116	6	21	7	2	0.24	0.29	0.74	—	1	68	2.42	383	0.15	58	16	5
Vegetarian vegetable soup (vegan)	8	ounce(s)	226	92	3	14	2	4	0.77	1.67	1.30	—	0	37	1.32	503	0.55	38	24	1
Boca burger																				
All American flamed grilled patty	1	item(s)	71	110	14	6	4	4	1.00	—	—	0	3	150	1.80	370	—	—	0	—
Boca meatless ground burger	½	cup(s)	57	70	11	7	4	1	0.00	—	—	—	0	80	1.44	220	—	—	0	—
Breakfast links	2	item(s)	45	100	10	6	5	4	0.50	0.50	2.00	0	0	60	1.44	330	—	—	0	—
Breakfast patties	2	item(s)	38	80	8	6	3	4	0.50	1.00	3.00	0	0	60	1.44	260	—	—	0	—
Vegan original patty	1	item(s)	71	90	13	4	3	1	0.00	0.50	0.60	0	0	80	1.80	350	—	—	1	—
Gardenburger																				
Black bean burger	1	item(s)	71	80	8	11	4	2	0.00	—	—	0	0	40	1.44	330	—	—	0	—
Chik'n grill	1	item(s)	71	100	13	5	3	3	0.00	—	—	—	0	60	3.60	360	—	—	0	—
Meatless breakfast sausage	1	item(s)	43	50	5	2	2	4	0.00	—	—	—	0	20	0.72	120	—	—	0	—
Meatless meatballs	6	item(s)	85	110	12	8	4	5	1.00	—	—	0	0	60	1.80	400	—	—	0	—
Original	3	ounce(s)	85	132	7	19	4	4	1.80	1.80	—	0	24	72	0.00	672	—	12	0	8
Morningstar Farms																				
America's Original Veggie Dog links	1	item(s)	57	80	11	6	1	1	0.00	0.00	0.00	0	0	0	0.72	580	—	—	0	—
Better n Eggs egg substitute	¼	cup(s)	57	20	5	0	0	0	0.00	0.00	0.00	0	0	20	0.63	90	—	24	0	—
Breakfast links	2	item(s)	45	80	9	3	2	3	0.50	0.50	2.00	0	0	0	1.44	320	—	—	0	—
Breakfast strips	1	item(s)	16	60	2	2	1	5	0.50	1.00	3.00	0	0	0	0.27	220	—	—	0	—
Garden veggie patties	1	item(s)	67	100	10	9	4	3	0.50	0.50	1.50	0	0	40	0.72	350	—	—	0	—
Spicy black bean veggie burger	1	item(s)	78	150	11	16	5	5	0.50	1.50	2.50	0	0	40	1.80	470	—	—	0	—

MIXED FOODS, SOUPS, SANDWICHES

Mixed Dishes

Food	Amt	Unit	Wt	Cal	C1	C2	C3	C4	C5	C6	C7	C8	C9	C10	C11	C12	C13	C14	C15
Bean burrito	1	item(s)	149	327	17	33	6	15	8.30	4.73	0.85	0	38	331	2.95	514	0.01	115	4	18
Beef & vegetable fajita	1	item(s)	223	397	23	35	3	18	5.50	7.53	3.45	—	45	84	3.74	757	0.80	23	27	—
Chicken & vegetables w/broccoli, onion, bamboo shoots in soy based sauce	1	cup(s)	162	287	22	6	1	19	5.13	7.65	4.68	—	84	22	1.38	962	1.12	13	8	—
Chicken cacciatore	1	cup(s)	230	266	28	5	1	14	3.98	5.78	3.11	0	103	45	2.21	451	0.00	15	8	22
Chicken Waldorf salad	½	cup(s)	100	178	14	6	1	11	1.76	3.18	5.05	0	42	20	0.78	246	0.62	15	2	11
Fettuccine alfredo	1	cup(s)	222	247	11	42	1	3	1.61	0.79	0.43	0	9	153	1.88	386	0.00	103	1	35
Hummus	½	cup(s)	123	218	6	25	5	11	1.38	6.04	2.56	—	0	60	1.93	298	0.92	73	10	3
Lasagna w/ ground beef	1	cup(s)	237	288	18	25	2	15	7.47	4.84	0.84	68	222	1.93	493	0.22	50	10	22
Macaroni & cheese	1	cup(s)	200	393	15	40	1	19	8.18	6.72	2.66	—	30	323	2.26	800	0.72	12	<1	17
Meat loaf	1	slice(s)	115	244	17	7	<1	16	6.15	6.89	0.83	0	85	54	2.09	423	0.00	20	<1	5
Potato salad	½	cup(s)	125	179	3	14	2	10	1.79	3.10	4.67	—	85	24	0.81	661	—	9	13	22
Spaghetti & meatballs w/ tomato sauce, prepared	1	cup(s)	248	330	19	39	3	12	3.90	4.40	2.20	—	89	124	3.70	1009	—	—	22	3

Soups

Food	Amt	Unit	Wt	Cal	C1	C2	C3	C4	C5	C6	C7	C8	C9	C10	C11	C12	C13	C14	C15
Spicy thai noodles (pad thai)	8	ounce(s)	231	222	9	36	3	6	0.83	3.33	1.83	0	37	32	1.58	598	0.36	44	22	3
Sushi w/ vegetables in seaweed	6	piece(s)	156	182	3	41	1	<1	0.10	0.11	0.11	—	0	20	1.54	153	0.12	10	2	—
Tuna salad	½	cup(s)	103	192	16	10	0	9	1.58	2.96	4.23	0	13	17	1.03	412	0.00	8	2	42
Chicken noodle, condensed, prepared w/water	1	cup(s)	241	75	4	9	1	2	0.65	1.11	0.55	—	7	17	0.77	1106	0.10	22	<1	6
Cream of chicken, condensed, prepared w/milk	1	cup(s)	248	191	7	15	<1	11	4.64	4.46	1.64	—	27	181	0.67	1047	—	7	1	8
Cream of mushroom, condensed, prepared w/milk	1	cup(s)	248	203	6	15	<1	14	5.13	2.98	4.61	—	20	179	0.60	918	1.24	10	2	4
Manhattan clam chowder, condensed, prepared w/water	1	cup(s)	244	78	2	12	1	2	0.38	0.38	1.29	—	2	27	1.63	578	0.34	10	4	9
Minestrone, condensed, prepared w/water	1	cup(s)	241	82	4	11	1	3	0.55	0.70	1.11	—	2	34	0.92	911	—	36	1	8
New England clam chowder, condensed, prepared w/milk	1	cup(s)	248	164	9	17	1	7	2.95	2.26	1.09	—	22	186	1.49	992	0.45	10	3	13
Split pea	1	cup(s)	165	85	4	19	2	<1	0.07	0.03	0.18	0	0	30	1.25	608	0.00	61	9	<1
Tomato, condensed, prepared w/milk	1	cup(s)	248	161	6	22	3	6	2.90	1.61	1.12	—	17	159	1.81	744	1.24	17	68	2
Tomato, condensed, prepared w/water	1	cup(s)	244	85	2	17	<1	2	0.37	0.44	0.95	—	0	12	1.76	695	2.32	15	66	<1
Vegetable beef, condensed, prepared w/water	1	cup(s)	244	78	6	10	<1	2	0.85	0.81	0.12	—	5	17	1.12	791	0.37	10	2	4
Vegetarian vegetable, condensed, prepared w/water	1	cup(s)	241	72	2	12	—	2	0.29	0.82	0.72	—	0	22	1.08	822	—	10	1	4

Sandwiches

Food	Amt	Unit	Wt	Cal	C1	C2	C3	C4	C5	C6	C7	C8	C9	C10	C11	C12	C13	C14	C15
Bacon, lettuce, & tomato w/mayonnaise	1	item(s)	164	349	11	34	2	19	4.54	7.22	6.07	—	20	76	2.54	837	1.16	31	15	—
Cheeseburger, large, plain	1	item(s)	185	609	30	47	0	33	14.84	12.74	2.44	—	96	91	5.46	1589	—	74	0	39
Cheeseburger, large, w/bacon, vegetables, & condiments	1	item(s)	195	608	32	37	2	37	16.24	14.49	2.71	—	111	162	4.74	1043	—	86	2	33
Club w/bacon, chicken, tomato, lettuce, & mayonnaise	1	item(s)	246	555	31	48	3	26	5.94	—	—	—	72	116	4.05	855	1.53	48	9	—
Cold cut submarine w/cheese & vegetables	1	item(s)	228	456	22	51	2	19	6.81	8.23	2.28	—	36	189	2.51	1651	—	87	12	31
Egg salad	1	item(s)	126	273	10	29	1	13	2.96	3.97	4.79	—	217	107	2.60	494	0.13	82	1	24
Hamburger, double patty, large, w/condiments & vegetables	1	item(s)	226	540	34	40	0	27	10.52	10.33	2.80	—	122	102	5.85	791	—	77	1	26
Hamburger, large, plain	1	item(s)	137	425	23	32	2	23	8.38	9.88	2.14	—	71	74	3.58	474	—	60	0	27
Hot dog w/bun, plain	1	item(s)	98	242	10	18	2	15	5.11	6.85	1.71	—	44	24	2.31	670	—	48	<.1	26
Pastrami	1	item(s)	134	331	14	27	2	18	6.18	8.74	1.02	—	51	68	2.64	1335	0.27	21	2	—
Peanut butter & jelly	1	item(s)	93	333	11	42	3	15	3.00	6.87	3.82	—	1	68	2.11	409	2.02	37	<1	—

FAST FOOD

Arby's

Food	Amt	Unit	Wt	Cal	C1	C2	C3	C4	C5	C6	C7	C8	C9	C10	C11	C12	C13	C14	C15
Au jus sauce	1	serving(s)	85	5	<1	1	<1	<.1	0.02	—	—	—	0	0	0.00	386	—	—	0	—
Beef 'n cheddar sandwich	1	item(s)	198	480	23	43	2	24	8.00	—	—	—	90	100	3.60	1240	—	—	1	—
Curly fries, medium	1	serving(s)	128	400	5	50	4	20	5.00	—	—	—	0	0	1.80	990	—	—	15	—
Market Fresh grilled chicken Caesar salad w/o dressing	1	serving(s)	338	230	33	8	3	8	3.50	—	—	—	80	200	1.80	920	—	—	42	—
Roast beef deluxe sandwich, light	1	item(s)	182	296	18	33	6	10	3.00	5.00	2.00	—	42	130	4.50	826	—	—	8	—
Roast beef sandwich, giant	1	item(s)	228	480	32	41	3	23	10.00	—	—	—	110	60	5.40	1440	—	—	0	—

Food Description	Qty	Measure	Wt (g)	Ener (cal)	Prot (g)	Carb (g)	Dietary Fiber (g)	Fat (g)	Fat Breakdown (g) Sat	Mono	Poly	Trans	Chol (mg)	Calc (mg)	Iron (mg)	Sodi (mg)	Vit E (mg)	Folate (mcg)	Vit C (mg)	Selenium (mcg)
FAST FOOD (continued)																				
Roast beef sandwich, regular	1	item(s)	157	350	21	34	2	16	6.00	—	—	—	85	60	3.60	950	—	—	0	—
Roast chicken deluxe sandwich, light	1	item(s)	194	260	23	33	3	5	1.00	—	—	—	40	100	2.70	1010	—	—	2	—
Burger King																				
BK Broiler chicken sandwich	1	item(s)	258	550	30	52	3	25	5.00	—	—	—	105	60	3.60	1110	—	—	6	—
Croissanwich w/ sausage, egg, & cheese	1	item(s)	157	520	19	24	1	39	14.00	—	—	1.93	210	300	4.50	1090	—	—	0	—
Fish Fillet sandwich	1	item(s)	185	520	18	44	2	30	8.00	—	—	1.12	55	150	2.70	840	—	—	1	—
French fries, medium, salted	1	item(s)	117	360	4	46	4	18	5.00	—	—	4.50	0	20	0.72	640	—	—	9	—
Onion rings, medium	1	serving(s)	91	320	4	40	3	16	4.00	—	—	3.50	0	97	0.00	460	—	—	0	—
Whopper	1	item(s)	291	710	31	52	4	43	13.00	—	—	1	85	150	6.30	980	—	—	9	—
Whopper w/ cheese	1	item(s)	316	800	36	53	4	50	18.00	—	—	2	110	250	6.30	1420	—	—	9	—
Chick Fil-A																				
Chargrilled chicken garden salad	1	item(s)	275	180	22	9	3	6	3.00	—	—	0	70	150	0.72	660	—	—	30	—
Chargrilled deluxe chicken sandwich	1	item(s)	195	290	27	31	2	7	1.50	—	—	0	70	80	1.80	990	—	—	5	—
Chicken biscuit w/ cheese	1	item(s)	151	450	19	43	2	23	7.00	—	—	2.85	45	150	2.70	1430	—	—	0	—
Chicken salad sandwich	1	item(s)	153	350	20	32	5	15	3.00	—	—	0	65	150	1.80	880	—	—	0	—
Chick-n-Strips	4	item(s)	127	290	29	14	1	13	2.50	—	—	0	65	20	0.36	730	—	—	1	—
Coleslaw	1	item(s)	105	210	1	14	2	17	2.50	—	—	0	20	40	0.36	180	—	—	27	—
Dairy Queen																				
Banana split	1	item(s)	369	510	8	96	3	12	8.00	3.00	0.50	0	30	250	1.80	180	—	—	15	—
Chocolate chip cookie dough blizzard, small	1	item(s)	319	720	12	105	0	28	14.00	—	—	2.50	50	350	2.70	370	—	—	1	—
Chocolate malt, small	1	item(s)	418	650	15	111	0	16	10.00	—	—	0.50	55	450	1.80	370	—	—	2	—
Vanilla soft serve	½	cup(s)	94	140	3	22	0	5	3.00	—	—	0	15	150	0.72	70	—	—	0	—
Domino's																				
Classic hand tossed pizza																				
America's favorite feast, 12"	2	slice(s)	205	508	22	57	4	22	9.20	—	—	—	49	202	3.70	1221	—	—	1	—
Pepperoni feast, extra pepperoni & cheese, 12"	2	slice(s)	196	534	24	56	3	25	10.92	—	—	—	57	279	3.36	1349	—	—	<1	—
Vegi feast, 12"	2	slice(s)	203	439	19	57	4	16	7.09	—	—	—	34	279	3.44	987	—	—	1	—
Thin crust pizza																				
Extravaganzza, 12"	¼	item(s)	159	425	20	34	3	24	9.41	—	—	—	53	245	1.95	1408	—	—	1	—
Pepperoni, extra pepperoni & cheese, 12"	¼	item(s)	159	420	20	32	2	24	10.46	—	—	—	54	316	1.34	1362	—	—	<1	—
Vegi, 12"	¼	item(s)	159	338	16	34	3	17	7.08	—	—	—	34	317	1.42	1047	—	—	1	—
Ultimate deep dish pizza																				
America's favorite, 12"	2	slice(s)	235	617	26	59	4	33	12.88	—	—	—	58	334	4.43	1573	—	—	1	—
Pepperoni, extra pepperoni & cheese, 12"	2	slice(s)	235	629	26	57	4	34	13.57	—	—	—	61	332	4.25	1650	—	—	1	—
Vegi, 12"	2	slice(s)	235	547	22	59	4	26	10.19	—	—	—	41	333	4.33	1334	—	—	2	—
In-n-Out Burger																				
Cheeseburger w/ mustard & ketchup	1	item(s)	268	400	22	41	3	18	9.00	—	—	—	55	200	3.60	1080	—	—	15	—
Chocolate shake	1	item(s)	425	690	9	83	0	36	24.00	—	—	—	95	300	0.72	350	—	—	0	—
Double-Double cheeseburger w/ mustard & ketchup	1	item(s)	328	590	37	42	3	32	17.00	—	—	—	115	350	5.40	1510	—	—	15	—
French fries	1	item(s)	125	400	7	54	2	18	5.00	—	—	—	0	20	1.80	245	—	—	0	—
Hamburger w/ mustard & ketchup	1	item(s)	243	310	16	41	3	10	4.00	—	—	—	35	40	3.60	720	—	—	15	—
Jack in the Box																				
Chicken club salad	1	item(s)	535	310	28	15	5	16	6.00	—	—	0	65	300	3.60	890	—	—	54	—
Hamburger	1	item(s)	104	250	12	30	2	9	3.50	—	—	0.88	30	100	3.60	610	—	—	0	—
Jack's Spicy Chicken sandwich	1	item(s)	253	580	24	53	3	31	6.00	—	—	2.81	60	150	1.80	950	—	—	9	—
Jumbo Jack hamburger w/ cheese	1	item(s)	294	690	26	60	3	38	16.00	—	—	1.55	75	250	4.50	1360	—	—	9	—
Sourdough Jack	1	item(s)	244	700	30	36	3	49	16.00	—	—	2.98	80	200	4.50	1220	—	—	9	—
Jamba Juice																				
Banana berry smoothie	24	fluid ounce(s)	719	470	5	112	5	2	0.50	—	—	—	5	200	1.08	85	0.32	33	15	0
Chocolate mood smoothie	24	fluid ounce(s)	612	690	16	142	2	8	4.50	—	—	—	25	500	1.08	280	0.00	9	6	4
Jamba powerboost smoothie	24	fluid ounce(s)	730	440	6	103	7	2	0.00	—	—	—	0	1100	1.44	40	17.71	640	294	70

Item	Amount	Unit																
Orange juice, freshly squeezed	16	fluid ounce(s)	496	220	3	52	1	1	0.00	—	—	0	60	1.08	0	—	—	246	0
Protein berry pizzaz smoothie	24	fluid ounce(s)	710	440	20	92	6	2	0.00	—	—	0	1100	2.62	240	—	—	60	4
Kentucky Fried Chicken (KFC)																			
Extra Crispy chicken, breast	1	item(s)	162	470	34	19	0	28	8.00	—	4.50	135	19	1.44	1230	—	—	1	—
Hot & spicy chicken, whole wing	1	item(s)	55	180	11	9	0	11	3.00	—	0	60	10	0.72	420	—	—	1	—
Original Recipe chicken, drumstick	1	item(s)	59	140	14	4	0	8	2.00	—	1	75	10	0.70	440	—	—	1	—
Long John Silver's																			
Baked cod	1	serving(s)	101	120	22	1	0	5	1.00	—	—	90	20	0.72	240	—	—	—	—
Batter dipped fish sandwich	1	item(s)	177	440	17	48	3	20	5.00	—	—	35	60	3.60	1120	—	—	0	—
Clam chowder	1	item(s)	227	220	9	23	1	10	4.00	—	—	25	150	0.72	810	—	—	9	—
Crunchy shrimp basket	21	item(s)	114	340	12	32	2	19	5.00	—	—	105	500	1.80	720	—	—	1	—
McDonald's																			
Big Mac hamburger	1	item(s)	216	590	24	47	3	34	11.00	—	1.48	85	300	4.50	1090	—	—	4	—
Cheeseburger	1	item(s)	121	350	15	36	2	14	6.00	—	1.02	45	250	2.70	830	—	—	2	—
Chicken McNuggets	4	item(s)	72	210	10	12	1	13	2.50	—	1.13	35	20	0.72	460	—	—	2	—
Egg McMuffin	1	item(s)	138	300	18	29	2	12	4.50	—	0.42	235	300	2.70	830	0.72	—	1	—
Filet-o-fish sandwich	1	item(s)	156	470	15	45	1	26	5.00	—	1.11	50	200	1.80	890	—	—	1	—
French fries, small	1	serving(s)	68	210	3	26	2	10	1.50	—	2.30	0	10	0.36	135	—	—	9	—
Fruit n' yogurt parfait	1	item(s)	338	380	10	76	2	5	2.00	—	0.18	15	300	1.80	240	—	—	24	—
Hash browns	1	item(s)	53	150	1	14	1	8	1.50	—	2	0	10	0.36	330	—	—	2	—
Honey sauce	1	item(s)	14	45	0	12	0	0	0.00	0.00	—	0	0	0.18	0	—	—	—	—
McSalad Shaker garden salad	1	item(s)	149	100	7	4	2	6	3.00	—	—	75	150	1.08	120	—	—	15	—
McSalad Shaker grilled chicken caesar salad	1	item(s)	163	100	17	3	2	3	1.50	—	—	40	100	1.08	240	—	—	12	—
Newman's Own creamy Caesar salad dressing	1	item(s)	59	150	2	4	0	18	3.50	—	0.29	20	60	0.18	500	15.40	—	1	—
Plain hotcakes w/syrup & margarine	3	item(s)	228	600	9	104	0	17	3.00	—	4	20	100	4.50	770	—	—	1	—
Quarter Pounder hamburger	1	item(s)	172	430	23	37	2	21	8.00	—	1.01	70	200	4.50	840	—	—	2	—
Quarter Pounder hamburger w/cheese	1	item(s)	200	530	28	38	2	30	13.00	—	1.51	95	350	4.50	1310	—	—	2	—
Sausage McMuffin w/egg	1	item(s)	164	450	20	29	2	28	10.00	—	0.59	255	300	2.70	930	0.72	—	1	—
Vanilla milkshake	8	fluid ounce(s)	227	254	9	40	0	7	4.28	1.98	—	27	331	0.23	215	0.11	16	0	5
Pizza Hut																			
Pepperoni Lovers stuffed crust pizza	1	slice(s)	171	480	23	44	3	24	11.00	—	1.05	65	300	2.70	1300	—	—	4	—
Pepperoni Lovers thin 'n crispy pizza	1	slice(s)	94	270	13	22	2	14	7.00	—	0.51	40	200	1.44	700	—	—	2	—
Personal Pan supreme pizza	1	slice(s)	73	170	8	19	1	7	3.00	—	0.95	15	80	1.86	400	—	—	4	—
Veggie Lovers stuffed crust pizza	1	slice(s)	181	370	17	45	3	14	7.00	—	0.53	35	250	2.70	980	—	—	12	—
Veggie Lovers thin 'n crispy pizza	1	slice(s)	110	190	8	23	2	7	3.00	—	0.54	15	150	1.44	480	—	—	12	—
Starbucks																			
Cappuccino, tall	12	fluid ounce(s)	360	120	7	10	0	6	4.00	—	0	25	250	0.00	95	—	—	1	—
Cinnamon spice mocha, tall nonfat w/o whipped cream	12	fluid ounce(s)	360	170	11	32	0	0	0.50	0.00	0	5	300	0.72	150	—	—	0	—
Frappuccino, tall chocolate	12	fluid ounce(s)	360	290	13	52	1	5	1.00	0.16	0	3	400	1.80	300	—	—	5	—
Latte, tall w/nonfat milk	12	fluid ounce(s)	360	123	12	17	0	1	0.40	0.02	0	6	420	0.18	174	—	18	4	—
Latte, tall w/whole milk	12	fluid ounce(s)	360	212	11	17	0	11	6.90	0.42	0	46	400	0.18	165	—	17	3	—
Macchiato, tall caramel w/whole milk	12	fluid ounce(s)	360	190	6	27	0	7	4.00	—	0	25	200	0.36	105	—	—	1	—
Tazo chai black tea, tall nonfat	12	fluid ounce(s)	360	170	6	37	0	0	0.00	0.00	0	5	200	0.36	95	—	—	0	—
Subway																			
Chocolate chip cookie	1	item(s)	48	209	3	29	0	10	3.50	—	1.07	12	0	1.00	135	—	—	0	—
Classic Italian B.M.T. sandwich, 6", white bread	1	item(s)	250	453	21	40	3	24	8.00	—	0	56	100	2.70	1740	—	—	24	—
Meatball sandwich, 6", white bread	1	item(s)	284	501	23	46	4	25	10.00	—	0.75	56	100	3.60	1350	—	—	24	—
Roast beef sandwich, 6", white bread	1	item(s)	220	264	18	39	3	5	1.00	—	0	20	40	3.60	840	—	—	24	—
Roasted chicken breast sandwich, 6", white bread	1	item(s)	234	311	25	40	3	6	1.50	—	0	48	60	3.60	880	—	—	24	—
Tuna sandwich, 6", white bread	1	item(s)	252	419	18	39	3	21	5.00	—	—	42	100	2.70	1180	—	—	24	—
Turkey breast sandwich, 6", white bread	1	item(s)	220	254	16	39	3	4	1.00	—	0	15	40	2.70	1000	—	—	24	—
Taco Bell																			
7-layer burrito	1	item(s)	283	533	18	67	10	22	8.00	—	3	25	300	3.59	1360	—	—	5	—
Beef burrito supreme	1	item(s)	248	443	18	51	7	18	8.00	—	2	40	200	2.70	1330	—	—	9	—
Grilled chicken burrito	1	item(s)	198	393	19	49	3	13	4.00	—	—	40	151	1.44	1240	—	—	2	—
Taco	1	item(s)	78	177	8	13	3	10	4.00	—	0.50	25	60	1.08	350	—	—	2	—
Veggie fajita wrap supreme	1	item(s)	255	473	11	55	3	22	7.00	—	—	30	150	1.44	990	—	—	6	—

CONVENIENCE MEALS

Food Description	Qty	Measure	Wt (g)	Ener (cal)	Prot (g)	Carb (g)	Dietary Fiber (g)	Fat (g)	Fat Breakdown (g)				Chol (mg)	Calc (mg)	Iron (mg)	Sodi (mg)	Vit E (mg)	Folate (mcg)	Vit C (mg)	Selenium (mcg)
									Sat	Mono	Poly	Trans								
Budget Gourmet																				
Cheese manicotti w/meat sauce	1	item(s)	284	420	18	38	4	22	11.00	6.00	1.34	—	85	300	2.70	810	—	31	0	—
Chicken w/fettuccine	1	item(s)	284	380	20	33	3	19	10.00	—	—	—	85	100	2.70	810	—	—	0	—
Light beef stroganoff	1	item(s)	248	290	20	32	3	7	4.00	—	—	—	35	40	1.80	580	—	19	2	—
Light sirloin of beef in herb sauce	1	item(s)	269	260	19	30	5	7	4.00	2.30	0.31	—	30	40	1.80	850	—	38	6	—
Light vegetable lasagna	1	item(s)	298	290	15	36	5	9	1.79	0.89	0.60	—	15	283	3.03	780	—	75	59	—
Healthy Choice																				
Chicken enchilada suprema meal	1	item(s)	320	360	13	59	8	7	3.00	2.00	2.00	—	30	40	1.44	580	—	—	4	—
Lemon pepper fish meal	1	item(s)	303	280	11	49	5	5	2.00	1.00	2.00	—	30	40	0.36	580	—	—	30	—
Traditional salisbury steak meal	1	item(s)	354	360	23	45	5	9	3.50	4.00	1.00	—	45	80	2.70	580	—	—	21	—
Traditional turkey breasts meal	1	item(s)	298	330	21	50	4	5	2.00	1.50	1.50	—	35	40	1.44	600	—	—	0	—
Zucchini lasagna	1	item(s)	383	280	13	47	5	4	2.50	—	—	—	10	200	1.80	310	—	—	0	—
Stouffers																				
Cheese enchiladas with mexican rice	1	serving(s)	276	370	12	48	5	14	5.00	—	—	—	25	200	1.44	890	—	—	12	—
Chicken pot pie	1	item(s)	284	740	23	56	4	47	18.00	12.41	10.48	—	65	150	2.70	1170	—	—	2	—
Homestyle beef pot roast & potatoes	1	item(s)	252	270	16	25	3	12	4.50	—	—	—	35	20	1.80	820	—	—	6	—
Homestyle roast turkey breast w/stuffing & mashed potatoes	1	item(s)	273	300	16	34	2	11	3.00	—	—	—	35	40	0.72	1190	—	—	0	—
Lean Cuisine Everyday Favorites chicken chow mein w/rice	1	item(s)	255	210	12	33	2	3	1.00	1.00	0.50	0	30	20	0.36	620	—	—	0	—
Lean Cuisine Everyday Favorites lasagna w/meat sauce	1	item(s)	291	300	19	41	3	8	4.00	2.00	0.50	0	30	200	1.08	650	—	—	5	—
Weight Watchers																				
Smart Ones chicken enchiladas suiza entree	1	serving(s)	255	270	15	33	2	9	3.50	—	—	—	50	250	1.08	660	—	—	4	—
Smart Ones garden lasagna entree	1	item(s)	312	270	14	36	5	7	3.50	—	—	—	30	350	1.80	610	—	—	6	—
Smart Ones pepperoni pizza	1	item(s)	158	390	23	46	4	12	4.00	—	—	—	45	450	1.80	650	—	—	5	—
Smart Ones spicy penne pasta & ricotta	1	item(s)	289	280	11	45	4	6	2.00	—	—	—	5	150	2.70	400	—	—	6	—
Smart Ones spicy Szechuan style vegetables & chicken	1	item(s)	255	220	11	39	3	2	0.50	—	—	—	10	150	1.80	730	—	—	2	—

Notes

Chapter 1

Notes

1. World Health Organization, *Global Strategy on Diet, Physical Activity, and Health,* http://who.int/dietphysicalactivity/en/, downloaded June 4, 2009.
2. U.S. Department of Health and Human Services, Office of the Surgeon General, *Disease Prevention,* http://surgeongeneral.gov/publichealthpriorities.html#disease, downloaded June 5, 2009.
3. U.S. Department of Health and Human Services, Centers for Disease Control and Prevention, National Center for Health Statistics, *National Vital Statistics Reports, Deaths: Preliminary Data for 2011* 61, no. 6 (October 10, 2012).
4. A. S. Go, et al., "AHA Statistical Update: Heart Disease and Stroke Statistics—2013 Update," *Circulation* 127 (2013): e6-e245.
5. American Cancer Society, *2013 Cancer Facts and Figures* (New York: ACS, 2013).
6. American College of Sports Medicine, *ACSM's Guidelines for Exercise Testing and Prescription* (Baltimore: Wolters Kluwer/Lippincott Williams & Wilkins, 2014).
7. National Academy of Sciences, Institute of Medicine, *Dietary Reference Intakes for Energy, Carbohydrates, Fiber, Fat, Fatty Acids, Cholesterol, Protein and Amino Acids (Macronutrients)* (Washington, DC: National Academies Press, 2005).
8. U.S. Department of Health and Human Services and Department of Agriculture, *Dietary Guidelines for Americans, 2005* (Washington, DC: DHHS, 2005).
9. W. L. Haskell, et al., "Physical Activity and Public Health: Updated Recommendation for Adults from the American College of Sports Medicine and the American Heart Association," *Medicine & Science in Sports & Exercise* 39 (2007): 1423-1434.
10. U.S. Department of Health and Human Services, *Physical Activity and Health: A Report of the Surgeon General* (Atlanta, GA: Centers for Disease Control and Prevention, National Center for Chronic Disease Prevention and Health Promotion, 1996).
11. U.S. Department of Health and Human Services, *2008 Physical Activity Guidelines for Americans,* http://health.gov/paguidelines, downloaded October 15, 2008.
12. See Haskell, et al., note 9.
13. American College of Sports Medicine, *Exercise Is Medicine,* http://www.exerciseismedicine.org/, downloaded March 4, 2011.
14. U.S. Department of Health and Human Services, *Healthy People 2020* (Washington, DC: 2010).
15. W. W. K. Hoeger, L. Bond, L. Ransdell, J. M. Shimon, and S. Merugu, "One-Mile Step Count at Walking and Running Speeds," *ACSM's Health & Fitness Journal* 11, no. 1 (2008): 14-19.
16. E. G. Wilmot, C. L. Edwardson, F. A. Achana, M. J. Davies, T. Gorely, L. J. Gray, K. Khunti, T. Yates, and S. J. H. Biddle. "Sedentary Time in Adults and the Association with Diabetes, Cardiovascular Disease and Death: Systematic Review and Meta-Analysis," *Diabetologia* 55 (2012): 2895-2905.
17. H. G. Koenig, "The Healing Power of Faith," *Bottom Line/Health* 18 (May 2004): 3-4.
18. L. Dossey, "Can Spirituality Improve Your Health?" *Bottom Line/Health* 15 (July 2001): 11-13.
19. R. S. Paffenbarger, Jr., R. T. Hyde, A. L. Wing, and C. H. Steinmetz, "A Natural History of Athleticism and Cardiovascular Health," *Journal of the American Medical Association* 252 (1984): 491-495.
20. S. N. Blair, H. W. Kohl III, R. S. Paffenbarger, Jr., D. G. Clark, K. H. Cooper, and L. W. Gibbons, "Physical Fitness and All-Cause Mortality: A Prospective Study of Healthy Men and Women," *Journal of the American Medical Association* 262 (1989): 2395-2401.
21. S. Mandic, et al., "Characterizing Differences in Mortality at the Low End of the Fitness Spectrum," *Medicine & Science in Sports & Exercise* 41 (2009): 1573-1579.
22. E. S. Ford, et al., "Healthy Living is Better Revenge," *Archives of Internal Medicine* 169 (2009): 1355-1362.
23. S. Kodama, et al., "Cardiorespiratory Fitness as a Quantitative Predictor of All-Cause Mortality and Cardiovascular Events in Healthy Men and Women," *Journal of the American Medical Association* 301 (2010): 2024-2035.
24. D. P. Swain, "Moderate- or Vigorous-Intensity Exercise: What Should We Prescribe?" *ACSM's Health & Fitness Journal* 10, no. 5 (2007): 7-11.
25. P. T. Williams, "Physical Fitness and Activity as Separate Heart Disease Risk Factors: A Meta-analysis," *Medicine & Science in Sports & Exercise* 33 (2001): 754-761.
26. D. P. Swain and B. A. Franklin, "Comparative Cardioprotective Benefits of Vigorous vs. Moderate Intensity Aerobic Exercise," *American Journal of Cardiology* 97 (2006): 141-147.
27. I. Lee, et al., "Effect of Physical Inactivity on Major Non-communicable diseases worldwide: An Analysis of Burden of Disease and Life Expectancy," *The Lancet* 380 (2012): 219-229.
28. P. C. Hallal, et al., "Global Physical Activity Levels: Surveillance, Progress, Pitfalls, and Prospects," *The Lancet* 380 (2012): 247-257.
29. Cooper Institute, Texas Youth Fitness Study (Dallas, TX), http://www.cooperinstitute.org/youth/documents/Texas%20Youth%20Fitness%20Study%20—%20Charts.pdf, downloaded March 9, 2011.
30. J. J. Ratey and E. Hagerman, *Spark: The Revolutionary New Science of Exercise and the Brain* (New York: Little, Brown and Company, 2008).

Suggested Readings

Bouchard, C., S. N. Blair, and W. Haskell. *Physical Activity and Health.* Champaign, IL: Human Kinetics, 2012.

Hoeger, W. W. K., and S. A. Hoeger. *Principles and Labs for Fitness and Wellness.* Belmont, CA: Wadsworth/Cengage Learning, 2014.

Hoeger, W. W. K., and S. A. Hoeger. *Fitness and Wellness.* Belmont, CA: Wadsworth/Cengage Learning, 2015.

National Academy of Sciences, Institute of Medicine. *Dietary Reference Intakes for Energy, Carbohydrates, Fiber, Fat, Fatty Acids, Cholesterol, Protein and Amino Acids (Macronutrients).* Washington, DC: National Academies Press, 2005.

Haskell, W. L., et al., "Physical Activity and Public Health: Updated Recommendation for Adults from the American College of Sports Medicine and the American Heart Association," *Medicine & Science in Sports & Exercise* 39 (2007): 1423-1434.

U.S. Department of Health and Human Services. *2008 Physical Activity Guidelines for Americans,* available at http://www.health.gov/paguidelines.

U.S. Department of Health and Human Services, Public Health Service. *Healthy People 2020,* available at http://www.healthypeople.gov.

Chapter 2
Notes

1. J. Annesi, "Using Emotions to Empower Members for Long-Term Exercise Success," *Fitness Management* 17 (2001): 54-58.
2. P. T. Katzmarzyk, et al., "Sitting Time and Mortality from All Causes, Cardiovascular Disease, and Cancer," *Medicine & Science in Sports & Exercise* 41 (2009): 998-1005.
3. D. W. Dunstan, et al., "Television Viewing Time and Mortality: The Australian Diabetes, Obesity, and Lifestyle Study (AusDiab)," *Circulation* 121 (2010): 384-391.
4. Television Bureau of Advertising, "Time Spent Viewing per TV Home: Per Day Annual Averages," http://www.tvb.org/nav/build_frameset.asp?url5/rcentral/index.asp, downloaded March 26, 2005.
5. R. Boynton-Jarret, T. N. Thomas, K. E. Peterson, J. Wiecha, A. M. Sobol, and S. L. Gortmaker, "Impact of Television Viewing Patterns on Fruit and Vegetable Consumption among Adolescents," *Pediatrics* 113 (2003): 1321-1326.
6. League of California Cities Planners Institute, Pasadena Conference Center (April 13-15, 2005).
7. J. Pucher and C. Lefevre, *The Urban Transport Crisis in Europe and North America* (London: Macmillan Press Ltd., 1996).
8. S. Gerrior, L. Bente, and H. Hiza, "Nutrient Content of the U.S. Food Supply, 1909-2000," Washington, D.C.: Home Economics Research Report No. 56 (U.S. Department of Agriculture, Center for Nutrition Policy and Promotion, 2004), p. 74, http://www.usda.gov/cnpp/nutrient_content.html, downloaded April 18, 2005.
9. Marion Nestle, *Food Politics* (Berkeley: University of California Press, 2002), pp. 1, 8, 22.
10. "Food Prepared Away from Home Is Increasing and Found to Be Less Nutritious," *Nutrition Research Newsletter* 21, no. 8 (August 2002): 10(2); A. Clauson, "Shares of Food Spending for Eating Reaches 47 Percent," *Food Review* 22 (1999): 20-22.
11. "A Diner's Guide to Health and Nutrition Claims on Restaurant Menus," (Washington, DC: Center for Science in the Public Interest, 1997), http://www.cspinet.org/reports/dinersgu.html, downloaded March 25, 2005.
12. L. R. Young and M. Nestle, "Expanding Portion Sizes in the U.S. Marketplace: Implications for Nutrition Counseling," *Journal of the American Dietetic Association* 103, no. 2 (February 2003): 231.
13. American Institute for Cancer Research, "As Restaurant Portions Grow, Vast Majority of Americans Still Belong to 'Clean Plate Club,' New Survey Finds," AICR News Release, January 15, 2001.
14. T. V. E. Kral, L. S. Roe, J. S. Meengs, and D. E. Wall, "Increasing the Portion Size of a Packaged Snack Increases Energy Intake," *Appetite* 39 (2002): 86.
15. J. A. Ello-Martin, L. S. Roe, J. S. Meengs, D. E. Wall, and B. J. Rolls, "Increasing the Portion Size of a Unit Food Increases Energy Intake" *Appetite* 39 (2002): 74.
16. B. Wansink, "Can Package Size Accelerate Usage Volume?" *Journal of Marketing* 60 (1996): 1-14.
17. National Alliance for Nutrition and Activity (NANA), From Wallet to Waistline: The Hidden Costs of Super Sizing, http://www.preventioninstitute.org/portionsizerept.html, downloaded June 10, 2010.
18. S. H. A. Holt, N. Sandona, and J. C. Brand-Miller, "The Effects of Sugar-Free vs. Sugar-Rich Beverages on Feelings of Fullness and Subsequent Food Intake," *International Journal of Food Sciences and Nutrition* 51, no. 1 (January 2000): 59.
19. "Wellness Facts," *University of California at Berkeley Wellness Letter* (Palm Coast, FL: The Editors, May 2004).
20. G. S. Howard, D. W. Nance, and P. Myers, *Adaptive Counseling and Therapy* (San Francisco: Jossey-Bass, 1987).
21. J. O. Prochaska, J. C. Norcross, and C. C. DiClemente, *Changing for Good* (New York: William Morrow, 1994).

Suggested Readings

Brehm, B. *Successful Fitness Motivation Strategies*. Champaign, IL: Human Kinetics, 2004.

Burgand, M., and K. Gallagher. "Self-Monitoring: Influencing Effective Behavior Change in Your Clients," *ACSM's Health & Fitness Journal* 10, no. 1 (2006): 14-19.

Hagger, M. S., and N. L. D. Chatzisarantis, editors. *Intrinsic Motivation and Self-Determination in Exercise and Sport*. Champaign, IL: Human Kinetics, 2007.

Prochaska, J. O., J. C. Norcross, and C. C. DiClemente. *Changing for Good*. New York: William Morrow, 1994.

Rodgers, W. M., and C. C. Loitz. "The Role of Motivation in Behavior Change," *ACSM's Health & Fitness Journal* 13, no 1 (2009): 7-12.

White, M. W., E. L. Mailey, and E. McAuley. "Leading a Physically Active Lifestyle," *ACSM's Health & Fitness Journal* 14, no. 1 (2010): 8-15.

Chapter 3
Notes

1. S. Park, A., F. Subar, A. Hollenbeck, and A. Schatzkin, "Dietary Fiber Intake and Mortality in the NIH-AARP Diet and Health Study," *Archives of Internal Medicine* 2011 171, no. 12 (2011):1061-1068, doi: 10.1001/archinternmed.2011.
2. National Academy of Sciences, Institute of Medicine, *Dietary Reference Intakes for Energy, Carbohydrates, Fiber, Fat, Protein and Amino Acids (Macronutrients)* (Washington, DC: National Academies Press, 2002).
3. "Saturated Fat: Not Quite so Bad After All?" *University of California at Berkeley Wellness Letter* (June 2010).
4. Editors of Environmental Nutrition *Healthy Eating: Essential Information for Living Longer and Living Better* (Norwalk, CT: Belvoir Media Group LLC, 2008).
5. J. L. Breslow, "n-3 Fatty Acids and Cardiovascular Disease," *American Journal of Clinical Nutrition* 83 (2006): 1477S-1482S.
6. P. E. Bowen, "Evaluating the Health Claim of Flaxseed and Cancer Prevention," *Nutrition Today* 36 (2001): 144-158; "Flax Facts," *University of California at Berkeley Wellness Letter* (May 2002).
7. A. Pan, et al., "Red Meat Consumption and Mortality: Results from 2 Prospective Cohort Studies," *Archives of Internal Medicine* 172 (2012): 555-563.
8. See note 2.
9. "Soy and Breast Cancer," *University of California at Berkeley Wellness Letter* (June 2007).
10. A. Trichopoulou, et al., "Adherence to a Mediterranean Diet and Survival in a Greek Population," *New England Journal of Medicine* 348 (2003): 2599-2608.
11. R. Estrutch, "Primary Prevention of Cardiovascular Disease with a Mediterranean Diet," *New England Journal of Medicine* 368 (2013): 1279-1290.
12. G. Kojda and R. Hambrecht, "Molecular Mechanism of Vascular Adaptations to Exercise: Physical Activity as an Effective Antioxidant Therapy?" *Cardiovascular Research* 67 (2005): 187-197.
13. G. Bjelakovic, et al., "Mortality in Randomized Trials of Antioxidant Supplements for Primary and Secondary Prevention," *Journal of the American Medical Association* 297 (2007): 842-857.
14. S. Saverio, et al., "Effects of Long-Term Selenium Supplementation on the Incidence of Type 2 Diabetes: A Randomized Trial," *Annals of Internal Medicine* 147 (2007): 217-223.
15. M. L. Neuhouser, et al., "Multivitamin Use and Risk of Cancer and Cardiovascular Disease in the Women's Health Initiative Cohorts," *Archives of Internal Medicine* 169 (2009): 294-304.

16. "Vitamin D May Help You Dodge Cancer: How to Be Sure You Get Enough," *Environmental Nutrition* 30, no. 6 (2007): 1, 4.
17. Vitamin D Council, Understanding Vitamin D Cholecalciferol, http://www.vitamindcouncil.org, downloaded June 19, 2009.
18. American Dietetic Association, "Position of the American Dietetic Association: Nutrient Supplementation," *Journal of the American Dietetic Association* 109 (2009): 2073-2085.
19. Writing Group for the Women's Health Initiative, "Risks and Benefits of Combined Estrogen and Progestin in Healthy Postmenopausal Women: Principal Results from the Women's Health Initiative Randomized Controlled Trial," *Journal of the American Medical Association* 288 (2002): 321-333.
20. U.S. Department of Health and Human Services and U.S. Department of Agriculture, *Dietary Guidelines for Americans 2010* (Washington, DC: U.S. Government Printing Office, 2010).

Suggested Readings

Benardot, D. *Advanced Sports Nutrition*. Champaign, IL: Human Kinetics, 2012.

Fink, H. H., A. E. Mikesky, and L. A. Burgoon. *Practical Applications in Sports Nutrition*. Burlington, MA: Jones & Bartlett Learning, 2012.

McArdle, W. D., F. I. Katch, and V. L. Katch. *Sports & Exercise Nutrition*. Baltimore: Lippincott Williams & Wilkins, 2012.

National Academy of Sciences, Institute of Medicine. *Dietary Reference Intakes for Energy, Carbohydrates, Fiber, Fat, Protein and Amino Acids (Macronutrients)*. Washington, DC: National Academies Press, 2002.

Rolfes, S. R., K. Pinna, and E. N. Whitney. *Understanding Normal and Clinical Nutrition*. Belmont, CA: Wadsworth/Cengage Learning, 2011.

Sizer, F. S., and E. N. Whitney. *Nutrition: Concepts and Controversies*. Belmont, CA: Wadsworth/Cengage Learning, 2011.

Whitney, E. N., and S. R. Rolfes. *Understanding Nutrition*. Belmont, CA: Wadsworth/Cengage Learning, 2011.

Chapter 4

Notes

1. W. W. K. Hoeger, D. Gonzalez, L. B. Ransdell, and J. Gao, "A Comparison of Air Displacement Plethysmography and Hydrostatic Weighing Techniques for Assessment of Percent Body Fat in Adults by Gender and BMI Category," *International Journal of Body Composition Research* 9 (2010): 89-94.
2. E. W. Demerath, et al., "Comparison of Percent Body Fat Estimates Using Air Displacement Plethysmography and Hydrodensitometry in Adults and Children," *International Journal of Obesity* 26 (2002): 389-397.
3. J. Stevens, J. Cai, E. R. Pamuk, D. F. Williamson, M. J. Thun, and J. L. Wood, "The Effect of Age on the Association Between Body Mass Index and Mortality," *New England Journal of Medicine* 338 (1998): 1-7.
4. E. E. Calle, M. J. Thun, J. M. Petrelli, C. Rodriguez, and C. W. Heath, "Body-Mass Index and Mortality in a Prospective Cohort of U.S. Adults," *New England Journal of Medicine* 341 (1999): 1097-1105.
5. K. M. Flegal, et al., "Cause-Specific Excess Deaths Associated with Underweight, Overweight, and Obesity," *Journal of the American Medical Association* 298 (2007): 2028-2037.
6. K. M. Flegal, M. D. Carrol, R. J. Kuczmarski, and C. L. Johnson, "Overweight and Obesity in the United States: Prevalence and Trends, 1960–1994," *International Journal of Obesity and Related Metabolic Disorders* 22 (1998): 39-47.
7. C. Bouchard, G. A. Bray, and V. S. Hubbard, "Basic and Clinical Aspects of Regional Fat Distribution," *American Journal of Clinical Nutrition* 52 (1990): 946-950; G. Hu, et al., "Joint Effects of Physical Activity, Body Mass Index, Waist Circumference, and Waist-to-Hip Ratio on the Risk of Heart Failure," *Circulation* 121 (2010): 237-244; D. Canoy, et al., "Body Fat Distribution and Risk of Coronary Heart Disease in Men and Women in the European Prospective Investigation into Cancer and Nutrition in Norfolk Cohort," *Circulation* 116 (2007): 2933-2943; J. P. Després, I. Lemieux, and D. Prudhomme, "Treatment of Obesity: Need to Focus on High Risk Abdominally Obese Patients," *British Medical Journal* 322 (2001): 716-720.
8. T. Pischon, et al., "General and Abdominal Adiposity and Risk of Death in Europe," *New England Journal of Medicine* 359 (2008): 2105-2120.
9. National Heart, Lung, and Blood Institute, National Institutes of Health, *The Practical Guide: Identification, Evaluation, and Treatment of Overweight and Obesity in Adults* (NIH Publication No. 00-4084) (Washington, DC: U.S. Government Printing Office, 2000).
10. M. B. Snijder, et al., "The Prediction of Visceral Fat by Dual-Energy X-ray Absorptiometry in the Elderly: A Comparison with Computed Tomography and Anthropometry," *International Journal of Obesity* 26 (2002): 984-993.
11. I. Janssen, P. T. Katzmarzyk, and R. Ross, "Waist Circumference and Not Body Mass Index Explains Obesity-Related Health Risk," *American Journal of Clinical Nutrition* 79 (2004): 379-384.
12. M. Ashwell, "Charts Based on Body Mass Index and Waist-to-Height Ratio to Assess the Health Risks of Obesity," *The Open Obesity Journal* 3 (2011): 78-84.
13. M. Ashwell, P. Gunn, and S. Gibson, "Waist-to-Height ratio is a Better Screening Tool than Waist Circumference and BMI for Adult Cardiometabolic Risk Factors: Systematic Review and Meta-Analysis," *Obesity Review* 13 (2012): 275-286.
14. M. Ashwell, et al., "Waist-to-Height Ratio Is More Accurate than Body Mass Index to Quantify Reduced Life Expectancy," *European Congress on Obesity* 2013; Abstract T3T4:P.013.

Suggested Readings

Heymsfield, S. B., T. G. Lohman, Z. Wang, and S. B. Going. *Human Body Composition*. Champaign, IL: Human Kinetics, 2005.

Heyward, V. H., and D. Wagner. *Applied Body Composition Assessment*. Champaign, IL: Human Kinetics, 2004.

Parr, R., and S. Haight. "Abdominal Visceral Fat: The New Direction in Body Composition," *ACSM's Health & Fitness Journal* 10, no. 4 (2006): 26-30.

Chapter 5

Notes

1. "Wellness Facts," *University of California at Berkeley Wellness Letter* (Palm Coast, FL: The Editors, May 2004).
2. C. L. Ogden, et al., "Prevalence of Overweight and Obesity in the U.S.," *Journal of the American Medical Association* 295 (2006): 1549-1555.
3. J. Stein, "The Epidemic of Obesity," *Journal of Clinical Endocrinology & Metabolism* 89 (2004): 2522-2525.
4. A. H. Mokdad, J. S. Marks, D. F. Stroup, and J. L. Gerberding, "Actual Causes of Death in the United States, 2000," *Journal of the American Medical Association* 291 (2004): 1238-1241.
5. R. Sturm and K. B. Wells, "Does Obesity Contribute as Much to Morbidity as Poverty or Smoking?" *Public Health* 115 (2001): 229-235.
6. E. E. Calle, et al., "Overweight, Obesity, and Mortality from Cancer in a Prospectively Studied Cohort of U.S. Adults," *New England Journal of Medicine* 348 (2003): 1625-1638.
7. A. Peeters, et al., "Obesity in Adulthood and Its Consequences for Life Expectancy: A Life-Table Analysis," *Annals of Internal Medicine* 138 (2003): 24-32.
8. K. R. Fontaine, et al., "Years of Life Lost Due to Obesity," *Journal of the American Medical Association* 289 (2003): 187-193.

9. American College of Sports Medicine, "Position Stand: Appropriate Physical Activity Intervention Strategies for Weight Loss and Prevention of Weight Regain for Adults," *Medicine & Science in Sports & Exercise* 41 (2009): 459-471.
10. S. Thomsen, "A Steady Diet of Images," *BYU Magazine* 57, no. 3 (2003): 20-21.
11. S. Lichtman, et al., "Discrepancy Between Self-Reported and Actual Caloric Intake and Exercise in Obese Subjects," *New England Journal of Medicine* 327 (1992): 1893-1898.
12. J. H. Wilmore, D. L. Costill, and W. L. Kenney, *Physiology of Sport and Exercise* (Champaign, IL: Human Kinetics, 2008).
13. C. D. Gardner, et al., "Comparison of the Atkins, Zone, Ornish, and LEARN Diets for Change in Weight and Related Risk Factors among Overweight Premenopausal Women," *Journal of the American Medical Association* 297 (2007): 969-977; G. D. Foster, et al., "A Randomized Trial of a Low-Carbohydrate Diet for Obesity," *New England Journal of Medicine* 348 (2003): 2082-2090.
14. American Psychiatric Association, *Diagnostic and Statistical Manual of Mental Disorders* (Washington, DC: APA, 1994).
15. See note 14.
16. R. L. Leibel, M. Rosenbaum, and J. Hirsh, "Changes in Energy Expenditure Resulting from Altered Body Weight," *New England Journal of Medicine* 332 (1995): 621-628.
17. R. J. Shepard, *Alive Man: The Physiology of Physical Activity* (Springfield, IL: Charles C. Thomas, 1975), pp. 484-488.
18. A. Eliasson, et al., "Sleep Is a Critical Factor in the Maintenance of Healthy Weight," paper presented at American Thoracic Society International Conference, San Diego, CA, (2009).
19. S. Pattel, et al., "Sleep Your Way to Weight Loss?" paper presented at American Thoracic Society International Conference, San Diego, CA (2006).
20. K. Knutson, "Impact of Sleep and Sleep Loss on Glucose Homeostasis and Appetite Regulation," *Sleep Medicine Clinic* 2 (2007): 187-197.
21. S. Taheri, et al., "Short Sleep Duration is Associated with Reduced Leptin, Elevated Ghrelin, and Increased Body Mass Index," *PLoS Medicine* 1 (2004): e62, doi:10.1371/journal.pmed.0010062.
22. W. C. Miller, D. M. Koceja, and E. J. Hamilton, "A Meta-Analysis of the Past 25 Years of Weight Loss Research Using Diet, Exercise, or Diet Plus Exercise Intervention," *International Journal of Obesity* 21 (1997): 941-947.
23. National Academy of Sciences, Institute of Medicine, *Dietary Reference Intakes for Energy, Carbohydrates, Fiber, Fat, Protein and Amino Acids (Macronutrients)* (Washington, DC: National Academies Press, 2002).
24. J. G. Thomas, et al., "The National Weight Control Registry: A Study of Successful Losers," *ACSM's Health & Fitness Journal* 15, no. 2 (2011): 8-12.
25. E. T. Poehlman, et al., "Effects of Endurance and Resistance Training on Total Daily Energy Expenditure in Young Women: A Controlled Randomized Trial," *Journal of Clinical Endocrinology and Metabolism* 87 (2002): 1004-1009; L. M. Van Etten, et al., "Effect of an 18-Wk Weight-Training Program on Energy Expenditure and Physical Activity," *Journal of Applied Physiology* 82 (1997): 298-304; W. W. Campbell, M. C. Crim, V. R. Young, and W. J. Evans, "Increased Energy Requirements and Changes in Body Composition with Resistance Training in Older Adults," *American Journal of Clinical Nutrition* 60 (1994): 167-175; Z. Wang, et al., "Resting Energy Expenditure: Systematic Organization and Critique of Prediction Methods," *Obesity Research* 9 (2001): 331-336.
26. J. R. Karp and W. L. Wescott, "The Resting Metabolic Rate Debate," *Fitness Management* 23, no. 1 (2007): 44-47.
27. A. Tremblay, J. A. Simoneau, and C. Bouchard, "Impact of Exercise Intensity on Body Fatness and Skeletal Muscle Metabolism," *Metabolism* 43 (1994): 814-818.
28. T. S. Church, et al. "Changes in Weight, Waist Circumference and Compensatory Responses with Different Doses of Exercise Among Sedentary, Overweight Postmenopausal Women," *PLoS ONE* 4, no. 2 (2009): e4515, doi:10.1371/journal.pone.0004515.
29. I. Lee, et al., "Physical Activity and Weight Gain Prevention," *Journal of the American Medical Association* 303 (2010): 1173-1179.
30. T. A. Hagobian and B. Braun, "Physical Activity and Hormonal Regulation of Appetite: Sex Differences and Weight Control," *Exercise and Sport Sciences Reviews*," 38 (2010): 25-30.
31. M. L. Klem, R. R. Wing, M. T. McGuire, H. M. Seagle, and J. O. Hill, "A Descriptive Study of Individuals Successful at Long-Term Maintenance of Substantial Weight Loss," *American Journal of Clinical Nutrition* 66 (1997): 239-246.
32. See note 24; U.S. Department of Health and Human Services, Department of Agriculture, *Dietary Guidelines for Americans 2005* (Washington, DC: DHHS, 2005).
33. W. W. K. Hoeger, C. Harris, E. M. Long, and D. R. Hopkins, "Four-Week Supplementation with a Natural Dietary Compound Produces Favorable Changes in Body Composition," *Advances in Therapy* 15, no. 5 (1998): 305-313; W. W. K. Hoeger, et al., "Dietary Supplementation with Chromium Picolinate/L-Carnitine Complex in Combination with Diet and Exercise Enhances Body Composition," *Journal of the American Nutraceutical Association* 2, no. 2 (1999): 40-45.
34. D. Mozaffarian, et al., "Changes in Diet and Lifestyle and Long-Term Weight Gain in Women and Men," *New England Journal of Medicine* 364 (2011): 2392-2404.
35. N. A. Christakis and J. H. Fowler, "The Spread of Obesity in a Large Social Network over 32 Years," *New England Journal of Medicine* 357 (2007): 370-379.

Suggested Readings

American College of Sports Medicine. "Position Stand: Appropriate Physical Activity Intervention Strategies for Weight Loss and Prevention of Weight Regain for Adults," *Medicine & Science in Sports & Exercise* 41 (2009): 459-471.

American Diabetes Association and American Dietetic Association. *Exchange Lists for Meal Planning*. Chicago: American Dietetic Association and American Diabetes Association, 2008.

National Academy of Sciences, Institute of Medicine. *Dietary Reference Intakes for Energy, Carbohydrates, Fiber, Fat, Protein and Amino Acids (Macronutrients)*. Washington, DC: National Academies Press, 2002.

Chapter 6
Notes
1. R. B. O'Hara, et al., "Increased Volume Resistance Training: Effects upon Predicted Aerobic Fitness in a Select Group of Air Force Men," *ACSM's Health & Fitness Journal* 8, no. 4 (2004): 16-25.
2. American College of Sports Medicine, *ACSM's Guidelines for Exercise Testing and Prescription* (Philadelphia: Wolters Kluwer/Lippincott Williams & Wilkins, 2014).
3. U.S. Department of Health and Human Services, *Physical Activity and Health: A Report of the Surgeon General* (Atlanta, GA: Centers for Disease Control and Prevention, National Center for Chronic Disease Prevention and Health Promotion, 1996).
4. American College of Sports Medicine, "Position Stand: Quantity and Quality of Exercise for Developing and Maintaining Cardiorespiratory, Musculoskeletal, and Neuromotor Fitness in Apparently Healthy Adults: Guidance for Prescribing Exercise" *Medicine & Science in Sports & Exercise* 43 (2011): 1334-1359.
5. See note 2.
6. See note 2.
7. S. E. Gormley, et al., "Effect of Intensity of Aerobic Training on VO_{2max}," *Medicine & Science in Sports & Exercise* 40 (2008): 1336-1343.

8. R. L. Gellish, et al., "Longitudinal Modeling of the Relationship Between Age and Maximal Heart Rate," *Medicine & Science in Sports & Exercise* 39 (2007): 822-829.
9. See note 3.
10. D. P. Swain, "Moderate or Vigorous Intensity Exercise: Which Is Better for Improving Aerobic Fitness?" *Preventive Cardiology* 8, no. 1 (2005): 55-58.
11. P. T. Williams, "Physical Fitness and Activity as Separate Heart Disease Risk Factors: A Meta-analysis," *Medicine & Science in Sports & Exercise* 33 (2001): 754-761.
12. D. P. Swain and B. A. Franklin, "Comparative Cardioprotective Benefits of Vigorous vs. Moderate Intensity Aerobic Exercise," *American Journal of Cardiology* 97, no. 1 (2006): 141-147.
13. R. F. DeBusk, U. Stenestrand, M. Sheehan, and W. L. Haskell, "Training Effects of Long versus Short Bouts of Exercise in Healthy Subjects," *American Journal of Cardiology* 65 (1990): 1010-1013.
14. National Academy of Sciences, Institute of Medicine, *Dietary Reference Intakes for Energy, Carbohydrates, Fiber, Fat, Protein and Amino Acids (Macronutrients)* (Washington, DC: National Academies Press, 2002).
15. U.S. Department of Health and Human Services, Department of Agriculture, *Dietary Guidelines for Americans 2005* (Washington, DC: DHHS, 2005).
16. W. Dunstan, et al., "Television Viewing Time and Mortality: The Australian Diabetes, Obesity, and Lifestyle Study (AusDiab)," *Circulation* 121 (2010): 384-391.
17. P. T. Katzmarzyk, et al., "Sitting Time and Mortality from All Causes, Cardiovascular Disease, and Cancer," *Medicine & Science in Sports & Exercise* 41 (2009): 998-1005.

Suggested Readings

ACSM's Guidelines for Exercise Testing and Prescription. Philadelphia: Wolters Kluwer/Lippincott Williams & Wilkins, 2014.

ACSM's Resource Manual for Guidelines for Exercise Testing and Prescription. Philadelphia: Wolters Kluwer/Lippincott Williams & Wilkins, 2012.

Hoeger, W. W. K., and S. A. Hoeger. *Fitness & Wellness*. Belmont, CA: Wadsworth/Cengage Learning, 2015.

Hoeger, W. W. K., and S. A. Hoeger. *Principles and Labs for Fitness & Wellness*. Belmont, CA: Wadsworth/Cengage Learning, 2014.

Karvonen, M. J., E. Kentala, and O. Mustala. "The Effects of Training on the Heart Rate: A Longitudinal Study," *Annales Medicinae Experimetalis et Biologiae Fenniae* 35 (1957): 307-315.

McArdle, W. D., F. I. Katch, and V. L. Katch. *Exercise Physiology: Energy, Nutrition, and Human Performance*, 5th ed. Philadelphia: Wolters Kluwer/Lippincott Williams & Wilkins, 2010.

Wilmore, J. H., and D. L. Costill. *Physiology of Sport and Exercise*. Champaign, IL: Human Kinetics, 2012.

Chapter 7
Notes

1. American College of Sports Medicine, *ACSM's Guidelines for Exercise Testing and Prescription* (Baltimore: Wolters Kluwer/Lippincott Williams & Wilkins, 2014).
2. C. Castaneda, et al., "A Randomized Controlled Trial of Resistance Exercise Training to Improve Glycemic Control in Older Adults with Type 2 Diabetes," *Diabetes Care* 25 (2002): 2335-2341.
3. G. B. Forbes, "The Adult Decline in Lean Body Mass," *Human Biology* 48 (1976): 161-173; W. R. Frontera, et al., "A Cross-sectional Study of Muscle Strength and Mass in 45 to 78 Yr-Old Men and Women," *Journal of Applied Physiology* 71 (1991): 644-650; W. R. Frontera, et al., "Aging of Skeletal Muscle: A 12-Yr Longitudinal Study," *Journal of Applied Physiology* 88 (2000): 1321-1326.
4. M. D. Peterson, A. Sen, and P. M. Gordon, "Influence of Resistance Exercise on Lean Body Mass in Aging Adults: A Meta-Analysis," *Medicine & Science in Sports & Exercise* 43 (2011): 249-258.
5. W. W. Campbell, M. C. Crim, V. R. Young, and W. J. Evans, "Increased Energy Requirements and Changes in Body Composition with Resistance Training in Older Adults," *American Journal of Clinical Nutrition* 60 (1994): 167-175.
6. W. J. Evans, "Exercise, Nutrition and Aging," *Journal of Nutrition* 122 (1992): 796-801.
7. P. E. Allsen, *Strength Training: Beginners, Body Builders and Athletes* (Dubuque, IA: Kendall/Hunt, 2009).
8. See note 5.
9. American College of Sports Medicine, "Progression Models in Resistance Training for Healthy Adults," *Medicine & Science in Sports & Exercise* 41 (2009): 687-708.
10. B. M. Hather, P. A. Tesch, P. Buchanan, and G. A. Dudley, "Influence of Eccentric Actions on Skeletal Muscle Adaptations to Resistance Training," *Acta Physiologica Scandinavica* 143 (1991): 177-185; C. B. Ebbeling and P. M. Clarkson, "Exercise-Induced Muscle Damage and Adaptation," *Sports Medicine* 7 (1989): 207-234.
11. W. W. K. Hoeger, D. R. Hopkins, S. L. Barette, and D. F. Hale, "Relationship Between Repetitions and Selected Percentages of One Repetition Maximum: A Comparison Between Untrained and Trained Males and Females," *Journal of Applied Sport Science Research* 4, no. 2 (1990): 47-51.
12. W. J. Kraemer and M. S. Fragala, "Personalize It: Program Design in Resistance Training," *ACSM's Health & Fitness Journal* 10, no. 4 (2006): 7-17.
13. See note 9.

Suggested Readings

American College of Sports Medicine, "Progression Models in Resistance Training for Healthy Adults," *Medicine & Science in Sports & Exercise* 41 (2009): 687-708.

Hesson, J. L. *Weight Training for Life*. Belmont, CA: Wadsworth/Cengage Learning, 2012.

Heyward, V. H. *Advanced Fitness Assessment and Exercise Prescription*. Champaign, IL: Human Kinetic Press, 2010.

Hoeger, W. W. K., and S. A. Hoeger. *Principles and Labs for Fitness and Wellness*. Belmont, CA: Wadsworth/Cengage, 2014.

Kraemer, J. K., and N. A. Ratamess. "Fundamentals of Resistance Training: Progression and Exercise Prescription," *Medicine & Science in Sports & Exercise* 36 (2004): 674-688.

Kraemer, W. J., and S. J. Fleck. *Optimizing Strength Training*. Champaign, IL: Human Kinetic Press, 2007.

Chapter 8
Notes

1. R. Artal, and M. O'Toole, "Guidelines of the American College of Obstetricians and Gynecologists for Exercise During Pregnancy and the Postpartum Period," *British Journal of Sports Medicine* 37 (2003): 6-12.
2. "Stretch Yourself Younger," *Consumer Reports on Health* 11 (August 1999): 6-7.
3. D. R. Hopkins and W. W. K. Hoeger, "A Comparison of the Sit and Reach and the Modified Sit and Reach in the Measurement of Flexibility for Males," *Journal of Applied Sports Science Research* 6 (1992): 7-10; W. W. K. Hoeger and D. R. Hopkins, "A Comparison between the Sit and Reach and the Modified Sit and Reach in the Measurement of Flexibility in Women," *Research Quarterly for Exercise and Sport* 63 (1992): 191-195; W. W. K. Hoeger, D. R. Hopkins, S. Button, and T. A. Palmer, "Comparing the Sit and Reach with the Modified Sit and Reach in Measuring Flexibility in Adolescents," *Pediatric Exercise Science* 2 (1990): 156-162.

4. American College of Sports Medicine, "Quantity and Quality of Exercise for Developing and Maintaining Cardiorespiratory, Musculoskeletal, and Neuromotor Fitness in Apparently Healthy Adults: Guidance for Prescribing Exercise," *Medicine & Science in Sports & Exercise* 43 (2011): 1334-1359.
5. American College of Sports Medicine, *ACSM's Guidelines for Exercise Testing and Prescription* (Philadelphia: Wolters Kluwer/ Lippincott Williams & Wilkins, 2014).
6. See note 4.
7. K. B. Fields, C. M. Burnworth, and M. Delaney, "Should Athletes Stretch before Exercise?" *Gatorade Sports Science Institute: Sports Science Exchange* 30, no. 1 (2007): 1-5.
8. S. B. Thacker, J. Gilchrist, D. F. Stroup, and C. D. Kimsey Jr., "The Impact of Stretching on Sports Injury Risk: A Systematic Review of the Literature," *Medicine & Science in Sports & Exercise* 36 (2004): 371-378.
9. D. G. Behm, et al., "Short Duration of Static Stretching When Combined with Dynamic Stretching Do Not Impair Repeated Sprints and Agility," *Journal of Sport Science and Medicine* 10 (2011): 408-416.
10. D. B. J. Andersson, L. J. Fine, and B. A. Silverstein, "Musculoskeletal Disorders," *Occupational Health: Recognizing and Preventing Work-Related Disease*, B. S. Levy and D. H. Wegman, editors (Boston: Little, Brown, 1995)
11. M. R. Bracko, "Can We Prevent Back Injuries?" *ACSM's Health & Fitness Journal* 8, no. 4 (2004): 5-11.
12. H. B. Albert, et al., "Antibiotic Treatment in Patients with Chronic Low Back Pain and Vertebral Bone Edema (Modic Type 1 Changes): A Double-Blind Randomized Clinical Controlled Trial of Efficacy," *European Spine Journal* 22 (2013): 690-696.
13. H. B. Albert, et al., "Antibiotic Treatment in Patients with Chronic Low Back Pain And Vertebral Bone Edema (Modic Type 1 Changes): A Double-Blind Randomized Clinical Controlled Trial of Efficacy," *European Spine Journal* 22 (2013): 697-707.
14. R. Deyo, "Chiropractic Care for Back Pain: The Physician's Perspective," *HealthNews* 4 (September 10, 1998).
15. B. W. Nelson, et al., "Can Spinal Surgery Be Prevented by Aggressive Strengthening Exercise? A Prospective Study of Cervical and Lumbar Patients," *Archives of Physical Medicine and Rehabilitation* 80 (1999): 20-25.
16. See note 11.
17. K. Williams, et al., "Evaluation of the Effectiveness and Efficacy of Iyegar Yoga Therapy on Chronic Low Back Pain," *Spine* 34 (2009): 2066-2076.
18. J. A. Hides, G. A. Jull, and C. A. Richardson, "Long-Term Effects of Specific Stabilizing Exercises for First-Episode Low Back Pain," *Spine* 26 (2001): E243-E248.
19. "Position Yourself to Stay Well," *Consumer Reports on Health* 18 (February 2006): 8-9.
20. A. Brownstein, "Chronic Back Pain Can Be Beaten," *Bottom Line/Health* 13 (October 1999): 3-4.

Suggested Readings

Alter, M. J. *Science of Flexibility*. Champaign, IL: Human Kinetic Press, 2004.
Bracko, M. R. "Can We Prevent Back Injuries?" *ACSM's Health & Fitness Journal* 8, no. 4 (2004): 5-11.
Hoeger, W. W. K. *The Assessment of Muscular Flexibility: Test Protocols and National Flexibility Norms for the Modified Sit-and-Reach Test, Total Body Rotation Test, and Shoulder Rotation Test*. Rockton, IL: Figure Finder Collection Novel Products, 2010.
Liemohn, W., and G. Pariser. "Core Strength: Implications for Fitness and Low Back Pain," *ACSM's Health & Fitness Journal* 6, no. 5 (2002): 10-16.
McAtee, R. E., and J. Charland. *Facilitated Stretching*. Champaign, IL: Human Kinetics, 2007.
Nelson, A. G., J. Kokkonen, and J. M. McAlexander. *Stretching Anatomy*. Champaign, IL: Human Kinetics, 2007.

Chapter 9

Notes

1. W. Hoeger, T. A. Spitzer-Gibson, N. Kaluhiokalani, J. Kokonnen, "Comparison of Physiologic Responses to Self-Paced Water Aerobics and Self-Paced Treadmill Running," *Journal of the International Council for Health, Physical Education, Recreation, Sport, and Dance* 30, no. 4 (2004): 27-30.
2. W. W. K. Hoeger, T. S. Gibson, J. Moore, and D. R. Hopkins, "A Comparison of Selected Training Responses to Low Impact Aerobics and Water Aerobics," *National Aquatics Journal* 9 (1993): 13-16.
3. E. J. Marcinick, J. Potts, G. Schlabach, S. Will, P. Dawson, and B. F. Hurley, "Effects of Strength Training on Lactate Threshold and Endurance Performance," *Medicine & Science in Sports & Exercise* 23 (1991): 739-743.
4. B. Klika and C. Jordan, "High-Intensity Circuit Training Using Body Weight: Maximum Results with Minimal Investment," *ACSM's Health & Fitness Journal* 17, no. 3 (2013): 8-13.
5. American College of Sports Medicine, and American Diabetes Association, "Joint Position Statement: Exercise and Type 2 Diabetes," *Medicine & Science in Sports & Exercise* 42 (2010): 2282-2303.
6. American College of Obstetricians and Gynecologists, "Exercise During Pregnancy and the Postpartum Period. ACOG Committee Opinion No. 267," *International Journal of Gynecology and Obstetrics* 77 (2002): 79-81.
7. University of California at Berkeley, *The Wellness Guide to Lifelong Fitness* (New York: Random House, 1993): 198.
8. W. J. Chodzko-Zajko, et al., "Exercise and Physical Activity for Older Adults," *Medicine & Science in Sports & Exercise* 41 (2009): 1510-1530.
9. F. W. Kash, J. L. Boyer, S. P. Van Camp, L. S. Verity, and J. P. Wallace, "The Effect of Physical Activity on Aerobic Power in Older Men (A Longitudinal Study)," *Physician and Sports Medicine* 18, no. 4 (1990): 73-83.
10. W. S. Evans, "Exercise, Nutrition and Aging," *Journal of Nutrition* 122 (1992): 796-801.
11. See note 8.
12. J. M. Moore and W. W. K. Hoeger, "Game On! Preparing Your Clients for Recreational Sports," *ACSM's Health & Fitness Journal* 9, no. 3 (2005): 14-19.
13. J. R. Karp, "Interval Training: The New and Better Way to Train Your Clients?" *IDEA Fitness Journal* 8, no. 2 (2011): 31-34.

Suggested Readings

American College of Obstetricians and Gynecologists. "Exercise During Pregnancy and the Postpartum Period. ACOG Committee Opinion No. 267." *International Journal of Gynecology and Obstetrics* 77 (2002): 79-81.
Clark, N. *Nancy Clark's Sports Nutrition Guidebook*. Champaign, IL: Human Kinetics, 2008.
Pfeiffer, R. P., and B. C. Mangus. *Concepts of Athletic Training*. Boston: Jones and Bartlett, 2012.

Chapter 10

Notes

1. U.S. Department of Health and Human Services, Centers for Disease Control and Prevention, National Center for Health Statistics, *National Vital Statistics Reports, Deaths: Preliminary Data for 2011* 61, no. 6 (October 10, 2012).
2. R. S. Paffenbarger, Jr., R. T. Hyde, A. L. Wing, I. Lee, D. L. Jung, and J. B. Kampert, "The Association of Changes in Physical-Activity Level and Other Lifestyle Characteristics with Mortality Among Men," *New England Journal of Medicine* 328 (1993): 538-545.
3. D. P. Swain and B. A. Franklin, "Comparative Cardioprotective Benefits of Vigorous vs. Moderate Intensity Aerobic Exercise," *American Journal of Cardiology* 97, no. 1 (2006): 141-147.

4. G. Samitz, M. Egger, and M. Zwahlen, "Domains of Physical Activity and All-Cause Mortality: Systematic Review and Dose-Response Meta-Analysis of Cohort Studies," *International Journal of Epidemiology* 40 (2011):1382-1400.
5. S. C. Moore, et al., "Leisure Time Physical Activity of Moderate to Vigorous Intensity and Mortality: A Large Pooled Cohort Analysis," *PLOS Medicine* 9, no. 11 (2012): e1335, doi:10.1371/journal.pmed.001001335.
6. "Lipid Research Clinics Program: The Lipid Research Clinic Coronary Primary Prevention Trial Results," *Journal of the American Medical Association* 251 (1984): 351-364.
7. "HDL on the Rise," *HealthNews* (September 10, 1999).
8. R. Singa, et al., "Meat Intake and Mortality: A Prospective Study of Over Half a Million People," *Archives of Internal Medicine* 169 (2009): 562-571.
9. A. E. Buyken, et al., "Modifications in Dietary Fat Are Associated with Changes in Serum Lipids of Older Adults Independently of Lipid Medication," *Journal of Nutrition* 140 (2010): 88-94.
10. C. M. Albert, et al., "Blood Levels of Long-Chain n-3 Fatty Acids and the Risk of Sudden Death," *New England Journal of Medicine* 346 (2002): 1113-1118.
11. A. H. Lichtenstein, et al., "Diet and Lifestyle Recommendations Revision 2006: A Scientific Statement from the American Heart Association Nutrition Committee," *Circulation* 114 (2006): 82-96.
12. E. B. Rimm, A. Ascherio, E. Giovannucci, D. Spiegelman, M. J. Stampfer, and W. C. Willett, "Vegetable, Fruit, and Cereal Fiber Intake and Risk of Coronary Heart Disease Among Men," *Journal of the American Medical Association* 275 (1996): 447-451.
13. National Cholesterol Education Program Expert Panel, "Summary of the Third Report of the National Cholesterol Education Program (NCEP) Expert Panel on Detection, Evaluation, and Treatment of High Blood Cholesterol in Adults (Adult Treatment Panel III)," *Journal of the American Medical Association* 285 (2001): 2486-2497.
14. P. W. Siri-Tarino, Q. Sun, F. B. Hu, and R. M. Krauss, "Meta-Analysis of Prospective Cohort Studies Evaluating the Association of Saturated Fat with Cardiovascular Disease," *American Journal of Clinical Nutrition* 91 (2010): 535-546.
15. P. W. Siri-Tarino, Q. Sun, F. B. Hu, and R. M. Krauss, "Saturated Fat, Carbohydrate, and Cardiovascular Disease," *The American Journal of Clinical Nutrition* 91 (2010): 502-509.
16. D. Mozaffarian, R. Micha, and S. Wallace, "Effects on Coronary Heart Disease of Increasing Polyunsaturated Fat in Place of Saturated Fat: A Systematic Review of Meta-Analysis of Randomized Controlled Trials," *PLoS Medicine* 7 (2010): 7:e1000252.
17. A. Jula, et al., "Effects of Diet and Simvastatin on Serum Lipids, Insulin, and Antioxidants in Hypercholesterolemic Men," *Journal of the American Medical Association* 287 (2002): 598-605.
18. "The Homocysteine-CVD Connection," *HealthNews* (October 25, 1999).
19. P. M. Ridger, et al., "Rosuvastatin to Prevent Vascular Events in Men and Women with Elevated C-Reactive Protein," *New England Journal of Medicine* 359 (2008): 2195-2207.
20. D. M. Nathan, "Navigating the Choices for Diabetes Prevention," *New England Journal of Medicine* 362 (2010): 1533-1535; The Accord Study Group, "Effects of Combination Lipid Therapy in Type 2 Diabetes Mellitus," *New England Journal of Medicine* 362 (2010): 1563-1574; The Accord Study Group, "Effects of Intensive Blood Pressure Control in Type 2 Diabetes Mellitus," *New England Journal of Medicine* 362 (2010): 1575-1585.
21. H. K. Choi, et al., "Dairy Consumption and Risk of Type 2 Diabetes Mellitus in Men," *Archives of Internal Medicine* 165 (2005): 997-1003.
22. G. M. Reaven, T. K. Strom, and B. Fox, *Syndrome X: Overcoming the Silent Killer That Can Give You a Heart Attack* (Englewood Cliffs, NJ: Simon & Schuster, 2000).
23. A. V. Chobanian, et al., "The Seventh Report of the Joint National Committee on Prevention, Detection, Evaluation, and Treatment of High Blood Pressure," *Journal of the American Medical Association* 289 (2003): 2560-2571.
24. "Shake the Salt Habit to Reduce Your Risk of Stroke and Heart Disease," *Health & Nutrition Letter* (March 2010).
25. P. Strazzullo, L. D'Elia, N-B Kandala, and F. P. Cappuccio, "Salt Intake, Stroke, and Cardiovascular Disease: Meta-Analysis of Prospective Studies," *British Medical Journal* 339 (2009): b4567.
26. K. Bibbins-Domingo, et al., "Projected Effect of Dietary Salt Reductions on Future Cardiovascular Disease," *New England Journal of Medicine* 362 (2010): 590-599.
27. "Salt Takes a Licking," *University of California at Berkeley Wellness Letter* (April 2010).
28. L. S. Pescatello, et al., "Exercise and Hypertension Position Stand," *Medicine & Science in Sports & Exercise* 36 (2004): 533-553.
29. G. Kelley, "Dynamic Resistance Exercise and Resting Blood Pressure in Adults: A Meta-analysis," *Journal of Applied Physiology* 82 (1997): 1559-1565; G. A. Kelley and Z. Tran, "Aerobic Exercise and Normotensive Adults: A Meta-Analysis," *Medicine & Science in Sports & Exercise* 27 (1995): 1371-1377; G. Kelley and P. McClellan, "Antihypertensive Effects of Aerobic Exercise: A Brief Meta-Analytic Review of Randomized Controlled Trials," *American Journal of Hypertension* 7 (1994): 115-119.
30. R. Collins, et al., "Blood Pressure, Stroke, and Coronary Heart Disease; Part 2, Short-term Reductions in Blood Pressure: Overview of Randomized Drug Trials in Their Epidemiological Context," *The Lancet* 335 (1990): 827-838.
31. G. A. Kelley and K. S. Kelley, "Progressive Resistance Exercise and Resting Blood Pressure: A Meta-Analysis of Randomized Controlled Trials," *Hypertension* 35 (2000): 838-843.
32. F. W. Kash, J. L. Boyer, S. P. Van Camp, L. S. Verity, and J. P. Wallace, "The Effect of Physical Activity on Aerobic Power in Older Men (A Longitudinal Study)," *Physician and Sports Medicine* 18, no. 4 (1990): 73-83.
33. S. G. Sheps, "High Blood Pressure Can Often Be Controlled Without Medication," *Bottom Line/Health* (November 1999).
34. J. E. Donnelly, et al., "Appropriate Physical Activity Intervention Strategies for Weight Loss and Prevention of Weight Regain for Adults," *Medicine & Science in Sports & Exercise* 41 (2009): 459-471.
35. C. A. Slentz, et al., "Inactivity, Exercise, and Visceral Fat. STRRIDE: A Randomized, Controlled Study of Exercise Intensity and Amount," *Journal of Applied Physiology* 99 (2005): 1613-1618.
36. S. Kenchaiah, et al., "Body Mass Index and Vigorous Physical Activity and the Risk of Heart Failure among Men," *Circulation* 119 (2009): 44-52.
37. M. Guarneri, "What Most People Don't Know about Heart Disease," *Bottom Line/Health* 21 (July 2007): 11-12.
38. B. A. Franklin, "Sex Can Cause a Heart Attack," *Bottom Line/Health* 27 (March 2013): 1-3.
39. See note 38.

Suggested Readings

American Heart Association. *2011 Heart and Stroke Facts Statistical Update*. Dallas, TX: AHA, 2011.

American Heart Association. *Heart and Stroke Facts*. Dallas, TX: AHA, 2011.

National Cholesterol Education Program Expert Panel. "Summary of the Third Report of the National Cholesterol Education Program (NCEP) Expert Panel on Detection, Evaluation, and Treatment of High Blood Cholesterol in Adults (Adult Treatment Panel III)," *Journal of the American Medical Association* 285 (2001): 2486-2497.

Chapter 11:

Notes

1. American Cancer Society, *Cancer Facts & Figures 2013* (New York: ACS, 2013).

2. L. H. Kushi, et al., "American Cancer Society Guidelines on Nutrition and Physical Activity for Cancer Prevention: Reducing the Risk for Cancer with Healthy Food Choices and Physical Activity, CA," *A Cancer Journal for Clinicians* 56, no. 5 (2006): 254-281.
3. J. E. Enstrom, "Health Practices and Cancer Mortality Among Active California Mormons," *Journal of the National Cancer Institute* 81 (1989): 1807-1814.
4. A. S. Ford, et al., "Healthy Living is the Best Revenge: Findings from the European Prospective Investigation into Cancer and Nutrition—Potsdam Study," *Archives of Internal Medicine* 169 (2009): 1355-1362.
5. See note 1.
6. Y. Park, et al., "Dietary Fiber Intake and Risk of Colorectal Cancer," *Journal of the American Medical Association* 294 (2005): 2849-2857.
7. V. W. Setiawan, et al., "Protective Effect of Green Tea on the Risks of Chronic Gastritis and Stomach Cancer," *International Journal of Cancer* 92 (2001): 600-604.
8. L. Mitscher, and V. Dolby, *The Green Tea Book—China's Fountain of Youth* (New York: Avery Press, 1997).
9. "Curbing Cancer's Reach: Little Things That Might Make a Big Difference," *Environmental Nutrition* 29, no. 6 (2006): 1, 6.
10. S. C. Larsson, L. Bergkvist, and A. Wolk, "Consumption of Sugar-Sweetened Foods and the Risk of Pancreatic Cancer in a Prospective Study," *American Journal of Clinical Nutrition* 84 (2006): 1171-1176.
11. N. E. Allen, et al., "Moderate Alcohol Intake and Cancer Incidence in Women," *Journal of the National Cancer Institute* 101 (2009): 296-305.
12. See note 1.
13. E. E. Calle, C. Rodriguez, K. Walker-Thurmond, and M. J. Thun, "Overweight, Obesity, and Mortality from Cancer in a Prospectively Studied Cohort of U.S. Adults," *New England Journal of Medicine* 348 (2003): 1625-1638.
14. American Cancer Society, *1995 Cancer Facts & Figures* (New York: ACS, 1995).
15. S. E. Whitmore, W. L. Morison, C. S. Potten, and C. Chadwick, "Tanning Salon Exposure and Molecular Alterations," *Journal of the American Academy of Dermatology* 44 (2001): 775-780.
16. C. A. Thomson, and P. A. Thomson, "Healthy Lifestyle and Cancer Prevention," *ACSM's Health & Fitness Journal* 12, no. 3 (2008): 18-26.
17. S. W. Farrell, et al., "Cardiorespiratory Fitness, Different Measures of Adiposity, and Cancer Mortality in Men," *Obesity* 15 (2007): 3140-3149.
18. L. Byberg, et al., "Total Mortality After Changes in Leisure Time Physical Activity in 50 Year Old Men: 35 Year Follow-up of Population Based Cohort," *British Medical Journal* (2009): 338, doi:10.1136.
19. E. L. Giovannucci, "A Prospective Study of Physical Activity and Incident and Fatal Prostate Cancer," *Archives of Internal Medicine* 165 (2005): 1005-1010.
20. L. Ratnasinghe, et al., *Exercise and Breast Cancer Risk: A Multinational Study* (Beltsville, MD: Genomic Nanosystems, BioServe Biotechnologies, Ltd.), http://www.bioserve.com/downloads/posters/Poster-Exercise-and-Reduced-Breast-Cancer-Risk-A-Multinational-Study.pdf, downloaded July 1, 2013.
21. C. W. Matthews, et al., "Physical Activity and Risk of Endometrial Cancer: A Report from the Shanghai Endometrial Cancer Study," *Cancer Epidemiology Biomarkers & Prevention* 14 (2005): 779-785.
22. M. D. Holmes, et al., "Physical Activity and Survival After Breast Cancer Diagnosis," *Journal of the American Medical Association* 293 (2005): 2479-2486.
23. J. R. Ruiz, "Muscular Strength and Adiposity as Predictors of Adulthood Cancer Mortality in Men," *Cancer Epidemiology, Biomarkers & Prevention* 18 (2009): 1468-1476.
24. D. Servan-Schreiber, "The Anticancer Life Plan," *Bottom Line Health* 23, no. 5 (May 2009).

Suggested Readings

American Cancer Society. *Cancer Facts & Figures 2013*. New York: ACS, 2013.

World Cancer Research Fund and American Institute for Cancer Research. *Food, Nutrition, Physical Activity and the Prevention of Cancer: A Global Perspective*. Washington, DC: WCRF/AICR, 2007.

"Dietary Do's and Don'ts from the Latest Research on Cancer Prevention," *Tufts University Health & Nutrition Letter* 27, no. 5 (July 2009).

U.S. Department of Health and Human Services, National Institutes of Health, National Cancer Institute. *Reducing Environmental Cancer Risk: What We Can Do Now*. Washington, DC: President's Cancer Panel, April 2010.

Chapter 12

Notes

1. H. Selye, *Stress without Distress* (New York: Signet, 1974).
2. E. Gullete, et al., "Effects of Mental Stress on Myocardial Ischemia during Daily Life," *Journal of the American Medical Association* 277 (1997): 1521-1525; C. A. Lengacher, et al., "Psychoneuroimmunology and Immune System Link for Stress, Depression, Health Behaviors, and Breast Cancer," *Alternative Health Practitioner* 4 (1998): 95-108.
3. R. J. Kriegel, and M. H. Kriegel, *The C Zone: Peak Performance Under Stress* (Garden City, NY: Anchor Press/Doubleday, 1985).
4. See note 2; J. Moses, et al., "The Effects of Exercise Training on Mental Well-Being in the Normal Population: A Controlled Trial," *Journal of Psychosomatic Research* 33 (1989): 47-61; C. Shang, "Emerging Paradigms in Mind–Body Medicine," *Journal of Complementary and Alternative Medicine* 7 (2001): 83-91.
5. See note 1.
6. M. Samuels, "Use Your Mind to Heal Your Body," *Bottom Line/Health* 19 (February 2005): 13-14.
7. S. Bodian, "Meditate Your Way to Much Better Health," *Bottom Line/Health* 18 (June 2004): 11-13.
8. D. Mueller, "Yoga Therapy," *ACSM's Health & Fitness Journal* 6 (2002): 18-24.
9. S. C. Manchanda, et al., "Retardation of Coronary Atherosclerosis with Yoga Lifestyle Intervention," *Journal of the Association of Physicians of India* 48 (2000): 687-694.

Suggested Readings

Girdano, D. A., D. E. Dusek, and G. S. Everly. *Controlling Stress and Tension*. San Francisco: Benjamin Cummings, 2009.

Greenberg, J. S. *Comprehensive Stress Management*. New York: McGraw-Hill, 2008.

Olpin, M., and M. Hesson. *Stress Management for Life*. Belmont, CA: Wadsworth/Cengage Learning, 2010.

Schwartz, M. S., and F. Andrasik. *Biofeedback: A Practitioner's Guide*. New York: Guilford Press, 2004.

Selye, H. *The Stress of Life*. New York: McGraw-Hill, 1978.

Chapter 13

Notes

1. U.S. Department of Health and Human Services: Office of Applied Studies, *Results from the 2011 National Survey on Drug Use and Health: National Findings*, http://nsduhweb.rti.org, downloaded June 20, 2013.
2. W. W. K. Hoeger, L. W. Turner, and B. Q. Hafen, *Wellness: Guidelines for a Healthy Lifestyle* (Belmont, CA: Wadsworth/Thomson Learning, 2007).
3. R. Goldberg, *Drugs Across the Spectrum* (Belmont, CA: Wadsworth/Cengage Learning, 2014).
4. See note 3.

5. U.S. Department of Health and Human Services, *Drug Use Among Racial/Ethnic Minorities* (Bethesda, MD: DHHS, National Institutes of Health, National Institute on Drug Abuse, Division of Epidemiology, Services & Prevention Research, 2003).
6. "A Snapshot of Annual High-Risk College Drinking Consequences," http://www.collegedrinkingprevention.gov/statssummaries/snapshot.aspx, downloaded June 25, 2013.
7. C. A. Presley, J. S. Leichliter, and P. W. Meilman, *Alcohol and Drugs on American College Campuses: Findings from 1995, 1996, and 1997 (A Report to College Presidents)* (Carbondale: Southern Illinois University, 1999).
8. See note 1.
9. U.S. Department of Agriculture, *Tobacco Outlook Report* (Washington, DC: U.S. Department of Agriculture, Market and Trade Economics Division, Economic Research Service, 2007).
10. American Cancer Society, *Cancer Facts & Figures—2013* (New York: ACS, 2013).
11. U.S. Public Health Service, *The Health Consequences of Involuntary Exposure to Tobacco Smoke: A Report of the Surgeon General—Executive Summary* (Rockville, MD: U.S. Department of Health and Human Services, 2006).
12. American Cancer Society, *World Smoking & Health* (Atlanta, GA: ACS, 1993).
13. American Heart Association, *AHA Public Affairs/Coalition on Smoking: Health Position* (Dallas, TX: AHA, 1996).
14. U.S. Department of Health and Human Services, *Nicotine Addiction, A Report of the Surgeon General* (Atlanta, GA: U.S. Department of Health and Human Services, Centers for Disease Control and Prevention, National Center for Chronic Disease Prevention and Health Promotion, 1988).
15. R. H. Zwick, et al., "Exercise in Addition to Nicotine Replacement Therapy Improves Success Rates in Smoking Cessation," *Chest* 130, no. 4 (2006): 145S.

Suggested Readings

American Cancer Society. *2013 Cancer Facts & Figures*. New York: ACS, 2013.

Doweiko, H. E. *Concepts of Chemical Dependency*. Belmont, CA: Wadsworth/Cengage Learning, 2012.

Goldberg, R. *Drugs Across the Spectrum*. Belmont, CA: Wadsworth/Cengage Learning, 2014.

U.S. Department of Health and Human Services. *A Report of the Surgeon General: How Tobacco Smoke Causes Disease: The Biology and Behavioral Basis for Smoking-Attributable Disease*. Rockville, MD, USDHHS, 2010.

U.S. Public Health Service. *The Health Consequences of Involuntary Exposure to Tobacco Smoke: A Report of the Surgeon General—Executive Summary*. Rockville, MD: U.S. Department of Health and Human Services, 2006.

Chapter 14

Notes

1. Centers for Disease Control and Prevention, "Sexually Transmitted Diseases," http://www.cdc.gov/STD/, downloaded June 29, 2013.
2. See note 1.
3. See note 1.
4. See note 1.
5. See note 1.
6. See note 1.
7. R. Horowitz, et al., "Herpes Simplex Virus Infection in a University Health Population: Clinical Manifestations, Epidemiology, and Implications," *The Journal of American College Health* 59, no. 2 (2011): 69-74.
8. See note 1.
9. World Health Organization, "Global Summary of the AIDS Epidemic, 2010," http://www.who.int/hiv/data/2011_epi_core_en.png, downloaded July 1, 2013.

Suggested Readings

Blona, R., and J. Levitan. *Healthy Sexuality*. Belmont, CA: Wadsworth/Thomson Learning, 2006.

Centers for Disease Control and Prevention. "Sexually Transmitted Diseases Treatment Guidelines 2010," *Morbidity and Mortality Weekly Report, Recommendations and Reports* 59, no. RR-12 (July 1, 2013): 1-110.

Hoeger, W. W. K., L. W. Turner, and B. Q. Hafen. *Wellness: Guidelines for a Healthy Lifestyle*. Belmont, CA: Wadsworth/Thomson Learning, 2007.

Chapter 15

Notes

1. M. Makary, "Surprising Dangers in the Hospital," *Bottom Line Health* 27, no. 2 (2013): 5-6
2. R. J. Donatelle, *Access to Health* (San Francisco: Benjamin Cummings, 2008).
3. National Institutes of Health, National Center for Complementary and Alternative Medicine, *2007 Statistics on CAM Use in the United States*, http://nccam.nih.gov/news/camstats/2007/index.htm, downloaded June 20, 2013.
4. National Center for Complementary and Alternative Medicine, National Institutes of Health, CAM Basics: What Is Complementary and Alternative Medicine?, http://nccam.nih.gov/health/whatiscam/, downloaded June 20, 2013.
5. National Institutes of Health, National Center for Complementary and Alternative Medicine, Statistics on CAM Costs, http://nccam.nih.gov/news/camstats/2007/index.htm, downloaded June 20, 2013.
6. D. M. Eisenberg, et al., "Trends in Alternative Medicine Use in the United States, 1990–1997," *Journal of the American Medical Association* 280, no. 18 (1998): 1569-1575.
7. *Dynamics of Fitness: The Body in Action*, Film (Pleasantville, NY: Human Relations Media, 1980).

Suggested Readings

American College of Sports Medicine. *ACSM's Health/Fitness Facility Standards and Guidelines*. Champaign, IL: Human Kinetics, 2011.

American College of Sports Medicine. *ACSM's Resources for Guidelines for Exercise Testing and Prescription*. Philadelphia: Wolters Kluwer/Lippincott Williams & Wilkins, 2010.

American College of Sports Medicine. *ACSM's Resources for the Personal Trainer*. Philadelphia: Lippincott Williams & Wilkins, 2009.

Roizen, M. F. *Real Age: Are You as Young as You Can Be?* New York: Cliff Street Books, 1999.

Answer Key

Chapter 1
1. c 2. e 3. d 4. a 5. e 6. d 7. c 8. b 9. a 10. b

Chapter 2
1. a 2. a 3. e 4. d 5. c 6. d 7. a 8. b 9. e 10. e

Chapter 3
1. b 2. e 3. c 4. d 5. d 6. a 7. a 8. c 9. a 10. e

Chapter 4
1. e 2. b 3. d 4. a 5. b 6. e 7. b 8. b 9. e 10. e

Chapter 5
1. b 2. c 3. e 4. a 5. b 6. e 7. a 8. c 9. d 10. e

Chapter 6
1. a 2. d 3. c 4. c 5. c 6. e 7. b 8. d 9. c 10. c

Chapter 7
1. c 2. d 3. a 4. b 5. d 6. a 7. c 8. c 9. e 10. e

Chapter 8
1. b 2. e 3. a 4. a 5. b 6. e 7. c 8. b 9. e 10. d

Chapter 9
1. d 2. a 3. b 4. e 5. d 6. b 7. a 8. e 9. a 10. e

Chapter 10
1. e 2. b 3. a 4. e 5. e 6. e 7. e 8. e 9. e 10. a

Chapter 11
1. b 2. a 3. a 4. e 5. e 6. e 7. b 8. e 9. b 10. e

Chapter 12
1. a 2. c 3. c 4. e 5. e 6. e 7. a 8. a 9. b 10. c

Chapter 13
1. e 2. a 3. c 4. d 5. d 6. d 7. d 8. e 9. e 10. e

Chapter 14
1. c 2. b 3. e 4. e 5. d 6. a 7. a 8. d 9. e 10. c

Chapter 15
1. e 2. c 3. b 4. d 5. e 6. a 7. e 8. c 9. e 10. a

Glossary

Action stage Stage of change in the transtheoretical model in which the individual is actively changing a negative behavior or adopting a new, healthy behavior.

Actions (for behavioral change) Steps required to reach a goal.

Activities of daily living Everyday behaviors that people normally do to function in life (cross the street, carry groceries, lift objects, do laundry, sweep floors).

Acupuncture Chinese medical system that requires body piercing with fine needles during therapy to relieve pain and treat ailments and diseases.

Addiction Compulsive and uncontrollable behavior(s) or use of substance(s).

Adenosine triphosphate (ATP) A high-energy chemical compound that the body uses for immediate energy.

Adequate Intake (AI) The recommended amount of a nutrient intake when sufficient evidence is not available to calculate the EAR and subsequent RDA.

Adipose tissue Fat cells in the body.

Advanced glycation end products (AGEs) Derivatives of glucose-protein and glucose lipid interactions that are linked to aging and chronic diseases.

Aerobic Describes exercise that requires oxygen to produce the necessary energy (ATP) to carry out the activity.

Aerobics A series of exercise routines performed to music.

AIDS (Acquired immunodeficiency syndrome) Any of a number of diseases that arise when the body's immune system is compromised by HIV; the final stage of HIV infection.

Air displacement Technique to assess body composition by calculating the body volume from the air replaced by an individual sitting inside a small chamber.

Alcohol (ethyl alcohol) A depressant drug that affects the brain and slows down central nervous system activity; has strong addictive properties.

Alcoholism Disease in which an individual loses control over drinking alcoholic beverages.

Altruism Unselfish concern for the welfare of others.

Alveoli Air sacs in the lungs where gas exchange (oxygen and carbon dioxide) takes place.

Amenorrhea Cessation of regular menstrual flow.

Amino acids Chemical compounds that contain nitrogen, carbon, hydrogen, and oxygen; the basic building blocks the body uses to build different types of protein.

Amotivational syndrome A condition characterized by loss of motivation, dullness, apathy, and no interest in the future.

Amphetamines A class of powerful central nervous system stimulants.

Anabolic steroids Synthetic versions of the male sex hormone testosterone, which promotes muscle development and hypertrophy.

Anaerobic Describes exercise that does not require oxygen to produce the necessary energy (ATP) to carry out the activity.

Anaerobic threshold The highest percentage of the VO_{2max} at which an individual can exercise (maximal steady state) for an extended time without accumulating significant amounts of lactic acid (accumulation of lactic acid forces an individual to slow down the exercise intensity or stop altogether).

Android obesity Obesity pattern seen in individuals who tend to store fat in the trunk or abdominal area.

Angina pectoris Chest pain associated with coronary heart disease.

Angiogenesis Formation of blood vessels (capillaries).

Angioplasty A procedure in which a balloon-tipped catheter is inserted, then inflated, to widen the inner lumen of the artery.

Anorexia nervosa An eating disorder characterized by self-imposed starvation to lose weight and maintain very low body weight.

Anthropometric measurement Techniques to measure body girths at different sites.

Antibodies Substances produced by the white blood cells in response to an invading agent.

Antioxidants Compounds such as vitamins C and E, beta-carotene, and selenium that prevent oxygen from combining with other substances in the body to form harmful compounds.

Aquaphobic Having a fear of water.

Arrhythmias Irregular heart rhythms.

Arterial-venous oxygen difference (a-vO_{2diff}) The amount of oxygen removed from the blood as determined by the difference in oxygen content between arterial and venous blood.

Atherosclerosis Fatty/cholesterol deposits in the walls of the arteries leading to formation of plaque.

Atrophy Decrease in the size of a cell.

Autogenic training A stress management technique using a form of self-suggestion, wherein an individual is able to place himself or herself in an autohypnotic state by repeating and concentrating on feelings of heaviness and warmth in the extremities.

Ayurveda Hindu system of medicine based on herbs, diet, massage, meditation, and yoga to help the body boost its own natural healing.

Ballistic (dynamic) stretching Exercises performed with jerky, rapid, bouncy movements.

Basal metabolic rate (BMR) The lowest level of oxygen consumption (and energy requirement) necessary to sustain life.

Behavior modification The process of permanently changing negative behaviors to positive behaviors that will lead to better health and well-being.

Benign Noncancerous.

Binge-eating disorder An eating disorder characterized by uncontrollable episodes of eating excessive amounts of food within a relatively short time.

Bioelectrical impedance Technique to assess body composition by running a weak electrical current through the body.

Biofeedback A stress management technique in which a person learns to influence physiological responses that are not typically under voluntary control or responses that typically are regulated but for which regulation has broken down as a result of injury, trauma, or illness.

Blood lipids (fat) Cholesterol and triglycerides.

Blood pressure A measure of the force exerted against the walls of the vessels by the blood flowing through them.

Bod Pod Commercial name of the equipment used to assess body composition through the air displacement technique.

Body composition The fat and nonfat components of the human body; important in assessing recommended body weight.

Body mass index (BMI) Technique to determine thinness or excessive fatness that incorporates height and weight to estimate critical fat values at which the risk for disease increases.

Bradycardia Slower heart rate than normal.

Breathing exercises A stress management technique wherein the individual concentrates on "breathing away" the tension and inhaling fresh air to the entire body.

Bulimia nervosa An eating disorder characterized by a pattern of binge eating and purging in an attempt to lose weight and maintain low body weight.

Calorie The amount of heat necessary to raise the temperature of one gram of water one degree centigrade; used to measure the energy value of food and cost (energy expenditure) of physical activity.

Cancer Group of diseases characterized by uncontrolled growth and spread of abnormal cells.

Capillaries Smallest blood vessels carrying oxygenated blood to the tissues in the body.

Carbohydrate loading Increasing intake of carbohydrates during heavy aerobic training or prior to aerobic endurance events that last longer than 90 minutes.

Carbohydrates A classification of a dietary nutrient containing carbon, hydrogen, and oxygen; the major source of energy for the human body.

Carcinogens Substances that contribute to the formation of cancers.

Carcinoma in situ Encapsulated malignant tumor that has not spread.

Cardiac output Amount of blood pumped by the heart in one minute.

Cardiomyopathy A disease affecting the heart muscle.

Cardiorespiratory endurance The ability of the lungs, heart, and blood vessels to deliver adequate amounts of oxygen to the cells to meet the demands of prolonged physical activity.

Cardiorespiratory training zone Recommended training intensity range, in terms of exercise heart rate, to obtain adequate cardiorespiratory endurance development.

Cardiovascular disease (CVD) The array of conditions that affect the heart and the blood vessels.

Carotenoids Pigment substances in plants, that are often precursors to vitamin A. More than 600 carotenoids are found in nature, about 50 of which are precursors to vitamin A, the most potent being beta-carotene.

Catecholamines "Fight-or-flight" hormones, including epinephrine and norepinephrine.

Cellulite Term frequently used in reference to fat deposits that "bulge out"; caused by the herniation of subcutaneous fat within fibrous connective tissue, giving it a padded-like appearance.

Chiropractics Health care system that proposes that many diseases and ailments are related to misalignments of the vertebrae and emphasizes the manipulation of the spinal column.

Chlamydia A sexually transmitted infection, caused by a bacterial infection, that can cause significant damage to the reproductive system.

Cholesterol A waxy substance, technically a steroid alcohol, found only in animal fats and oil; used in making cell membranes, as a building block for some hormones, in the fatty sheath around nerve fibers, and other necessary substances.

Chronic diseases Illnesses that develop as a result of an unhealthy lifestyle and last a long time.

Chronological age Calendar age.

Chylomicrons Triglyceride-transporting molecules.

Circuit training Alternating exercises by performing them in a sequence of three to six or more.

Cirrhosis A disease characterized by scarring of the liver.

Clinical study A research study in which the investigator intervenes (makes certain changes or uses certain interventions or programs) to prevent or treat a disease.

Cocaine 2-beta-carbomethoxy-3-betabenozoxytropane, the primary psychoactive ingredient derived from coca plant leaves.

Cold turkey Eliminating a negative behavior all at once.

Complementary and alternative medicine (CAM) A group of diverse medical and health care systems, practices, and products that are not presently considered to be part of conventional medicine; also called unconventional, or nonallopathic, or integrative medicine.

Complex carbohydrates Carbohydrates formed by three or more simple sugar molecules linked together; also referred to as polysaccharides.

Concentric Describes shortening of a muscle during muscle contraction.

Contemplation stage Stage of change in the transtheoretical model in which the individual is considering changing behavior within the next 6 months.

Contraindicated exercises Exercises that are not recommended because they may cause injury to a person.

Controlled ballistic stretching Exercises done with slow, short, gentle, and sustained movements.

Conventional Western medicine Traditional medical practice based on methods that are tested through rigorous scientific trials; also called allopathic medicine.

Cool-down Tapering off an exercise session slowly.

Core strength training A program designed to strengthen the abdominal, hip, and spinal muscles (the core of the body).

Coronary heart disease (CHD) Condition in which the arteries that supply the heart muscle with oxygen and nutrients are narrowed by fatty deposits, such as cholesterol and triglycerides.

C-reactive protein (CRP) A protein whose blood levels increase with inflammation, at times hidden deep in the body; elevation of this protein is an indicator of potential cardiovascular events.

Creatine An organic compound derived from meat, fish, and amino acids that combines with inorganic phosphate to form creatine phosphate.

Creatine phosphate (CP) A high-energy compound that the cells use to resynthesize ATP during all-out activities of very short duration.

Cross-training A combination of aerobic activities that contribute to overall fitness.

Cruciferous vegetables Plants that produce cross-shaped leaves (cauliflower, broccoli, cabbage, Brussels sprouts, kohlrabi), which seem to have a protective effect against cancer.

Daily Values (DVs) Reference values for nutrients and food components used in food labels.

Dentist Practitioner who specializes in diseases of the teeth, gums, and oral cavity.

Deoxyribonucleic acid (DNA) Genetic substance of which genes are made; molecule that contains cell's genetic code.

Diabetes mellitus A disease in which the body doesn't produce or utilize insulin properly.

Diastolic blood pressure Pressure exerted by blood against walls of arteries during relaxation phase (diastole) of the heart; lower of the two numbers in blood pressure readings.

Dietary fiber A complex carbohydrate in plant foods that is not digested but is essential to digestion.

Dietary Reference Intake (DRI) A general term that describes four types of nutrient standards that establish adequate amounts and maximum safe nutrient intakes in the diet: Estimated Average

Requirement (EAR), Recommended Dietary Allowance (RDA), Adequate Intake (AI), and Tolerable Upper Intake Level (UL).

Disaccharides Simple carbohydrates formed by two monosaccharide units linked together, one of which is glucose. The major disaccharides are sucrose, lactose, and maltose.

Distress Negative stress; unpleasant or harmful stress, which causes health and performance to deteriorate.

Dopamine A neurotransmitter that affects emotional, mental, and motor functions.

Dual energy x-ray absorptiometry (DXA) Method to assess body composition that uses very low-dose beams of x-ray energy to measure total body fat mass, fat distribution pattern, and bone density.

Dynamic constant external resistance (DCER) See Fixed resistance.

Dynamic stretching Stretching exercises that require speed of movement, momentum, and active muscular effort to help increase the range of motion about a joint or group of joints.

Dynamic training Strength-training method referring to a muscle contraction with movement.

Dysmenorrhea Painful menstruation.

Eccentric Describes lengthening of a muscle during muscle contraction.

Ecosystem A community of organisms interacting with each other in an environment.

Elastic elongation Temporary lengthening of soft tissue.

Electrocardiogram (ECG or EKG) A recording of the electrical activity of the heart.

Electrolytes Substances that become ions in solution and are critical for proper muscle and neuron activation (include sodium, potassium, chloride, calcium, magnesium, phosphate, and bicarbonate, among others).

Emotional eating The consumption of large quantities of food to suppress negative emotions.

Emotional wellness The ability to understand your own feelings, accept your limitations, and achieve emotional stability.

Endorphins Morphine-like substances released from the pituitary gland (in the brain) during prolonged aerobic exercise; thought to induce feelings of euphoria and natural well-being.

Energy-balancing equation A principle holding that as long as caloric input equals caloric output, the person will not gain or lose weight. If caloric input exceeds output, the person gains weight; if output exceeds input, the person loses weight.

Environmental wellness The capability to live in a clean and safe environment that is not detrimental to health.

Enzymes Catalysts that facilitate chemical reactions in the body.

Essential fat Minimal amount of body fat needed for normal physiological functions; constitutes about 3 percent of total weight in men and 12 percent in women.

Estimated Average Requirement (EAR) The amount of a nutrient that meets the dietary needs of half the people.

Estimated Energy Requirement (EER) The average dietary energy (caloric) intake that is predicted to maintain energy balance in a healthy adult of defined age, gender, weight, height, and level of physical activity, consistent with good health.

Estrogen Female sex hormone essential for bone formation and conservation of bone density.

Eustress Positive stress: Health and performance continue to improve, even as stress increases.

Exercise A type of physical activity that requires planned, structured, and repetitive bodily movement with the intent of improving or maintaining one or more components of physical fitness.

Exercise intolerance Inability to function during exercise because of excessive fatigue or extreme feelings of discomfort.

Explanatory style The way people perceive the events in their lives, from an optimistic or a pessimistic perspective.

Fast-twitch fibers Muscle fibers with greater anaerobic potential and fast speed of contraction.

Fats A classification of nutrients containing carbon, hydrogen, some oxygen, and sometimes other chemical elements.

Fighting spirit Determination; the open expression of emotions, whether negative or positive.

Fight-or-flight Physiological response of the body to stress that prepares the individual to take action by stimulating the body's vital defense systems.

FITT-VP An acronym used to describe the cardiorespiratory exercise prescription variables: frequency, intensity, time (duration), type (mode), volume, and progression.

Fixed resistance Type of exercise in which a constant resistance is moved through a joint's full range of motion (dumbbells, barbells, machines using a constant resistance).

Flexibility The achievable range of motion at a joint or group of joints without causing injury.

Folate One of the B vitamins.

Fortified foods Foods that have been modified by the addition or increase of nutrients that either were not present or were present in insignificant amounts with the intent of preventing nutrient deficiencies.

Free weights Barbells and dumbbells.

Frequency Number of times per week a person engages in exercise.

Functional capacity The ability to perform the ordinary and unusual demands of daily living without limitations and excessive fatigue or injury.

Functional foods Foods or food ingredients containing physiologically active substances that provide specific health benefits beyond those supplied by basic nutrition.

Functional independence Ability to carry out activities of daily living without assistance from other individuals.

General adaptation syndrome (GAS) A theoretical model that explains the body's adaptation to sustained stress that includes three stages: alarm reaction, resistance, and exhaustion/recovery.

Genetically modified (GM) foods Foods whose basic genetic material (DNA) is manipulated by inserting genes with desirable traits from one plant, animal, or microorganism into another one either to introduce new traits or to enhance existing ones.

Genital herpes A sexually transmitted infection caused by a viral infection of the herpes simplex virus types 1 and 2. The virus can attack different areas of the body but typically causes blisters on the genitals.

Genital warts A sexually transmitted infection caused by a viral infection.

Gonorrhea A sexually transmitted infection caused by a bacterial infection.

Girth measurements Technique to assess body composition by measuring circumferences at specific body sites.

Glucose intolerance A condition characterized by slightly elevated blood glucose levels.

Glycemic index A measure that is used to rate the plasma glucose response of carbohydrate-containing foods with the response produced by the same amount of carbohydrate from a standard source, usually glucose or white bread.

Glycogen Manner in which carbohydrates (glucose molecules) are stored in the human body, predominately in the liver and muscles.

Goals The ultimate aims toward which effort is directed.

Gynoid obesity Obesity pattern seen in people who store fat primarily around the hips and thighs.

Hatha yoga A form of yoga that incorporates specific sequences of static-stretching postures to help induce the relaxation response.

Health A state of complete well-being—not just the absence of disease or infirmity.

Health fitness standards The lowest fitness requirements for maintaining good health, decreasing the risk for chronic diseases, and lowering the incidence of muscular-skeletal injuries.

Health promotion The science and art of enabling people to increase control over their lifestyles to move toward a state of wellness.

Health-related fitness Fitness programs that are prescribed to improve the individual's overall health.

Heart rate reserve (HRR) The difference between maximal heart rate and resting heart rate.

Heat cramps Muscle spasms caused by heat-induced changes in electrolyte balance in muscle cells.

Heat exhaustion Heat-related fatigue.

Heat stroke Emergency situation resulting from the body being subjected to high atmospheric temperatures.

Hemoglobin Protein–iron compound in red blood cells that transports oxygen in the blood.

Herbal medicine Unconventional system that uses herbs to treat ailments and diseases.

Heroin A potent drug that is a derivative of opium.

High-density lipoproteins (HDL) Cholesterol-transporting molecule in the blood ("good" cholesterol) that helps clear cholesterol from the blood.

High-impact aerobics Exercises incorporating movements in which both feet are off the ground at the same time momentarily.

High-intensity interval training (HIIT) Training program that involves high- to very high-intensity (80 to 90 percent of maximal capacity) intervals, each followed by a low-to-moderate intensity recovery interval. Usually 1:3 or lower work-to-recovery ratio is used.

HIV (Human immunodeficiency virus) Virus that leads to acquired immunodeficiency syndrome (AIDS).

Homeopathy System of treatment based on the use of minute quantities of remedies that in large amounts produce effects similar to the disease being treated.

Homeostasis A natural state of equilibrium; the body attempts to maintain this equilibrium by constantly reacting to external forces that attempt to disrupt this fine balance.

Homocysteine An amino acid that, when allowed to accumulate in the blood, may lead to plaque formation and blockage of arteries.

Human papillomavirus (HPV) A group of viruses that can cause sexually transmitted infections.

Hydrostatic weighing Underwater technique to assess body composition; considered the most accurate of the body composition assessment techniques.

Hypertension Chronically elevated blood pressure.

Hypertrophy An increase in the size of the cell, as in muscle hypertrophy.

Hypokinetic diseases "Hypo" denotes "lack of"; therefore, illnesses related to a lack of physical activity.

Hyponatremia A low sodium concentration in the blood caused by overhydration with water.

Hypotension Low blood pressure.

Hypothermia A breakdown in the body's ability to generate heat; a drop in body temperature below 95°F.

Imagery Mental visualization of relaxing images and scenes to induce body relaxation in times of stress or as an aid in the treatment of certain medical conditions such as cancer, hypertension, asthma, chronic pain, and obesity.

Immunity The function that guards the body from invaders, both internal and external.

Insulin A hormone secreted by the pancreas; essential for proper metabolism of blood glucose (sugar) and maintenance of blood glucose level.

Insulin resistance Inability of the cells to respond appropriately to insulin.

Integrative medicine The combination of the practices and methods of alternative medicine with conventional Western medicine.

Intensity In cardiorespiratory exercise, how hard a person has to exercise to improve or maintain fitness.

Intensity (for flexibility exercises) Degree of stretch when doing flexibility exercises.

International units (IU) Measure of nutrients in foods.

Interval training A system of exercise wherein a short period of intense effort is followed by a specified recovery period according to a prescribed ratio; for instance, a 1:3 work-to-recovery ratio.

Isokinetic training Strength-training method in which the speed of the muscle contraction is kept constant because the equipment (machine) provides an accommodating resistance to match the user's force (maximal) through the range of motion.

Isometric training Strength-training method referring to a muscle contraction that produces little or no movement, such as pushing or pulling against an immovable object.

Iyegar yoga Form of yoga that aims to develop flexibility, strength, balance, and stamina using props (belts, blocks, blankets, and chairs) to aid in the correct performance of asanas, or yoga postures.

Lactic acid End product of anaerobic glycolysis (metabolism).

Lactovegetarians Vegetarians who eat foods from the milk group.

Lapse (v.) To slip or fall back temporarily into unhealthy behavior(s); (n.) short-term failure to maintain healthy behaviors.

Lean body mass Body weight without body fat.

Learning theories Behavioral modification perspective stating that most behaviors are learned and maintained under complex schedules of reinforcement and anticipated outcomes.

Life expectancy How many years a person is expected to live.

Life Experiences Survey A questionnaire used to assess sources of stress in life.

Lipoproteins Lipids covered by proteins; these transport fats in the blood. Types are LDL, HDL, and VLDL.

Locus of control A concept examining the extent to which a person believes that he or she can influence the external environment.

Low-density lipoprotein (LDL) Cholesterol-transporting molecule in the blood ("bad" cholesterol) that tends to increase blood cholesterol.

Low-impact aerobics Exercises in which at least one foot is in contact with the ground or floor at all times.

Lymphocytes Immune system cells responsible for waging war against disease or infection.

Magnetic therapy Unconventional treatment that relies on magnetic energy to promote healing.

Maintenance stage Stage of change in the transtheoretical model in which the individual maintains behavioral change for up to five years.

Malignant Cancerous.

Mammogram Low-dose x-rays of the breasts used as a screening technique for the early detection of breast cancer.

Marijuana A psychoactive drug prepared from a mixture of crushed leaves, flowers, small branches, stems, and seeds from the hemp plant *Cannabis sativa*.

Massage therapy The rubbing or kneading of body parts to treat ailments.

Maximal heart rate (MHR) Highest heart rate for a person, related primarily to age.

Maximal oxygen uptake (VO$_{2max}$) Maximum amount of oxygen the body is able to utilize per minute of physical activity, commonly expressed in (mL/kg/min) the best indicator of cardiorespiratory or aerobic fitness.

MDA A hallucinogenic drug that is structurally similar to amphetamines.

MDMA A synthetic hallucinogenic drug with a chemical structure that closely resembles MDA and methamphetamine; also known as Ecstasy.

Meditation A stress management technique used to gain control over one's attention by clearing the mind and blocking out the stressor(s) responsible for the increased tension.

Mediterranean diet Typical diet of people around the Mediterranean region, focusing on olive oil, red wine, grains, legumes, vegetables, and fruits, with limited amounts of meat, fish, milk, and cheese.

Megadoses For most vitamins, 10 times the RDA or more; for vitamin A, 5 times the RDA.

Melanoma The most virulent, rapidly spreading form of skin cancer.

Mental wellness A state in which your mind is engaged in lively interaction with the world around you.

MET Short for metabolic equivalent, the rate of energy expenditure at rest; 1 MET is the equivalent of a VO$_2$ of 3.5 mL/kg/min.

Metabolic fitness A component of physiological fitness that denotes reduction in the risk for diabetes and cardiovascular disease through a moderate-intensity exercise program in spite of little or no improvement in cardiorespiratory fitness.

Metabolic profile A measurement of plasma insulin, glucose, lipid, and lipoprotein levels to assess risk for diabetes and cardiovascular disease.

Metabolic syndrome An array of metabolic abnormalities that contribute to the development of atherosclerosis triggered by insulin resistance. These conditions include low HDL cholesterol, high triglycerides, high blood pressure, and an increased blood-clotting mechanism.

Metabolism All energy and material transformations that occur within living cells; necessary to sustain life.

Metastasis The movement of cells from one part of the body to another.

Methamphetamine A potent form of amphetamine.

Minerals Inorganic nutrients essential for normal body functions; found in the body and in food.

Mitochondria Structures within the cells where energy transformations take place.

Mode Form or type of exercise.

Moderate physical activity Activity that uses 150 calories of energy per day, or 1,000 calories per week.

Monosaccharides The simplest carbohydrates (sugars), formed by five- or six-carbon skeletons. The three most common monosaccharides are glucose, fructose, and galactose.

Morbidity A condition related to or caused by illness or disease.

Motivation The desire and will to do something.

Motor neurons Nerves connecting the central nervous system to the muscle.

Motor unit The combination of a motor neuron and the muscle fibers that neuron innervates.

Muscular endurance The ability of a muscle to exert submaximal force repeatedly over time.

Muscular fitness A term used in reference to the general health, strength, and endurance of a person's muscular system.

Muscular strength The ability of a muscle to exert maximum force against resistance (for example, 1 repetition maximum [or 1 RM] on the bench press exercise).

Myocardial infarction Heart attack; damage to or death of an area of the heart muscle as a result of an obstructed artery to that area.

Myocardium Heart muscle.

Naturopathic medicine Unconventional system of medicine that relies exclusively on natural remedies to treat disease and ailments.

Negative resistance The lowering or eccentric phase of a repetition during a strength-training exercise.

Neustress Neutral stress; stress that is neither harmful nor helpful.

Nicotine Addictive compound found in tobacco leaves.

Nitrosamines Potentially cancer-causing compounds formed when nitrites and nitrates, which prevent the growth of harmful bacteria in processed meats, combine with other chemicals in the stomach.

Nonexercise activity thermogenesis (NEAT) Energy expended doing everyday activities not related to exercise.

Nonmelanoma skin cancer Cancer that spreads or grows at the original site but does not metastasize to other regions of the body.

Nonresponders Individuals who exhibit small or no improvements in fitness as compared with others who undergo the same training program.

Nurse Health care practitioner who assists in the diagnosis and treatment of health problems and provides many services to patients in a variety of settings.

Nutrient density A measure of the amount of nutrients and calories in various foods.

Nutrients Substances found in food that provide energy, regulate metabolism, and help with growth and repair of body tissues.

Nutrition Science that studies the relationship of foods to optimal health and performance.

Obesity An excessive accumulation of body fat, usually at least 30 percent greater than recommended body weight.

Observational study A research study in which the investigator does not intervene to make changes but only observes the outcomes based on a particular lifestyle pattern.

Occupational wellness The ability to perform your job skillfully and effectively under conditions that provide personal and team satisfaction and adequately reward each individual.

Oligomenorrhea Irregular menstrual cycles.

Omega-6 fatty acids Polyunsaturated fatty acids found primarily in corn and sunflower oils and most oils in processed foods.

Omega-3 fatty acids Polyunsaturated fatty acids found primarily in cold-water seafood, flaxseeds, and flaxseed oil. Thought to lower blood cholesterol and triglycerides.

Oncogenes Genes that initiate cell division.

One repetition maximum (1 RM) The maximum amount of resistance an individual is able to lift in a single effort.

Ophthalmologist Medical specialist concerned with diseases of the eye and prescription of corrective lenses.

Opportunistic infections Infections that arise in the absence of a healthy immune system, which would fight them off in healthy people.

Optometrist Health care practitioner who specializes in the prescription and adaptation of lenses.

Oral surgeon A dentist who specializes in surgical procedures of the oral–facial complex.

Orthodontist A dentist who specializes in the correction and prevention of teeth irregularities.

Osteopath A medical practitioner with specialized training in musculoskeletal problems who uses diagnostic and therapeutic methods of conventional medicine in addition to manipulative measures.

Osteoporosis A condition of softening, deterioration, or loss of bone mineral density that leads to disability, bone fractures, and even death from medical complications.

Overload principle Training concept that the demands placed on a system (cardiorespiratory or muscular) must be increased systematically and progressively over time to cause physiological adaptation (development or improvement).

Overtraining An emotional, behavioral, and physical condition marked by increased fatigue, decreased performance, persistent muscle soreness, mood disturbances, and feelings of "staleness" or "burnout" as a result of excessive physical training.

Overweight An excess amount of weight against a given standard, such as height or recommended percent body fat.

Ovolactovegetarians Vegetarians who include eggs and milk products in their diet.

Ovovegetarians Vegetarians who allow eggs in their diet.

Oxygen free radicals Substances formed during metabolism that attack and damage proteins and lipids, in particular the cell membrane and DNA, leading to diseases such as heart disease, cancer, and emphysema.

Oxygen uptake (VO_2) The amount of oxygen the human body uses.

Passive stretching Stretching exercises performed with the aid of an external force applied by either another individual or an external apparatus.

Pedometer An electronic device that senses body motion and counts footsteps. Some pedometers also record distance, calories burned, speeds, "aerobic steps," and time spent being physically active.

Pelvic inflammatory disease (PID) An overall designation referring to the effects of other STIs, primarily chlamydia and gonorrhea.

Percent body fat Proportional amount of fat in the body based on the person's total weight; includes both essential fat and storage fat; also termed fat mass.

Periodization A training approach that divides the season into cycles (macrocycles, mesocycles, and microcycles) using a systematic variation in intensity and volume of training to enhance fitness and performance.

Peripheral vascular disease Narrowing of the peripheral blood vessels.

Peristalsis Involuntary muscle contractions of intestinal walls that facilitate excretion of wastes.

Personal trainer A health/fitness professional who evaluates, motivates, educates, and trains clients to help them meet individualized, healthy lifestyle goals.

Physical activity Bodily movement produced by skeletal muscles; requires expenditure of energy and produces progressive health benefits. Examples include walking, taking the stairs, dancing, gardening, doing yard work, house cleaning, snow shoveling, washing the car, and all forms of structured exercise.

Physical activity perceived exertion (H-PAPE) A perception scale to monitor or interpret the intensity of aerobic exercise.

Physical fitness The ability to meet the ordinary as well as the unusual demands of daily life safely and effectively without being overly fatigued and still have energy left for leisure and recreational activities.

Physical fitness standards A fitness level that allows a person to sustain moderate-to-vigorous physical activity without undue fatigue and the ability to closely maintain this level throughout life.

Physical wellness Good physical fitness and confidence in your personal ability to take care of health problems.

Physician assistant Health care practitioner trained to treat most standard cases of care.

Physiological age The biological and functional capacity of the body as it should be in relation to the person's maximal potential at any given age in the lifespan.

Phytonutrients Compounds found in fruits and vegetables that block formation of cancerous tumors and disrupt the progress of cancer.

Pilates A training program that uses exercises designed to help strengthen the body's core by developing pelvic stability and abdominal control; exercises are coupled with focused breathing patterns.

Plastic elongation Permanent lengthening of soft tissue.

Plyometric exercise Explosive jump training, incorporating speed and strength training to enhance explosiveness.

Plyometric training A form of aerobic exercise that requires forceful jumps or springing off the ground immediately after landing from a previous jump.

Positive resistance The lifting, pushing, or concentric phase of a repetition during a strength-training exercise.

Prayer Sincere and humble communication with a higher power.

Precontemplation stage Stage of change in the transtheoretical model in which an individual is unwilling to change behavior.

Preparation stage Stage of change in the transtheoretical model in which the individual is getting ready to make a change within the next month.

Primary care physician A medical practitioner who provides routine treatment of ailments; typically, the patient's first contact for health care.

Primordial prevention Prevention of the development of risk factors for disease.

Principle of individuality Training concept holding that genetics plays a major role in individual responses to exercise training and these differences must be considered when designing exercise programs for different people.

Probiotics Healthy bacteria that help break down foods and prevent disease-causing organisms from settling in the intestines.

Problem-solving model Behavioral modification model proposing that many behaviors are the result of making decisions as the individual seeks to solve the problem behavior.

Processed foods A food which has been chemically altered from its natural state through additives such as flavors, flavor enhancers, colors, binders, preservatives, stabilizers, emulsifiers, fillers, and so on, or which has been manufactured through combination or other methods.

Processes of change Actions that help you achieve change in behavior.

Progressive muscle relaxation A stress management technique that involves sequential contraction and relaxation of muscle groups throughout the body.

Progressive resistance training A gradual increase of resistance used during strength training over a period of time.

Proprioceptive neuromuscular facilitation (PNF) Mode of stretching that uses reflexes and neuromuscular principles to relax the muscles being stretched.

Proteins A classification of nutrients consisting of complex organic compounds containing nitrogen and formed by combinations of amino acids; the main substances used in the body to build and repair tissues.

Quackery/fraud The conscious promotion of unproven claims for profit.

Range of motion Entire arc of movement of a given joint.

Recommended body weight Body weight at which there seems to be no harm to human health; healthy weight.

Recommended Dietary Allowance (RDA) The daily amount of a nutrient (statistically determined from the EARs) that is considered adequate to meet the known nutrient needs of almost 98 percent of all healthy people in the United States.

Recovery time Amount of time the body takes to return to resting levels after exercise.

Registered dietitian (RD) A person with a college degree in dietetics who meets all certification and continuing education requirements of the American Dietetic Association or Dietitians of Canada.

Relapse (v.) To slip or fall back into unhealthy behavior(s) over a longer time; (n.) longer-term failure to maintain healthy behaviors.

Relapse prevention model Behavioral modification model based on the principle that high-risk situations can be anticipated through the development of strategies to prevent lapses and relapses.

Repetitions Number of times a given resistance is performed.

Resistance Amount of weight lifted.

Resistance training See Strength training.

Responders Individuals who exhibit improvements in fitness as a result of exercise training.

Resting heart rate (RHR) Heart rate after a person has been sitting quietly for 15 to 20 minutes.

Resting metabolic rate (RMR) The energy requirement to maintain the body's vital processes in the resting state.

Resting metabolism Amount of energy (expressed in milliliters of oxygen per minute or total calories per day) an individual requires during resting conditions to sustain proper body function.

Reverse cholesterol transport A process in which HDL molecules attract cholesterol and carry it to the liver, where it is changed to bile and eventually excreted in the stool.

Ribonucleic acid (RNA) Genetic material that guides the formation of cell proteins.

RICE An acronym used to describe the standard treatment procedure for acute sports injuries: rest, ice (cold application), compression, and elevation.

Risk factors Lifestyle and genetic variables that may lead to disease.

Sarcopenia Age-related loss of lean body mass, strength, and function.

Sedentary Description of a person who is relatively inactive and whose lifestyle is characterized by a lot of sitting.

Sedentary Death Syndrome (SeDS) Cause of death attributed to a lack of regular physical activity.

Self-efficacy One's belief in the ability to perform a given task.

Self-esteem A sense of positive self-regard and self-respect.

Semivegetarians Vegetarians who include milk products, eggs, and fish and poultry in the diet.

Set A fixed number of repetitions; one set of bench presses might be 10 repetitions. Even two-a-day workouts are common. The frequency depends on the amount of resistance, number of sets performed per session, and the person's ability to recover from the previous exercise bout (see Table 7.5). The latter often is dictated by level of conditioning.

Setpoint Weight control theory that the body has an established weight and strongly attempts to maintain that weight.

Sexually transmitted infections (STIs) Communicable diseases spread through sexual contact.

Shin splints Injury to the lower leg characterized by pain and irritation in the shin region of the leg.

Side stitch A sharp pain in the side of the abdomen.

Simple carbohydrates Formed by simple or double sugar units with little nutritive value; divided into monosaccharides and disaccharides.

Sitting disease A term coined by the scientific community to refer to the detrimental health effects caused by excessive sitting throughout most days of the week.

Skill-related fitness Fitness components important for success in skillful activities and athletic events; encompasses agility, balance, coordination, power, reaction time, and speed.

Skinfold thickness Technique to assess body composition by measuring a double thickness of skin at specific body sites.

Slow-sustained stretching Exercises in which the muscles are lengthened gradually through a joint's complete range of motion.

Slow-twitch fibers Muscle fibers with greater aerobic potential and slow speed of contraction.

SMART (goals) An acronym in reference to specific, measurable, attainable, realistic, and time-specific goals.

Social cognitive theory Behavioral modification model holding that behavior change is influenced by the environment, self-efficacy, and characteristics of the behavior itself.

Social wellness The ability to relate well to others, both within and outside the family unit.

Specific adaptation to imposed demand (SAID) training Training principle stating that, for improvements to occur in a specific activity, the exercises performed during a strength-training program should resemble as closely as possible the movement patterns encountered in that particular activity.

Specificity of training Principle that training must be done with the specific muscle(s) the person is attempting to improve.

Sphygmomanometer Inflatable bladder contained within a cuff and a mercury gravity manometer (or aneroid manometer) from which blood pressure is read.

Spiritual wellness The sense that life is meaningful, that life has purpose, and that some power brings all humanity together; the ethics, values, and morals that guide you and give meaning and direction to life.

Spontaneous remission Inexplicable recovery from incurable disease.

Spot reducing Fallacious theory proposing that exercising a specific body part will result in significant fat reduction in that area.

Static stretching (slow-sustained stretching) Exercises in which the muscles are lengthened gradually through a joint's complete range of motion.

Step aerobics A form of exercise that combines stepping up and down from a bench with arm movements.

Sterols Derived fats, of which cholesterol is the best-known example.

Storage fat Body fat in excess of essential fat; stored in adipose tissue.

Strength training A program designed to improve muscular strength and/or endurance through a series of progressive resistance (weight) training exercises that overload the muscle system and cause physiological development.

Stress The mental, emotional, and physiological response of the body to any situation that is new, threatening, frightening, or exciting.

Stress electrocardiogram An exercise test during which the workload is increased gradually until the individual reaches maximal fatigue, with blood pressure and 12-lead electrocardiographic monitoring throughout the test.

Stress Events Scale A questionnaire used to assess sources of stress in life.

Stressor Stress-causing event.

Stretching Moving the joints beyond the accustomed range of motion.

Stroke Condition in which a blood vessel that feeds the brain ruptures or is clogged, leading to blood flow disruption to the brain.

Stroke volume Amount of blood pumped by the heart in one beat.

Structured interview Assessment tool used to determine behavioral patterns that define Type A and B personalities.

Subcutaneous fat Deposits of fat directly under the skin.

Subluxation Partial dislocation of a joint.

Substrates Substances acted on by an enzyme (examples: carbohydrates, fats).

Sun protection factor (SPF) Degree of protection offered by ingredients in sunscreen lotion; at least SPF 15 is recommended.

Supplements Tablets, pills, capsules, liquids, or powders that contain vitamins, minerals, antioxidants, amino acids, herbs, or fiber that individuals take to increase their intake of these nutrients.

Suppressor genes Genes that deactivate the process of cell division.

Synergistic action The effect of mixing two or more drugs, which can be much greater than the sum of two or more drugs acting by themselves.

Synergy A reaction in which the result is greater than the sum of its two parts.

Syphilis A sexually transmitted infection caused by a bacterial infection.

Systolic blood pressure (SBP) Pressure exerted by blood against walls of arteries during forceful contraction (systole) of the heart; higher of the two numbers in blood pressure readings.

Tachycardia Faster than normal heart rate.

Tai chi A self-paced form of exercise often described as "meditation in motion" because it promotes serenity through gentle, balanced, low-impact movements that bring together the mind, body, and emotions.

Tar Chemical compound that forms during the burning of tobacco leaves.

Techniques of change Methods or procedures used during each process of change.

Telomerase An enzyme that allows cells to reproduce indefinitely.

Telomeres A strand of molecules at both ends of a chromosome.

Termination/adoption stage Stage of change in the transtheoretical model in which the individual has eliminated an undesirable behavior or maintained a positive behavior for more than five years.

Thermogenic response Amount of energy required to digest food.

Tolerable Upper Intake Level (UL) The highest level of nutrient intake that seems safe for most healthy people, beyond which exists an increased risk of adverse effects.

Trans fatty acid Solidified fat formed by adding hydrogen to monounsaturated and polyunsaturated fats to increase shelf life.

Transtheoretical model Behavioral modification model proposing that change is accomplished through a series of progressive stages in keeping with a person's readiness to change.

Triglycerides Fats formed by glycerol and three fatty acids; also called free fatty acids.

Type A Behavior pattern characteristic of a hard-driving, overambitious, aggressive, at times hostile, and overly competitive person.

Type B Behavior pattern characteristic of a calm, casual, relaxed, and easygoing individual.

Type C Behavior pattern of individuals who are just as highly stressed as Type A people but do not seem to be at higher risk for disease than Type B.

Type 1 diabetes Insulin-dependent diabetes mellitus (IDDM), a condition in which the pancreas produces little or no insulin; also known as juvenile diabetes.

Type 2 diabetes Non–insulin-dependent diabetes mellitus (NIDDM), a condition in which insulin is not processed properly; also known as adult-onset diabetes.

Ultraviolet A (UVA) rays Ultraviolet rays that pass deeper into the skin and are believed to cause skin damage and skin cancers.

Ultraviolet B (UVB) rays Ultraviolet rays that cause sunburn and lead to skin cancers.

Underweight Extremely low body weight.

Upper Intake Level (UL) The highest level of nutrient intake that seems safe for most healthy people, beyond which exists an increased risk of adverse effects.

Variable resistance Training using special machines equipped with mechanical devices that provide differing amounts of resistance through the range of motion.

Vegans Vegetarians who eat no animal products at all.

Vegetarians Individuals whose diet is of vegetable or plant origin.

Very low calorie diet A diet that allows an energy intake (consumption) of only 800 calories or less per day.

Very low density lipoproteins (VLDLs) Triglyceride, cholesterol, and phospholipid-transporting molecules in the blood.

Vicarious experiences Developing a belief that one can perform a task by observing peers of similar ability perform that task.

Vigorous activity Any exercise that requires a MET level equal to or greater than 6 METs (21 mL/kg/min). One MET is the energy expenditure at rest, 3.5 mL/kg/min, and METs are defined as multiples of this resting metabolic rate. (Examples of activities that require a 6 MET level include aerobics, walking uphill at 3.5 mph, cycling at 10 to 12 mph, playing doubles in tennis, and vigorous strength training.)

Vigorous exercise CR exercise that requires an intensity level of approximately 70 percent of capacity.

Vitamins Organic nutrients essential for normal metabolism, growth, and development of the body.

Volume (in strength training) The sum of all the repetitions performed multiplied by the resistances used during a strength-training session.

Volume (of training) The total amount of training performed in a given work period (day, week, month, or season).

Waist circumference (WC) A waist girth measurement to assess potential risk for disease based on intra-abdominal fat content.

Waist-to-Height Ratio (WHtR) A waist-to-height ratio assessment equally applicable to tall and short persons used to determine potential risk for disease based on excessive body weight.

Warm-up Starting a workout slowly.

Water The most important classification of essential body nutrients, involved in almost every vital body process.

Weight-regulating mechanism (WRM) A feature of the hypothalamus of the brain that controls how much the body should weigh.

Wellness The constant and deliberate effort to stay healthy and achieve the highest potential for well-being. It encompasses seven dimensions—physical, emotional, mental, social, environmental, occupational, and spiritual—and integrates them all into a quality life.

Workload Load (or intensity) placed on the body during physical activity.

Yoga A school of thought in the Hindu religion that seeks to help the individual attain a higher level of spirituality and peace of mind.

Index

Note: Pages numbers in bold are exercises.

Abdominal breathing technique, 426
Abdominal crunch
  with stability ball, **276–277**
  with weights, **267**
  without weights, **239–240**, 263
Abdominal curl-up, **304**
Abdominal muscles, 232
Acceptable goals, 63
Accidents, deaths from, 6
ACSM. *See* American College of Sports Medicine (ACSM)
Action stage, 57
Actions, purpose of, 62
Activities of daily living (ADLs)
  definition of, 235
  eating associated, 46
  muscle fitness and, 234
  requirements of, 44
Acupuncture, 495
Addiction
  definition of, 437
  factors of, 436
  marijuana, 440
  risk factors for, 438
  treatments for, 449–450
  types of, 437–438
Addictive behaviors
  behavior assessment, 465
  changing, 58
  FAQs, 436
  knowledge assessment, 466
  personal profile, 437
  questionnaires, 447 (Activity 13.1)
Adductor stretch, **301**
Adenosine triphosphate (ATP)
  definition of, 113
  function of, 196–197
  recovery time and, 249
  synthesis of, 112
Adenosine triphosphate (ATP)-creatine phosphate (CP) system, 112, 249
Adequate intake (AI), 87–88
Adipose tissue, 76, 76–77
ADLs. *See* Activities of daily living (ADLs)
Adoption stage, 58
Adults
  activity guidelines and, 11
  activity levels of, 12
  exercise guidelines for, 9
Advanced glycation end products (AGEs), 102, 103
Aerobic activity, 309. *See also* Cardiorespiratory (CR) endurance; Cardiorespiratory (CR) exercise
  benefits of, 197–199
  blood pressure and, 364–365
  body composition and, 144, 236
  cardiovascular protection from, 194, 195–196
  choices of, 307–313
  for diabetics, 316–317
  fitness benefits of, 222–224
  forms of, 309
  heart rate monitoring during, 216
  intensity of, 213–214
  light-intensity, 194
  MET level, 223–224
  moderate-intensity, 214, 216
  periodization program for, 330
  personal trainers for, 501–502
  selected, ratings for, 223
  for sports conditioning, 326–327
  training pattern for, 215
  training zone, 214
  vigorous-intensity, 214, 216
  in water, 310
  weight management and, 167–168
African-American diet, 103
AGES. *See* Advanced glycation end products (AGEs)
Aging. *See also* Older adults
  CHD risk and, 367
  diet history and, 165
  dietary guidelines for, 119
  EER and, 173
  exercise and, 324–326
  flexibility and, 282
  heart disease risk and, 340
  metabolic rate and, 164
  muscle fitness and, 234
  physical activity and, 486
  sedentary lifestyle and, 164, 486
  types of, 486
  values and, 44
  VO_{2max} uptake, 208
AIDS (acquired immunodeficiency syndrome)
  characterization of, 474
  clinical trials for, 481
  incidence of, 474, 479
  prevention guidelines, 482–483
  risky behavior, 478
  screening guidelines, 469
  self-quiz on, 475–476 (Activity 14.1)
  trends in, 479
  wise dating and, 479
Alarm reaction, 406
Alcohol
  cancer risk of, 380, 445
  osteoporosis risk of, 116
  social acceptance of, 444
  standard drink, 444
  use questionnaire, 447 (Activity 13.2)
Alcohol abuse
  accidents and, 6
  among students, 445–446
  consequences of, 445
  CRP levels and, 358
  long-term risks, 446
  overcoming, 449
  prevalence of, 444
  signs of, 446, 449
Alcoholism, 445
All-out interval training, 328
Allopathic medicine. *See* Conventional Western medicine
Alpha-linolenic acid (ALA), 81
Altruism, 18, 20
Alveoli, 197, 451
Amenorrhea, 117, 319
American College of Sports Medicine (ACSM), 500
American Heart Association
  CVD risk, 368
  mercury level recommendations, 73
  sodium recommendations, 362
  sugar recommendations, 72
  supplementation recommendations, 109
American Medication Association (AMA), 9
Amino acids, 82
Amotivational syndrome, 440–441
Amphetamines, 441
Anabolic steroids
  definition of, 235
  detrimental effects of, 235
  use of, 235–236
Anaerobic exercise, definition of, 197
Anaerobic threshold, 221
Anaerobic, definition of, 197
Android obesity, 133
Anger management, 413
Angina pectoris, 349
Angiogenesis, 374, 375
Angioplasty, 341, 343
Anorexia nervosa, 158–159
Antibodies, 403
Antihypertensive medicine, 362
Antioxidants
  benefits of, 106
  definition of, 106
  free radical absorption by, 378
  phytonutrients *vs.*, 73
  supplements, 105–106
Appetite, 165
Aquaphobic, 127
Arachidonic acid (AA), 81
Arby's, 91, 523–524
Architecture, health effects of, 44
Arm curl, **264, 271, 300**
Arousal, emotional, 59
Arrhythmias, 367
Arterial-venous oxygen difference, 202
Ashwell Shape Chart, 143
Asian foods, 104
Aspirin therapy, 367, 372
Asthma, 314–315, 315
Astrand-Ryhming, 204–205, 207
Atherosclerosis, 349, 362
Athletes
  endurance, 113–114, 117–118
  carbohydrate loading by, 113
  cardio fitness of, 199
  creatine supplementation by, 114–115
  dietary needs of, 113
  exhaustion stage, 406
  overtraining by, 327–328
Atkins Diet, 155
ATP. *See* Adenosine triphosphate (ATP)
Atrophy, 245
Autogenic training, 428–429
Automobile driving, 45–46
Ayurveda, 495

Back extension, **275, 277**
Back extension stretch, **303**
Back pain. *See* Low-back pain
Backache syndrome, 290
Balanced diet
  athletes and, 113
  daily food plan for, 96
  government recommendations for, 118–119
  healthy plate for, 97
  nutrients in, 92, 96
  vegetarianism, 100–102
Ballistic stretching, 287
Barefoot running, 319–320
Basal metabolic rate (BMR), 162, 168
Behavior
  changing, 42
  environmental influences on, 44–47
  future goals, 505, 508 (Activity 15.4)
  stressful, 408, 411–412
Behavior analysis, 59
Behavior modification. *See also* Change
  consciousness-raising in, 58
  knowledge assessment, 69
  personal profile, 43

547

Behavior modification *(continued)*
  progress form, 190
  repetition and, 50
  self-efficacy and, 52–53
  stages of, 63
  success factors for, 53–54
  success steps to, 60
  weight loss plan, 179 (Activity 5.2)
  weight management, 177
Behavior modification planning
  anger management, 413
  blood chemistry test guidelines, 354
  breakfast choices, 176
  calories and fats in selected foods, 91
  cancer risk reduction, 376, 383, 398
  cancer-fighting diet, 377
  change stages, 64–65 (Activity 2.2)
  common time killers, 416
  CVD risk reduction, 368
  daily physical activity increase, 200
  date drinking strategies, 449
  de-stress technique, 427
  for diabetes, 360
  dietary fiber intake, 79
  eating on the run, 164
  exercise compliance, 225
  financial fitness, 23–24
  food contamination avoidance, 111
  good stress management, 428
  healthy
    diet guidelines for, 110
    lifestyle habits for, 28
    restaurant dining for, 104
  hypertension prevention, 364
  LDL lowering guidelines, 355
  low-back pain prevention, 294
  nutritious foods selection, 100
  overtraining signs, 329
  pesticide avoidance, 111
  physically inactive people, 220
  smoking cessation, 463–465
  STI protection, 480
  strength training, 253
  stress symptoms, 422
  super foods, 96
  thirty-second body scan, 424
  type A changes, 412
  weight loss strategies, 180–181
  weight management, 140, 167
Bench jump, **239**
Bench press, **266**
Benign tumors, 373
Bent-arm fly, **272**
Bent-arm pull over, **275**
Bent-leg curl up, **239, 263**
Bent-over lateral raise, **267**
"Berlin patient," 480
Best Life Diet, 155
Better Business Bureau (BBB), 499

Bias, Len, 440
Bicycle ergometer, 205
Biggest Loser Diet, 155
Bile acid sequestrans, 357
Binge cycle, 442
Bioelectrical impedance, 129–130
Biofeedback
  application of, 424
  definition of, 425
  instruments used in, 424–425
Bladder cancer, 396
Blood lipids, 349, 362
Blood pressure
  assessment of, 30–31
  definition of, 361
  diastolic, 361
  guidelines, 361
  high (*See* Hypertension)
  log for, 38 (Activity 1.4)
  lowering of, 198
  mean, 31
  measures of, 31
  mortality based on, 363
  physical activity and, 363–364
  systolic, 31, 361
BMI. *See* Body mass index (BMI)
Boca burgers, 522
Body composition
  aerobic exercise and, 144
  aerobic/strength training and, 236
  assessments of
    air displacement, 127–128
    Ashwell Shape Chart, 143
    bioelectrical impedance, 129–130
    BMI, 130–133, 135–138
    DXA, 126
    girth measurement, 128, 132–135
    hydrostatic weighing, 127, 143
    log for, 141 (Activity 4.2)
    SEE, 126
    skinfold thickness, 128–132, 143
    training for, 124
    trends in, 124
    waist circumference, 133
    waist-to-height ratio, 137–138
  definition of, 125
  EER and, 173
  FAQs, 124
  fats and, 126
  frequent dieting and, 165
  importance of, 125
  knowledge of, 144–145
  personal profile, 125
  personal program for, 331–332
  for sports participation, 326
  typical, change in adults, 144
Body fat
  burning, exercise-intensity and, 168–170, 194
  burning, swimming and, 173
  calorie equivalence to, 161
  girth measurement for, 136

percentages, classification, 139
risk factors, 140
subcutaneous, 128–129, 140
types of, 126–127
visceral, 140
Body mass index (BMI)
  calculation of, 130
  CHD risk and, 365
  definition of, 131
  determination of, 137
  disease risk and, 142 (Activity 4.2)
  mortality risk and, 135
  obesity defined by, 149
  popularity of, 130–131
  uses for, 132–133
  weakness of, 133
Body Pod, 127
Body rotation, **300**
Body scan, 424
Body weight
  average, 150
  calorie balancing and, 118
  classification, 139–140
  healthy, maintaining, 28
  monitoring of, 165–166
  recommended
    criteria for, 124
    definition of, 125
    determination of, 139, 141 (Activity 4.1)
    maintenance plan for, 140
  tolerable, 152
Body-based practices, 495
Bodyweight training, 314
Bone density
  diet and, 115–116
  exercise and, 116–117
  test for, 117
Boredom, 417
Bradycardia, 30–31
Brain function
  exercise and, 25–26
  habits and, 50–51
  stress and, 403
BRCA1/BRCA2 gene, 390, 393
Breakfast, 175–176
Breast cancer
  early detection of, 393
  exercise and, 382
  risk factors, 390, 393
  self-examine, 384
Breast feeding, 119
Breathing exercises, 426–427
Budget Gourmet, 526
Burger King, 91, 524

C-reactive protein (CRP), 357–358
Caffeine
  addiction to, 437
  as energy booster, 437–438
  in energy drinks, 72
Calcium supplements
  cancer prevention and, 378
  for osteoporosis prevention, 116
  for vegetarians, 101

Calf press, **268**
Caloric expenditures. *See also* Estimated energy requirement (EER)
  calculation of, 76
  computation of, 178 (Activity 5.1)
  estimating, 173–174
  in HITT, 327
  selected physical activities, 175
  strength training and, 168
  weight loss and, 173
Calories
  balancing, 118
  calculation of, 76
  consumption times, 178
  definition of, 77
  fat, 79, 161
  nutritional analysis and, 90
  recommended intake, 163
  sedentary people need, 167
  time of day consumed, 148
Cancer
  bladder, 396
  breast, 382, 390–394
  cervical, 393–394
  colon/rectum, 384
  deaths from, 375
  definition of, 373
  early detection, 383
  early signs of, 382 (Activity 11.2)
  endometrial, 394–395
  esophageal, 396
  incidents of, 5, 374–376
  kidney, 396
  leukemia, 397
  lung, 384
  lymphoma, 397
  oral, 396
  ovarian, 397
  pancreatic, 396
  process of, 373–374
  promoters of, 383
  prostrate, 395
  risk factors
    assessment of, 384, 387–389
    environmental contaminants, 376
    excessive body fat, 140
    excessive sun exposure, 381–382
    food additives, 383–384
    genetics, 384
    soy products, 102
    tobacco products, 381
  risk profile, 391–392 (Activity 11.3)
  skin, 389–390
  stomach, 396
  survival, 376
  testicular, 395
  thyroid, 397
  tobacco use and, 451
  warning signs of, 384
Cancer prevention
  behavior assessment, 399
  dietary changes, 377–380

FAQs, 272
guidelines, 375
healthy lifestyles, 375–376
knowledge assessment, 399
lifestyle factors, 6, 385 (Activity 11.1), 398
personal profile, 373
physical activity and, 382–383
selenium and, 107
vitamin D for, 107
Canola oil, 80
Capillaries, 198–199
Carbohydrate loading, 113
Carbohydrates
calories in, 76, 90
complex, 77
definition of, 77
glucose levels and, 154
glycemic index and, 73
simple, 76
types of, 76
Carcinogens, 378–379
Carcinoma in situ, 375
Cardiac output
definition of, 199
function of, 198
in trained athlete, 199
Cardio/resistance training program, 328
Cardiomyopathy, 445
Cardiorespiratory (CR) endurance
activities benefiting, 197–199
assessment of, 201–206
behavior assessment of, 228
behavior modification plan for, 212 (Activity 6.3)
definition of, 22, 195
development of, 219
FAQs, 194–195
inactivity and, 347
knowledge assessment of, 228–229
personal profile, 195
personal program for, 331
physiology of, 196–197
prolonged exercise and, 197
VO_2 classification, 208
Cardiorespiratory (CR) exercise. *See also* Aerobic activity
apps for, 215–216
frequency of, 221
intensity guidelines, 213–214
lifetime program, 224
prescription for, 217–218 (Activity 6.4), 222
rate of progression, 221–222
readiness for, 206, 211–213, 211 (Activity 6.2)
recommended duration of, 219–221
record form, 226–227 (Activity 6.5)
volume, 221
Cardiorespiratory training zone, 214–215
Cardiorespiratory training zone, 214

Cardiovascular disease (CVD). *See also* Coronary heart disease (CHD)
alcohol use and, 445
atherosclerosis, 349
behavior assessment, 368
body fat and, 140
characterization of, 5
definition of, 343
factors of, 342
hypertension, 361–365
incidence of, 342
knowledge assessment, 368–369
physical inactivity and, 347–348
prevalence of, 342
prevention of, 340
risk profile for, 341
risk reduction plan, 368
types of, 342
Cardiovascular system
energy drinks effects on, 194–195
nuts benefits for, 101
tobacco's effects of, 451
Carotenoids, 377–378
Cat, The, **304**
Catecholamines, 366–367
CDC. *See* Centers for Disease Control (CDC)
Cell division, 373
Cellulite, 171–172
Cellulose, 78
Centers for Disease Control (CDC)
HIV testing recommendations, 480
physical activity report by, 233–234
prescription drug abuse classification, 436
STI screening recommendations, 469
Cervical cancer, 393–394
Change. *See also* Behavior modification
addictive behaviors, 58
barriers to, 51–52
categories of, 54
difficulty of, 42
helping relationships in, 60
imitating tips, 51–52
process of, 58–61, 65 (Activity 2.2)
rewards and, 60–61
stages of
action, 57
applicable processes, 56
behavioral modification for, 64 (Activity 2.2)
contemplation, 57
online tracking of, 63
precontemplation, 57–58
preparation, 57
termination, 58
techniques of, 61
theories of, 54–58

toxic environment and, 43–46
triggers for, 42
Chest fly, **272**
Chest press, **266**
Chest stretch, **300**
Chick Fil-A, 524
Children
cycling by, 46
exercise guidelines for, 9
healthy eating habits for, 119–120
Chinese cuisine, 104
Chiropractics, 495
Chlamydia, 470, 471
Chocolate, 340–341
Cholesterol. *See also* High-density lipoprotein (HDL); Low-density lipoprotein (LDL); Triglycerides
counteracting, 351–352
definition of, 349
lowering, medications for, 356
metabolic syndrome and, 360
in selected foods, 351
testing guidelines, 354
Chronic diseases, 3, 13
Chronic lower respiratory disease (CLRD), 6
Chronological age, 486, 489
Chylomicrons, 356
Cigarette smoking. *See also* Smoking cessation; Tobacco use
cancer risk of, 381, 451
cardiovascular effects of, 451
CHD risk and, 365–366
daily log for, 462 (Activity 13.6)
deaths from, 450–451
exercise and, 319
health risks from, 28
popularity of, 450
psychological dependency on, 454
reasons for, 454–455, 461 (Activity 13.5)
secondhand, 451–452
Cinogens, 378
Circuit training
advantage of, 250
definition of, 251
history of, 314
intensity of, 314–315
Cirrhosis, 445
Classical periodization, 245
Clinical study, 102, 103
Clothing
exercise, 319, 322
sun-protective, 382
CLRD. *See* Chronic lower respiratory disease (CLRD)
Club drugs, 441–442
Cocaine
characterization of, 440
crack, 440
effects of, 441
Cold turkey, 455, 459–460

Colds, 322
Colon/rectum cancer, 384
Commitment, 59
Community resources, 503–504 (Activity 15.2)
Competence, problems of, 53
Complacency, risks of, 51
Complementary and Alternative medicine (CAM). *See also* National Center for Complementary and Alternative Medicine (NCCAM)
costs of, 496
definition of, 490
fraud in, 497–500
health philosophies of, 495–496
shortcomings of, 496
standard scrutiny of, 495
therapies of, 490, 495
Complex carbohydrates, 77, 359–360
Complexity, 51
Compound fats, 78, 92
Comprehensive fitness programming
aerobic activities, 307–313
behavior assessment of, 333
example of, 330–332
FAQs, 306
knowledge assessment of, 333
new trends in, 313–315
overtraining in, 327–328
personal plan for
components of, 331–332
log, 334–337 (Activity 9.1)
overview of, 330–331
specific considerations for
appropriate clothing, 319, 322
arthritic people, 315–316
asthmatics, 315–316
colds/flu, 322
diabetics, 316
first aid measures, 320
footwear, 319–320
glucose levels, 317
injuries, 322–324
menstrual cycles and, 318–319
physical highs, 315
pregnancy, 317–318
sports participation, 326–330
strength training, 317
time of day, 320
weather conditions, 319
Compulsive exercisers, 437
Concentric resistance, 246–247
Confidence, problems of, 53–54
Consciousness-raising, 58
Consumer Product Safety Commission (CPS), 499
Consumers
educating, 497–498
Internet information and, 498–499
protection organizations, 499

Contemplation stage, 57
Contraindicated exercises, 290–291
Controlled ballistic stretching, 288–289
Convenience meals, nutrition values of, 526
Conventional Western medicine
 advances in, 488
 alternative practices referrals, 496–497
 definition of, 489
 hospital selection, 489–490
 standard scrutiny of, 495
Cool downs, 220–221
Core strength training, 314
Core values, 50–51
Coronary heart disease (CHD). See also Myocardial infarction
 angina pectoris in, 349
 chocolate and, 340–341
 ECG and, 348–349
 fat consumption and, 81
 homocysteine levels and, 356
 incidences of, 5
 LCHP diets and, 156
 nutritional factors in, 76
 premature, 367
 prevalence of, 342
 prevention of, 347–349
 resveratrol and, 340
 risk factors for
  abnormal cholesterol profile, 349–356
  age, 367
  analysis, 345–346 (Activity 10.1)
  chronic inflammation, 357–358
  cigarette smoking, 365–366
  diabetes, 358–360
  emotional-related, 367
  gum disease, 367
  leading, 344–345
  low-birth rate, 367
  medical history, 367
  metabolic syndrome, 360
  nutritional, 76
  obesity, 151, 365
  sleep apnea, 367
 risk profile for, 342–344
 treatments, 367
 type A personalities and, 411
Countering, 59
Cox-2 enzyme, 372
Crack cocaine, 440
Creatine, 115
Creatine phosphate, 115, 249
Creatine supplementation, 114–115
Criterion referenced. See Health fitness standards
Cross-country skiing, 312
Cross-training, 312, 329
CRP. See C-reactive protein (CRP)
Cruciferous vegetables, 377–378

Cuban cuisine, 104
Cycling
 benefits of, 310
 government commitment to, 45–46
 guidelines for, 311
 physical barriers to, 45
 stationary, 311–312

Daily food plan, 96
Daily steps, 11–12
Daily values (DV), 86–87
Dairy products. See Milk and milk products
Dairy Queen, 524
DASH diet, 155, 365
DCER. See Dynamic constant external resistance (DCER)
Death
 leading causes of, 3–6
 life-style related, 7
 physical inactivity and, 20
 smoking related, 450–451
Death rates
 cancer, 375
 by physical fitness groups, 20
 studies of, 19
Deep breathing, 426
Delegation, 416
Dentists, 489
Derived fats, 78, 82
Dextrins, 77
Diabetes mellitus
 CHD and, 358–360
 definition of, 359
 exercise precautions for, 316–317
 metabolic syndrome and, 360–361
 prevalence of, 359
 prevention of, 359–360
 tests for, 358–359
 types of, 316
Diastolic blood pressure (DBP), 31, 361
Dietary fat. See also Cholesterol; Oils; Trans fatty acid
 as cancer risk factor, 379
 chemical structure of, 90
 classification of, 79
 compounds, 82
 derived, 82
 excretion of, 78
 in foods, 351
 moderate intake of, 353
 partially hydrogenated, 352–353
 saturated, 351, 354–356
 unsaturated, 351–352
Dietary fiber
 cancer prevention and, 378
 characterization of, 77
 consumption of, 77–78
 definition of, 77
 food content, 78
Dietary Guidelines for Americans, 8

Dietary Reference Intakes (DRI)
 age and gender based, 88
 definition of, 87
 on food labels, 86–87
 values in, 87
 vitamin D, 107
Diets. See also Balanced diet
 for athletes, 113
 cancer risk and, 372
 cancer-fighting, 377
 cost factors and, 47
 diabetes prevention, 359–360
 environmental influence on, 46–47
 ethnic, 103–104
 high fiber, 77
 Mediterranean, 103, 156
 NAS guidelines, 86
 red meat in, 83
 for strength development, 251–253
 weight loss
  body composition and, 165
  books on, 154
  crash, 154
  crazes, 153–154
  effective, 146
  1,800 calorie plan, 185 (Activity 5.3)
  extreme, 146
  fad, recognizing, 158
  1,500 calorie plan, 184 (Activity 5.3)
  food choices, 177
  food logs for, 176, 182
  LCHP, 154–157
  metabolism and, 164–165
  outcome comparison, 164
  percentages, 150–151
  popular, 155–157
  2,000 calorie plan, 186 (Activity 5.3)
  very low calorie, 162–163
  view of, 163
  yo-yo, 153
  well-balanced, 86
Dips, **239, 263, 275**
Disaccharides
 breakdown of, 77
 definition of, 77
 major, 76
Disease risk
 BMI and, 126, 142 (Activity 4.2)
 WC and, 138, 142 (Activity 4.2)
Disease, See also specific conditions
 spontaneous remission, 408
Distractions, 417
Distress, 405
DNA, 373
Docosahexaenoic acid (DHA), 81
Domino's, 524
Dopamine, 50, 441–442
Double-knee-to-chest stretch, **302**

"Do You Want to Quit" Test
 categories in, 456
 need for, 455–456
 questions in, 458 (Activity 13.4)
Dramatic release, 59
Drug abuse. See Substance abuse
Drugs. See also Medications
 alcohol, 444–449
 club, 441–442
 definition of, 438
 licit, 439–444
 tobacco products, 450–454
Dual energy x-ray absorptiometry (DXA), 126–127
Duration
 CR exercises, 219–221
 exercise for weight management, 168–170
 fat burning exercises, 173
DXA. See Dual energy x-ray absorptiometry (DXA)
Dynamic constant external resistance (DCER), 246–247
Dynamic stretching, 287–288
Dynamic training, 246–247
Dysmenorrhea, 281, 318–319

Earle, Richard, 42
Eating disorders
 anorexia nervosa, 158–159
 binge-eating, 160
 bulimia, 159–160
 emotional eating, 160–161
 overview of, 158
 treatment for, 161
Eating out, 46
Eccentric resistance, 246–247
ECG. See Electrocardiogram (ECG/EKG)
Ecosystem, 19
Education
 increasing, 28
 values and, 47–48
 wellness, 29–30
EKG. See Electrocardiogram (ECG/EKG)
Elastic elongation, 282–283
Elastic-band resistive, 255
Elastic-band resistive exercise, **254**
Electrocardiogram (ECG/EKG), 348–349
Electrolytes, 115
Electronic cigarettes, 460
Elliptical training, 312–313
Emotional arousal, 59
Emotional eating, 160–161
Emotional health, 403
Emotional wellness, 17
Endometrial cancer, 394–395
Endorphins, 315, 423
Endurance athletes
 carbohydrate loading by, 113–114
 iron deficiency in, 117–118
Energy (ATP) production, 112

Energy drinks
  caffeine in, 195
  heart rate and, 194–195
  sugar in, 72
  work capacity and, 194
Energy-balance equation in, 161–162
Environment
  awareness of, 28, 43
  cancer risks in, 376
  control of, 59–60
Environmental influences
  diet and nutrition, 46–47
  exercising control over, 48–49 (Activity 2.1)
  physical activity, 44–46
Environmental wellness, 18–19
Enzymes, 82
Ephedra, 496
Epigallocatechin (EGCG), 378
Equipment, *See* Exercise equipment
Esophageal cancer, 396
Estimated average requirement (EAR), 87
Estimated energy requirement (EER)
  adjustments to, 161
  age-based, 173
  body composition-based, 173
  definition of, 87
Estrogen, 115
Ethnic diets, 103–104, 105
Eustress, 405
"Exercise Is Medicine" program, 9
Exercise. *See also* Physical activity
  addiction to, 437
  brain function and, 25–26
  CHD prevention and, 347–348
  choices in, 307
  cigarette smoking and, 319
  compliance, 225
  cool-down, 220–221
  definition of, 7, 201
  dropout rate, 42
  eating before, 306
  economic benefits of, 26–27
  energy drinks and, 194–195
  equipment, 502
  functional, 315
  H-PAPE during, 216, 219
  immediate benefits of, 25
  light-intensity, 169–170
  long-term benefits of, 26
  lower back, 294–295
  moderate-intensity, 169, 172
  nutritional requirements following, 306
  during pregnancy, 317–318
  related injuries, 322–324
  safety measures for, 29–30
  stretching and, 289–290
  vigorous-intensity
    fat burned in, 168–169
    lifestyle effects on, 172
    precautions for, 170
  warm-up, 220–221
  weight management and duration, 168–170, 173
  guidelines for, 167
  importance of, 167–168
  intensity, 168–170
  limits of, 148
  research on, 166
  time required, 166
Exercise equipment
  free weights, 246–248
  machines, 247
  purchasing, 502
Exercise volume, 221
Exercise-induced asthma (EIA), 315
Experiences, self-efficacy and, 52
Explanatory style, 406–408
Extra virgin olive oil, 80

Fad diets, 158
Fartlek training, 328
Fast-food restaurants, 46, 523–524
Fast-twitch fibers, 244, 245
Fat. *See* Body fat
Fat mass and obesity associated (FTO) gene, 170
Fat-soluble vitamins, 84
Fat-burning enzymes, 199
Fats (lipids)
  athletes use of, 113
  in balanced diet, 92, 96
  body's use of, 78–79
  calories in, 79, 90
  content, selected foods, 95
  definition of, 79
  in food, computation, 92
  major types of, 76
  in nuts, 101
Fatty acids
  free (*See* Triglycerides)
  omega-3, 80–81
  omega-6, 80–81
  omega-9, 82
  storage of, 356
Federal Physical Activity Guidelines for Americans
  age-based, 9
  duration recommendations, 219
  issuance of, 8
Fiber
  classification of, 78
  common types of, 78
  diet high in, 77
  excessive intake of, 78
Fight-or-flight mechanism, 422–423
Fighting spirit, 408
Financial fitness, 23–24
First aid measures, 320
Fish
  cardiac benefits of, 73
  contaminants in, 73
  fatty acids in, 81
  omega acids in, 81
"Fit and fat" debate, 170–171
Fitness. *See also* Lifetime fitness
  community resources for, 503–504 (Activity 15.2)
  FAQs, 2
  flexibility categories, 287
  lifetime commitment to, 224, 228
  personal profile, 4
  reliable information on, 499
  standards, 21–22
FITT-VP, 213
Five-minute de-stress technique, 427
Fixed-resistance
  definition of, 247
  free weights *vs.*, 247
  movement with, 246
Flaxseeds, 81
Flexibility
  aging and, 282
  assessment of
    log for, 296 (Activity 8.1)
    Shoulder Rotation Test, 283, 285–286
    Sit-and-Reach Test, 283, 285
    test interpretation, 283, 287
    Total Body Rotation Test, 283–284, 286
  behavior assessment of, 299
  benefits of, 281–282
  decline in, 281
  definition of, 281
  development guidelines, 289
  factors affecting, 282
  FAQs, 280
  fitness categories for, 287
  knowledge assessment of, 299
  low-back conditioning and, 295, 297–298 (Activity 8.2)
  personal profile, 281
  personal program for, 331
  prescription principles, 287–290
  for sports participation, 326
Flu, 322
Folate, 109–110, 357
Food labels
  design of, 89
  fats listed on, 80
  nutrient recommendations on, 86–87
  sodium listed on, 373
  sugar listed on, 72
Food pyramids, 103
Foods, *See also* Fast-food restaurants
  addiction to, 437
  AGEs in, 102
  Asian, 104
  benefits of, 109
  calories in, 91
  cholesterol in, 350
  choosing wisely, 174
  contamination of, 110–111
  daily intake record, 183–189 (Activity 5.3)
  description of, 516–526
  energy derived from, 112
  fat in, 91, 95
  fortified, 110
  functional, 109–110
  genetically modified, 111–112
  glycemic index, 156
  high protein, 177
  Hispanic, 104
  iron levels in, 118
  low-fat, 177
  nutritious, selection of, 100
  nutritional values of, 516–526
  organic, 110–111
  overabundance of, 46
  packaging of, 47
  potassium levels in, 363
  pre-exercise, 306
  probiotics in, 102
  processed, 352–353
  selenium levels in, 107
  sodium levels in, 363
  soul, 104
  super, 96
  top antioxidant, 109
  trans fats in, 340, 352–353
  vitamin D in, 107
Fortified foods, 110
Free radicals. *See* Oxygen-free radicals
Free weights
  advantages of, 247–248
  definition of, 247
  movement with, 246
  resistance machines *vs.*, 247
Frequency
  aerobic activity, 221
  strength training, 244, 250
  stretching, 289
Friendships, 28
Fruits, 92, 109
FTO gene. *See* Fat mass and obesity associated (FTO) gene
Functional capacity, 488–489
Functional fitness, 315
Functional foods, 109–110
Functional independence, 325

Gamma-linolenic acid (GLA), 81
Gardenburgers, 522
Gender differences
  anabolic steroid use, 235–236
  body weight, 151, 182
  in flexibility, 282
  life expectancy, 5
  nutrient intake recommendations, 88
  strength training, 234–235
General adaptation syndrome (GAS), 406–407
Genetic factors
  breast cancer, 390
  cancer-associated, 373, 384
  HDL, 951
  morbidity and, 6
  in obesity, 168, 170–172
Genetically modified (GM) foods, 111–112

Genetically modified organisms (GMOs), 111
Genital herpes, 472–473
Genital warts, 471
Ghrelin, 165
Girth measurement
  body fat estimates, 136
  conversion constants, 134–135
  definition of, 129
  limitations of, 128
  procedures for, 133
Glucose
  athletes use of, 113
  excess, 76
  intolerance, 360
  levels, tests for, 358–359
  physical activity and, 112
Gluteal stretch, **303**
Gluten sensitivity, 72
Glycemic index
  definition of, 154
  diet based on, 155–156
  function of, 73, 360
Glycemic Index Diet, 155–156
Glycemic load, 73
Glycogen
  athletes use of, 113
  average stores of, 153
  definition of, 77
  storage of, 113–114
Goals
  acceptable, 63
  behavior change and, 59
  defined, 61
  evaluation of, 68
  measurable, 63
  priorities and, 420 (Activity 12.6)
  self-evaluation of, 505
  specificity in, 61–62
  time specific, 68
Goal setting
  behavioral, future, 505, 508 (Activity 15.4)
  long- and short-term, planning, 419 (Activity 12.5)
  personal training and, 502
  wellness, 39 (Activity 1.5)
Golgi tendon, 288
Gonorrhea, 470, 471
Gratification, 51
Gum disease, 367
Gums, 78
Gynoid obesity, 133

H-PAPE. *See* Physical activity perceived exertion (H-PAPE)
Habits
  brain function and, 50–51
  dietary, changing, 148
  formation of, 50
  modifying, 182
  values and, 50
Hamstring roll, **278**
Hand Grip Strength Test, 237
Happiness, 17
Hatha yoga, 431

HDL. *See* High-density lipoprotein (HDL)
Health
  categories of, WHtR and, 138
  definition of, 3
  factors affecting, 7
  fitness and, 2
  history questionnaire, 36–37 (Activity 1.3)
  philosophies, 495
Health care, 26–27. *See also* Complementary and Alternative medicine (CAM); Conventional Western medicine
Health fitness standards
  attaining, 21–22
  categories of, 21
  definition of, 21
  motor skill components, 21
Health information
  deception in, 497–498
  Internet sources, 498–499
  refereed scientific journals, 499–500
  reliable sources of, 499
  reliable websites for, 500
Health promotion, 14
Health-related fitness, 20–21
Health/fitness clubs, 500–501
Healthy Choice, 526
Healthy Habits, 5
Healthy People Initiative, 10
Healthy plate, 97
Heart attack. *See* Myocardial infarction
Heart disease. *See* Coronary heart disease (CHD)
Heart rate. *See also* Maximal heart rate (MHR)
  monitoring of, 216
  recovery, 324
  while cycling, 310–311
Heart rate reserve (HRR), 213
Heat cramps, 320
Heat exhaustion, 320–321
Heat illness, 320–321
Heat stroke, 320–321
Heel cord stretch, **301**
Heel raise, **264**
Helping relationships, 60
Helplessness, 51
Hemoglobin, 117, 197
Hemoglobin A_{1c}, 360
Herbal medicine, 495–496
Heroin, 443–444
Herpes simplex viruses, 472–473
Heterocyclic amines (HCAs), 379
High-density lipoprotein (HDL)
  characterization of, 79
  CHD and, 80, 82
  definition of, 349
  increasing, benefits of, 351
  omega-6 and, 81
  subgroups of, 350
  tobacco's effects of, 451
High-fructose corn syrup (HFCS), 72

High-impact aerobics (HIA), 309
High-intensity interval training (HITT)
  benefits of, 306
  definition of, 313
  sample programs, 328
  for sports conditioning, 327
Hiking, 308
Hill, Jan, 42
Hip abduction and adduction, **269**
Hip flexor stretch, **302**
Hispanic foods, 104
HITT. *See* High-intensity interval training (HITT)
HIV (human immunodeficiency virus)
  characterization of, 474
  diagnosis, 477
  myths about, 478–479
  people living with, 477
  PEP, 474, 477
  prevention guidelines, 482–483
  risky behavior, 478
  screening guidelines, 469
  self-quiz on, 475–476 (Activity 14.1)
  testing for, 479–480
  transmission of, 477–479
  treatment of, 480
  trends in, 479
Holistic therapy, 496
Homeopathy, 495
Homeostatsis, 406–407
Homocysteine, 356
Hormones, 165
Hospital, searching for, 489–490
Human papilloma virus
  cervical cancer from, 393–394
  characterization of, 471
  types of, 471
  vaccines for, 471–472
Hunger cues, 46–47
Hydrostatic weighing, 127, 143
Hypertension
  atherosclerosis and, 362
  definition of, 361
  essential, 362
  incidence of, 361
  obesity and, 363
  pathology of, 361–362
  prevention of, 362–364
  sodium consumption and, 362
  standards, 361
  treatments of, 362
Hypertrophy, 234
Hypokinetic diseases
  definition of, 21, 197
  risks of, 20–21
  types of, 196
Hyponatremia, 114, 115, 321
Hypotension, 361
Hypothermia, 321–322

Immune system
  explanatory style and, 407
  function of, 403
  stress and, 404

Immunity, 403
In-n-Out Burger, 524
Indifference, 51
Individuality, principle of, 200–201
Inflammation, 357–358
Inhalant abuse, 444
Injuries, exercise-related
  common causes of, 322–323
  muscle cramps, 324
  muscle soreness/stiffness, 323–324
  reference guide for, 323
  shin splints, 324–325
  side stitches, 324–325
  sports injuries, 323
Insoluble fiber, 78
Insulin, 359
Insulin resistance, 358, 359
Integrative medicine, 497
Intellectual wellness. *See* Mental wellness
Intensity
  aerobic, 213–214, 216
  circuit training, 314–315
  definition of, 213
  fat burning and, 168–170, 194
  lifestyle effects on, 172
  precautions for, 170
  resistance *vs.*, 248
  stretching, 288–289
  weight management, 168–170
Intermediate-density lipoprotein (IDL), 350
International unit (IU), 106
Internet
  addiction to, 437
  health advice on, 498–499
Interval training, 312
Invincibility, illusions of, 51–52
Iron deficiency, 105, 117
Isokinetic training, 247
Isometric training
  benefits of, 246
  definition of, 247
  distinction of, 246–247
Iyegar yoga, 294–295

Jack in the Box, 524
Jack knives, **278**
Jamba Juice, 524–525
Jogging/running
  barefoot, 319–320
  calories burned from, 12
  overview of, 308

Kentucky Fried Chicken (KFC), 525
Kidney cancer, 396

L-Carnitine, 83
Lactic acid, 112–113
Lactobacillus bulgaricus, 102
Lapse, 55
Lat pull-down, **269**
Lateral plank, **265**
Lateral trunk flexion, **276**

LCHP. *See* Low-carbohydrate/high protein (LCHP) diets
LDL. *See* Low-density lipoprotein (LDL)
Lean body mass, 125
Learning theories, 54
Leg abduction/adduction, **265, 269**
Leg curl, **263, 268**
Leg extension, **271**
Leg press, **267**
Leisure time, 45
Leptin, 165
Leukemia, 397
Life expectancy. *See also* Longevity
  definition of, 3
  gender differences, 5
  global percentages, 4
  physical activity and, 347
  physiological age and, 488, 491–494 (Activity 15.1)
  questionnaire, 491–494
  sedentary lifestyles and, 488
  U.S. ranking, 4–5
Lifestyles. *See also* Sedentary lifestyles
  cancer prevention and, 6, 375–376, 398
  exercise intensity and, 172
  health and fitness benefits, 22
  healthy habits for, 28
  mortality and, 5–6
  risk factors and, 6–7
  SCD risk and, 344
  wellness questionnaire, 33–35 (Activity 1.2)
  wellness, self-assessment, 509–510 (Activity 15.5)
Lifetime fitness
  behavior assessment, 511
  FAQs, 486
  future challenges of, 505–506, 511
  guidelines for, 498
  gym membership and, 500–501
  implementation of, 487
  knowledge assessment, 511–512
  life expectancy and, 488
  personal profiles, 487
Linoleic acid (LA), 81
Lipoproteins, 82–83. *See also* High-density lipoprotein (HDL); Low-density lipoprotein (LDL)
Locus of control, 53
Long-distance athletic events, 113–114
Longevity. *See also* Life expectancy
  factors determining, 3, 4
  personal profile, 487
  physical activity and, 19–20
Low-back pain
  causes of, 290–291
  chronic, 294

cycling and, 310
disease/injury indicators, 292
incidences of, 290
prevention of, 293–294
stress and, 295
stretching for, 303
treatments for
  flexibility development, 297–298 (Activity 8.2)
  spinal manipulation, 292
  strengthening program, 294–295
  stress management, 295
  time as, 294
Low-carbohydrate/high protein (LCHP) diets, 154–157
Low-density lipoprotein (LDL)
  characterization of, 79
  CHD and, 80, 82
  definition of, 349
  lowering of, 353–355
  omega-6 and, 81
  phenotype B, 356
  release of, 349–350
Low-impact aerobics (LIA), 309
Lower back stretch, **303**
Lung cancer, 384, 387
Lymphocytes, 403–404
Lymphoma, 397

Ma huang, 496
Macrocycles, 329
Magnetic therapy, 495
Maintenance stage, 57–58
Malignant, 373
Mammograms, 393
Manipulative practices, 495
Marijuana
  active ingredients, 439–440
  characterization of, 439
  effects of, 440
Massage therapy, 495
Mastery experiences, 52
Maximal heart rate (MHR)
  definition of, 201
  during swimming, 309
  training zone, 214
Maximal oxygen uptake VO_{2max}
  age-based correction factors, 208
  ATP generation and, 112
  definition of, 197
  expression of, 22
  increase in, 197
  prediction equation for, 203–204
  tests for
    Astrand-Ryhming, 204–205, 207
    1.0 mile run, 203–204
    1.5-mile run, 202–203
    result interpretation, 206
    results log, 209–210 (Activity 6.1)
    step, 204–205
    12-minute swim, 205, 208
McDonald's, 91, 525

MDMA, 442, 442–443
Mean blood pressure, 31
Measurable goals, 61
Meats, consumption of, 83
Medications. *See also* specific drugs
  antihypertensive, 362
  cholesterol-lowering, 356–357
  nonmedical use of, 439
Meditation
  benefits of, 428–429
  initial routine for, 429
  mindfulness, 430
  mindless, 429–430
Mediterranean diet, 103, 156
Mediterranean diet pyramid, 103
Megadoses, 105
Melanoma, 381
Menopausal hormone therapy (MHT), 117
Mental wellness, 17
Mercury toxicity, 73
Mesocycles, 329
Metabolic equivalents (METs), 222–223
Metabolic profile, 22
Metabolic syndrome, 360–361
Metabolism
  definition of, 235
  diet and, 164–165
  muscle fitness and, 234
  weight management and, 162
Metastasis, 375
Methamphetamine
  binge cycle in, 442
  characterization of, 441
  effects of, 441–442
METs. *See* Metabolic equivalents (METs)
Microcycles, 329
Milk and milk products
  diabetes prevention with, 359–360
  nutritional value of, 509
  osteoporosis prevention with, 92
Mind-body connection, 403
Mind-body medicine, 495
Mindfulness meditation, 430
Mindless meditation, 429
Minerals, 85
Mitochondria, 198–199
Mixed dishes, 523
Mode, 216
Moderate physical activity
  benefits of, 8, 9
  definition of, 7
  recommendations for, 8
Moderate-impact aerobics (MIA), 309
Modified dip, **239, 263**
Modified push up, **239**
Monitoring, 59
Monosaccharides, 76–77
Monosaturated fatty acids (MUFA), 80
Monounsaturated fatty acids, 79

Morbidity
  definition of, 7
  smoking related, 450–451
Morningstar Farms, 522
Mortality rates
  BMI and, 135
  environmental influences on, 44–45
  hypertension and, 363
  underweight and, 129
Motivation, 42, 53
Motor neurons, 244
Motor unit, 244–245
Mucilages, 78
Multiple-joint exercises, 250
Multivitamins, 107
Muscles
  activation of, 250
  cramps in, 324
  major, 252
  progressive relaxation of, 425–426
  soreness/stiffness, 323–324
  spindles, 288
  types of, 244
Muscular endurance
  assessment, 242–243
  definition of, 237
  establishment of, 236
  FAQs, 232
  healthy backs and, 294
  periodization program for, 332
  tests for, 237–241
Muscular fitness
  ADLs and, 234
  aerobic fitness *vs.*, 232
  circuit training and, 250
  definition of, 233
  factors affecting, 244–245
  need for, 233
  personal program for, 331
Muscular strength
  definition of, 237
  determination of, 236
  FAQs, 232
  overload principle in, 244
  periodization program for, 332
  tests for, 236–241
MyPlate
  record form, 98 (Activity 3.3)
  vegetarian, 101
Myocardial infarction, 343, 367

NAS. *See* National Academy of Science (NAS)
National Academy of Science (NAS), 86
National AIDS Hotline, 479
National Alliance for Nutrition, 47
National Center for Complementary and Alternative Medicine (NCCAM)
  establishment of, 490
  heath information from, 497
  therapy categories of, 495
National Health Objectives. *See* Healthy People initiative

National Institutes of Health (NIH), 480, 497
National Physical Activity Plan
 establishment of, 10
 implementation of, 11
 vision for, 10–11
Natural products, 495
Naturopathic medicine, 495
NCCAM. *See* National Center for Complementary and Alternative Medicine (NCCAM)
NEAT. *See* Nonexercise activity thermogenesis (NEAT)
Neck stretches, **300**
Negative caloric balance, 173
Negative resistance, 246–247
Neural function, 244
Neuropeptide Y, 366
Neustress, 408
Niacins, 356
Nicotine, 451, 453
Nicotine-substitution products, 460
Nicotinic acid, 357
Nitrosamines
 cancer risk in, 378
 cancer risk of, 379
 definition of, 379
Nonexercise activity thermogenesis (NEAT), 13, 221
Nonresponders
 definition of, 201
 responders vs., 199–201
 studies of, 200
Nonsteroidal anti-inflammatory drug (NSAID), 372
Nurses, 489
Nutrient density, 76–77
Nutrients. *See also* specific types
 analysis of, 88, 90
 in balanced diet, 92, 96
 consumption of, 74, 76
 daily intake, 93 (Activity 3.1), 94 (Activity 3.2)
 definition of, 74
 essential, 76
 post-exercise, 306
 proportions in body, 86
 recommendations for, 119
 standards for, 86–88
 supplementation (*See* Supplements)
 vegetarians deficient in, 100–101
Nutrition
 for athletes, 113–115
 behavior modification plan, 99 (Activity 3.4)
 definition of, 74
 environmental influence on, 46–47
 exercising control over, 49 (Activity 2.1)
 FAQs, 72–73
 healthy living and, 119–120
 misinformation about, 97

personal habits, 74
reliable information on, 499
Nuts, 101, 107

Obesity
 cancer risks of, 380
 definition of, 125
 epidemic of, 46, 149–150
 genetic factors in, 168
 health consequences of, 151
 hypertension and, 363
 overweight *versus*, 151–152
 patterns of, 133
 trends in, 135
 U.S. trends in, 150
Observational study, 103
Occupational wellness, 18–19
Oils
 characterization of, 92
 nutritional information for, 509
 types of, 79, 82
 use of, 80
Okinawan diet, 103
Older adults. *See also* Aging
 dietary guidelines for, 119
 exercise guidelines for, 9
 functional independence of, 325
 nutrient intake recommendations, 88
 physical inactivity among, 282, 325
 physical training for, 324–326
 supplement needs of, 105
 VO_{2max}, 325
Oligomenorrhea, 117
Olive oil, 80
Omega eicosapentaenoic acid (EPA), 81
Omega-3 fatty acids
 cancer prevention with, 379
 definition of, 81
 good health and, 80–81
Omega-6 fatty acids
 consumption of, 81
 definition of, 81
 good health and, 80–81
 health risks from, 81
Omega-9 fatty acids, 82
Oncogenes, 373
1.0 mile run, 203—204
1.5-mile run, 202–203
One repetition (1 RM)
 definition of, 237
 determination of, 236
 number performed, 248–249
Ophthalmologists, 489
Optometrists, 489
Oral cancer, 396
Oral surgeon, 489
Ornish diet, 155
Orthodontists, 489
Osteopaths, 489
Osteoporosis
 definition of, 115
 incidence of, 115

LCHP diets and, 156
 prevention of
  exercise and, 116–117
  supplements for, 115–116
 risky activities for, 223
 treatments for, 117
Ovarian cancer, 397
Overload principle, 244–245
"Overtimes," 417
Overtraining
 definition of, 327
 effects of, 328
 prevention of, 245
 signs and symptoms of, 329
Overweight
 activity choices for, 172
 cancer risks of, 380
 definition of, 125
 fit and, 170–171
 health consequences of, 151
 obesity *versus*, 151–152
 swimmers, 309–310
 trends in, 135
Ovovegetarians, 100
Oxygen-free radicals
 absorption of, 378
 antioxidants and, 106–107
 body's defense against, 106
 definition of, 107
Oxygen uptake (VO_2), 197

Palpitations, 194
Pancreatic cancer, 379, 396
PAR-Q. *See* Physical Activity Readiness Questionnaire (PAR-Q)
Passive stretching, 287
Pectins, 78
Pedometers, 11–12
Peer support, 60
Pelvic clock, **304**
Pelvic inflammatory disease (PID), 470, 471
Pelvic tilt, **265, 304**
Periodization
 concept behind, 329
 contraindications for, 330
 cycles of, 329
 definition of, 329
 for muscular fitness, 332
 sample sequence of, 329–330
 types of, 245, 328–329
Peristalsis, 78–79
Personal fitness programming
 components of, 331–332
 log for, 334–337 (Activity 9.1)
 overview of, 330–331
 success in, 332
Personal trainers
 certification of, 501
 credentials of, 501–502
 definition of, 501
 selection of, 502
Pesticides, 110–111
Phenotype B, 356
Phillip Morris, 453–454

Physical activity. *See also* Exercise; Moderate physical activity
 aging and, 486
 for asthmatics, 314–315
 benefits of, 19–20
 best, 306
 blood pressure and, 363–364
 calories expended during, 175
 cancer prevention and, 372, 382–383
 cardiorespiratory loss from, 347
 daily log for, 15–16 (Activity 1.1)
 daily, monitoring of, 11–12, 14
 definition of, 7, 201
 diabetes prevention and, 359
 energy substrates for, 112
 environment influence on, 44–46
 exercise benefits lost to, 228
 exercising control over, 49 (Activity 2.1)
 federal guidelines for, 8–10
 glycogen and, 113
 importance of, 7–8
 increasing, 200–201
 long-distance events, 113–114
 minimizing, 13
 modern conveniences and, 44
 most popular, 308
 national plan for, 10–14
 in older adults, 282, 325
 programs, participation in, 28
 stress management and, 422–424
 stress reduction by, 367
 technology's impact on, 196
 vigorous, 20
Physical activity perceived exertion (H-PAPE) scale, 216
Physical activity pyramid, 222
Physical Activity Readiness Questionnaire (PAR-Q)
 health history, 36–37 (Activity 1.3)
 HITT programs, 328
 purpose of, 29
Physical fitness
 assessment of, 199–201
 definition of, 21
 health-related components of, 21
 premature mortality and, 19
 profile of, 504
 types of, 20–21
Physical fitness programs
 benefits of, 2
 comprehensive, 24
 health benefits of, 24–25
Physical fitness standards
 benefits of, 22, 23
 definition of, 22
 health fitness standards vs., 21
Physical inactivity
 chronic disease and, 13
 CVD and, 347–348

deaths from, 20
economic costs of, 26–27
epidemic of, 2–3
modern technology and, 2–3
studies on, 2
weight management and, 166
Physical wellness, 17
Physician assistant, 489
Physicians
complaints about, 497
selection of, 489
specialties of, 489
Physiological age
chronological age *vs.*, 486
definition of, 487
life expectancy and, 488
questionnaire, 491–494 (Activity 15.1)
Phytochemicals. *See* Phytonutrients
Phytoestrogens, 380
Phytonutrients
antioxidants *vs.*, 73
cancer prevention and, 378
definition of, 92, 379
PID. *See* Pelvic inflammatory disease (PID)
Pilates, 253–254, 422
Pilates, Joseph, 254
Pizza Hut, 525
Plank (stability ball), **276**
Plastic elongation, 282–283
Plyometric training, 309
Plyometrics, 251
PNF. *See* Proprioceptive neuromuscular facilitation (PNF)
Polycyclic aromatic hydrocarbons (PAHs), 379–380
Polyunsaturated fatty acids (PUFA), 79–80
Positive outlook, 59
Positive resistance, 246–247
Post-exposure prophylaxis (PEP), 474, 477
Post-sex heart attack, 367
Postpartum women, 9
Posture, 293, 295
Prayer, 18, 20
Precancerous cells, 374
Precontemplation stage, 55, 57
Pregnancy
dietary guidelines for, 119
exercise guidelines for, 9, 317–318
smoking during, 450–451
Preparation stage, 57
Prescription drugs. *See* Medications
Prevention. *See also* Cancer prevention
AIDS, 482–483
CHD, 347–349
CVD, 340
diabetes, 359–360
HIV, 482–483
hypertension, 362–364

lapses/relapses, 55
low-back pain, 294
osteoporosis, 115–118
overtraining, 245
primordial, 14
STIs, 481–482
Primary care physician, 489
Primordial prevention, 14
Principle of individuality, 200–201
Probiotics, 102
Problem-solving model, 54–55
Processed foods
cancer risk of, 379–380
nutritional information on, 522–524
trans fats in, 352–353
Processes of change, 58–60
Procrastination, 51
Progression, rate of, 221–222
Progressive muscle relaxation
definition of, 425
development of, 425
example of, 425–426
Progressive resistance training, 233
Prone plank, **266**
Proprioceptive neuromuscular facilitation (PNF), 288
Proprioceptors, 288
Proteins
amino acids in, 82
classification of, 82
consumption of, 82–83
definition of, 83
intake recommendations, 113, 177
for osteoporosis prevention, 116
in soy products, 102
Prostate cancer, 395
Psychotherapeutic drugs, 439
Psyllium, 354
Puerto Rican cuisine, 104
Pull up, **264**
Push-up, **262, 277**

Quackery
debunking, 498–500
definition of, 497
media role in, 497–498
protection against, 497–500
Quad stretch, **301**
Questionnaires
addictive behaviors, 447 (Activity 13.1)
alcohol use, 447 (Activity 13.2)
health history, 36–37 (Activity 1.3)
life expectancy/physiological age, 491–494 (Activity 15.1)
PAR-Q, 36–37 (Activity 1.3)
stress vulnerability, 414 (Activity)
wellness lifestyles, 33–35 (Activity 1.2)

Racquet sports, 313
Range of motion, 246–247
Rapid heart rate. *See* Palpitations; Tachycardia
Rationalization, 51
Recommended body weight
criteria for, 124
definition of, 125
determination of, 139
Recommended Dietary Allowance (RDA)
age and gender based, 88
definition of, 87
on food labels, 86–87
for vitamin E, 106
Recovery heart rate, 324
Recovery time, 199
Red meat consumption, 83
Registered dietitian (RD), 109
Relapse
action stage and, 57
defined, 55
precontemplation stage and, 58
Relapse prevention model, 55
Relaxation techniques
autogenic training, 428
biofeedback, 424–425
body scan, 424
breathing exercises, 426–427
five-minute de-stress, 427
meditation, 428–430
overview of, 424
progress muscle relaxation, 425–426
selection of, 431
visual imagery, 427–428
REM (rapid eye movement), 404
Repetitions, 289
Resistance
definition of, 249
guidelines for, 250
intensity *vs.*, 248
moderate, 249
stressor, 406
types of, 246–247
Resistance training. *See* Strength training
Responders, 199–201
Rest intervals, 249
Restaurant food
calories in, 46
nutritional information on, 523–525
sodium in, 363
Resting heart rate (RHR)
assessment of, 30
decrease in, 197–198
definition of, 197
guidelines, 31
log for, 38 (Activity 1.4)
ratings, 30
in trained athlete, 199
Resting metabolic rate (RMR), 161
Resting metabolism, 234–235
Resveratrol, 340

Reverse cholesterol transport, 351
Reverse crunch, **265**
Reverse periodization, 245
Reverse supine plank, **277**
RICE, 323
Risk factors
addiction, 438
BMI as, 135
body fat as, 140
CHD, 344–346
cigarette smoking as, 28
complacency as, 51
CVD, 342–344
definition of, 343
lifestyle-related, 6–7
omega-6 consumption as, 81
osteoporosis, 116, 223
RNA, 373
Rogers, Don, 440
Role models, 47, 50
Rotary torso, **270**
Rowing, 312
Rowing torso, **262**
Rubberized wet suits, 171–172
Running. *See* Jogging/running

Safety measures
cardiovascular, 30–31
during exercise, 29–30
PAR-Q, 28
Sandwiches, nutrition values of, 523
Sarcopenia, 234–235
Saturated fats
characterization of, 79
chemical structure of, 80
replacement of, 354–356
Saturated fatty acids, 80
Schultz, Johannes, 428
Scientific journals, refereed, 499–500
Seated back, **268**
Seated leg curl, **274**
Secondhand smoke, 452
Sedentary, 3
Sedentary death syndrome (SeDS), 3
Sedentary lifestyles, 168. *See also* Physical inactivity
aging and, 164, 486
caloric needs of, 167
flexibility decline and, 282
lean tissue decline from, 82, 125
life expectancy and, 488
nutritional needs for, 113
SEE. *See* Standard error estimate (SEE)
Selective estrogen receptor modulators (SERMs), 117
Selenium, 107, 378
Self-analysis, 59
Self-efficacy, 52–53
Self-esteem, 407–408
Self-reevaluation, 59
Selye, Hans, 405

Semivegetarians, 100
Setpoint
  example of, 162
  lowering, 163
  theory of, 162, 162–163
Sets
  definition of, 249
  guidelines for, 250
  intervals between, 249–250
Sexually transmitted infection (STI). See also AIDS (acquired immunodeficiency syndrome); HIV (human immunodeficiency virus)
  behavior assessment, 483
  chlamydia, 470
  definition of, 469
  genital herpes, 472
  gonorrhea, 470
  HPV, 471–472
  knowledge assessment, 484
  personal profile survey, 469
  PID, 470
  prevalence of, 469
  prevention guidelines, 481–482
  protection from, 480
  STD vs., 468
  syphilis, 473
  trichomoniasis, 473
  wise dating and, 479
Shoeless running, 319–320
Shoulder hyperextension, **301**
Shoulder press, **272**
Shoulder rotation stretch, **301**
Shoulder Rotation Test
  indications of, 283
  percentile ranks for, 286
  procedure for, 285
Side stitches, 324–325
Side stretches, **300**
Sighing, 426
Simple carbohydrates, 76–77. See also Sugar
Simple fats, 78–79
Single-joint exercises, 250
Single-knee-to-chest stretch, **302**
Sit-and-reach stretch, **302**
Sit-and-Reach Test, 283, 285
Sitting adductor stretch, **301**
Sitting disease, 13, 221
Sitting time
  activities related to, 45–46
  death rates, 44
  life expectancy and, 348
Skill-related fitness, 20–21
Skin cancer
  prevention of, 381–382
  risk factors, 389
  self-exam for, 390
  types of, 381
  warning signs of, 390
Skinfold thickness measurement
  percentage estimates, 130–132
  practicality of, 143
  principle of, 128
  procedure for, 129
  training for, 128

Sleep
  deprivation of, 165, 404
  enhancing quality of, 404–405
  weight management and, 165
Sleep apnea, 367
Sleep debt, 404
Slow-sustained stretching. See Static stretching
Slow-twitch fibers, 244, 245
SMART goals
  components of, 61–63
  defined, 61
  evaluation of, 68
  identification, 61–62
  setting, 66–67 (Activity 2.3)
Smoking cessation
  behavior modification plan for, 463–465
  cold turkey, 455, 459–460
  difficulty of, 455
  gradual approach to, 460
  life after, 460, 463
  nicotine-substitution products for, 460
  peer support for, 60
  reasons for, 461 (Activity 13.5)
  steps for, 456, 459
  test for, 455–456
Snacking, 28
Social cognitive theory, 54–55
Social liberation, 58–59
Social support, 413
Social wellness, 18–19
Sodium, 362–363
Soft drinks, 116
Soluble fiber, 78
Soul food. See African-American diet
Soups, nutrition values of, 523
South Beach Diet, 155
Soy products, 102, 380
Specific adaptation to imposed demand (SAID) training, 245
Specificity of training, 245
Sphygmomanometer, 30–31
Spice, 444
Spinal manipulation, 495
Spiritual wellness
  benefits of, 18
  definition of, 19
  practices for, 20
Spontaneous remission, 408
Sports. See also Athletes
  acute injuries in, 323
  base fitness conditioning for, 326
  periodization for, 328–329
  specific conditioning for, 326–327
  specific/pre-exercise stretching, 289
Spot reducing, 171–172
Squat, **278**
Stability exercise balls
  abdominal crunch on, **276–277**
  back extension on, **277**
  benefits of, 313–314

  plank on, **276**
  strength training with, 254–255, 276–278
Stair climbing, 312–313
Standard error estimate (SEE), 126
Starbucks, 525
Starch, 77
Static stretching, 287
Statins, 356, 358
Stationary cycling, 311–312
Step aerobics, 309
Step test, 204–205
Step-up, **262**
Step-wise intensity interval training, 328
Sterol regulatory element-binding proteins (SREBPs), 340
Sterols, 82
STIs. See Sexually transmitted infection (STI)
Stomach cancer, 396
Storage fat, 126, 127
Stouffers, 526
Strength training, behavior assessment 261
  for abdominal, 232
  behavior modification plan for, 253
  calories expenditures in, 168
  cancer prevention and, 383
  circuit, 250
  definition of, 233
  for diabetics, 316–317
  dietary guidelines for, 251–253
  flexibility and, 280
  frequency of, 250
  gains from, 251
  gender difference, 234–235
  guidelines, 250
  gym membership and, 500–501
  knowledge assessment, 261
  modes of, 245–248, 314
  periodization for, 245, 330
  personal trainers for, 501–502
  popularity of, 308
  prescription, 244–245
  principles of, 245
  progressive, 233
  resistance in, 248–249
  rest intervals, 249
  sets in, 249–250
  specificity of, 244
  for sports participation, 326–327
  variations in, 250
  volume, 245
  weight management and, 167–168
Strength training programs
  circuit-based, 250
  core-based, 253
  elastic-band resistive, **254**, 255
  guidelines for, 250
  overview of, 251
  personalized, setting up, 256, 257–258 (Activity 7.2)

  Pilates, 253–254
  plyometrics, 251
  record form, 259–260 (Activity 7.3)
  stability balls, 254–255
  with weights, 266–276
Stress
  adaptation to, 406
  behavior patterns and, 408, 411–412
  body's response to, 405
  brain's role in, 403
  CHD risk from, 366–367
  common symptoms, 422
  coping with, 417, 429
  definition of, 405
  events scale, 409–410 (Activity 12.1)
  explanatory style and, 406–407
  fighting spirit and, 408
  harmful effects of, 402–403
  immune system and, 403–404
  knowledge assessment, 434
  low-back pain and, 295
  lowering, 28
  profile, 415 (Activity 12.3)
  response, 422
  self-assessment, 433 (12.9)
  self-esteem and, 407–408
  sources of, 408
  vulnerability to, 412–413
  vulnerability questionnaire, 414 (Activity 12.2)
Stress electrocardiogram, 348–349
Stress Events Scale, 408
Stress management. See also Relaxation techniques; Time management
  behavior assessment, 434
  coping strategies, 429
  effective strategies for, 402
  experience, 432 (Activity 12.8)
  FAQs, 402
  good characteristics of, 428
  personal survey, 403
  physical activity in, 422–424
  yoga as, 430–431
Stressors
  college students', 408
  definition of, 405
  responses to, 406, 422
Stretch reflex, 288
Stretching
  best time for, 289–290
  contraindicated, 290–291
  definition of, 281
  frequency of, 289
  injury prevention by, 280
  intensity of, 288–289
  modes of, 287–288
  pain from, 280
  physiological response to, 288
  repetitions, 289
  sports-specific/pre-exercise, 289

Index

Stretching exercises
  basic, 300–303
  contraindicated, 290–291
  for lower back, 303
Stroke, 342–343
Stroke volume
  definition of, 199
  endurance and, 201
  function of, 198
  measurement of, 202
  in trained athletes, 199
Structured interview, 411
Subcutaneous fat, 128–129, 140
Subluxation, 281
Substance abuse
  characterization of, 438
  criminal behavior and, 438–439
  early stages of, 436
  overview of, 437
Substrates, 74
Subway, 91, 525
Sudden cardiac death (SCD)
  characterization of, 344
  risk for, 352
  stress and, 366
Sugar
  cancer risk from, 379
  in energy drinks, 72
  health effects of, 72
Sun exposure
  excessive, 108
  excessive, avoiding, 381–382
  vitamin D and, 107–108
Sun protection factor (SPF), 381–382
Sunscreen lotions, 381–382
Super foods, 96
Supine bridge, **304**
Supine plank, **276**
Supplements
  age and, 105
  antioxidants, 106
  cancer risks of, 380
  creatine, 114
  definition of, 105
  minerals, 101, 106–107
  overview of, 105–106
  vitamins, 106–108
Suppressor genes, 373
Supramaximal interval training, 328
Surgeon General's Report, 450, 455
Swimming
  benefits of, 309
  specificity training principles in, 310
  sun protection and, 382
  weight loss limits of, 173
Synergistic action, 445
Synergy, 109
Syphilis, 473
Systolic blood pressure (SBP), 31, 361

Tachycardia, 194, 440–441
Taco Bell, 91, 525

Tai chi
  definition of, 423
  performance of, 431
  stress management with, 422
Tar, 451
Tea drinking, 378–379
Techniques of change, 61, 62
Technology, 2–3
Television viewing, 45, 437
Telomerase, 373
Telomeres, 373
Tempo training, 328
Termination stage, 58
Testicular cancer, 395
THC (delta-9-tetrahydrocannabinol), 439–440
Thermogenic response, 320
Thirst, 85
Thirty-second body scan, 424
Thyroid cancer, 397
Time killers, 416, 418 (Activity 12.4)
Time management
  goal planning, 419 (Activity 12.5)
  goals and priorities, 420 (Activity 12.6)
  overview of, 413
  skills, 416–417, 421 (Activity 12.7)
  steps to, 413, 416
Time specific goals, 68
Timing, 58
Tobacco use. *See also* Cigarette smoking
  health care costs of, 453
  health consequences, awareness of, 452–453
  products of, 453
  trends in, 453–454
Tolerable Upper Intake Levels (UL), 87–88
Top-priority tasks, 416
Total Body Rotation Test, 284, 286
Traffic-calming strategies, 45
Training volume, 245
Trans fatty acid
  controversy over, 340
  definition of, 81
  effects of, 352
  in food, 352
  labeling of, 352–353
Transportation alternatives, 45–46
Transtheoretical model, 55
Triceps extension, **270–271**
Triceps stretch, **302**
Trichomoniasis, 473
Triglycerides
  definition of, 351
  elevated, 356
  guidelines, 355
  lowering, 351–352
  metabolic syndrome and, 360
Trimethylamine-N-oxide (TMAO), 83
Trunk rotation stretch, **303**

Tumors, types of, 373
Tweaking stage, 442
12-minute swim test, 205, 208
25-Hydroxyvitamin D test, 108
2010 Dietary Guidelines for Americans, 118–119
Type 1 diabetes, 359–360
Type 2 diabetes, 359–360
Type A personalities
  bases of, 408
  changing, 412
  characterization of, 411
Type B personalities, 408, 411
Type C personality, 411

U.S. Pharmacopoeia (USP), 109
Ultraviolet A rays (UVA), 381, 389
Ultraviolet B rays (UVB), 381, 389
Underweight, 133, 139
Undulating periodization, 245
Unilateral eccentric knee flexion, **271**
Unsaturated fatty acids
  bond formation in, 79–80
  chemical structure of, 80
  classification of, 79
  oils rich in, 80
Upper back stretch, **303**
Upright rowing, **274**

Value marketing, 47
Values
  age-related change, 44
  core, 50
  defined, 47
  establishment of, 47–48
Variable resistance, 247
Variable-resistance, 246–247
Vegans, 100
Vegetables
  antioxidants in, 109
  cancer fighting, 377–378
  phytonutrients in, 92, 109
Vegetarianism
  definition of, 100
  healthful, 100–101
  products for, 522
  types of, 100
Very low calorie diet, 162–163
Very low density proteins, 349
Vibrators, 172
Vicarious experiences, 52–53
Vigorous activity, 20–21
Vigorous exercise, 213
Virgin olive oil, 80
Visceral (VSC) fat, 140
Visual imagery, 427–428
Vitamin B inf12/inf, 116
Vitamin C, 107, 352
Vitamin D
  cancer protection with, 378
  characterization of, 107
  deficiency rate, 108
  good sources of, 108
Vitamin E, 106, 352
Vitamin K, 116

Vitamins
  antioxidant effects of, 378
  classification of, 84
  definition of, 85
  functions of, 84
  supplements, 106–108
Volumetrics eating plans, 155

Waist circumference (WC), 137, 142 (Activity 4.2)
Waist-to-height ratio (WHtR), 137–138
Walking
  calories burned from, 12
  as conditioning activity, 307–308
  daily, recommendations for, 44
  government commitment to, 45–46
  in water, 308
Wall squat, **278**
Warm-ups, 220–221, 289
Water
  consumption of, 85–86
  definition of, 85
  functions of, 85
  heat stroke and, 321
  walking in, 308
Water aerobics, 310
Water soluble vitamins, 84
WC. *See* Waist circumference (WC)
Weight. *See* Body weight
Weight gain
  food choices for, 177
  healthy, 171
  healthy plan for, 187–188 (Activity 5.4)
  stress and, 366
Weight loss. *See also under* Diets; Eating disorders
  behavior modification plan, 179 (Activity 5.2)
  breakfast and, 175–176
  caloric intake and, 175
  effective, 146
  extreme, 146
  friendship factors, 182
  gender factors, 182
  metabolism and, 164–165
  myths of, 171–172
  physiology of, 161–163
  during pregnancy, 318
  relapse causes, 182
  sensible approach to, 172–182
  stretching and, 280
  truth of, 182
Weight management
  assumptions about, 161
  behavior assessment of, 191
  behavior modification for, 140, 177
  calorie consumption and, 148
  energy-balance equation in, 161–162
  exercise and
    duration, 168–170
    guidelines for, 167

Weight management *(continued)*
    importance of, 167–168
    intensity, 168–170
    limits of, 148
    research on, 166
    time required, 166
  extreme loss and, 152
  FAQs, 148
  knowledge assessment of, 191
  lifetime, personal profile, 149
  measuring progress, 189–190 (Activity 5.5)
  metabolism and, 162
  regular monitoring in, 165–166
  setpoint theory of, 162–163
  sleep and, 165

Weight Watchers, 155, 526
Weight-regulating mechanism, 162–163
Wellness
  challenges of, 27–28
  community resources for, 503–504 (Activity 15.2)
  components, evaluation of, 505, 507 (Activity 15.3)
  continuum, 17
  definition of, 14
  dimensions of, 14, 17, 39 (Activity 1.5)
  FAQs, 2
  lifestyle questionnaire, 29, 33–35 (Activity 1.2)
  lifestyle self-assessment, 509–510 (Activity 15.5)
  lifestyles, 486
  personal profile, 4
  premature mortality and, 19
  reliable information on, 499
  sleep and, 404–405
  types of, 17–20
Western medicine. *See* Conventional Western medicine
Whole grains, 92
WHtR. *See* Waist-to-height ratio (WHtR)
"Why do You Smoke" Test
  development of, 454
  factors in, 455–456

questions in, 457 (Activity 13.3)
Workload, 198–199

Yo-yo diets, 153
Yoga
  application of, 430–431
  back benefits of, 294
  benefits of, 313
  code of ethics, 430
  definition of, 423
  stress management and, 422
  styles of, 431
Yogurt, 102

Zocor®, 356
The Zone Diet, 155

Tear-Out Cards

On the following pages, you will find a selection of tear-out cards, correlated with each chapter of the text.

For Easy Reference cards

The "For Easy Reference" cards contain key information that you will want to remember, both to succeed in your class, and to monitor your own health and behavior. Tear these out and carry them in your backpack, tape them by your desk, or put them anywhere you find handy so that you can easily reference this important health information.

Check Yourself cards

The "Check Yourself" cards contain "to-do" lists of healthy habits and behaviors. Check off those items you have already accomplished or guidelines you routinely follow. Let the unchecked boxes serve as a reminder of what you need to work on. Continue to track your progress, and experience the feeling of satisfaction when all the boxes have been checked!

CHAPTER 1 FOR EASY REFERENCE
Health-Related Components of Physical Fitness

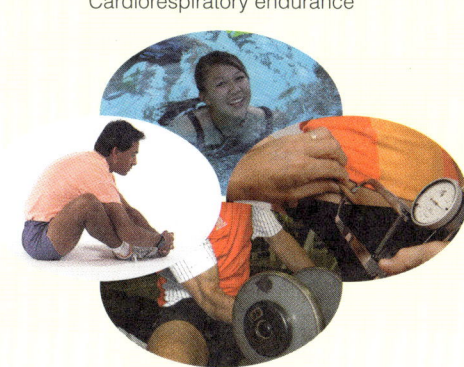

- Cardiorespiratory endurance
- Muscular flexibility
- Body composition
- Muscular fitness (strength and endurance)

Photos © Fitness & Wellness, Inc.

CHAPTER 1 CHECK YOURSELF
Healthy Lifestyle Habits

Research indicates that adhering to the following 12 lifestyle habits will significantly improve health and extend life.

☐ 1. Participate in a lifetime physical activity program.
☐ 2. Do not smoke cigarettes.
☐ 3. Eat right.
☐ 4. Avoid snacking.
☐ 5. Maintain recommended body weight through adequate nutrition and exercise.
☐ 6. Sleep seven to eight hours every night.
☐ 7. Lower your stress levels.
☐ 8. Be wary of alcohol.
☐ 9. Surround yourself with healthy friendships.
☐ 10. Be informed about the environment.
☐ 11. Increase education.
☐ 12. Take personal safety measures.

CHAPTER 1 FOR EASY REFERENCE
Health-Related Components of Physical Fitness—Key Definitions

- **Cardiorespiratory endurance** The ability of the lungs, heart, and blood vessels to deliver adequate amounts of oxygen to the cells to meet the demands of prolonged physical activity.
- **Body composition** The fat and non-fat components of the human body; important in assessing recommended body weight.
- **Muscular strength** The ability of a muscle to exert maximum force against resistance (for example, 1 repetition maximum [or 1 RM] on the bench press exercise).
- **Muscular endurance** The ability of a muscle to exert submaximal force repeatedly over time.
- **Flexibility** The achievable range of motion at a joint or group of joints without causing injury.

CHAPTER 1 FOR EASY REFERENCE
Estimated Number of Steps to Walk or Jog a Mile

	Pace (min/mile)				
	Walking			Jogging	
Height	20	15	12	10	8
Women					
5'0"	2,371	2,054	1,997	1,710	1,423
5'4"	2,315	1,998	1,943	1,656	1,369
5'8"	2,258	1,941	1,889	1,602	1,315
6'0"	2,202	1,885	1,835	1,548	1,261
Men					
5'2"	2,310	1,993	1,970	1,683	1,396
5'6"	2,253	1,937	1,916	1,629	1,342
5'10"	2,197	1,880	1,862	1,575	1,288
6'2"	2,141	1,824	1,808	1,521	1,234

Prediction Equations (pace in min/mile and height in inches):
Walking
Women: Steps/mile = 1,949 + [(63.4 × pace) − (14.1 × height)]
Men: Steps/mile = 1,916 + [(63.4 × pace) − (14.1 × height)]
Running
Women and Men: Steps/mile = 1,084 + [(143.6 × pace) − (13.5 × height)]
SOURCE: Werner W. K. Hoeger et al., "One- mile step count at walking and running speeds." *ACSM's Health & Fitness Journal*, Vol 12(1):14–19, 2008.

CHAPTER 2 FOR EASY REFERENCE
Stages of Change: Model of Progression and Relapse

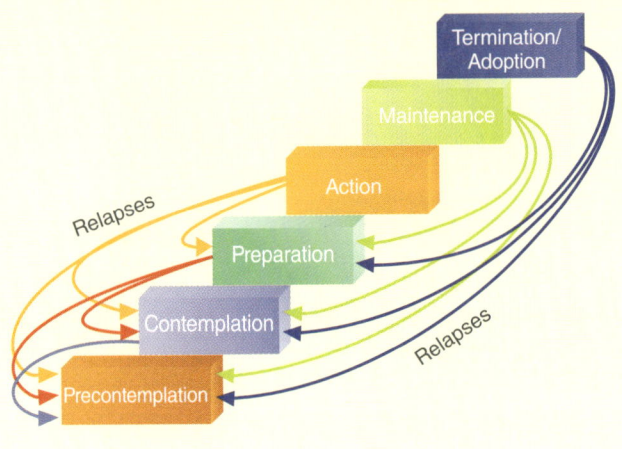

CHAPTER 2 CHECK YOURSELF
Steps for Successful Behavior Modification

- ❏ 1. Acknowledge that you have a problem.
- ❏ 2. Describe the behavior to change (increase physical activity, stop overeating, quit smoking).
- ❏ 3. List advantages and disadvantages of changing the specified behavior.
- ❏ 4. Decide positively that you will change.
- ❏ 5. Identify your stage of change.
- ❏ 6. Set a realistic goal (SMART goal), completion date, and sign a behavioral contract.
- ❏ 7. Define your behavioral change plan: List processes of change, techniques of change, and actions that will help you reach your goal.
- ❏ 8. Implement the behavior change plan.
- ❏ 9. Monitor your progress toward the desired goal.
- ❏ 10. Periodically evaluate and reassess your goal.
- ❏ 11. Reward yourself when you achieve your goal.
- ❏ 12. Maintain the successful change for good.

CHAPTER 3 FOR EASY REFERENCE
Computation for Fat Content in Food

Nutrition Facts
Serving Size 1 cup (240 ml)
Servings Per Container 4

Amount Per Serving	
Calories 120	Calories from Fat 45

	% Daily Value*
Total Fat 5g	8%
Saturated Fat 3g	15%
Trans Fat 0g	0%
Cholesterol 20mg	7%
Sodium 120mg	5%
Total Carbohydrate 12g	4%
Dietary Fiber 0g	0%
Sugars 12g	
Protein 8g	

| Vitamin A | 10% | • | Vitamin C | 4% |
| Calcium | 30% | • | Iron | 0% |

* Percent Daily Values are based on a 2,000 calorie diet. Your daily values may be higher or lower depending on your calorie needs:

		Calories	2,000	2,500
Total Fat	Less than		65g	80g
Sat Fat	Less than		20g	25g
Cholesterol	Less than		300mg	300mg
Sodium	Less than		2,300mg	2,300mg
Total Carbohydrate			300g	375g
Fiber			25g	30g

Calories per gram:
Fat 9 • Carbohydrate 4 • Protein 4

Percent fat calories = (grams of fat × 9) ÷ calories per serving × 100

5 grams of fat × 9 calories per grams of fat = 45 calories from fat

45 calories from fat ÷ 120 calories per serving × 100 = 38% fat

CHAPTER 3 FOR EASY REFERENCE
Good Sources of Vitamin D

Food	Amount	IU*
Multivitamins (most brands)	daily dose	400
Salmon	3.5 oz	360
Mackerel	3.5 oz	345
Sardines (oil/drained)	3.5 oz	250
Shrimp	3.5 oz	200
Orange juice (D-fortified)	8 oz	100
Milk (any type/D-fortified)	8 oz	100
Margarine (D-fortified)	1 tbsp	60
Yogurt (D-fortified)	6–8 oz	60
Cereal (D-fortified)	¾–1 c	40
Egg	1	20

*IU = international units

CHAPTER 3 FOR EASY REFERENCE
Caloric and Fat Content of Selected Fast Foods

	Calories	Total Fat (grams)	Saturated Fat (grams)	Percent Fat Calories
Burgers				
McDonald's Big Mac	590	34	11	52
McDonald's Big N' Tasty with Cheese	590	37	12	56
McDonald's Quarter Pounder with Cheese	530	30	13	51
Burger King Whopper	760	46	15	54
Burger King Bacon Double Cheeseburger	580	34	18	53
Burger King BK Smokehouse Cheddar Griller	720	48	19	60
Burger King Whopper with Cheese	850	53	22	56
Burger King Double Whopper	1,060	69	27	59
Burger King Double Whopper with Cheese	1,150	76	33	59
Wendy's Baconator	830	51	22	55

Continued on back

CHAPTER 3 FOR EASY REFERENCE
Caloric and Fat Content of Selected Fast Foods

	Calories	Total Fat (grams)	Saturated Fat (grams)	Percent Fat Calories
Mexican				
Taco Bell Crunchy Taco	170	10	4	53
Taco Bell Taco Supreme	220	14	6	57
Taco Bell Soft Chicken Taco	190	7	3	33
Taco Bell Bean Burrito	370	12	4	29
Taco Bell Fiesta Steak Burrito	370	12	4	29
Taco Bell Grilled Steak Soft Taco	290	17	4	53
Taco Bell Double Decker Taco	340	14	5	37
French Fries				
Wendy's, biggie (5½ oz)	440	19	7	39
McDonald's, large (6 oz)	540	26	9	43
Burger King, large (5½ oz)	500	25	13	45

Continued on back

CHAPTER 3 CHECK YOURSELF
Selecting Nutritious Foods

Do you regularly follow the habits below?

To select nutritious foods:

☐ 1. Given the choice between whole foods and refined, processed foods, choose the former (apples rather than apple pie, potatoes rather than potato chips). No nutrients have been refined out of the whole foods, and they contain less fat, salt, and sugar.

☐ 2. Choose the leaner cuts of meat. Select fish or poultry often, beef seldom. Ask for broiled, not fried, to control your fat intake.

☐ 3. Use both raw and cooked vegetables and fruits. Raw foods offer more fiber and vitamins, such as folate and thiamin, that are destroyed by cooking. Cooking foods frees other vitamins and minerals for absorption.

☐ 4. Include milk, milk products, or other calcium sources for the calcium you need. Use low-fat or non-fat items to reduce fat and calories.

☐ 5. Learn to use margarine, butter, and oils sparingly. A little gives flavor, a lot overloads you with fat and calories, and increases disease risk.

CHAPTER 3 CHECK YOURSELF
"Super" Foods

The following "super" foods that fight disease and promote health should be included often in your diet. Are you eating these foods regularly?

☐ Acai berries
☐ Avocados
☐ Bananas
☐ Barley
☐ Beans
☐ Beets
☐ Blueberries
☐ Broccoli
☐ Butternut squash
☐ Carrots
☐ Flaxseeds
☐ Goji berries
☐ Grapes
☐ Kale
☐ Kiwifruit
☐ Lentils
☐ Nuts (Brazil, walnuts)
☐ Oats and oatmeal
☐ Olives and olive oil
☐ Onions
☐ Oranges
☐ Peppers
☐ Pomegranates
☐ Quinoa
☐ Salmon (wild)
☐ Soy
☐ Strawberries
☐ Spinach
☐ Sweet potatoes
☐ Tea (green, black, red)
☐ Tomatoes
☐ Walnuts
☐ Watermelon
☐ Yogurt

Continued on back

CHAPTER 3 FOR EASY REFERENCE
Caloric and Fat Content of Selected Fast Foods

Sandwiches	Calories	Total Fat (grams)	Saturated Fat (grams)	Percent Fat Calories
Arby's Regular Roast Beef	350	16	6	41
Arby's Super Roast Beef	470	23	7	44
Arby's Roast Chicken Club	520	28	7	48
Arby's Market Fresh Roast Beef & Swiss	810	42	13	47
McDonald's Crispy Chicken	430	21	8	43
McDonald's Filet-O-Fish	470	26	5	50
McDonald's Chicken McGrill	400	17	3	38
Wendy's Chicken Club	470	19	4	36
Wendy's Breast Fillet	430	16	3	34
Wendy's Grilled Chicken	300	7	2	21
Burger King Specialty Chicken	560	28	6	45
Subway Veggie Delight*	226	3	1	12
Subway Turkey Breast	281	5	2	16
Subway Sweet Onion Chicken Teriyaki	374	5	2	12
Subway Steak & Cheese	390	14	5	32
Subway Cold Cut Trio	440	21	7	43
Subway Tuna	450	22	6	44

Shakes	Calories	Total Fat (grams)	Saturated Fat (grams)	Percent Fat Calories
Wendy's Frosty, medium (16 oz)	440	11	7	23
McDonald's McFlurry, small (12 oz)	610	22	14	32
Burger King, Old Fashioned Ice Cream Shake, medium (22 oz)	760	41	29	49
Hash Browns				
McDonald's Hash Browns (2 oz)	130	8	4	55
Burger King, Hash Browns, small (2½ oz)	230	15	9	59

*6-inch sandwich with no mayo

SOURCE: Adapted from Restaurant Confidential. Copyright © 2002 by the Center for Science in the Public Interest. Used by permission of Workman Publishing Co., Inc., New York. All rights reserved.

CHAPTER 3 CHECK YOURSELF
Guidelines for a Healthy Diet

- ❏ Base your diet on a large variety of foods.
- ❏ Consume ample amounts of green, yellow, and orange fruits and vegetables.
- ❏ Eat foods high in complex carbohydrates, including at least three 1-ounce servings of whole-grain foods per day.
- ❏ Obtain most of your vitamins and minerals from food sources.
- ❏ Eat foods rich in vitamin D.
- ❏ Maintain adequate daily calcium intake and consider a bone supplement with vitamin D_3.
- ❏ Consume protein in moderation.
- ❏ Limit meat consumption to 3 to 6 ounces per day.
- ❏ Limit daily fat, trans fat, and saturated fat intake.
- ❏ Limit cholesterol consumption to less than 300 mg per day.
- ❏ Limit sodium intake to 2,300 mg per day.
- ❏ Limit sugar intake.
- ❏ If you drink alcohol, do so in moderation (one daily drink for women and two for men).
- ❏ Consider taking a daily multivitamin (preferably one that includes vitamin D_3).

CHAPTER 3 CHECK YOURSELF
Selecting Nutritious Foods

- ❏ 6. Vary your choices. Eat broccoli today, carrots tomorrow, and corn the next day. Eat Chinese today, Italian tomorrow, and broiled fish with brown rice and steamed vegetables the third day.
- ❏ 7. Load your plate with vegetables and unrefined starchy foods. A small portion of meat, poultry, or fish is all you need for protein.
- ❏ 8. When choosing breads and cereals, choose the whole-grain varieties.

To select nutritious fast foods:

- ❏ 9. Choose the broiled sandwich with lettuce, tomatoes, and other goodies—and hold the mayo—rather than the fish or chicken patties coated with breadcrumbs and cooked in fat.
- ❏ 10. Select a salad—and use more plain vegetables than those mixed with oily or mayonnaise-based dressings.
- ❏ 11. Order chili with more beans than meat. Choose a soft bean burrito over tacos with fried shells.
- ❏ 12. Drink low-fat milk rather than a cola beverage.

When choosing from a vending machine:

- ❏ 13. Choose cracker sandwiches over chips and pork rinds (virtually pure fat). Choose peanuts, pretzels, and popcorn over cookies and candy.
- ❏ 14. Choose milk and juices over cola beverages.

CHAPTER 4 FOR EASY REFERENCE
Disease Risk According to Body Mass Index (BMI) and Waist-to-Height Ratio (WHtR).

Body Mass Index		
BMI	Disease Risk	Classification
<18.5	Increased	Underweight
18.5–21.99	Low	Acceptable
22.0–24.99	Very Low	Acceptable
25.0–29.99	Increased	Overweight
30.0–34.99	High	Obesity I
35.0–39.99	Very High	Obesity II
≥40.00	Extremely High	Obesity III

Waist-to-Height Ratio		
Category	WHtR (Waist/Height)	Disease Risk
Take Care	<.4	Increased
Acceptable (OK)	.4–.5	Very low
Take Care	.5–.7	Increased
Take Action	>.7	Highest

CHAPTER 4 CHECK YOURSELF
Tips for Lifetime Weight Management

- ❑ Accumulate 60 to 90 minutes of physical activity daily.
- ❑ Exercise at a brisk aerobic pace for a minimum of 20 minutes three times per week.
- ❑ Strength train two to three times per week.
- ❑ Consume an adequate amount of protein with each meal (between .33 and .40 g per kg of body weight three times per day).
- ❑ Manage daily caloric intake by keeping in mind long-term benefits (recommended body weight) instead of instant gratification (overeating).
- ❑ "Junior-size" instead of "super-size."
- ❑ Regularly monitor body weight, body composition, body mass index, and waist circumference.
- ❑ Do not allow increases in body weight (percent fat) to accumulate; deal immediately with the problem through moderate reductions in caloric intake and maintenance of physical activity and exercise habits.

CHAPTER 5 CHECK YOURSELF
Physical Activity Guidelines for Weight Management

The following physical activity guidelines are recommended to effectively manage body weight:

- ❑ 30 minutes of physical activity on most days of the week if you do not have difficulty maintaining body weight (more minutes and/or higher intensity if you choose to reach a high level of physical fitness).
- ❑ 60 minutes of daily activity if you want to prevent weight gain.
- ❑ Between 60 and 90 minutes each day if you are trying to lose weight or attempting to keep weight off following extensive weight loss (30 pounds of weight loss or more). Be sure to include some high-intensity/low-impact activities at least twice a week in your program.

CHAPTER 6 FOR EASY REFERENCE
Cardiorespiratory Exercise Prescription

Intensity of Exercise

1. Estimate your own maximal heart rate (MHR)

   MHR = 207 − (.70 × age)

   MHR = 207 − ☐ × ☐ = ☐ bpm

2. Resting Heart Rate (RHR) = ☐ bpm

3. Heart Rate Reserve (HRR) = MHR − RHR

   HRR = ☐ − ☐ = ☐ beats

4. Training Intensities (TI) = HRR × TI + RHR

   30 Percent TI = ☐ × .30 + ☐ = ☐ bpm

   40 Percent TI = ☐ × .40 + ☐ = ☐ bpm

   60 percent TI = ☐ × .60 + ☐ = ☐ bpm

   90 Percent TI = ☐ × .90 + ☐ = ☐ bpm

5. Light-Intensity Cardiorespiratory Training Zone:

   ☐ (30% TI) to ☐ (40% TI)

6. Moderate-Intensity Cardiorespiratory Training Zone:

   ☐ (40% TI) to ☐ (60% TI)

7. Vigorous-Intensity Cardiorespiratory Training Zone:

   ☐ (60% TI) to ☐ (90% TI)

CHAPTER 6 FOR EASY REFERENCE
Cardiorespiratory Exercise Guidelines

Mode: Moderate- or vigorous-intensity aerobic activity (examples: walking, jogging, stair climbing, elliptical activity, aerobics, water aerobics, cycling, stair climbing, swimming, cross-country skiing, racquetball, basketball, and soccer)

Intensity: 30% to 90% of heart rate reserve (the training intensity is based on age, health status, initial fitness level, exercise tolerance, and exercise program goals)

Duration: Be active 20 to 90 minutes. At least 20 minutes of continuous vigorous-intensity or 30 minutes of moderate-intensity aerobic activity (the latter may be accumulated in segments of at least 10 minutes in duration each over the course of the day)

Frequency: 3 to 5 days per week for vigorous-intensity aerobic activity to accumulate at least 75 minutes per week, or 5 days per week of moderate-intensity aerobic activity for a minimum total of 150 minutes weekly

Rate of progression:
- Start with three training sessions per week of 15 to 20 minutes
- Increase the duration by 5 to 10 minutes per week and the frequency so that by the fourth or fifth week you are exercising five times per week
- Progressively increase frequency, duration, and intensity of exercise until you reach your fitness goal prior to exercise maintenance

SOURCE: Adapted from American College of Sports Medicine, *ACSM's Guidelines for Exercise Testing and Prescription* (Philadelphia: Wolters Kluwer/Lippincott Williams & Wilkins, 2014).

CHAPTER 7 FOR EASY REFERENCE
Strength-Training Guidelines

Mode: Select 8 to 10 dynamic strength-training exercises that involve the body's major muscle groups and include opposing muscle groups (chest and upper back, abdomen and lower back, front and back of the legs).

Resistance: Sufficient resistance to perform 8 to 12 repetitions maximum for muscular strength and 15 to 25 repetitions to near fatigue for muscular edurance. Older adults and injury prone individuals should use 10 to 15 repetitions with moderate resistance (50% to 60% of their 1 RM).

Sets: 2 to 4 sets per exercise with 2 to 3 minutes recovery between sets for optimal strength development. Less than 2 minutes per set if exercises are alternated that require different muscle groups (chest and upper back) or between muscular endurance sets.

Frequency: 2 to 3 days per week on nonconsecutive days. More frequent training can be done if different muscle groups are exercised on different days. (Allow at least 48 hours between strength-training sessions of the same muscle group.)

SOURCE: Adapted from American College of Sports Medicine, *ACSM's Guidelines for Exercise Testing and Prescription* (Philadelphia: Wolters Kluwer/Lippincott Williams & Wilkins, 2014).

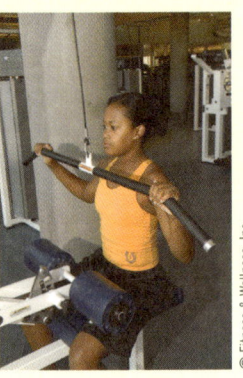

CHAPTER 7 CHECK YOURSELF
Healthy Strength Training

- ❏ Make a progressive resistance strength-training program a priority in your weekly schedule.
- ❏ Strength train at least once a week; even better, twice a week.
- ❏ Find a facility where you feel comfortable training and where you can get good professional guidance.
- ❏ Learn and use proper technique for each exercise.
- ❏ Train with a friend or group of friends.
- ❏ Consume a pre-exercise snack consisting of a combination of carbohydrates and some protein about 30 to 60 minutes before each strength-training session.
- ❏ Use a minimum of 8 to 10 exercises that involve all major muscle groups of your body.
- ❏ Perform at least one set of each exercise to near muscular fatigue.
- ❏ To enhance protein synthesis, consume one post-exercise snack with a 4-to-1 gram ratio of carbohydrates to protein immediately following strength training; and a second snack one hour thereafter.
- ❏ Allow at least 48 hours between strength-training sessions that involve the same muscle groups.

CHAPTER 8 FOR EASY REFERENCE
Flexibility Development Guidelines

Mode: Static, dynamic, proprioceptive neuromuscular facilitation (PNF), or controlled ballistic stretching to include all major muscle/tendon groups of the body.

Intensity: To the point of feeling tightness in the stretched area or mild discomfort.

Repetitions: Repeat each exercise 2 to 4 times, holding the final position between 10 and 30 seconds each, with a target of 60 seconds of total stretching for each exercise performed.

Frequency: At least 2 or 3 days per week but ideally 5 to 7 days per week.

SOURCE: Adapted from American College of Sports Medicine, *ACSM's Guidelines for Exercise Testing and Prescription* (Philadelphia: Wolters Kluwer/Lippincott Williams & Wilkins, 2014).

CHAPTER 8 CHECK YOURSELF
Tips to Prevent Low Back Pain

- ❏ Be physically active.
- ❏ Maintain recommended body weight (excess weight strains the back).
- ❏ Stretch often using spinal exercises through a functional range of motion.
- ❏ Regularly strengthen the core of the body using sets of 10 to 12 repetitions to near fatigue with isometric contractions when applicable.
- ❏ Lift heavy objects by bending at the knees and carry them close to the body. Place one foot forward, and keep your knees slightly bent while standing.
- ❏ Avoid sitting (over 50 minutes) or standing in one position for lengthy periods of time.
- ❏ Maintain correct posture.
- ❏ Sleep on your back with a pillow under the knees or on your side with the knees drawn up and a small pillow between the knees.
- ❏ Try out different mattresses of firm consistency before selecting a mattress.
- ❏ Warm up properly using mild stretches before engaging in physical activity.
- ❏ Practice adequate stress management techniques.
- ❏ Don't smoke (it reduces blood flow to the spine, increasing back pain risk).

CHAPTER 9 FOR EASY REFERENCE
Contraindications to Exercise During Pregnancy

Stop exercise and seek medical advice if you experience any of the following symptoms:

- Unusual pain or discomfort, especially in the chest or abdominal area
- Cramping, primarily in the pelvic or lower back areas
- Muscle weakness, excessive fatigue, or shortness of breath
- Abnormally high heart rate or a pounding (palpitations) heart rate
- Decreased fetal movement
- Insufficient weight gain
- Amniotic fluid leakage
- Nausea, dizziness, or headaches
- Persistent uterine contractions
- Vaginal bleeding or rupture of the membranes
- Swelling of ankles, calves, hands, or face

CHAPTER 10 FOR EASY REFERENCE
American Heart Association Guidelines for Cardiovascular Risk Reduction

- ❏ Consume an overall healthy diet.
- ❏ Aim for a healthy body weight.
- ❏ Aim for recommended levels of LDL cholesterol, HDL cholesterol, and triglycerides.
- ❏ Aim for a normal blood pressure.
- ❏ Aim for normal blood glucose levels.
- ❏ Be physically active.
- ❏ Avoid use of and exposure to tobacco products.

CHAPTER 10 FOR EASY REFERENCE
Blood Pressure Guidelines (mm Hg)

Rating	Systolic	Diastolic
Normal	<120	<80
Prehypertension	121–139	81–89
Stage 1 hypertension	140–159	90–99
Stage 2 hypertension	≥160	≥100

SOURCE: National High Blood Pressure Education Program.

Continued on back

CHAPTER 10 FOR EASY REFERENCE
Signs of Heart Attack and Stroke

Any or all of the following signs may occur during a heart attack or a stroke. If you experience any of these and they last longer than a few minutes, call 911 and seek medical attention immediately. Failure to do so may cause irreparable damage and even result in death.

Warning Signs of a Heart Attack

- Chest pain, discomfort, pressure, or squeezing that lasts for several minutes. These feelings may go away and return later.
- Pain or discomfort in the shoulders, neck, or arms or between the shoulder blades
- Chest discomfort with shortness of breath, lightheadedness, cold sweats, nausea and/or vomiting, a feeling of indigestion, sudden fatigue or weakness, fainting, or sense of impending doom

Warning Signs of Stroke

- Sudden weakness or numbness of the face, arm, or leg—particularly on one side of the body
- Sudden severe headache
- Sudden confusion, dizziness, or difficulty with speech and understanding
- Sudden difficulty walking; loss of balance or coordination
- Sudden visual difficulty

CHAPTER 10 CHECK YOURSELF
Leading Coronary Heart Disease Risk Factors

- ❏ Physical Inactivity
- ❏ Abnormal blood lipids (cholesterol and triglycerides)
- ❏ Smoking
- ❏ Excessive body weight (high body mass index)
- ❏ Hypertension
- ❏ Elevated homocysteine
- ❏ Inflammation
- ❏ Diabetes
- ❏ Tension and stress
- ❏ Personal/family history of heart disease
- ❏ Abnormal electrocardiograms
- ❏ Age

CHAPTER 10 CHECK YOURSELF
Dietary Guidelines to Lower LDL Cholesterol

- ❏ Minimize the use of simple and refined carbohydrates and processed foods.
- ❏ Consume between 25 and 38 grams of fiber daily.
- ❏ Increase consumption of vegetables, fruits, whole grains, and beans.
- ❏ Do not consume more than 200 mg of dietary cholesterol a day.
- ❏ Consume 3 ounces of red meat three times per week or less.
- ❏ Do not eat commercially baked foods.
- ❏ Avoid foods that contain trans fatty acids or hydrogenated fat.
- ❏ Eat two to three meals of omega-3–rich fish per week.
- ❏ Consume 25 grams of soy protein a day.
- ❏ Drink low-fat milk and use low-fat dairy products.
- ❏ Do not use coconut oil, palm oil, or cocoa butter.
- ❏ Limit egg consumption to fewer than three eggs per week.
- ❏ Use margarines and salad dressings that contain stanol.
- ❏ Bake, broil, grill, poach, or steam food instead of frying.
- ❏ Avoid fatty sauces made with butter, cream, or cheese.
- ❏ Maintain recommended body weight.

CHAPTER 10 FOR EASY REFERENCE
Diagnosis of Metabolic Syndrome

Components	Men	Women
Waist circumference	>40 inches	>35 inches
Blood pressure	>130/85 mm Hg	>130/85 mm Hg
Fasting blood glucose	>110 mg/dL	>110 mg/dL
Fasting HDL cholesterol	<40 mg/dL	<50 mg/dL
Fasting triglycerides	>150 mg/dL	>150 mg/dL

Note: Metabolic syndrome is identified by the presence of at least three of the above components.

CHAPTER 11 CHECK YOURSELF
Tips for a Healthy Cancer Fighting Diet

- ❑ Eat a predominantly vegetarian diet.
- ❑ Eat six to eight servings of fruits and vegetables every day.
- ❑ Increase the consumption of broccoli, cauliflower, kale, turnips, cabbage, kohlrabi, Brussels sprouts, hot chili peppers, red and green peppers, carrots, sweet potatoes, winter squash, spinach, garlic, onions, strawberries, tomatoes, pineapple, and citrus fruits in your regular diet.
- ❑ Eat vegetables raw or quickly cooked by steaming or stir-frying.
- ❑ Substitute tea and fruit and vegetable juices for coffee and soda.
- ❑ Eat whole-grain breads.
- ❑ Include soy products in the diet.
- ❑ Use whole-wheat flour instead of refined white flour in baking.
- ❑ Use brown (unpolished) rice instead of white (polished) rice.
- ❑ Use primarily unsaturated fats (olive and canola oils, nuts, seeds, avocado, fish, and flaxseeds).
- ❑ Maintain recommended body weight.

CHAPTER 11 CHECK YOURSELF
Lifestyle Factors That Decrease Cancer Risk

Do you have these healthy lifestyle factors working in your favor?

Factor	Function
❑ Physical activity	Controls body weight, may influence hormone levels, strengthens the immune system.
❑ Fiber	Contains anti-cancer substances, increases stool movement, blunts insulin secretion.
❑ Fruits and vegetables	Contain phytonutrients and vitamins that thwart cancer.
❑ Recommended weight	Helps control hormones that promote cancer.
❑ Healthy grilling	Prevents formation of carcinogenic substances.
❑ Tea	Contains polyphenols that neutralize free radicals.
❑ Spices	Provide phytonutrients and strengthen the immune system.
❑ Vitamin D	Disrupts abnormal cell growth.
❑ Monounsaturated fat	May contribute to cancer cell destruction.

CHAPTER 12 FOR EASY REFERENCE
Stressors in the Lives of College Students

Adapted from W. W. K. Hoeger, L. W. Turner, and B. Q. Hafen. *Wellness Guidelines for a Healthy Lifestyle.* Wadsworth/Thomson Learning, 2007.

Photo © Fitness & Wellness, Inc.

CHAPTER 12 CHECK YOURSELF
Common Symptoms of Stress

Check those symptoms you experience regularly.

- ❑ Headaches
- ❑ Muscular aches (mainly in neck, shoulders, and back)
- ❑ Grinding teeth
- ❑ Nervous tic, finger tapping, toe tapping
- ❑ Increased sweating
- ❑ Increase in or loss of appetite
- ❑ Insomnia
- ❑ Nightmares
- ❑ Fatigue
- ❑ Dry mouth
- ❑ Stuttering
- ❑ High blood pressure
- ❑ Tightness or pain in the chest
- ❑ Impotence
- ❑ Hives
- ❑ Dizziness
- ❑ Depression
- ❑ Irritation
- ❑ Anger
- ❑ Hostility
- ❑ Fear, panic, anxiety
- ❑ Stomach pain, flutters
- ❑ Nausea
- ❑ Cold, clammy hands
- ❑ Poor concentration
- ❑ Pacing
- ❑ Restlessness
- ❑ Rapid heart rate
- ❑ Low-grade infection
- ❑ Loss of sex drive
- ❑ Rash or acne

CHAPTER 12 CHECK YOURSELF
Tips to Manage Anger

- ❏ Commit to change and gain control over the behavior.
- ❏ Remind yourself that chronic anger leads to illness and disease and may eventually kill you.
- ❏ Recognize when feelings of anger are developing and ask yourself the following questions:
  - Is the matter really that important?
  - Is the anger justified?
  - Can I change the situation without getting angry?
  - Is it worth risking my health over it?
  - How will I feel about the situation in a few hours?
- ❏ Tell yourself, "Stop, my health is worth it" every time you start to feel anger.
- ❏ Prepare for a positive response: Ask for an explanation or clarification of the situation, walk away and evaluate the situation, exercise, or use appropriate stress management techniques (breathing, meditation, imagery) before you become angry and hostile.
- ❏ Manage anger at once; do not let it build up.
- ❏ Never attack anyone verbally or physically.
- ❏ Keep a journal and ponder the situations that cause you to be angry.
- ❏ Seek professional help if you are unable to overcome anger by yourself: You are worth it.

CHAPTER 13 CHECK YOURSELF
Addictive Behavior Questionnaire

- ❏ 1. Are you a compulsive person?
- ❏ 2. Are you a person of excesses?
- ❏ 3. Do you depend heavily on others or are you completely independent of others?
- ❏ 4. Are you unable to stop using drugs or limit their use to required situations only?
- ❏ 5. Has drug misuse ever created a problem between you and friends or relatives?
- ❏ 6. Have family members or friends ever sought help for problems associated with your misuse of drugs?
- ❏ 7. Have you ever sought help for drug misuse?
- ❏ 8. Do you tend to associate with people who exhibit the same behaviors or take the same drugs you do?
- ❏ 9. Has the misuse of drugs affected the way you function in life (school, work, recreation)?
- ❏ 10. Have you unsuccessfully tried to cut back or stop the misuse of drugs?

CHAPTER 14 CHECK YOURSELF
Protecting Yourself and Others from STI's

Are you sexually active? If you are not, read the following items to better educate yourself regarding intimacy. If you are sexually active, continue through all the questions below.

- ❏ Do you plan ahead before you get into a sexual situation?
- ❏ Do you know whether your partner now has or has ever had an STI? Are you comfortable asking your partner this question?
- ❏ Are you in a mutually monogamous sexual relationship and you know that your partner does not have an STI?
- ❏ Do you have multiple sexual partners? If so, do you *always* practice safe sex?
- ❏ Do you avoid alcohol and drugs in situations where you may end up having planned or unplanned sex?
- ❏ Do you abstain from sexual activity if you know or suspect that you have an STI? Do you seek medical care and advice as to when you can safely resume sexual activity?

CHAPTER 15 CHECK YOURSELF
Healthy Lifestyle Guidelines

- ❏ 1. Accumulate a minimum of 30 minutes of moderate-intensity physical activity at least five days per week.
- ❏ 2. Exercise aerobically in the proper cardiorespiratory training zone at least three times per week for a minimum of 20 minutes.
- ❏ 3. Strength train at least once a week (preferably twice per week) using a minimum of eight exercises that involve all major muscle groups of the body.
- ❏ 4. Perform flexibility exercises that involve all major joints of the body at least two to three times per week.
- ❏ 5. Eat a healthy diet that is rich in whole-wheat grains, fruits, and vegetables and is low in saturated and trans fats.
- ❏ 6. Eat a healthy breakfast every day.
- ❏ 7. Do not use tobacco in any form, avoid secondhand smoke, and avoid all other forms of substance abuse.
- ❏ 8. Maintain healthy body weight (achieve a range between the high-physical fitness and health-fitness standards for percent body fat).
- ❏ 9. Get 7 to 8 hours of sleep per night.
- ❏ 10. Get 10 to 20 minutes of safe sun exposure on most days of the week.
- ❏ 11. Manage stress effectively.
- ❏ 12. Limit daily alcohol intake to two or less drinks per day if you are a man or one drink or less per day if you are a woman (or do not consume any alcohol at all).
- ❏ 13. Seek proper medical evaluations as necessary.